Biochromatography

Biochromatography

Theory and practice

Edited by
M. A. Vijayalakshmi

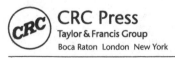

CRC Press
Taylor & Francis Group
Boca Raton London New York

CRC Press is an imprint of the
Taylor & Francis Group, an **informa** business
A TAYLOR & FRANCIS BOOK

CRC Press
Taylor & Francis Group
6000 Broken Sound Parkway NW, Suite 300
Boca Raton, FL 33487-2742

First issued in paperback 2020

© 2002 by Taylor & Francis Group, LLC
CRC Press is an imprint of Taylor & Francis Group, an Informa business

No claim to original U.S. Government works

ISBN-13: 978-0-367-45503-3 (pbk)
ISBN-13: 978-0-415-26903-2 (hbk)

Visit the Taylor & Francis Web site at
http://www.taylorandfrancis.com

and the CRC Press Web site at
http://www.crcpress.com

Typeset in 10/12 pt Baskerville
by Newgen Imaging Systems (P) Ltd, Chennai, India.

British Library Cataloguing in Publication Data
A catalogue record for this book is available
from the British Library

Library of Congress Cataloging in Publication Data
A catalog record has been requested

I would like to thank, from the depth of my heart, Prof J. Porath who initiated me into this field, guided and encouraged me throughout, and my colleague and friend Prof E. Sulkowski for his sustained interest and advice. I dedicate this book to them.

Contents

Contributors

Francisco Batista Viera Catedra de Bioquimica, Facultad de Zuimica, Gral, Flores 2124, Casilla de Correo 1157, Montevideo, Uruguay.

E. Boschetti Biosepra S.A, 35 Avenue Jean Jaurés, 92390 Villeneuve la Garenne, France.

J. M. S. Cabral Instituto Superior Tecnico, Departamento de Engenharia Quimica, Secçao de Biotecnologia, Avenue Rouisco Pais, 1096 Lisboa Codex, Portugal.

Gargi Choudhary Berlex Biosciences, 15049 San Pablo Avenue, Richmond, CA 94804-0099, USA.

Yannis D. Clonis Enzyme Technology Laboratory, Department of Agricultural Biotechnology, The Agricultural University of Athens, Iera Odos 75, GR 11855 Athens, Greece.

Peter A. G. Cormack Department of Pure and Applied Chemistry, University of Strathclyde, Thomas Graham Building, 295 Cathedral Street, Glasgow, Scotland.

Henri Debray Laboratoire de Chimie Biologique, Universié des Sciences et Technologies de Lille 1, UMR CNRS 8576, 59655 Villeneuve d'Ascq Cedex, France.

Kjell-Ove Eriksson Amersham Biosciences, Björkgatan 30, 751 84 Uppsala, Sweden.

Igor Yu. Galaev Department of Biotechnology, Center for Chemistry and Chemical Engineering, Lund University, P.O. Box 124, Lund S-221 00, Sweden.

F. A. P. Garcia Departmento de Engenharia Quimica, Universidade de Coimbra, 3000 Coimbra, Portugal.

P. Girot Biosepra S. A., 35 avenue Jean Jaurés, 92390 Villeneuve la Garenne, France.

Karsten Haupt INTS U76 INSERM, 6 rue Alexandre Cabarel, 75739 Paris Cedex 15, France.

Milton T. W. Hearn Center for Bioprocess Technology, Department of Biochemistry and Molecular Biology, Monash University, Wellington Road, Clayton, 3168 Victoria, Australia.

Csaba Horváth Department of Chemical Engineering, Yale University, Mason Lab., P.O. 208286, 9 Hill House Avenue, Newhaven CT 06520, USA.

Herbert P. Jennissen Institut für Physiologische Chemie, Universität GHS Essen, Hufeland str. 55, D 45122 Essen, Germany.

Nikos E. Labrou Enzyme Technology Laboratory, Department of Agricultural Biotechnology, The Agricultural University of Athens, Iera Odos 75, GR 11855 Athens, Greece.

C. Legallais Université de Technologie de Compiègne, Département de Génie Biologique, UMR CNRS 6600, BP 20.529, 60205 Compiègne Cedex, France.

Xiao-Chuan Liu Department of Chemistry, Indiana State University, Terre Haute, IN 47809.

Charles Lutsch Director of the Department of Protein Purification, Pasteur Mérieux Connaught, 1541, Av. Marcel Merieux, 69280 Marcy l'Etoile, France.

Bo Mattiasson Department of Biotechnology, Center for Chemistry and Chemical Engineering, Lund University, P.O. Box 124, S-22100 Lund, Sweden.

Jean Montreuil Laboratoire de Chimie Biologique, Université des Sciences et Technologies de Lille 1, UMR CNRS 111, 59655 Villeneuve d'Ascq Cedex, France.

Ph. Moriniére Service d'Hémodialyse, Centre Hospitalier Universitaire d'Amiens, Hôpital Sud, Avenue René Laennec, Salouel 80054 Amiens Cedex, France.

Klaus Mosbach Lund University, Pure and Applied Biochemistry, Chemical Center, P.O. Box 124, S-22100 Lund, Sweden.

Nadir T. Mrabet Université Henri Poincaré Nancy l, Faulté de Medecine, Department of Cellular and Molecular Pathology in Nutrition, 54506 Vandoeuvre-Lès-Nancy Cedex, France.

Sven Oscarsson Institutionen för Biologioch Kemitecnik, Box 325, 631 05 Eskilterna, Sweden.

Olivier Pitiot Pasteur Mérieus Connaught, 1541, Av. Marcel Merieux, 69280 – Marcy l'Etoile, France.

J. Porath University of Arizona, Separation Science Center, Tucson, Arizona 85721, USA.

D. M. F. Prazeres Instituto Superior Tecnico, Departamento de Engenharia Quimica, Secçao de Biotecnologia, Avenue Rouisco Pais, 1096 Lisboa Codex, Portugal.

Robert K. Scopes School of Biochemistry, Faculty of Science and Technology, La Trobe University, Bundoora, Victoria 3083, Australia.

William H. Scouten Biotechnology Center, Utah State University, Logan UT 84322, USA.

Gérard Strecker Laboratoire de Chimie Biologique, Université des Sciences et Technologies de Lille 1, UMR CNRS 111, 59655 Villeneuve d'Ascq Cedex, France.

Jaroslava Turková Institute of Organic Chemistry and Biochemistry, Academy of Sciences of the Czech Republic, Flemingovo namestri 2, Czech Academy of Science, 16610 Prague 6, Czech Republic.

Mookambeswaran A. Vijayalakshmi Université de Technologie de Compiègne, LIMTechS – UPRES A CNRS 6022, Centre de Recherches, BP 20.529, 60205 Compiègne Cedex, France.

Nicolas Voute Biosepra, 35 Avenue Jean Jaurés, 92390 Villeneuve la Garenne, France.

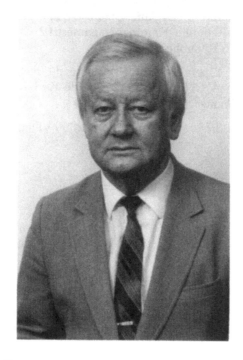

To my friend, Prof. Eugene Sulkowski

Acknowledgements

The preparation of this book started a few years ago. I would like to thank all the authors for their co-operation from the planning stage to the final phase of getting it in print, with patience. Unfortunately, one of the authors, my good friend, J. Turkova, passed away last year and I am deeply sorrowed and am indebted to her.

I would like to thank Harwood Academic Publishers (now Taylor and Francis), particularly Dr Edmar Weitenberg, a former member to have prompted and encouraged me to undertake this tough project. I also would like to thank Dr (Ms) Claire Rhodes in Reading for her sustained interest, encouragement and collaboration. The present colleagues from Taylor and Francis have made it possible to at last see the book published. I would like to express my thanks to all of them.

I would like to put on record my most sincere thanks to Prof E. Sulkowski, Roswell Park Cancer Institute, Buffalo, NY, USA, who has been behind the scene doing a good part of my editing job. I would like to thank all my coworkers at LIMTechS, France, for their sustained help all through these years. My special thanks are due to Miss Daniela Todorova, my PhD student for her precious collaboration in organising and following up the work with other colleagues, Mrs Laurence Alegria, my secretary, Mr Olivier Pitiot and Mr Yannick Coffinier, both my PhD students.

Finally, I would express my thanks to my deceased mother (who passed away during the preparation of this book) and to my two brothers and their wives who have constantly encouraged me and helped me to stand up to any tough challenges, through their love and affection.

Preface

Biochromatography, which is one of the key aspects of biomolecule/protein separation, has now progressed to the extent that is no longer just a "purification tool", that one can now open a commercial catalogue and perform an efficient purification. The field of bioseparation/biochromatography, cannot any more be considered as simply technical, but emerges as a Science: the bioseparation sciences.

Today the development of the concept of bioseparation is, to a considerable extent, based on (1) the knowledge of the molecular properties of biomolecules (e.g. proteins) and (2) the knowledge of the physicochemical and thermodynamic nature of the molecular interactions involved in chromatographic operations.

The advanced knowledge of proteins has helped the development of chromatographic methods, and the same chromatographic methods, in their turn, became very useful complementary tools for the study of protein structure and structural modifications. The Immobilized Metal-ion Affinity Chromatography is one of the best examples to illustrate this view point.

In this book we attempt to emphasize the potentials of biochromatographic methods in protein studies, starting with their purification. Specific discussions on the mechanism(s) of protein retention on many of the "pseudobioaffinity" adsorbents are highlighted in order to be able to use these tools more efficiently in protein studies.

While the main body of the book deals with biochromatography, the importance of upstream and downstream steps in protein purification is evoked.

In order to provide students, teachers and research workers in different biofields (biotechnology, biomedicine etc.) with a concise and a practical treatise, I have included both the well established basic chromatographic methods and also emerging methods with high potential. In each case, both theoretical and practical aspects are discussed so as to enable the reader to put them into practice in an efficient manner.

The field of bioseparation in general, and biochromatography in particular, is advancing so rapidly that no single person will be able to cover and describe, with confidence and authority, the wealth of techniques and methods which makes up the arsenal for protein separation and studies. In order to get the best description of each of the biochromatography methods presented in this volume, I have solicited contributions from the corresponding experts. Most of them graciously accepted my request to share their expertise with the readers.

Biochromatography has contributed enormously to biomolecule/protein separation, but its biomedical (i.e. clinical) applications have not followed suit, as one might expect. This is mainly due to a lack of dialogue between the scientists involved in these apparently distinct fields. I therefore tried to introduce a new feature, viz. the biomedical (clinical) applications of biochromatography, highlighting the common and specific traits to be considered for the clinical exploitation of developments in biochromatographic science.

The fulgurant evolution of biochromatography, particularly the affinity chromatographic systems, is mainly reflected today in the scientific progress in terms of scientific publications, meetings etc. In order for this evolution to be useful to industries, we try to cover the following aspects: (1) computer simulation to predict and plan the protein purification, (2) engineering aspects and (3) the regulatory aspects for the production of molecules of pharmaceutical interest.

Foreword

We are approaching the year 2003 when we intend to celebrate the centenary of the Russian scientist M. Tswett's invention that made separation of chlorophylls, carotenoids and other pigments in plant extracts possible. In some of his experiments light petroleum extracts were poured onto beds of powdered calcium carbonate and he "developed chromatograms" by washing the beds with the same or different solvents. Yellow and green zones appeared in the bed and the corresponding substances could be recovered by cutting the bed into sections or collected in the eluates of "flowing chromatograms". He called the method "chromatography"; a linguistic construction of dubious meaning! Tswett himself also separated colorless substances by adsorption followed by desorption in columns.

Since Tswett's time the concept, liquid chromatography, has undergone an immense expansion and chromatography has become an indispensable tool in the daily life of chemists and biologists. Liquid chromatography includes all procedures characterized by differential migration of sample components in a solution that is passing through a bed of particulate matter, whether the separation depends on adsorption, molecular sieving, liquid/liquid partitioning or a combination of these factors. Broader definitions are used to include separations in thin layers (planar chromatography). Under the name "covalent chromatography" we also find the technique to separate sample substances by covalent fixation to a solid support followed by an appropriate chemical release reaction. We also encounter electrochromatography – a hybrid between electrophoresis and adsorption chromatography.

With such a wide definition we have to admit that there were forerunners to Tswett: for example, F. Goppelroeder with his "capillary analysis". We may also argue that nature operates with chromatography on a giga scale as, for example, when iron becomes concentrated by mineral leaching in podzols.

Bioaffinity chromatography was pioneered long ago, but its full-fledged technology emerged rather recently. Conceptually, biochromatography is founded on the principle of steric complementarity combined with a multitude of affinity functions. Restrictions due to ligand immobilization and to the presence of "artificial solvents" (not the same as in the living systems) usually do not permit the high specificity and selectivity occurring in nature to be fully realized. In spite of that fact, bioaffinity chromatography has become an extremely powerful and useful tool for rapid separation of fragile biomolecules in biological extracts and fluids. However, the scarcity and lability of bioactive proteins limit their use as ligands in chromatography. Use of less selective but more robust small molecular ligands sometimes called "pseudobio affinity ligands", may often be preferable. The price for giving up extreme selectivity can usually be compensated for by combinatorial use of composite columns made up by many beds, each containing an adsorbent with its specified characteristic pseudobioaffinity. The beds may be arranged in sequence and, even more efficiently, in branched cascades. The number of affinity combinations are legion, and consequently extremely efficient separations may be obtained. Even isolation of particular trace substances from a complex mixture may therefore be achieved quickly and in a reproducible manner. Improved, safer technology will no doubt be available to meet pressing future demands for extreme purity of synthetic and modified macromolecular drugs for their use in therapy. To cope with the large scale operations it will become necessary to develop efficient displacement technologies. Extracorporeal processes with sorbents of very high selectivity and capacity will be forthcoming. The present state of the art in this fascinating branch of biochromatography is covered in this monograph.

This volume surveys many areas of biochromatography. The chapters are written by authors who have made major contributions in their fields of expertise. Up to ninety percent of the articles in the reference lists were published after 1980. This I take as a good omen that the history of chromatography is not at all approaching an end, but rather is still at an early stage.

Prof Jerker Porath,
University of Uppsala
and University of Arizona

Chapter 1

Upstream and downstream steps in biochromatography

Mookambeswaran A. Vijayalakshmi

Introduction

The "Biochromatography" or "chromatography of biological molecules" is a multidisciplinary field, involving the expertise development in:

1 Polymer chemistry, for the development of column packing materials/adsorbents with different composition, different derivatization and different particle sizes etc.
2 Mechanical designing of the columns with fluid mechanics knowledge.
3 Development of software for data handling, operation controls and even simulations.
4 Detection systems with optics, lasers, amperometrics etc.
5 Sophisticated physico-chemical analytical methods on-line or off-line such as ESI-MS.

The striking development of highly efficient and sophisticated microanalytical and preparative chromatography has led to tremendous progress in the study of proteins and peptides. Nevertheless, optimisation of upstream and downstream operations, in chromatography steps, such as finding the right conditions of extraction, sample preparation and suitable methods for monitoring the protein and biological activities remain crucial. Several manuals are available which cover the detailed operations of protein separation and purification covering relevant details of the extraction methods (Scopes, 1987; Ladish *et al.*, 1990; Janson and Ryden, 1989; *Methods in Enzymology*, 22, 34 and 204).

We can divide protein separation and purification into four broad steps: *extraction; fractional precipitation; purification and final polishing* (Fig. 1.1). Before these four steps the source identification and choice of raw material for the targetted protein is an important issue which in turn, will determine/orientate the choice of extraction methods.

Choice of sources of raw materials

In the case, particularly, of biochromatographic operations of proteins, the following questions have to be answered before designing any experimental set up (Fig. 1.2). What is the final targetted use of the protein? Is the protein for purification meant for basic studies on the protein, such as crystal structure or is it meant for large scale production to be used in agro food industry or pharmaceutical industry? If

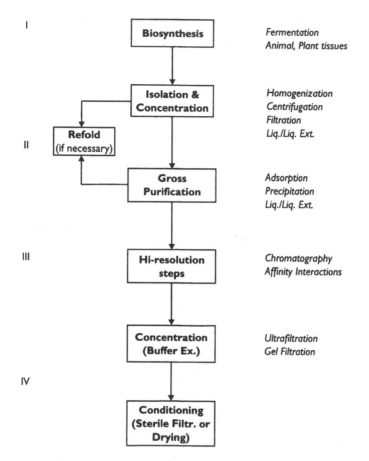

Figure 1.1 General purification scheme with the four major setps, in downstream processing.

the final use is pharmaceutical, then one has to take into consideration the high demand on the purity of the final product: 99.9–99.99%. In terms of choice of raw material, these questions have a high relevance. If we use animal sources e.g. albumin or IgG from animal/human sera, we have to seriously consider alternative sources to avoid the potential HIV, Hepatitis B, etc. contamination, from the raw material.

These alternative sources are mainly based on recombinant technology; human/animal proteins are expressed in micro-organisms or humanised cells or plant cells or whole plants, seeds, fruits etc. The use of the latter sources, also termed as Molecular Farming, is more recent and is quite promising in terms of cost effective and facile production of the raw material. But, here the purification, particularly the extraction steps prior to the chromatographic steps needs special care, both in terms of the enormous quantity of the raw material to be treated (leaves, seeds, fruits etc.) and also the composition of buffers (e.g. addition of polyvinylpyrolidone) for preventing the complexation of the target proteins with polyphenols.

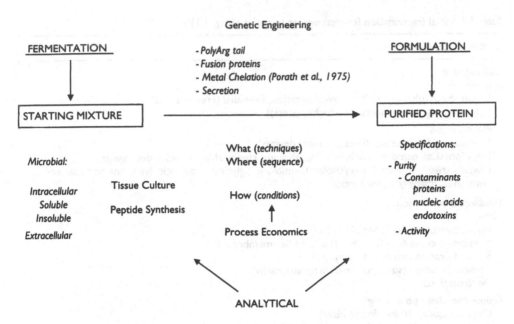

Figure 1.2 The multifaceted nature of protein purification process development. (From HO 1990 with permission.)

Extraction methods

The extraction step is meant for obtaining the target molecule (protein) in solution. It is obvious that certain raw materials of biological origin constitute an almost clear solution of the protein. Some of the examples are: blood sera, urine, milk, extracellular protein in the animal, bacterial, yeast, mammalian and plant cells culture media. The main upstream step in these cases is just the cell separation and concentration step by membrane (ultrafiltration) processes or by precipitation techniques.

In the case of insoluble raw materials such as animal or vegetal tissues and in the case of intracellular proteins produced in the cell culture systems, not only adequate extraction methods should be used to obtain the protein in its soluble form, but also specific additives such as protease inhibitors, reducing agents, polyphenol blockers (e.g. polyvinylpyrolidone) should be added to the extraction media.

A classification of extraction methods and their applicability to different raw materials is described in Table 1.1.

The use of detergents in the extraction step needs some special comments. The addition of detergents is used mainly for the extraction of membrane bound proteins, by reducing the hydrophobic interactions involved in the protein binding to the membranes. Some chaotopic agents can replace detergents for the same purpose. Some detergents may denature the proteins; hence attention has to be paid both for the choice of the detergents for extraction, their concentration and also whether to keep the presence of detergent in all the steps including the final chromatographic steps. This last point evokes the question of compatibility of the specific detergent added to the buffer and the chromatographic adsorption media chosen. Non-ionic detergents such as

Table 1.1 Initial fractionation (corresponding to step I of Fig. 1.1)

Isolation methods

Cell rupture
Mechanical
   Liquid shear (ultrasound, Mechanical agitation, Pressure (French press))
   Solid shear (grinding, pressure (Hughes press))
Non-mechanical
   Dessication (air, vaccum, freeze, solvent dryings)
   Lysis (physical: osmotic shock, freezing, thawing; chemical: pH shocks, detergents
   (Tween, triton, sodium desoxycholate), antibiotics, glycine; enzymatic: lysozyme and related
      enzymes, phage lysis, antibiotics

Solid/liquid separation
Filtration
   Membrane ultrafiltration/diafiltration
   Membrane cross-flow filtration (hollow fiber membrane)
   Sterile filtration (flat membrane)
   Particle filtration (size exclusion chromatography)
   Electrodialysis
Aquous two phase partitioning
   Organic/aquous (chloroform/water)
   Aquous/aquous (polyethylen glycol/dextran)
Centrifugation (is also associated with precipitation methods)
Precipitation
   pH
   Temperature
   Salts (ammonium sulfate, sodium sulfate)
   Polymers (polyethylen glycol)
   Organic solvents (butanol, acetone, lipidic solvents...)
   Affinity (homo, hetero multi biofunctional ligands supporting by soluble polymers)

Triton x-100 are usually more compatible with the different affinity adsorbants than the ionic detergents such as Sodium Dodecyl Sulfate (SDS). Moreover SDS can denature the protein and interfere with its biological activity. The ionic, non-ionic and zwitterionic nature of the specific detergent may have an impact both on protein surface as well as on the chromatographic adsorbent properties, thus influencing both adsorption and the elution of the protein in the chromatographic steps. Thus a fairly good knowledge of the chemical structure of the detergent to be chosen is very useful. The reader can get more information on the detergents and their physicochemical properties, in Hjelmeland's chapter in *Methods in Enzymology* vol. 124, 1986.

The optimum concentration of the detergent to be used, should invariably be below the critical micelle concentration, in order to avoid the protein being entrapped into the micelle and thus not able to interact with chromatographic adsorbent surfaces. However, in the electrokinetic chromatographic mode, the protein-detergent micelles are exploited for separating/studying the proteins as a function of their size (Landers, 1993).

The other additives to be used, including the buffers, during the extraction step and up to the chromatographic steps are enumerated in Table 1.2.

Table 1.2 Extraction medium

Agents

Buffers
   Sodium (acetate, bicarbonate,citrate, phosphate)
   Ammonium (acetate, bicarbonate)
   Tris (chloride, phosphate)
   Goods buffres (MOPS, MES, HEPES, EPPS)

Detergents
   Triton X-100 (non ionic, mild non denaturing)
   Nonidet (non ionic)
   Lubrol PX (non ionic)
   Octyl glucoside (non ionic)
   Tween 80 (non ionic)
   Sodium deoxycholate (anionic)
   Sodium dodecyl sulphate, SDS (anionic, strong denaturing)
   CHAPS (zwitterionic)

Reducing agents
   Mercaptoethanol
   1.4 Dithioerythritol, DTE
   1.4 Dithiotreitol, DTT

Precipitation agents
   Ammonium sulfate salt
   Sodium sulfate salt
   Organic solvent (ethanol, acetone)
   Polyethylen glycol

Proteolytic inhibitors
   Diisopropyl fluorophosphate, DFP (serine proteases)
   Phenylmethylsulfonylfluoride, PMSF (serine proteases)
   Ethylendiaminetetracetate, EDTA (metal-activated enzymes)
   Cystine reagents (cystine dependent proteases)
   Pepstatin A (acid proteases)

Fractionation techniques

This step is intended mainly for reducing the volume of the solution to be handled in further steps. It also reduces the total number of components present in the medium. The fractionation methods are mainly based on precipitation of the target protein by decreasing its solubility by modifying the salt concentration ("salting in" and "salting out" approaches); or by the addition of organic solvents or organic polymers. Temperature and/or pH variations leading to targetted denaturation of the contaminating proteins and precipitation of the desired protein may also be used as a fractionation step.

In the "salting out" approach the property of a particular salt (e.g. $(NH_4)_2 SO_4$) as an efficient precipitation agent is deduced from the so called Hofmeister series

anions : $PO_4^{3-} > SO_4^{2-} > CH_3COO^- > Cl^- > B^{2-} > NO_3^- > ClO_3^- > I^- > SCN$
i.e. PO_4^{3-} and SO_4^2 are the most effective precipitating agents.
Cations : $NH_4^+ > K^+ > Na^+ >$ guanidine $C(NH_2)_3^+$
i.e. NH_4^+ is the most efficient agent.

Hence it follows from the above that $(NH_4)_2 SO_4$ is a very good precipitation agent. Moreover, this salt ensures minimisation of any denaturation as it stabilises the native conformation of the protein to be precipitated.

Organic solvents promote the precipitation of proteins by disturbing the organised water molecules around the protein. Even though, it may, at first sight look like organic solvents may denature the proteins, two organic solvents namely, ethanol and acetone have been very successfully used for the selective precipitation of serum proteins, enzymes or hormones.

The ethanol precipitation of serum proteins known as the "COHN fractionation" method introduced in 1946 (Cohn, 1946) is used even today at all levels, may be with some modification (Taylor, 1956). This method, by a proper control of pH and temperature, enables one to prepare fractions particularly enriched in albumin, β globulins and γ globulins. In addition, the use of ethanol and subzero temperatures ensures certain safety against microbial and other contamination during the process.

The organic polymers such as polyethylene glycol (PEG) in the molecular weight range of 6000 to 20000 are able to precipitate the proteins by sequestrating the water molecules in a rather similar way to the organic solvents (Curling, 1980). PEG is the most widely used polymer due to its inocuity, non toxicity, low immunogeneicity etc.

In some cases inorganic polymers are used to concentrate the protein solutions. Here the phenomenon exploited is not a precipitation, but a physical adsorption. A case in study is the use of silica or cesium, Kieselger etc. to concentrate proteins from culture broth or even from urine. The adsorbed proteins are then stripped off using minimum quantity of buffers to be used in further steps.

Sample preparation from the precipitates

In the fractional precipitation step where the sample is concentrated, the precipitates are recovered either by simple centrifugation most often in laboratories or by liquid–liquid two phase partition (see Scopes, 1987 for more details of the technique) at larger scales. Then the precipitated protein fraction is solubilized in a minimum quantity of buffer and either used as such (if hydrophobic interaction chromatography is used as the first step) or desalted using either membrane process (ultrafiltration) or by desalting chromatography using a sephadex G25 gel filtration mode.

Organisation of different chromatographic steps in the protein fine purification

In this book more than ten different chromatographic approaches, based mainly on diffusion and adsorption principles are discussed in detail. A clear understanding of their underlying principles will enable one to set up the purification train as described in Fig. 1.1, schematising the different unit operations. The unit no. III englobes the chromatographic steps.

The sequential order in which these chromatographic operations should be set up, must take into account the minimisation of the total number of steps in a purification scheme. Increasing the number of steps not only results in increased investment and operational costs, but, also entails loss of the pure protein. In fact, at each step due to denaturation and product loss by strong adsorption etc. the yield of the pure product decreases (Hu *et al.*, 1985).

Monitoring the fractionation and purification

An important prerequisite for setting up a purification scheme is to have adequate assay procedures to follow the biological activity and protein content. The protein content can be monitored both by calorimetric assays, such as Lowry method (Lowry, 1951), Bradford method (Bradford, 1976), Biuret method (Smith *et al.*, 1985) or by bisinconinic acid (Sorenson and Brodbeck, 1986), and by UV monitoring at 280 nm or eventually with multiple wavelength detection.

The biological activity and protein contents should be recorded at each step, in order to follow the efficiency of purification and yield. A typical example of a purification table is shown in (Table 1.3).

Other methods of control such as in Fig. 1.3 should be performed, mainly at the final steps of purification.

Table 1.3 A typical table presenting the protein purification from a crude extract

Fraction	Protein (mg)	Activity (U)	Specific activity (U/mg)	Yield (%)	Purification factor
Crude extract					
(NH₄)SO₄ precipitation					
Dialysed extract					
Adsorption chromatography					
Unbound peak					
Retained and eluted peak					

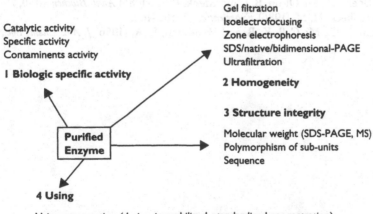

Figure 1.3 General process for the quality control of purified enzyme/protein.

Conventionally, the SDS-PAGE and Molecular Sieving by Gel filtration chromatography either using Sepharose®, Superose® at low pressure or HPLC-SEC approach using TSK range of gels are used. But with the advent of mass spectrometry techniques, particularly the electrospray ionic mass spectrometry (ESI-MS) the molecular heterogeneicity and molecular masses can be determined with high precision. In our lab, in the last few years, in the chromatographic steps, meant for fine purification, the fractions are routinely analysed by ESI-MS. This enabled us to identify the separation of subspecies/isoforms of the enzymes (Berna *et al.*, 1997).

References

Berna, P. P., Mrabet, N. T., Van Beeumen, J., Devreese, B., Porath, J. and Vijayalakshmi, M. A. (1997) *Biochem.*, **36**(51), 16355–16356.

Bradford, M. M. (1976) *Anal. Biochem.*, **72**, 248–254.

Cohn, E. J., Strong, L. E., Hughes, W. L., Mulford, D. J., Asworth, J. N., Melin, M. and Taylor, H. L. (1946) *J. Amer. Chem. Soc.*, **68**, 459–475.

Curling, J. M. (1980) *Methods of plasma protein fractionation*, Academic Press Ed.

Hjelmeland, L. M. (1986) In: *Methods in Enzymology*, **124**, 135–164.

Ho, S. V. (1990) Strategies for large scale protein purification. In: *Protein purification: from molecular mechanisms to large-scale processes.* (Ladish, Willson, Painton and Builder, eds), American Chemical Society, Washington, USA, 14–34.

Hu, W. S. and Wang, D. I. C. (1985) In: Mammalian cell technology (Thilly, W. G. and Addison-Wesley, eds.), Menlo Park, CA.

Jansen, J. C. and Ryden, L. (1989) Protein purification: principles, high resolution methods and applications. VCH publishers Inc.

Ladish, M. R., Willson, R. C., Painton, C. D. and Builder, S. E. (1990) Protein purification: from molecular mechanisms to large scale processes. American Chemical Society, pp. 20–22.

Landers, J. P. (1993) *TIBS*, **18**, 409–414.

Lowry, O. H. (1951) *J. Biol. Chem.*, **193**, 265–267.

Scopes, R. K. (1987) Protein purification principles and pratice, Springer-Verlag.

Smith, P. K., Krohn, R. I., Hermanson, G. T., Mallia, A. K., Gartner, F. H., Provenzano, M. D., Fujimoto, E. K., Goeke, N. M., Olson, B. J. and Klenk, D. C. (1985) *Anal. Biochem.*, **150**, 76–85.

Sorenson, L. and Brodbeck, H. M. (1986) *Experientia*, **42**, 161–162.

Taylor, H. L., Bloom, F. C., Mc Call, K. B. and Hyndman, L. A. (1956) *J. Am. Chem. Soc.*, **78**, 1356–1358.

Chapter 2

Gel filtration

Kjell-Ove Eriksson

Introduction

In gel filtration molecules separate according to size as they pass through the column. They are separated due to the varying degree of steric exclusion from the pores of the packing material. The pores within the beads are such that not the whole pore volume is accessible for large molecules, while smaller molecules can penetrate into all pores. Accordingly, larger molecules elute earlier than smaller ones in gel filtration.

Separation by gel filtration was described by Lathve and Ruthven (Lathve and Ruthven, 1955); they used granulated starch as packing material. This packing material could only be used at very low flow rates. The technique came into prominence in 1959, when Porath and Flodin (Porath and Flodin, 1959) demonstrated gel filtration on dextran gels. This led to the introduction of the Sephadex® gels. Later, polyacrylamide (Hjerten and Mosbach, 1962) and agarose (Hjerten, 1962) were introduced as packing materials. In 1967 DeVries introduced the first totally rigid porous packing material for gel filtration, silica (DeVries *et al.*, 1967).

Over the years, several different names for the technique have been used. The name gel filtration chromatography is today the most commonly used for aqueous based size separation. This name is somewhat misleading since none of the different packing materials used are true gels and the separation principle is not filtration. Other names used for the technique are (size) exclusion chromatography (Pederson, 1962), molecular sieve chromatography (Hjerten and Mosbach, 1962) and gel permeation chromatography (Moore, 1964). Gel permeation chromatography is almost exclusively used in the area of polymer chemistry where the technique is widely used for polymer characterization.

In the area of peptide/protein purification and characterization gel filtration has three main areas of application: analytical (including molecular weight estimations), fractionation, and desalting (or group separation). The technique is used in small HPLC scale as well as in large industrial scale processes.

Separation principle

The separation in gel filtration is, ideally, only dependent on the size and shape of the different molecules to be separated and the pore size and shape of the packing material. The molecules distribute themselves between the volume outside the particles and the volume inside the pores. At a particular moment during the separation a certain fraction of each molecular species is found inside the pores (except for large molecules totally excluded from the pores). The smaller the molecule the larger this fraction is. Larger molecules do not have access to the entire pores due to steric hindrance, while smaller molecules have access to a larger portion of the pores. The smaller molecules thus spend longer time inside the pores compared to larger ones. The fraction of the molecules that are outside the particles move down the column with the same speed as the solvent itself. Thus, the larger molecules elute earlier than the smaller ones. The separation principle of gel filtration is illustrated in Fig. 2.1.

Selectivity is a term describing the actual degree of separation or difference in retention between different molecules in a sample on a chromatographic column. The selectivity of a gel filtration packing material is not altered by changing the composition of the mobile phase as long as this change does not influence the solute shape and size or the shape and size of the pore (structure) of the packing material. A selectivity curve can be obtained by plotting an expression of the solute size vs a function describing the elution volume of the solute.

The capacity factor, k', is widely used in chromatography to define the elution position of a particular solute with respect to the solvent front. (k' – a normalized measure of retention, equal to the retention time (or volume) of a given solute minus the void time (or volume, equal to the time or volume of a completely unretained peak) divided by the void time or volume.) In adsorption chromatography where the solute interacts with the stationary phase the k' values are positive. In gel filtration chromatography the solutes elute earlier than the solvent front, and thus k' is negative. The separation process in gel filtration is therefore not normally described by k' but rather with K_{av} (or K_D).

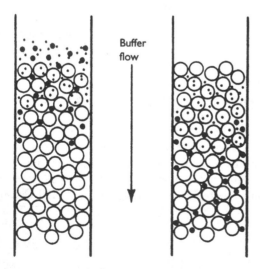

Buffer flow

Figure 2.1 Simplified drawing illustrating the principle of gel filtration. Large molecules are excluded from the pores of the particles and thus move rapidly through the column. Small molecules, which can diffuse into the pores, move down the column less rapidly. Reproduced with permission from Springer-Verlag (Scopes, 1982).

The volume of the mobile phase outside the beads is called the void volume (V_0), the volume occupied by the solvent inside the particles (the packing material or stationary phase) (V_i), and the volume occupied by the gel matrix (V_g). The total volume of the bed (V_c) is the sum of these:

$$V_c = V_0 + V_i + V_g \tag{1}$$

The elution volume of a solute is called (V_e). Using these parameters K_{av} can be defined:

$$K_{av} = \frac{V_e - V_0}{V_c - V_0} \tag{2}$$

A different approach is to define K_D:

$$K_D = \frac{V_e - V_0}{V_t - V_0} \tag{3}$$

where V_t is the elution volume of a molecule totally permeating the pores of the beads (particles). K_{av} is probably used more than K_D. Note that K_{av} is not a true distribution coefficient, while K_D is.

The size of a molecule is generally expressed as molecular mass or as the logarithm of the molecular mass, log M. Figure 2.2 shows a plot of K_{av} against log M for a gel filtration column. Note that in reality the curve is sigmoidal, and not linear over the separation range. Even if this is the most common way to plot the data one has to

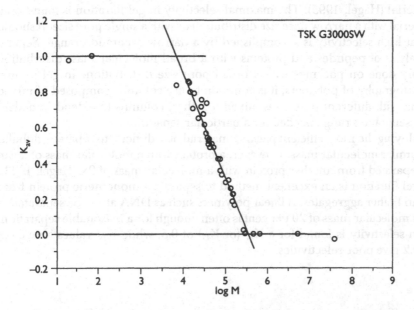

Figure 2.2 Plot of K_{av} vs log M for 37 standard proteins. The chromatography was performed at 1.0 ml/min with two 7.8 × 300 mm TSK G3000 SW columns in 10 mM phosphate buffer in 100 mM NaCl. Reproduced with permission from Marcel Dekker (Himmel *et al.*, 1995).

remember that it is the size of the molecule that determines the elution volume of a solute, and not the molecular mass. Only if the column is calibrated with homologous standard compounds of known molecular mass, one can find a relationship between molecular mass and molecular size. In the plot in Fig. 2.2 it is seen that there are solutes eluting at a K_{av} of 1.0, e.g. $V_e = V_c$. This indicates that there is an interaction between these solutes and the packing material.

Factors affecting the separation

Pore volume/size

Packing materials for gel filtration are available in many different sizes, i.e. packings suitable for peptide separations as well as for protein complexes and small virus particles. Normally manufacturers of the gel filtration media specify which molecular mass range (proteins or dextrans) that the different media are intended for. Rarely is the pore size given the exception being silica-based materials, where an apparent pore size some times is specified.

The total pore volume of the media (packing material) is a most important characteristic, since it is in this volume the separation of the solutes take place. The larger this volume is the higher the resolution in a particular separation. A very large pore volume, i.e. too low content of gel media will generally result in a more fragile or compressible material. The porosities are lower for silica packings compared to polymeric and carbohydrate packings (Gooding and Hagestam Freiser, 1991).

In gel filtration, the selectivity is a direct function of the pore size distribution of the packing material (Hagel, 1995). The maximal selectivity in gel filtration is found on a packing material with a narrow pore size distribution or with a single pore size. It should be noted that high selectivity is accomplished by a narrow separation range. Separation and analysis of peptides and proteins with a broad molecular mass distribution are preferably done on packings with a broad pore size distribution. In gel permeation chromatography of polymers, it is common to use columns composed of mixed media (media with different pore sizes mixed together) columns to extend (broaden) the effective separation range needed for a particular separation.

Even employing the most efficient packing material, it is difficult to separate globular proteins of similar molecular mass. However, a protein with a molecular mass of x can usually be separated from another protein with a molecular mass of 2x (Hagel, 1993). Therefore, gel filtration is an excellent method to separate a monomeric protein from its dimers and higher aggregates. If linear polymers such as DNA are to be separated, a difference in molecular mass of 20 per cent is often enough for a reasonable separation. An optimum selectivity is found for a K_{av} (or K_D) of 0.5, while K_{av} values above 0.9 and below 0.2 give poor selectivities.

Particle size

The column efficiency, or plate count, is more important in gel filtration than in adsorption chromatography of peptides and proteins, because the molecules are eluted isocratically instead of in a linear or step gradient. HPLC packing materials with a particle size of 5–10 μm give the highest efficiency (the sharpest, most narrow peaks). The disadvantage of such small particles is the high backpressure they generate. This is rarely a problem in analytical separations where a HPLC pump often is used, but for large scale separations the only cost effective choice of packing materials are those of 30 μm and larger. It is important to realize this limitation before scaling up a separation based on an analytical media (Himmel *et al.*, 1955). Many packing materials are available in several particle sizes (fine, medium and coarse).

Support materials

In gel filtration it is important that the separation is due strictly to size and that adsorption, if any, is suppressed. This is generally accomplished by choosing a mobile phase that eliminates, or minimizes, any adsorption phenomena of the solutes onto the support material. No single support can be said to be the ideal or ultimate support material for gel filtration. The support medium thus has to be chosen dependent upon the particular separation.

The relative surface area of peptides is larger than for proteins, and the interaction between peptides and gel filtration media is expected to be more extensive than between proteins and the media (Hagel, 1995). One important interaction, sometimes used for separation/purification, is the adsorption of tryptophan-containing peptides on gel filtration media (Eaker and Porath, 1967). The most common interactions are hydrophobic interaction and electrostatic (ionic) interactions.

Some important characteristics of a packing material for gel filtration chromatography are

1 Rigidity, to allow a practical flow rate
2 Macroporosity
3 High pore volume
4 Hydrophilic – no hydrophobic interaction
5 Neutral – no ionic interaction
6 Good packability
7 Chemical stability over a broad pH range and with different mobile phases

Silica

Silica gel has an amorphous structure, which is highly porous, with a large surface area. The silica surface contains silanol groups of different configurations giving a high affinity for polar solutes, which makes it an excellent choice for many applications for small molecules (normal phase chromatography). This high affinity for polar solutes makes underivatized silica an unsuitable packing material for gel filtration of peptides and proteins. By derivatization of the silica surface, almost all nonspecific interactions can be prevented. Simple silanes like 1,2-epoxy-3-propoxypropyl-triethoxy silane, first introduced for gel filtration by Regnier's group (Regnier and Noel, 1976), as well as a polymer type of coating (TSK-gel SW packings) have been used. Silica has a limited pH stability and can not be used at a pH much above 7.5. Silica is a rigid packing material that is used mostly in analytical and semipreparative separations in a HPLC mode. Gel filtration on silica was recently reviewed (Eksteen and Pardue, 1995).

Dextran and polyacrylamide

Dextran gels have been used extensively for a long time under the trade name Sephadex® and so has polyacrylamide under the name BioGel P©. The separation range (pore size) is dependent on the degree of crosslinking of the gels. The lower degree of crosslinking of the media, the larger the molecules that can be separated. One drawback of a low degree of crosslinking is the low rigidity that results. Highly crosslinked dextran and polyacrylamide, on the other hand, are rigid and work well for desalting applications, even on industrial scale. Both dextran and polyacrylamide are hydrophilic and thus have a low nonspecific interaction with peptides and proteins.

Agarose

Agarose is a polysaccharide produced by red seaweed. Small amounts of sulfate and methyl groups could be found in agarose. Agarose has a unique structure; the individual polysaccharide chains are aggregated to form stiff fibers. The separation range of agarose media is controlled by the agarose content. The agarose media are semi-rigid, especially after crosslinking. The crosslinking does not influence the pore size. The pores in agarose media are relatively large and agarose based gel filtration media are thus suitable for separation of larger proteins and their aggregates. The relative rigidity of this packing material makes it suitable for preparative separations. Agarose media are sold under the trade names Sepharose® and BioGel A©.

Composite materials

These materials are polymer gels, which have a rigid backbone and a second polymer with its linear structure determines the separation properties (separation range) (Janson, 1995). Several different products were/are available. Ultrogel™ AcA in which polyacrylamide was trapped inside agarose pores and Sephacryl® which is a composite gel made by covalently crosslinking allyl dextran with N,N'-methylene bisacrylamide. Superdex® is based on a highly crosslinked, rigid, agarose packing with pores containing grafted dextran chains. These media are useful in many different applications in both analytical and preparative separations/purifications of peptides and proteins.

Solvent

Ideally, there are only two limitations for the solvent used in gel filtration: the stability of the packing material and the stability and solubility of the solute.

Polymeric bonded phases, including carbohydrate and composite packing materials, are stable in almost all buffers (pH 2–13) and at all buffer concentrations (ionic strengths) that could be used in gel filtration of peptides and proteins. Silica based packings are sensitive to alkaline conditions: pH values above 7.5 should be avoided for silica, except for short periods (sample loading at alkaline pH). Therefore, the buffer (solvent) can be chosen to suit the requirements of the peptides proteins in such a way that biological activity and three-dimensional structure are retained. Certain peptides and proteins may need detergents or an addition of an organic solvent to the buffer for a maximal solubility. Some peptides need drastic conditions for gel filtration, such as 10 per cent formic acid, for a good result. It should be noted that the buffer (solvent) can be chosen to suit a subsequent chromatography step, for example a proper ionic strength and pH for a follow-up ion-exchange purification step.

Nonspecific interaction

There is no single ideal packing material for gel filtration chromatography. On all packing materials some adsorption may occur, depending on the buffer chosen and the properties of the peptides and proteins that are to be separated.

There are two main types of adsorption phenomena: hydrophobic and ionic (electrostatic) interactions. Both agarose and silica based packing materials contain negatively charged groups that can interact with positively charged amino acid side chains in peptides and proteins. To prevent this type of interaction between solute and packing material the ionic strength of the buffer should be increased or salt could be added to the buffer (0.1–0.2 M NaCl). Hydrophobic interaction is found on most packing materials, especially on heavily crosslinked carbohydrate based packings, at high ionic strengths. Additives that can prevent this are isopropanol, ethylene glycol and detergents (to be used below their critical micelle concentration, or (CMC). It should be noted that these adsorption effects rarely effect a particular separation to a great extent. In some cases they can even contribute to the improvement of a separation.

Column length

The length of the column is a significant parameter since the resolution in gel filtration is proportional to the square root of the column length (Rs is proportional to $\sqrt{L}$, resolution is a term describing the full degree of separation between two chromatographic peaks, defined as the difference in retention divided by the average of peak widths). Thus the longer the column is the greater the resolution. But since the resolution is proportional to the square root of the column length and not the column length itself the gain in resolution does not justify the use of columns much longer than 80 cm. Longer columns take excessive time to elute, with high back pressures, and the separated zones (solutes) get more diluted as the column length increases. Most separations are done on columns that are 60–80 cm in length. With modern HPLC packings that have smaller particle sizes, 5–10 μm, shorter columns are often used. A typical HPLC column for gel filtration is 20–40 cm in length. For desalting (group separation) much shorter columns can be used. Desalting of small protein samples can be done on columns not longer than 5 cm in length.

Flow rate

The useful flow rate in gel filtration is restricted by the low diffusion coefficients of proteins and peptides. Zone broadening results due to non-equilibrium between the mobile phase outside the particle and inside the pores. The larger the solute, the more slowly it diffuses into and out of the pores of the particles. This slow diffusion results in peaks that broaden quickly with increased flow rate. Figure 2.3 illustrates the effect of the flow rate on a separation of standard proteins. Note that the solutes with higher molecular mass are more affected than molecules with lower molecular mass (Ricker

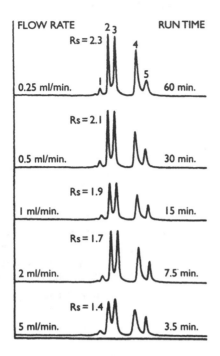

Figure 2.3 Effect of flow rate on resolution. A protein mixture was separated on a Zorbax GF-250 column (9.4 × 250 mm) in a 200 mM sodium phosphate buffer, pH 7.0. The flow rate was varied from 0.25 to 6.0 ml/min. All chromatograms are scaled relative to the flow rate used. Resolution between BSA (peak 2) and ovalbumin (peak 3) is shown. Reproduced with permission from Elsevier (Ricker and Sandoval, 1996).

and Sandoval, 1996). Gel filtration separations are normally performed at low flow rates and separation times are often 10 h or more for a column of 100 cm. HPLC columns packed with particles of small size such as 5 or 10 μm can be run faster, often with flow rates of 1.0–2.0 ml/min for a column with a diameter of 1.0 cm. Flow rates can be higher when smaller peptides are separated than when proteins are separated. For group separation (desalting) the flow rate can be high since the required resolution is between a protein (high molecular mass, totally excluded from the pores) and a salt (buffers etc. with low molecular mass).

Sample volume

Of the various mode of chromatography used to separate proteins and peptides, gel filtration has the lowest loading capacity in terms of sample volume. This limitation is due to the true isocratic nature of gel filtration. Depending on the resolution needed for a particular separation, it is recommended that sample volume not larger than 3–6 per cent of the total bed volume be applied. For high efficiency analytical gel filtration separations, the sample volume should be minimized and not exceed 0.5 per cent of the total bed volume (Hagel, 1985). The influence of the sample volume in gel filtration

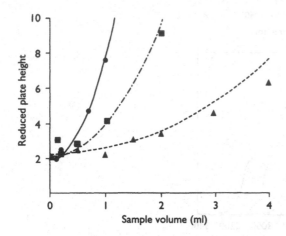

Figure 2.4 Effect of sample volume on the peak width, expressed as reduced plate height (*h*) for cytidine (reduced plate height is defined by: the plate height divided by the particle size). (●) Superose® 6 (10 × 500 mm column), (■) Superose 6 prep grade (10 × 530 mm) and (▲) Superose 6 prep grade (16 × 510 mm). Dots represents experimental data and lines represents a calculated relationship. Reproduced with permission from Elsevier (Hagel, 1985).

is illustrated in Fig. 2.4. For desalting, much larger volumes can be applied to the gel filtration column, often as much as one third of the total bed volume.

Sample concentration

In addition to sample volume the loading of a gel filtration column is restricted by the sample concentration. It has been observed that resolution at high sample concentrations is compromised. Non-uniform flow develops when the viscosity of the sample is too high. As a general rule, the viscosity of the sample relative to the eluent should be less than 1.5. This corresponds to a maximum concentration of 70 mg/ml of a globular protein such as human serum albumin (Hagel, 1989). Non uniform flow that arises from too high sample concentrations is often called "viscous fingering". Because of the opacity of most chromatography packing materials the phenomena has mostly been studied indirectly. The phenomena have recently been characterized directly by magnetic resonance imaging (Plante *et al.*, 1994). Figure 2.5 illustrates how sample concentration affects the flow profile in a gel filtration column.

Applications of gel filtration

There are three basic applications of gel filtration of peptides and proteins: analytical, fractionation and group separation/desalting.

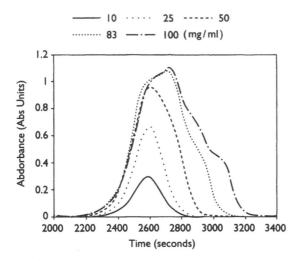

Figure 2.5 Gel filtration chromatograms of BSA at various sample concentrations. Sample volume: 0.5 ml, flow rate: 0.4 ml/min, column dimensions: 10 × 300 mm, packing: Toyopearl HW-65S (30 μm particle size). Reproduced with permission from Elsevier (Plante *et al.*, 1994).

Analytical gel filtration

The primary use of analytical gel filtration is the estimation of molecular masses of peptides and proteins. Other applications include the estimation of aggregation of proteins and as a technique for the determination of binding constants between proteins and low molecular mass ligands.

Molecular mass estimations of proteins and peptides by gel filtration can be made on a laboratory scale column (approximately 1 × 60 cm), as well as on a HPLC scale. Standard proteins with known molecular mass are used for the characterization of the column and for the construction of the calibration curve, K_{av} (or K_D) vs log molecular mass. As mentioned above, the standards must have the same shape as the analyte.

For an elongated protein molecule the estimated molecular mass will be too high when globular proteins are used as standards. When the molecular mass is estimated in a native buffer system (phosphate, Tris-HCl etc.) a degree of uncertainty is introduced into the result when a protein with unknown shape is analyzed. Combined with results from SDS-PAGE, the result from analytical gel filtration in a nondenaturing buffer can be used to determine the number of subunits in a particular protein.

In a denaturing solvent, a protein/peptide behaves like a random coil, provided that the disulfide bridges are reduced. Such solvents are 6 M guanidine hydrochloride and 8 M urea. Gel filtration in these solvents thus eliminates the shape of the protein as a factor influencing the chromatography. The molecular mass determination under these conditions can be done with high accuracy. Strictly speaking, it is not the molecular mass that is the determining factor for the elution of the proteins during gel filtration in denaturing solvents, but rather the number of amino acids in the protein. The results obtained are normally more accurate than results obtained with SDS-PAGE.

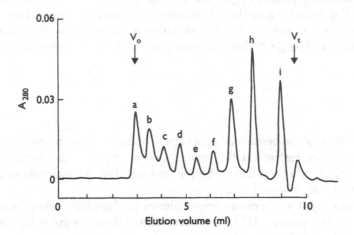

Figure 2.6 Gel filtration of model peptides and proteins on a column (6 × 345 mm) packed with 20 per cent agarose (10 μm particle size) in 6 M guanidine hydrochloride. Solutes were reduced and alkylated. Flow rate: 0.1 ml/min. Reproduced with permission from Elsevier (Eriksson and Hjerten, 1986).

This method has been used both on a laboratory scale (Davison, 1968 and Fish *et al.*, 1969) as well as on HPLC scale (Eriksson and Hjerten, 1986). An example of gel filtration in guanidine hydrochloride in HPLC scale is shown in Fig. 2.6.

As an alternative to guanidine hydrochloride or urea, SDS can be used as a denaturing agent in analytical gel filtration. In SDS (above CMC) proteins form a complex with detergent molecules (Lundahl *et al.*, 1986) and do not behave as random coils as in guanidine hydrochloride or urea. It has been used both on a laboratory scale (Page' and Godin, 1969) and HPLC scale (Eriksson, 1985), but are not as commonly used as guanidine hydrochloride.

It should be noted that for glycoproteins, the results obtained in analytical gel filtration are not as accurate as for non glycosylated proteins, neither in guanidine hydrochloride nor in SDS (Leach *et al.*, 1980). When SDS is used, it should be kept in mind that membrane proteins typically bind more detergent molecules than water-soluble proteins do.

When the gel filtration is used for the estimation of molecular mass, it is important to get an accurate value for K_{av} or K_D, therefore both V_0 and V_t have to be determined. For the determination of V_0, blue dextran (molecular mass 2 000 000) is often used. For gel filtration with media with the largest pores blue dextran is not the best choice due to the micro heterogeneity of the dextran. In this case a larger molecule or virus particle could be used. For determination of V_t, a small molecule that penetrates the entire pore volume is chosen. Molecules often used are acetone or NaCl etc. Acetone is a good choice since it can be monitored by an UV-detector.

Analytical gel filtration is almost always done on HPLC scale or with a laboratory scale column, although it can be predicted that microcolumns could be of importance in the future, especially in combination with mass spectrometry.

HPLC columns are normally packed by the manufacturer. For the best results the conditions specified by the manufacturer should be followed during operation. Laboratory scale columns with a diameter of 1–3 cm and with lengths of about 60 cm are slurry packed. For packing and usage of these columns, the manufacturer instructions should be followed.

Fractionation

Fractionation by gel filtration can be performed on a variety of scales. From preparation of a few mg of a protein (or even less) on a HPLC scale to very large process gel filtration applications where kilograms of a product can be purified per day. An example of a fractionation by gel filtration is given in Fig. 2.7.

The operation and packing of a laboratory scale column (1–5 cm in diameter and about 100 cm in length) and preparative HPLC columns follows the same guidelines as given for the analytical columns above.

Gel filtration is inherently a low capacity technique, and is therefore often used late in a protein (or peptide) purification process. Gel filtration is therefore used as a final, polishing, step in many purifications, to remove trace amounts of impurities and self aggregates of the product, and to buffer exchange (see below). However, it is also used at an earlier stage in many purification processes. This is exemplified by Marrs (Marrs, 1993), who describes an initial buffer exchange of raw plasma in a large scale albumin fractionation.

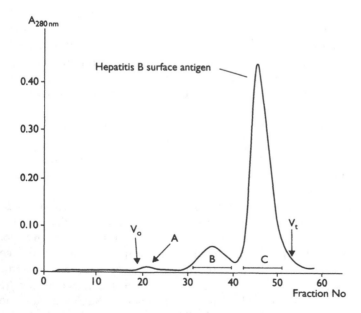

Figure 2.7 Gel filtration of a 9.5 ml sample containing recombinant hepatitis B surface antigen on a column packed with Sepharose® 4FF (column dimensions: 2.6 × 89 cm). Linear flow rate of 8.6 cm/h, buffer: 20 mM sodium phosphate containing 150 mM NaCl. Reproduced with permission from Kluwer (Belew et al., 1991).

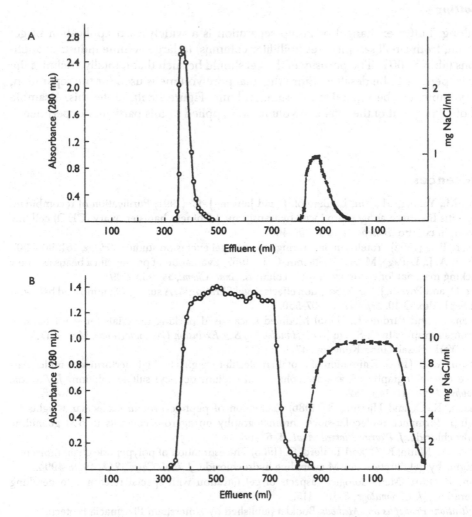

Figure 2.8 Buffer exchange/desalting of a large sample on Sephadex® G-25. Column: 4 × 85 cm, sample: (o) hemoglobin and (x) NaCl, sample volume in (A) 10 ml and in (B) 400 ml. Reproduced with permission from Elsevier (Flodin, 1960).

In process scale gel filtration, column diameters of up to 80 cm (and higher) are often used (Hagel and Janson, 1992). Column lengths of 60–80 cm are normally applied. If a column diameter larger than 10 cm is needed for capacity, columns connected in series (2–6 "stacked" columns) should be used, each with a bed height of 20–30 cm. Shorter columns allow a higher flow velocity during packing, resulting in beds with low v_0 values and less zone broadening (Janson, 1995). The higher packing velocity also prevents ongoing settling of the chromatographic bed. Stacked columns also limit the risk of a bed collapse, that can occur in a single column packed with a soft/semi rigid packing material.

Desalting

Desalting (buffer exchange) or group separation is a widely used application of gel filtration, from small sample sizes (milliliter columns) to large volume industrial applications (above 100 l). The porosity of the gel should be such that it totally excludes the protein/peptide to be desalted. Since the total pore volume is used for the separation, large volumes can be applied to a desalting column. Figure 2.8 illustrates this. A sample load of 37 per cent of the total bed volume was applied in this particular experiment.

References

Belew, M., Yafang, M., Bin, L., Berglöf, J. and Janson, J.-C. (1991) Purification of recombinant hepatitis B surface antigen produced by transformed Chinese hamster ovary (CHO) cell line grown in culture. *Bioseparation*, 1, 397–408.

Davison, P. F. (1968) Proteins in denaturing solvents: gel exclusion studies. *Science*, 161, 906–907.

DeVries, A. J., LePage, M. and Guillemin, C. L. (1967) Evaluation of porous silica beads as a new packing material for chromatographic columns. *Anal. Chem.*, 39, 935–939.

Eaker, D. and Porath, J. (1967) Sorption effects in gel filtration: I. A survey of amino acid behavior on Sephadex G-10. *Sep. Sci.*, 2, 507–550.

Eksteen, R. and Pardue, K. (1995) Modified silica-based packing materials for size exclusion chromatography. In C.-S. Wu (ed.), *Handbook of Size Exclusion Chromatography*, Marcel Dekker, New York, Basel, Hong Kong, pp. 47–101.

Eriksson, K.-O. (1985) Estimation of protein molecular weights by high performance molecular-sieve chromatography on agarose columns in sodium dodecyl sulfate solution. *J. Biochem. Biophys. Meth.*, 11, 145–152.

Eriksson, K.-O. and Hjerten, S. (1986) Estimation of peptide/protein molecular weights by high-performance molecular-sieve chromatography on agarose columns in 6 M guanidine hydrochloride. *J. Pharm. Biomed. Anal.*, 4, 63–68.

Fish, W. W., Mann, K. G. and Tanford, C. (1968) The estimation of polypeptide chain molecular weights by gel filtration in 6 M guanidine hydrochloride. *J. Biol. Chem.*, 244, 4989–4994.

Flodin, P. (1961) Methodological aspects of gel filtration with special reference to desalting operations. *J. Chromatogr.*, 5, 103–115.

Gel filtration: Principles and Methods. Booklet published by Amersham Pharmacia Biotech.

Gooding, K. M. and Hagestam Freiser, H. (1991) High-Performance size-exclusion chromatography of proteins. In C. T. Mant and R. S. Hodges (eds), *High-Performance Liquid Chromatography of Peptides and Proteins: Separation, Analysis and Conformation*, CRC, Boca Raton, Ann Arbor, Boston, London, pp. 135–144.

Hagel, L. (1985) Effect of sample volume on peak width in high-performance gel filtration chromatography. *J. Chrom.*, 324, 422–427.

Hagel, L. (1989) Gel filtration. In J.-C. Janson and L. Ryde'n (eds), *Protein Purification, Principles, High Resolution Methods, and Applications*. VCH, New York, Weinheim, Cambridge, pp. 63–106.

Hagel, L. (1993) Size-exclusion chromatography in an analytical perspective. *J. Chromatogr.*, 648, 19–25.

Hagel, L. (1996) Characteristics of modern media for aqueous size exclusion chromatography. In M. Potscka and P. L. Dubin (eds), *Strategies in Size Exclusion Chromatography, ACS Symposium Series 635.*, ACS, Washington, D.C., pp. 225–248.

Hagel, L. and Janson, J.-C. (1992) Size-exclusion chromatography. In E. Heftman (ed.), *Chromatography, 5th edition. Journal of Chromatography Library-Volume 51A.*, Elsevier, Amsterdam, Oxford, New York, Tokyo, pp. A267–A307.

Himmel, M. E., Baker, J. O. and Mitchell, D. J. (1995) Size exclusion chromatography of proteins. In C.-S. Wu (ed.), *Handbook of Size Exclusion Chromatography*, Marcel Dekker, New York, Basel, Hong Kong, pp. 409–428.

Hjerten, S. (1962) Chromatographic separation according to size of macromolecules and cell particles on columns of agarose suspensions. *Arch. Biochem. Biophys.*, 99, 466–475.

Hjerten S. and Mosbach, R. (1962) "Molecular-sieve" chromatography of proteins on columns of cross-linked polyacrylamide. *Anal. Biochem.*, 3, 109–118.

Janson, J.-C. (1995) Process scale size exclusion chromatography. In G. Subramanian (ed.), *Process Scale Liquid Chromatography*, VCH, Weinheim, New York, pp. 81–98.

Lathve, G. H. and Ruthven, C. R. J. (1956) The separation of substances and estimation of their relative molecular sizes by the use of columns of starch in water. *Biochem. J.*, 62, 665–674.

Leach, B. S., Collawn, Jr. J. F. and Fish, W. W. (1980) Behavior of glycopeptides with empirical molecular weight estimation methods. 2. In random coil producing solvents. *Biochemistry*, 19, 5741–5747.

Lundahl, P., Greijer, E., Sandberg, M., Cardell, S. and Eriksson, K.-O. (1986) A model for ionic and hydrophobic interactions and hydrogen-bonding in sodium dodecyl sulfate-protein complexes. *Biochim. Biophys. Acta*, 873, 20–26.

Marrs, S. B. (1993) Large scale albumin fractionation by chromatography. *Biotech. Blood Prot.*, 227, 169–173.

Moore, J. C. (1964) Gel permeation chromatography. I. A new method for molecular weight distribution of high polymers. *J. Polym. Sci.*, 132, 835–843.

Page', M. and Godin, C. (1969) On the determination of molecular weight of protein subunits on Sephadex G-200 in the presence of detergent. Glutamate dehydrogenase. *Can. J. Biochem.*, 47, 401–403.

Pederson, K. O. (1962) Exclusion chromatography. *Arch. Biochem. Biophys. Suppl.*, 1, 157–168.

Plante, L. D., Romano, P. M. and Fernandez, E. J. (1994) Viscous fingering in chromatography visualized via magnetic resonance imaging. *Chemical Engineering Sciences*, 49 (14), 2229–2241.

Porath, J. and Flodin, P. (1959) Gel filtration: a method for desalting and group separation. *Nature*, 183, 1657–1659.

Regnier, F. and Noel, R. (1976) Glycerolpropylsilane bonded phases in steric exclusion chromatography of biological macromolecules. *J. Chromat. Sci.*, 14, 316–320.

Ricker, R. D. and Sandoval, L. A. (1996) Fast reproducible size-exclusion chromatography of biological macromolecules. *J. Chromatogr. A*, 743, 43–50.

Scopes, R. (1982) *Protein Purification Principles and Practice*, Springer-Verlag, New York, Heidelberg, Berlin.

Chapter 3

Ion exchange interaction biochromatography

E. Boschetti and P. Girot

Introduction

Fractionation of protein mixtures by chromatography requires solid phases on which proteins are adsorbed reversibly without deterioration of their biological properties. Proteins are large size multifunctional polyelectrolytes and as such they can be adsorbed by electrostatic or coulombic interactions onto ionizable resins of opposite sign. This principle is extensively used and represents the most popular means to separate proteins from complex mixtures. Its effectiveness depends on a number of factors which have been studied in depth at theoretical and practical levels (Vermeulen *et al.*, 1984; Fernandez *et al.*, 1996). Since the interaction is based on electrical charges that can vary in sign, and strength, the possibilities of ion exchange in protein separation are numerous, and special conditions can be found to optimize operational parameters to obtain the best separation results for a particular protein mixture. A number of solid phase media are available today; they are made using various matrices to which ionizable groups are attached. Such diversity is firstly caused by the specificity that may vary from one matrix to another for the same ionic chemical group. Secondly, ion exchangers are also prepared to enhance various separation parameters such as binding capacity (Boschetti *et al.*, 1995), sorption kinetics (Muller, 1990), or speed (Afeyan *et al.*, 1990). Separation efficiency, mechanical stability or even the enhancement of diffusion (Coffman *et al.*, 1998) have recently been at the basis of new ion exchangers to reach better or more rapid separations.

In this review several practical aspects are presented with the aim to summarize for the chromatographer the information required to understand phenomena involved in ion exchange chromatography and to optimize the separation.

Matrices and ion exchange groups

Ion exchangers are composed of a solid porous structure supporting ionizable chemical groups. A wide variety of groups have been described and are classified into two categories: cationic and anionic.

Cationic chemical functions are substituted amines such as primary, secondary, tertiary and quaternary amino groups and also substituted pyridine groups. Anionic chemical functions are strong and weak acids such as sulfonates, sulfates, phosphates, carboxylates, boronates. Differentiation between weak and strong ionic groups is made on the basis of the pH range over which the groups display their electric charge.

All these ionizable functions are chemically attached to the polymeric solid material by means of a covalent bond. Attachment is obtained by chemical reactions (Peterson *et al.*, 1956); another method for the introduction of ionic groups on the matrix is a whole copolymerization of monomeric ionic molecules (Girot *et al.*, 1981).

Most generally ether, thioether and secondary amides are used as linkers. Table 3.1 summarizes the various most known ion exchange groups used for protein separation. The density of these functional groups on the polymeric matrix constitutes the ion exchange capacity which is measured by a simple ionic titration or by chemical analysis. Matrices of ion exchangers play a significant role in their behavior. The hydrophilic or hydrophobic dominant character of an ion exchanger is of primary importance for its selectivity as well as for the binding capacity of proteins.

There are three main categories of matrices: polysaccharide based polymers, synthetic ionic copolymers, mineral porous materials. Materials associating organic moieties with mineral structures are also well known since they represent an excellent advancement in high rigidity, high binding capacity and high density.

Table 3.2 summarizes the properties of various ion exchangers based on different matrices. They are characterized by the number and the nature of ionic groups, the

Table 3.1 Most common ionic groups used in ion exchange chromatography of proteins. These groups are anchored to the matrix of crosslinked polymeric material

Chemical group	Structure	pK	Anchorage to matrix
Sulphate	$-O-SO_3H$	<2	Ether linkage
Sulphonate	$-(CH_2)_n-SO_3H$	<2	Ether linkage
Phosphate	$-O-PO(OH)_2$	<2 and 6	Ether linkage
Carboxylate	$-(CH_2)_n-COOH$	3.5–4.2	Ether linkage
Tertiary amine	$-(CH_2)_n-N^+(CH_2)_2-(CH_2)_2-N(C_2H_5)_2$	8.5–9.5	Amido or ether linkage
Quarternary amine	$-(CH_2)_n-N^+(CH_3)_3$	>9	Amido or ether linkage

Table 3.2 Common ion exhangers for protein separation at preparative scale

Nature of the matrix	Composition	Trade name	Supplier	Ion exchange group
Polysaccharide	Agarose	Sepharose	Pharmacia Bio	DEAE, CM, Q, S
	Dextran	Sephadex	Pharmacia Bio	DEAE, CM, SP, QAE
	Cellulose	Sephacel	Pharmacia Bio	DEAE
		Cellulose fibers	Whatman	DEAE, CM, S
Synthetic	Acrylic	Trisacryl	BioSepra	DEAE, CM, QA, SP
		Macroprep	BioRad	CM, Q, S
	Vinylic	Fractogel	Merck	TMAE, DMAE, CM, SP
		Toyopearl	TosoHaas	QAE, DEAE, CM, SP
	Polystyrene	Resource	Pharmacia Bio	Q, S
		Poros	Perspective Bio	Q, S
Mineral composite	Silica	Spherosil	BioSepra	QMA
	Silica-dextran	Spherodex	BioSepra	DEAE, SP, CM
	Silica-acrylic pol.	HyperD	BioSepra	DEAE, CM, Q, S
	Silica-PEI	Matrex	Millipore	Mostly DEAE-type

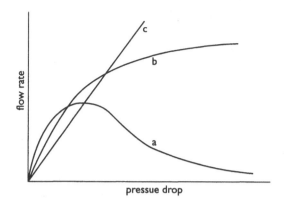

Figure 3.1 Variation of the flow rate as a function of pressure drop across a column of a soft ion exchanger "a", a semirigid sorbent "b", and rigid non compressible material. When the sorbent is soft the pressure at the top of the column compresses very significantly the gel and the flow rate diminishes to zero. On the contrary, with a rigid non compressible ion exchanger there is a linear relationship between the pressure drop and the flow rate.

protein binding capacity, the porosity, and the swelling properties which influence directly the flow rate at a given linear velocity.

Shrinking and swelling

Significant volumetric changes are present in soft and semirigid ion exchangers when exposed to different pH or ionic strength. In open columns these phenomena are visualized by variations in bed height; in closed columns the sorbent cannot physically expand and swelling results in large increase of the back pressure (Fig. 3.1) due to reduction of column void volume. Volume modifications are reduced when soft hydrogels are highly crosslinked or when they are constraint into rigid porous mineral particles.

Shrinkage of soft hydrogels in the presence of organic solvents such as ethanol in water is another possible reason for volumetric changes.

Porosity

When separating proteins, the size of the matrix pores can limit the diffusion rate of the proteins inside the gel network. In order to avoid sieving effects, the size of the pores should be larger than the protein diameter to oppose a minimal diffusional resistance. For physicochemical reasons the pores are not usually of the same dimension and their size can vary as a function of the environment. This undesired phenomenon can generate a protein trapping inside the matrix when shrinking occurs. Moreover, small pores do not offer an adequate accessibility for proteins to ionic charges within the network.

As a general rule, small and large pores co-exist in all macroporous matrices. While the protein access to the interior of the gel is restricted to largest pores, the ionic charges are randomly distributed in the matrix including small pores.

A special case of protein enhanced diffusion is described for soft hydrogels entrapped into rigid porous structures, where the size of the pores does not play a dominant role (Coffman *et al.*, 1998).

Binding capacity

In ion exchange chromatography, ionic groups are responsible for protein adsorption, however their high number is not synonymous with a high protein binding capacity of an ion exchanger. A limited number of ionic groups can allow for quite high binding capacity, but the opposite is not necessarily true (Boschetti, 1994). Binding capacity varies also as a function of ionic strength, pH, temperature and the nature of the counter ion.

Binding capacity is one of the most important parameters when considering scaling up operations where productivity is the ultimate important parameter. Binding capacity however, can be influenced by the flow rate on the columns, this is why one must distinguish static from dynamic binding capacity. Static capacity can be measured in batch mode by adding a large excess of protein to a given volume of buffered ion exchanger and then measure the amount of protein remaining in solution in the liquid phase after equilibration has been reached. The static capacity is then deducted from a simple mass balance.

Dynamic binding capacity is determined using breakthrough curves obtained by injecting a protein solution into a buffered column of ion exchanger at a given flow rate until outlet and inlet protein solutions are at the same concentrations (Chase, 1985). The positioning and slope of obtained curves can differ from one ion exchanger to another; the calculation of the dynamic binding capacity is measured mostly at 1–10% breakthrough (Janson *et al.*, 1987). Basic parameters that influence dynamic binding capacity at a given linear velocity are the size of the sorbent pores, the particle size of the sorbent, the flexibility of the polymer and the column bed height.

Figure 3.2 shows variation of the binding capacity versus flow rate of various ion exchangers.

Particle size

Small sorbent particles influence positively both resolution and variation of binding capacity versus flow rate. On preparative scale, however, using small particles will lead to a significant back pressure. This is always the case for soft and semirigid sorbents and cannot easily be predicted *a priori*. With rigid incompressible material, the phenomenon is at least predictable since there is a linear relation between the flow rate and the back pressure. Despite the interest to use small rigid beads at preparative scale for a better capacity and resolution, small particles are generally expensive and represent a large capital investment affecting the protein separation cost. Large-particle packings are less expensive, but give inferior performance. Economic models have been proposed for beads of various diameter assuming an identical sorbent life (Peskin *et al.*, 1992). For medium scale columns productivity data versus particle size showed that the use of 20–30 μm particle diameter is an ideal choice.

Dynamic binding capacity being higher compared to large particle diameter, the size of the column can be reduced for the same amount of protein to process; in this

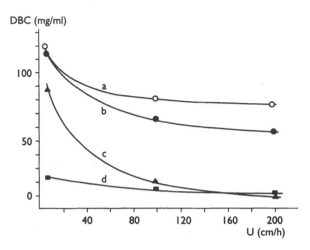

Figure 3.2 Variation of the dynamic binding capacity (DBC) of anion exchange materials as a function of the linear velocity (U). Binding capacity was measured at 10% breakthrough using a 10 mg/ml solution of bovine serum albumin at pH 8.6 in a 50 mM tris-buffer. A decrease in binding capacity when increasing the flow rate is related to mass transfer resistance phenomena. "a" represents a composite material constituted of a soft cationic hydrogel dispersed within the pores of a rigid ceramic material (Q-HyperD F Grade); "b" represents the behavior of a totally synthetic beaded Q polymer; "c" is an agarose gel containing quaternary amino groups and "d" represents a polystyrene based sorbent also carrying quaternary amino groups.

situation not only the resolution is better, but also the back pressure is significantly lower compared to small particle diameter, particularly with rigidly structured ion exchangers.

Ion exchange mechanism

As other chromatographic separation methods, ion exchange mechanism is based on the reversible adsorption of sample components. Ion exchange interaction occurs in an environment where the protein has an opposite net charge vis a vis the charge of the solid sorbent. The distribution of components of a mixture between the liquid and the solid phase depends on a number of parameters some of which are related to the nature and the structure of the solid ion exchanger. In order to predict the behavior of small molecules in ion exchange chromatography, mathematical models have been developed (Carta *et al.*, 1994; Vermeulen *et al.*, 1984; Wang, 1990).

All these models, however, are not directly applicable to complex molecules such as proteins because separations are often operated in various conditions (pH gradients, ionic strength gradients, displacements) which induce conformational changes and therefore result in an unpredictable behavior. Models taking into account all parameters would be of too large complexity and would not be applicable to all ion exchangers. However, as a general rule ionic sites of the ion exchanger are associated with a mobile counterion of the opposite charge and can be exchanged with other small or large ions of the same charge when present in the mobile phase. Models describing ion exchange chromatography are known as Stoichiometric Displacement Model (Kopaciewicz *et al.*,

1983; Velayudhan *et al.*, 1988), Steric Mass Action Law Model (Brooks *et al.*, 1992) and Modified Langmuir Isotherm Model (Antia *et al.*, 1989). In this book a specific chapter is dedicated to mathematical modeling of ion exchange mechanisms with the aim to use them for separation simulations (Voute, 1999).

On the mechanistic point of view, when components of a mixture are in contact with the ion exchanger an equilibrium is established between the liquid phase and the solid phase. A given distribution equilibrium is characteristic of a given molecule and depends on the concentration of the solutes. Species with higher affinity for the resin will attain a relatively higher concentration on the sorbent than low affinity species. An ion exchange reaction can be expressed by the general mass action law (Whitley *et al.*, 1989):

$$[\text{Prot}] + z[\text{R} \cdot \text{I}] = [\text{Rz} \cdot \text{Prot}] + z[\text{I}] \tag{1}$$

where [Prot] is the concentration of the protein in the solution, $[\text{R} \cdot \text{I}]$ is the resin associated with the counterion, [I] is the concentration of the counterion, $[\text{R} \cdot \text{Prot}]$ is the adsorbed protein on the resin and z is the effective charge of the protein.

Combining equilibrium constants with the concentrations of the protein and the counterion along with their multivalency, it is possible to define theoretical isotherms. In practice, however, it is very difficult to know the protein concentration on the stationary phase unless complex numerical models are used. Therefore, simpler models derived from Langmuir isotherms are often used to depict the ion exchange equilibrium.

Diffusion of macromolecule into a porous ion exchanger (see the section on Mass transfer mechanism) and non linear isotherms in the presence of relatively large amount of protein solute, result in a situation where the real equilibrium may not be reached in actual column operation.

In the presence of more than one protein in the mobile phase, competition between components occurs. In this situation, today ion exchange mechanism is mostly achieved by empirical models.

Separation of a mixture of protein components by ion exchange chromatography is the result of very complex interdependence of thermodynamic and kinetic phenomena which are highly modulated by the pore structure of the ion exchanger that influences the diffusion phenomena.

Mass transfer mechanism

Mass transfer, which describes how proteins diffuse into and out of a sorbent, has an important impact in ion exchange chromatography. It indicates how fast proteins can find the ionic binding sites within the matrix and therefore it dictates how fast an ion exchange column can be operated.

Four fundamental mass transfer phenomena occur in ion exchange chromatography.

● Axial dispersion
● Boundary layer mass transfer or diffusion from the mobile phase to the external surface of the particle
● Intraparticle diffusion in the liquid phase of the sorbent pores
● Adsorption on the ion exchange site

Axial dispersion is a combination of two mass transfer phenomena: (i) axial diffusion, which dominates at low flow rates and when Peclet number is $<\sim2.6$ (Equation 2) and (ii) convective diffusion, which dominates at higher flow rates when Peclet number is $>\sim2.6$. Peclet number Pe (also called reduced velocity) is commonly defined by the following equation:

$$Pe = \varepsilon_b v d_p / D_f \tag{2}$$

where ε_b is the interstitial void volume, v is the interstitial velocity, d_p is the particle diameter and D_f is the free solution diffusivity of the solute.

Axial diffusion causes slow broadening of any concentration gradient due to diffusion in the axial direction. Convective diffusion is caused by the random flow paths taken by solutes as they travel through a bed of randomly packed particles.

Axial and convective diffusion processes are generally lumped into a single Fickian diffusion term (Han et al., 1985). The primary contribution to this term is, however, the convective diffusion at the most commonly used chromatographic speeds.

Boundary layer mass transfer mechanism in liquid chromatography refers to a solute which moves from the flowing mobile phase toward the particle where it encounters a relatively stagnant layer of liquid. This stagnant layer through which the solute diffuses is relatively thin, and mass transfer through the boundary layer is often ignored. Under certain conditions, however, it dominates the mass transfer, especially during the initial part of loading, or in the case of solid diffusion at low concentration of solute or with large particles.

Once the solute is in the particle proper, it must move to find an available site. It does so by intraparticle diffusion which dominates over the other forms of mass transfer at velocities commonly used in liquid ion exchange chromatography. The effect of this mass transfer can be minimized with a smaller particle diameter. The height of a theoretical plate decreases by a factor of four for a factor of two in decrease of particle size. Unfortunately, for process liquid chromatography, this factor of two decrease in particle size is accompanied by a factor of four increase in pressure drop which is to some extent the limiting factor at large scale process.

Convection inside the microparticles can be caused by a large pressure drop across the particle, and typically occurs in very large pores of particles of small diameter. A practical result of this mechanism is that the chromatographic systems can be operated more quickly, but at very high velocities, mass transfer resistance to diffusion is still the limiting factor. Once the solute reaches an adsorption site, it may take time for the actual adsorption process to occur. In most ion exchange systems, however, the sorption kinetics are very fast compared to intraparticle diffusion. This mass transfer resistance may, however, dominate in some affinity systems.

Figure 3.3 depicts schematically the mass transfer phenomena by the variation of binding capacity of a medium size protein as a function of the linear velocity.

For more details on mass transfer mechanisms see review by Coffman et al., 1998.

Protein separation on ion exchangers

The choice of the most appropriate ion exchanger is a compulsory step that is dependent on a number of factors mostly related to the protein behavior.

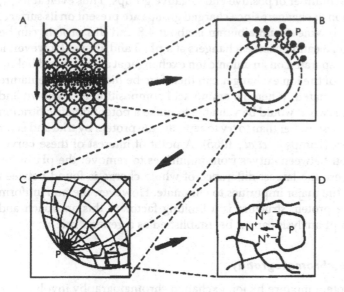

Figure 3.3 Schematic representation of single mass transfer phenomena described in the text. Axial dispersion of molecules is one of the well known peak broadening phenomena "a". The proteins to separate "P" are then transported to the surface of the sorbent where they encounter a thin film of liquid (boundary layer) which constitute a resistance to diffusion "b". During the diffusion event, protein molecules diffuse in the liquid moiety of the gel network ("c") and finally they have to reach the ionic complementary group where they interact electrostatically ("d").

On average all proteins are identical molecules in their composition. They are composed of hundred or thousand of the 20 different existing natural amino acids linked to each other. As a result of the relative content of individual amino acids, proteins contain positive and negative charges differently distributed within the protein structure. Charges can be found in specific zones, called clusters, or can be uniformly distributed in the tridimensional structure of the macromolecule.

What characterizes a protein is its isoelectric point, pI, which is the pH where the total net charge of the protein is zero. Above and below that pH the protein shows a net charge as a function of its ionizable amino acid content. In acidic proteins or proteins showing a low isoelectric point, aspartic acid and glutamic acid can be predominantly present. In proteins with a cationic net charge, lysine and arginine are playing the most dominant role.

In this situation acidic protein could be adsorbed and separated on cationic ion exchangers and basic proteins on anionic ion exchangers. However, since a protein contains both acidic and alkaline amino acids, its net charge depends on the environmental pH and the choice of the ion exchanger is rather made according to the net charge of the protein at a pH chosen for the separation. As a general rule a protein is negatively charged at high pH and is positively charged at low pH. The variation of the whole charge as a function of pH is governed by known mathematical equations (Tanford *et al.*, 1956) involving the valency of the ions, the Faraday's constant and the degree of dissociation. Although the net charge at a pH identical to pI is zero, it only means that there are equal number of positive and negative groups. Thus even at its pI, a protein may adsorb on ion exchangers since charged groups are present on its surface.

For example, the pI of bovine serum albumin is about 4.8 and this protein can be adsorbed and separated on a cationic ion exchangers at a pH 5 and above. However, it can also be adsorbed and separated on an anionic ion exchanger at a pH 4.5 and below. The choice of the pH and of the ion exchanger can therefore be dictated by the nature of the impurities to be eliminated. When the amino acid composition is unknown and the net charge is also unknown, it would be valuable to make a potentiometric titration curve of the protein of interest, rather than to try to separate the protein by trial and error on various ion exchangers (Lampson *et al.*, 1965). A point of interest of these curves is the possible comparison between curves from impurities to remove: the pH of the buffer can be chosen where the largest difference of whole charge is found between the protein to isolate and the major impurities to eliminate. However, the non uniform charge distribution in the protein structure is a limiting factor of this approach and rational approaches from pI analysis cannot be established as a general rule.

Classical ion exchange chromatography

The fractionation of a protein mixture by ion exchange chromatography involves five separate stages: sample loading, column washing, protein elution, column regeneration and re-equilibration to start another run (see Fig. 3.4).

Loading: Loading an ion exchange column consists of introducing the protein solution previously equilibrated in the appropriate buffer onto the column. Conditions have to be chosen to promote binding, adjusting the ionic strength and the pH of the buffer which is generally used for the equilibration of the column. When a protein is brought into contact with solid media having an opposite charge, an adsorption–desorption equilibrium is being established. Considering that any other external influencing parameters remain constant (e.g. temperature, ionic environment, pH) the partition of the protein between the liquid and the solid phase depends on the protein concentration. Ion exchange isotherms may be of a good help to discriminate between two different

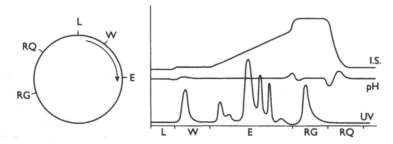

Figure 3.4 Schematic representation of a chromatographic ion exchange cycle (left) composed of five different phases: sample loading (L), washing phase (W), elution of the adsorbed proteins (E), column regeneration (RG) and finally column equilibration (RQ) to restart a new cycle. During this chromatographic cycle various events can be monitored at the column outlet (right) such as the variation of UV absorbance (UV) when proteins are desorbed, variations of ionic strength (I.S.) and pH. In the present case elution is performed by a salt gradient.

species depicted by the mass action law. Proteins are complex multivalent ions and higher interaction strength for ion exchangers is found with species having a higher number of accessible charged sites.

During the loading phase the total amount of protein brought into contact with the ion exchanger must not exceed the binding capacity of the sorbent.

Washing: A column washing is always necessary to evacuate non bound or weakly bound compounds; this operation is frequently performed using the equilibration buffer. Non bound compounds could also be the protein of interest as is the case when isolating immunoglobulins G from human plasma using DEAE columns (Corthier *et al.*, 1984).

Elution: Protein adsorption is the result of a complementarity between the ionic charges of both, protein and solid media; this interaction can be disrupted exploiting two distinct principles. The first is to act on the environmental pH that modifies the net charge of the protein or even changes its sign. This can be accomplished by developing pH gradients with appropriate buffers; the protein net charge is progressively modified and when it becomes of the same sign as the sorbent, it is released.

The adsorbed components out of the initial mixture are constituted by proteins of different isoelectric points and, when submitted to a pH gradient, they reach their electric neutrality at different pHs, therefore they are desorbed sequentially and thus are separated.

The second elution method is based on the use of competitive ions acting as eluents. The ions are progressively shielding the charged groups on the solid matrix. An increasing concentration of eluent ions in the buffer, releases bound proteins as a function of their net charge at a given pH. Proteins with different net charge are dissociated from the media at specific ionic strength are then separated. The first desorbed proteins are those that possess the lowest net charge at the working pH.

The nature of counter-ions is also to be considered when eluting proteins. The most common monovalent ions are chlorine ions for cationic resins and sodium ions for anionic resins. Counterions can, however, be polyvalent and their valence contributes to the effectiveness of the elution of the adsorbed protein species.

Two main types of elution are known: continuous gradients and step gradients. Continuous gradients are characterized by a progressive increase of the modifier that elutes the protein, or changes the pH and modifies the net charge of the protein. Continuous elution gradients are generally linear but they can be concave, convex and mixed. pH gradients can also be superimposed to salt gradients. The slope of linear continuous gradient is adjusted when optimizing separation conditions.

If a step elution gradient is made, discrete volumes of buffered solutions of defined salt concentration are sequentially injected into the column.

Most generally the optimal concentrations of salt of the various solutions are determined using a linear gradient elution first, and measuring the peak elution molarity. Isocratic elutions (elutions performed at constant buffer composition) are only occasionally used in ion exchange chromatography.

Regeneration: Separation of protein being accomplished, the column is washed with chemicals that have the property to remove all the non specifically or strongly adsorbed protein material. Sodium chloride of 1–2 M is frequently used, but many other regenerating solutions can be used as extensively described in the literature (Boschetti *et al.*, 1993).

Re-equilibration: Before reusing of the ion exchanger it is necessary to equilibrate it again with the initial buffer to permit the process of protein adsorption. This phase can be critical, since the amount of buffer could reach high values (Boschetti, 1994). If so, first it is advisable to use a concentrated buffer of the same composition and pH, followed by the dilute re-equilibration buffer.

Special aspects of ion exchange chromatography

Two particular aspects of ion exchange operations are considered in this section: ion exchange displacement chromatography and chromatofocusing.

Ion Exchange displacement chromatography, uses appropriate molecules as displacers to desorb species interacting with the solid phase (Peterson, 1978; Torres *et al.*, 1987). A distinction between the displacement and elution ion exchange chromatography with salt, and or pH gradients, is that the chemicals used as displacing agents remain always behind the displaced protein zone whereas with salt elution the ions move through the protein zone. This behavior is particularly important in that the eluted protein zones stay concentrated and components with low separation factor can be purified.

In ion exchange displacement chromatography, the first operating step consists in equilibrating the column with an appropriate buffer so that components of the mixture to be separated are adsorbed on the solid phase. This step is followed by the injection of a displacer solution composed of molecules having higher affinity for the ion exchanger than the protein components of the mixture. The components of the mixture are therefore progressively displaced and are eluted as zones of concentrated purified material. Once the breakthrough of the displacer occurs, all proteins are theoretically desorbed and the column is to be regenerated. This operation is performed by purging the displacer with high salt solutions, followed by a new equilibration of the column to start another separation run.

This ion exchange displacement mode takes advantage of the non linearity of the adsorption isotherm (Brooks *et al.*, in press); it is operated with large amount of feed stock and is adapted for processing large amount of proteins on relatively small columns.

The displacers used for protein desorption are generally macromolecules and are selected because of their higher affinity for the solid phase media than all protein species of the mixture therefore, they compete very effectively during the displacement steps. Among the most known displacers, ionizable dextrans have been described (Peterson, 1978; Gadam *et al.*, 1994; Jen *et al.*, 1991) for the purification of a number of proteins including antibodies and several serum proteins. Chondroitin sulfate has also been described for the separation of beta-galactosidase (Liao *et al.*, 1990). Other displacers used in ion exchange applications are protamine (Gerstner *et al.*, 1992a), heparin (Gerstner *et al.*, 1992b), pentosan polysulfate (Gadam *et al.*, 1994), methacrylic polyampholites (Patrickios *et al.*, 1995), protected amino acids (Kundu *et al.*, 1995b) and aminoglycosidic antibiotics (Kundu *et al.*, 1995a). More recently pentaerythritol-based dendrimers have also been successfully reported as displacers in ion exchange chromatography (Jayaraman *et al.*, 1995). In distinction to linear chain displacers they are low molecular weight three-dimensional molecules. They displayed good efficacy in displacing proteins.

In spite of its large potential, displacement ion exchange chromatography has some limitations mainly due to the difficult choice of effective and cheap displacers. Large molecular size displacers are difficult to eliminate from the purified proteins and require a follow-up chromatographic step. With the advent of low molecular weight displacers it should be easier to separate them by ultrafiltration or dialysis. Moreover, the extent of mixed zones is frequently underestimated and consequently the purity is lower than expected, as are the yields.

Isoelectric focusing using ion exchange media was first reported by Sluyterman *et al.*, 1978. This separation method known under the form of chromatofocusing is based on the ability of a pH gradient traveling through the column to change the sign of a charged protein adsorbed to an ion exchanger. By using ion exchange media with high buffering capacity, a pH gradient can be obtained when a buffer of a certain pH is injected into the column after a pre-equilibration with another buffer of a different pH. During the process of pH development single proteins change their charge.

The initial protein adsorption by ion exchange is followed by a pH gradient which changes the electric sign of the protein with consequent instant desorption. However, as the protein migrates the environmental buffer pH encountered reverses again the protein sign with consequent re-adsorption on the ion exchanger. By such a mechanism the protein adsorbs and desorbs along with the pH gradient fluctuation. In other words the protein is carried along the column by the flow rate of the eluent buffer until the pH becomes higher or lower than the pI of the protein resulting into rebinding phenomena.

A protein mixture may contain species of different isoelectric points. Thus, they move onto different distances before encountering the appropriate pH to interact with the ion exchanger; they elute, therefore, according to their isoelectric point.

The sorption–desorption phenomenon due to pH changes around the protein creates a certain focusing effect, since it opposes to the band broadening due to the diffusion effect. This peculiar aspect of ion exchange operation requires special ion exchangers with a high buffering capacity, and it needs special buffer compositions so as to create linear pH gradients.

Major factors affecting the resolution of chromatofocusing are the pH gradient slope, total charge of ion exchanger, the column packing, the nature of the counterion which should have a pKa at least two pH units below the lowest point of the pH gradient (Giri, 1990). Flow rate is, however, not very critical for the resolution.

Scaling up of ion exchange chromatography

Ion exchange chromatography is today used on both small laboratory and large production scale. The changeover from small scale to large scale is, however, still not completely rationalized and has somewhat different meaning. Process economy is, therefore, the driving force for the calculation of large scale purification protocols. Once the ion exchange process is optimized on laboratory scale, several parameters have to be modified to switch to a larger scale. The primary parameter is the volume of media needed for a given amount of load and is easily calculated when specific binding capacity is known for the expected linear flow rate. While linear scaling up procedures are simply a question of proportionality between the ion exchanger volume and the diameter of the column, they could have some limitations when dealing with very large columns. In such a configuration larger beads may be preferred to avoid too high back pressure developed if small particle size ion exchangers are used.

A process development step takes place between research laboratory procedures and the final large scale protocols.

At a research level the choice of the most appropriate ion exchanger is done primarily on the basis of its ability to resolve efficiently protein mixtures. At a process development level an optimization of separation conditions must occur involving studies of dynamic binding capacity, particle size choice, column length and the type of elution gradient.

The final changeover to large scale is done by enlarging the column diameter to reach a media volume corresponding to the amount of feed stock to process (Fig. 3.5). The importance of column length is directly related to the number of plates of the column since this determines the separation efficiency and the dilution factor. Long

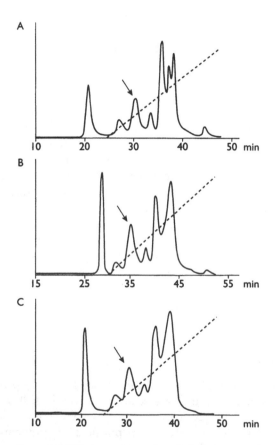

Figure 3.5 Representation of a method development approach for the separation of IgG from sweet whey. The first step is an analytical optimized separation of protein components by ion exchange on Q-HyperD 10 μm particle size (A) followed by an increase of the particle size to 35 μm in the same operating conditions. The last phase is the media volume increase using larger column diameter columns of the same length. Column dimensions: 4.3 mm I.D. × 100 mm for "A" and "B"; 10 mm I.D. × 100 mm for "C". Sample: IgG enriched sweet whey. Loading buffer 10 mM tris-HCL, pH 8.6; elution by salt gradient in the same buffer up to 0.4 M. Linear flow rate was 380 cm/h for all column (volumetric flow rate was 0.43 ml/min for small diameters and 2.15 ml/min for column "C"). The arrow represents the positioning of IgG peak.

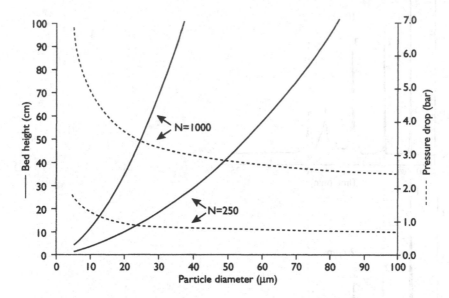

Figure 3.6 Variation of back pressure and equivalent bed heights as a function of particle diameter at constant column efficiency. Column efficiency was postulated here to be equivalent to 250 plates (N) or 1000 plates. All curves were calculated from the extended Van Deemter model and the Kozeny–Carman equation using the following parameters: $\varepsilon_O = 0.45$, $U_O = 300 \, cm/h$, $K = 2$, $D_S = 1.6 \times 10^{-8} \, cm^2/s$ and $\mu = 10^{-3} \, Pa/s$.

columns are in this case preferable. However, the length of a column is a critical factor for compressible material.

Ideally, ion exchange media used on laboratory scale are of 10–20 μm particle diameter and for large scale they are between 50 and 300 μm depending on to the size of the column. When switching from a small particle size to a large particle size the separation efficiency is decreased since the number of plates of the column decreases. To maintain constant the separation efficiency it is useful to increase the length of the column when using large particles. Interdependence of particle size, back pressure, number of plates is given on Fig. 3.6. Back pressure generated by longer columns is in this case compensated by the larger size of the ion exchange particles.

An important issue in scaling up of a process including particle diameter modification is the limited availability of the same media with different particle size.

An example of the impact of particle size on the separation of a protein mixture is given on Fig. 3.7.

Columns vs batches

Ion exchange mechanism can occur in a slurry where the media particles and the protein solutions are mixed in the presence of an appropriate buffer. The elimination of non bound species as well as the recovery of the desorbed proteins are, in this case, carried out by centrifugation or filtration.

This mode of extraction is used when the molecule of interest present in the initial liquid mixture is very dilute and when the volume of the utilized solid phase is small. It does not make sense actually to process very large volumes on small chromatographic

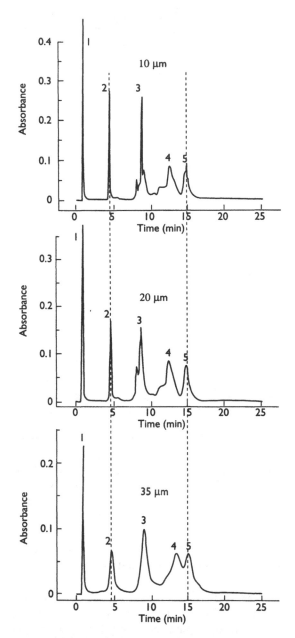

Figure 3.7 Chromatographic separation of the same protein sample on a chromatographic media constituted of particles of different diameter (10, 20 and 35 μm). Sample composition: cytochrome c (0.6 mg/ml), myoglobin (0.6 mg/ml), transferrin (2.35 mg/ml), ovalbumin (3.4 mg/ml) and human serum albumin (2.7 mg/ml); sample volume 50 μl; column: Q-HyperD 4.3 mm I.D. × 100 mm; adsorption buffer: 50 mM tris-HCl, pH 8.6; elution gradient 0.4 M NaCl in 20 min; flow rate 1 ml/min. The separation efficiency and, therefore, the resolution is dependent on the particle diameter; however, peak positioning remain strictly the same when the chemical composition of the solid phase is unchanged.

columns since the time spent for sample application would be too long compared to other steps of the chromatographic cycle (see also Fig. 3.4).

In batch adsorption, complex mixtures can be either clarified by filtration and centrifugation, or can contain insoluble material in suspension such as protein precipitates, cell debris or even living cells. The initial character of the feed stock dictates to some extent the mode of use of the solid phase designated to extract the target molecule.

Batch mode adsorption is a labor-intensive process and involves a number of discrete steps: agitation of solid particles within the crude extract, filtration to separate the solid phase, intensive washings, elution of the target molecule and regeneration of the solid phase. It also involves special mechanical devices for each single operation and is performed frequently in open vessels thus constituting a high risk of contamination by external agents.

A classical example of batch mode extraction is given by the separation of Prothrombin complex from human plasma (Prothrombin complex contains Factor IX clotting agent for hemophilia B disease) prior any other fractionation operation (Clark *et al.*, 1988).

To one liter of human plasma cryosupernatant few grams of dry DEAE-Sephadex are added, the suspension is stirred for a few hours and the gel separated by filtration. Another example is the removal of DNA molecules from purified protein preparations; the amount of such a material is most generally very small when compared to the protein concentration.

Solid phase batch extraction has also been described for the removal of proteins from nucleic acids preparations (McCormick, 1989).

At a laboratory scale the advantage of batch mode is the speed of the operation. However, since the mass transfer is less efficient and will require longer time, the separation efficiency is extremely poor and cannot be applied to a fractionation of a sample, but rather to an on-off separation.

A particular mode of the exploitation of ion exchange is the so called fluidized or expanded bed. This is an intermediate concept between the batch and the packed column modes. It is based on particles of sorbent suspended theoretically in a sort of steady state by an upward flow generated by the buffer stream (Draeger *et al.*, 1991; Spence *et al.*, 1994; Chang *et al.*, 1996). Protein fractionation is possible, but the number of plates that such a device generates is much less than a packed column, because of the large size of the beads and the large void volume between the beads. Dilution of the collected fractions is also one of the limiting factors, however fluid ion exchange beds allow to process unclarified feed stocks.

When cationic exchangers are utilized, adsorption of cell debris present in the feed stock may occur; this partially prevents the adsorption of proteins and contributes for column fouling.

Regulatory considerations in ion exchange biochromatography

Protein purification processes to achieve purity, high biological specific activity and consistency, have to be performed under strict validation rules. Cells from which expressed target protein is obtained, may release adventitious agents such as nucleic acids, cell wall components, viruses, which have to be totally eliminated at the early steps of the purification process. Additionally, the use of solid phase matrices, such as ion exchangers to accomplish the separation process, may generate other concerns triggering specific validation and hygienic rules.

While reversible, ion exchange media may adsorb tightly undesirable components from the feed stock which must be eliminated by harsh cleaning operations. For this purpose strong chemical agents are used that may damage polymeric matrices or alter ion exchange chemical groups giving rise to two distinct issues. The first is the progressive diminution of the adsorbing and separation properties of the chromatographic media, and the second is the production of chemical components that could contaminate the protein to be purified (for specific review, see Jungbauer *et al.*, 1994).

Extractable chemicals from the solid phase media

Extractable chemical components may originate from the synthesis of the ion exchanger that are not totally eliminated from the manufacturing process. They can come from the polymerization process, from the crosslinking processes, and from the grafting of ion exchange groups. Identification and quantification of all these chemical products is accomplished by using HPLC, gravimetric methods, spectroscopy, chemical, immunochemical and radiochemical assays. An easy approach has been reported on the extraction, identification, quantification and toxicity determination of chemicals used in the manufacturing of ion exchangers (Boschetti *et al.*, 1996).

Matrix deterioration

Several chemical and physical factors are responsible for the irreversible degradation of ion exchangers.

Strong acidic treatments are generally damaging for polysaccharide structures; osidic linkages are hydrolyzed and sugars or oligosaccharides are released.

Strong alkaline treatments degrade progressively silica based media by formation of sodium silicates. Degradation extent is proportional however to the surface area of the matrix. Alkaline treatments can degrade polysaccharides as well by complex chemical degradation reactions catalyzed by the presence of divalent cations under oxidizing conditions. Polyacrylamide gels are also sensitive to high pHs, but polyacrylamide based ion exchangers are not.

Among physical degrading agents heating cooling and attrition have to be carefully considered. Most of ion exchangers are stable when autoclaved at 120–130°C. Cationic groups can, however, be degraded after repeated autoclave treatments. Radiation damages are generally limited to substituted amines, but radiolytic action is more deleterious to polysaccharide based supports than with mineral or synthetic based ion exchangers. Compression actions due to tight column packing and attrition due to collisions between particles when agitated in suspension, may also damage ion exchangers. These treatments do not alter, however, the properties of the media but rather generate small particles which have deleterious effect on flow properties of the column.

Cleaning processes for ion exchangers

The repeated adsorption and desorption of proteins is frequently associated with irreversible, non specific binding of impurities. Therefore, cleaning or regeneration operations are an integral part of an ion exchange separation cycle.

Cleaning procedures cover two main aspects: the removal of undesired adsorbed material and inactivation of bacteria, yeasts and viruses, that are present within the chromatographic packing.

A number of possible solutions has been described to desorb an undesirable material. Most generally a separation cycle is followed by a washing cycle with buffer containing high salt concentrations.

Nevertheless, the removal of strongly retained material is often achieved only using more severe cleaning agents. Specific dedicated washings can be better designed when the nature of the impurity to be removed is known (see Table 3.3). To achieve effective cleaning conditions some general rules have to be followed. For instance, foul deposits are frequently found in a concentrated form at the top of the column. It makes sense then to reverse the flow direction when cleaning. This shortens the length of washing operations while minimizing unnecessary contamination of the rest of the bed. Abrupt changes of buffers increase the risk of precipitation of foul deposits therefore gradual changes are preferred.

When cell debris is clogging partially the void volume of packed beds it can be removed by selective fluidization of the packed bed. Fouling material is frequently less dense than the media beads and can be eliminated by back flushing with buffers or cleaning solutions. This procedure is particularly recommended when sorbents are relatively dense such as silica or mineral based ion exchangers and when fouling material is insoluble due to precipitation within the void volume (Van-Der-Wiel, 1989; Boschetti et al., 1990).

Acidic treatments are not very popular as cleaning solutions, since carbohydrates that constitute most of ion exchangers are not acid stable. However, it is known that, acidic cleaning agents are good dissociating agents. With the introduction of more and more acid stable sorbents the use of low pH washing regimes is of growing interest.

Table 3.3 Commonly used regeneration solutions for the removal of strongly adsorbed material on ion exchangers

Adsorbed material	Regeneration solution	Comments
Highly charged macromolecules	1–2 M NaCl or KCl Buffers pH 2–3 or 9–11	Avoid low temperature pH 3 with CM and SP; pH 9 with Q and DEAE
Hydrophobic proteins	Non ionic detergents Cationic detergents at pH 9–11 Anionic detergents at pH 3–4 0.01–1 M sodium hydroxide 60% ethanol-0.5 M acetic acid	Possible formation of foam For cationic media only For anionic media only Not for alkaline sensitive media Use with non shrinkable media
Protein aggregates	6–8 M urea or guanidine-HCl Detergents (see above) 50–80% acetic acid Various proteases	Not for native agarose gel See above Not for polysaccharide media Eliminate protease traces carefully
Metal complexes	Complexing agents e.g. EDTA Strong acids at pH 1	Use at low concentration Not for acid sensitive sorbents
Non polar lipids	Isopropanol up to 100%	Not for shrinkable sorbents
Complex pigments	Strong acids with ethanol	Not for acid sensitive sorbents

Organic acids alone or in combination with alcohols are preferred cleaning solutions for the removal of lipids and pigments (Veron et al., 1993).

Other common cleaning solutions are highly concentrated salts and alkaline agents; sodium hydroxide at various concentration is widely used. High pHs tend to solubilize a number of substances such as fatty acids, some protein aggregates and acidic pigments. Alkaline solutions are convenient because they are inexpensive and permit a quite good level of sanitization while contributing to the removal of pyrogenic substances.

Acidic and alkaline solutions can also be used in alternating cycles, or in combination with solvents and non ionic detergents to better remove hydrophobic material.

Concentrated solution of urea in sodium carbonate or mixed with sodium hydroxide are also recommended to clean ion exchange columns. To remove strongly bound non polar material, treatments with 70% ethanol in water or 30% isopropanol in water may be useful.

Finally diluted non ionic detergents may be used alone or in combination with alkaline solutions. Here all operations must be effected with care to avoid adsorption of detergents on the matrix that may contaminate the protein to be purified unless washed out by long ethanol treatments. This latter procedure can only be envisaged with non shrinkable ion exchangers in the presence of organic solvents.

Where fouling is the result of strong protein aggregation, mixture of proteases has been used successfully to clean and restore the binding capacity (Holdroyde et al., 1976; Allary et al., 1991).

Another aspect of column cleaning is sterilization. Several approaches have been described to inactivate microorganisms. Steam sterilization is probably the most effective, but cannot be used in packed columns. Sodium hydroxide has also been suggested to sterilize chromatographic media (Berglof et al., 1988), but other studies demonstrated the limitation of these treatments to non sporulated microorganisms (Girot et al., 1990). More effective ways to inactivate sporulated living cells have been described; they suggest the use of mixtures of alkaline solutions in association with ethanol (Boschetti et al., 1990). Irradiation with sterilizing doses (e.g. 2.5 M Rad) does not cause any serious decrease in the binding capacity of the ion exchangers.

Formaldehyde and glutaraldehyde can also be used, but their use is restricted to virgin or very well regenerated sorbents to avoid any crosslinking of protein traces present within the ion exchangers. Two percent Hibitane digluconate in the presence of 20% ethanol has also been suggested to sterilize the chromatographic packings.

Oxidizing agents such as hypochlorites, peracetates and hydrogen peroxide may also be efficiently used for sterilization, however, their use is restricted to stable ion exchangers (Jungbauer et al., 1994) and should not be applied to polysaccharide based sorbents.

Conclusion

Although ion exchange chromatography of proteins is today very popular and is used on both, laboratory and industrial scales with a high degree of success, it remains a complex separation methodology. Parameters contributing to its performance are very complex chemical interaction phenomena where the chemical nature of the matrix has a non negligible impact; additionally thermodynamic and kinetic phenomena are not yet very well understood. A variety of ion exchangers are, however, available and they satisfy most of protein separation applications.

Mathematical models adapted to the understanding of ion exchange chromatography are increasingly applicable and already help in the interpretation of molecular phenomena. Computer assisted simulation of separations has been accomplished (Voute, in this book) and it contributes to decrease of the empirical effort of technicians and engineers when defining conditions for separation protocols.

References

Afeyan, N., Gordon, M., Mazsarof, M., Varady, L., Foulton, S. P., Yang, Y. B. and Regnier, F. E. (1990) Flow through particles for the high performance liquid chromatography of biomolecules: perfusion chromatography. *J. Chromatogr.*, **519**, 1–29.

Allary, M., Saint Blancard, J., Boschetti, E. and Girot, P. (1991) Large scale production of human albumin: three years experience of an affinity chromatography process. *Bioseparation*, **2**, 167–175.

Antia, F. and Horvath, C. (1989) Gradient elution in non linear preparative liquid chromatography. *J. Chromatogr.*, **484**, 1–27.

Berglof, J. H., Adner, N. P. and Doversten, S. Y. (1988) Inactivation of microbial contamination in chromatographic separation media using sodium hydroxide. *Proc. XX Congr. Int. Soc. Blood. Trans.*, June 1988, London, UK.

Boschetti, E. (1994) Advanced sorbents for preparative protein separation purposes. *J. Chromatogr.*, **658**, 207–236.

Boschetti, E., Girot, P. and Guerrier, L. (1990) Silica-dextran sorbent composites and their cleaning in place. *J. Chromatogr.*, **523**, 35–42.

Boschetti, E., Girot, P., Guerrier, L. and Santambien, P. (1996) Quantification and in vitro toxicity studies of extractable chemicals from synthetic ion exchangers. *J. Biochem. Biophys. Meth.*, **32**, 15–25.

Boschetti, E., Guerrier, L., Girot, P. and Horvath, J. (1995) Preparative high performance liquid chromatography separation of proteins with HyperD ion exchange supports. *J. Chromatogr.*, **664**, 225–231.

Boschetti, E., Pouradier Duteil, X., Nguyen, C. and Moroux, Y. (1993) Concerns and solutions for a proper decontamination of chromatographic packing. *Chemistry Today*, **11**, 29–35.

Brooks, C. A. and Cramer, S. M. (1992) Steric mass action ion exchange: displacement profiles and induced salt gradients. *AIChE J.*, **38**, 1969–1978.

Brooks, C. A. and Cramer, S. M. (1996) Solute affinity in ion exchange displacement chromatography. *Chem. Eng. Sci.*, **51**, 3487–3860.

Carta, G. and Dinerman, A. (1994) Displacement chromatography of amino acids: effects of selectivity reversal. *AIChE J.*, **40**, 1618–1628.

Chang, Y. K. and Chase, H. A. (1996) Ion exchange purification of G6PDH from unclarified yeast cells homogenates using expanded bed adsorption. *Biotechnol. Bioeng.*, **49**, 204–216.

Chase, H. A. (1985) Factors important in the design of fixed bed adsorption processes for the purification of proteins, in *Discovery and Isolation of Microbial Products*, Verral M. S., (ed.), Ellis Horwood Ltd., pp. 129–147.

Clark, D. B., Menache, D., Gee, D. M., Miekka, S. I. and Drowan, W. (1988) Coagulation factor IX for replacement therapy in hemophilia B patients, in *Biotechnology of Plasma Proteins*, Stoltz J. F. and Rivat C. (eds), INSERM Press, Paris, 1988, pp. 315–323.

Coffman, J. L. and Boschetti, E. (1997) Enhanced diffusion chromatography and related sorbents for biopurification, in *Bioseparation*, Subramanian G. (ed.), WILEY-VCH Press, Weinheim, 1998, pp. 157–198.

Corthier, G., Boschetti, E. and Charley-Poulain, J. (1984) Improved method for IgG purification from various animal species by ion exchange chromatography. *J. Immunol. Meth.*, **66**, 75–79.

Draeger, N. M. and Chase, H. A. (1991) Liquid fluidized bed adsorption of proteins in the presence of cells. *Bioseparation*, **2**, 67–80.

Gadam, S. D. and Cramer, S. M. (1994) Salt effect in anion exchange displacement chromatography: comparison of pentosan polysulfate and dextran sulfate displacers. *Chromatographia*, **39**, 409–418.

Fernandez, M. A., Laughinghouse, W. S. and Carta, G. (1996) Characterization of protein adsorption by composite silica-polyacrylamide gel anion exchangers. *J. Chromatogr.*, **746**, 185–198.

Gerstner, J. A. and Cramer, S. M. (1992a). Cation exchange displacement chromatography of proteins with protamine displacers: Effect of induced salt gradient. *Biotechnology Progr.*, **8**, 540–545.

Gerstner, J. A. and Cramer, S. M. (1992b). Heparin as a non toxic displacer for anion exchange displacement chromatography of proteins. *Biopharm.*, **5**, 42–45.

Giri, L. (1990) Chromatofocusing. *Meth. Enzymol.*, **182**, 380–392.

Girot, P. and Boschetti, E. (1981) Physico-chemical and chromatographic properties of new ion exchangers. I. CM-Trisacryl. *J. Chromatogr.*, **213**, 389–396.

Girot, P., Moroux, Y., Pouradier Duteil, X., Nguyen, C. and Boschetti, E. (1990) Composite sorbents and their cleaning in place. *J. Chromatogr.*, **510**, 213–223.

Han, N. W., Bhakta, J. and Carbonell, R. G. (1985) Longitudinal and lateral dispersion in packed beds. Effect of column length and particle size distribution . *AIChE J.*, **31**, 277–288.

Holdroyde, M. J., Cheser, J. M. E., Trayer, I. P. and Walker, D. G. (1976) *Biochem. J.*, **153**, 351–359.

Janson, J. C. and Hedman, P. (1987) On the optimization of process chromatography of proteins. *Biotechnol. Prog.*, **3**, 9–13.

Jayaraman, G., Li, Y.-F. Moore, J. A. and Cramer, S. M. (1995) Ion exchange displacement chromatography of proteins. Dendritic polymers as novel displacers. *J. Chromatogr.*, **702**, 143–155.

Jen, S. C. D. and Pinto, N. G. (1991) Dextran sulfate as a displacer for the displacement chromatography of pharmaceutical proteins. *J. Chromatogr. Sci.*, **29**, 478–484.

Jungbauer, A. and Boschetti, E. (1994) Manufacture of recombinant proteins with safe and validated chromatographic sorbents. *J. Chromatogr.*, **662**, 143–179.

Jungbauer, J., Lettner, H. P., Guerrier, L. and Boschetti, E. (1994) Chemical sanitization in process chromatography. Part 2: In situ treatment of packed columns and long term stability of resins. *Biopharm.*, **7**, 37–42.

Kopaciewicz, W., Rounds, M., Fausnaugh, J. and Regnier, F. (1983) Retention model for high performance ion exchange chromatography. *J. Chromatogr.*, **266**, 3–21.

Kundu, A., Vunnum, S. and Cramer, S. M. (1995a). Antibiotics as low molecular mass displacers in ion exchange displacement chromatography. *J Chromatogr.*, **707**, 57–67.

Kundu, A., Vunnum, S., Jayaraman, G. and Cramer, S. M. (1995b). Protected amino acids as novel low molecular weight displacers in cation exchange displacement chromatography. *Biotechnol. Bioeng.*, **48**, 452–460.

Lampson, G. P. and Tytell, A. A. (1965) A simple method for estimating isoelectric points. *Anal. Biochem.*, **11**, 374–377.

Liao, A. W. and Horwath, C. (1990) Purification of β-galactosidase by combined frontal and displacement chromatography. *Ann. NY Acad. Sci.*, **589**, 182–191.

Mc Cormick, R. M. (1989) Solid phase extraction procedure for DNA purification. *Anal. Biochem.*, **181**, 66–74.

Muller, W. (1990) New ion exchangers for chromatography of biopolymers. *J. Chromatogr.*, **510**, 133–142.

Patrickios, C. J., Gadam, S. D., Cramer, S. D., Hertler, W. R. and Hatton, T. A. (1995) Novel acrylic block co-polymeric displacers for ion exchange separation of proteins. *Biotechnol. Progr.*, 11, 33–38.

Peskin, A. P. and Rudge, S. R. (1992) Optimization of large scale chromatography for biological applications. *Appl. Biochem. Biotechnol.*, 34, 49–59.

Peterson, E. A. and Sober, H. A. (1956) Chromatography of proteins. I. Cellulose ion exchange adsorbents. *J. Am. Chem. Soc.*, 78, 751–759.

Peterson, E. A. (1978) Ion exchange displacement chromatography of serum proteins using carboxymethyl dextran as displacers. *Anal. Biochem.*, 90, 767–784.

Sluyterman, L. A. A. and Elgersma, O. (1978) Chromatofocusing: isoelectric focusing on ion exchange columns. I. General principles. *J. Chromatogr.*, 150, 17–30.

Spence, C., Schaffer, C. A., Kessler, S. and Bailon, P. (1994) Fluidized bed receptor affinity chromatography. *Biomed. Chromatogr.*, 8, 236–241.

Tanford, C. and Havenstein, J. D. (1956) Hydrogen ion equilibria of ribonuclease. *J. Am. Chem. Soc.*, 78, 5287–5291.

Torres, A. R., Edberg, S. C. and Peterson, E. A. (1987) Preparative high performance liquid chromatography of proteins on an ion exchanger using unfractionated carboxymethyl dextran displacers. *J. Chromatogr.*, 389, 117–182.

Van-Der-Wiel, J. P. (1989) Continuous recovery of biproducts by adsorption. Thesis, Acad. Biochem. Centrum De Lier, Netherland, 1989.

Velayudhan, A. and Horvath, C. (1988) Preparative chromatography of proteins, analysis of the multivalent ion-exchange formalism. *J. Chromatogr.*, 443, 13–29.

Veron, J. L., Gattel, P., Pla, J., Fournier, P. and Grandgeorge, M. (1993) Combined Cohn/chromatography purification process for the manufacturing of high purity human albumin from plasma. Rivat, C. and Stoltz, J. F. (eds), John Libbey Eurotext, 1993, pp. 183–187.

Vermeulen, T., LeVan, M. D., Hiester, N. K. and Klein, G. (1984) Adsorption and ion exchange, *in Chemical Engineers' Handbook*, 6th edn, Perry, R. H., Green, D. W., Maloney, J. A. (eds), Mc Graw-Hill NY, 1984.

Voute, N., Computer-aided simulation of biochromatography, in this book.

Wang, L. (1990) Ion exchange in purification, *in Separation Process in Biotechnology*, Asenjo, J. (ed.), Marcel Dekker, New York, 1990.

Whitley, R., Wachter, R., Liu, F. and Wang, L. (1989) Ion exchange equilibria of lysozyme, myoglobin and bovine serum albumin. Effective valence and exchange capacity. *J. Chromatogr.*, 465, 137–156.

Chapter 4

Hydrophobic (interaction) chromatography of proteins

Herbert P. Jennissen

Introduction and historical aspects

Hydrophobic interactions have been described as "the unusually strong attraction between non-polar molecules and surfaces in water" (Israelachvili, 1985). For two contacting methane molecules the attraction energy is ca. 6-fold higher in water than the van der Waals interaction energy in vacuum. This energy, which has been estimated to be ca. -8.5 kJ mol^{-1} for two methane molecules (Ben-Naim *et al.*, 1973; Israelachvili, 1985) is due to the extrusion of ordered water on two adjacent hydrophobic surfaces into less-ordered bulk water with a concomitant increase in entropy. This entropy driven attraction between non-polar groups in water (Israelachvili, 1985; Israelachvili and Pashley, 1984; Kauzmann, 1959; Lewin, 1974; Tanford, 1973) is the basis for hydrophobic interaction chromatography as summarized in several reviews (Arakawa and Narhi, 1991; Eriksson, 1989; Halperin *et al.*, 1981; Hjerten, 1981; Hofstee and Otillio, 1978; Hubert and Dellacherie, 1993; Jennissen, 1988; Mohr and Pommerening, 1986; Ochoa, 1978; Oscarsson, 1997; Shaltiel, 1984; Yon, 1977). For an interesting distinction between definitions of "hydrophobicity" and "hydrophobic interactions" see the technical comment by Dill (Dill, 1990). Recently the terms ultra-hydrophilic and ultra-hydrophobic have extended the above range of definitions to new applications in the area of biomaterials (Jennissen, 2001).

Reversed-phase vs hydrophobic interaction chromatography

The chromatographic separation of proteins depends on the differential accumulation of molecules at certain sites within a chromatographic system. The term *reversed-phase chromatography* goes back to a paper by Howard and Martin 1950 who first separated long chain fatty acids by what they called "reversed phase partition" chromatography. The principle underlying this separation rested on the synthesis of a hydrophobic silica support (by treating it with dichlorodimethylsilane) which was capable of retaining non-polar liquid phases such as acetone, n-octane or paraffin (stationary liquid phase) when applied as the less polar phase in a solvent system. In this classical method the solutes are thus absorbed and separated (partitioned) in an apolar stationary liquid phase (i.e. a three dimensional system). Today the silica gels employed for reversed-phase HPLC of proteins and peptides are generally highly substituted with octadecyl, octyl or phenyl residues and therefore display a very high hydrophobicity capable of retaining liquid non-polar phases such as acetonitrile or methanol in water. In *hydrophobic interaction chromatography* the solutes applied in an aqueous phase are a*d*sorbed and separated directly on the apolar stationary solid phase (i.e. a two-dimensional system) in the majority of cases consisting of immobilized hydrophobic groups on a paracrystalline carbohydrate surface (e.g. agarose, cellulose see also (Jennissen, 1981, 1995)). The application of reversed phase chromatography and hydrophobic interaction chromatography is not restricted to proteins but also encompasses nucleic acids (Hjerten, 1981; Liautard, 1992).

In reverse phase chromatography of proteins there appears to be no clear theoretical boundary between partition and adsorption, since it is conceivable that a molecule the size of a protein may interact with the stationary liquid phase as well as with the stationary solid phase. As a rule the high hydrophobicity of a reverse phase matrix and the stationary organic phase make this procedure primarily suited for denatured proteins and peptides only. Thus due to the very well defined and reproducible methodological approach reversed-phase HPLC of proteins and peptides has become one of the most powerful analytical tools in protein and peptide chemistry. In hydrophobic interaction chromatography on the other hand the hydrophobicity is of a low or intermediate level obviating the organic stationary phase and (ideally) allowing the separation of proteins in their native states directly on the apolar stationary phase. The aim in this case is not so much analytical but moreover preparative and directed towards the purification of proteins in their native state. For practical purposes therefore a simple differentiation of reversed phase chromatography from hydrophobic interaction chromatography can be made on the basis that in the former an organic liquid stationary phase is present and in the latter there is not. For further details on these two chromatographic modes see also (Fausnaugh *et al.*, 1984; Pearson *et al.*, 1982).

The focus of this review is hydrophobic interaction chromatography, thus excluding reversed phase chromatography, although both methods indeed have a number of factors in common. Furthermore it is restricted to the separation of proteins excluding small molecular weight compounds and other classes of biomolecules such as nucleic acids. In addition a distinction between classical chromatography systems and HPLC will also not be made, since the difference between the two is essentially the bead or particle size which is mainly responsible for the higher performance.

The CNBr procedure

Hydrophobic chromatography was discovered on agarose gels containing covalently immobilized hydrophobic groups that were introduced by the CNBr procedure (for review (see Jennissen, 1995)). Therefore the CNBr method dominated all other coupling procedures for many years and is still in use today. For an understanding of the previous work in the field of hydrophobic interaction chromatography it is therefore necessary to briefly review the chemistry of the CNBr activation and coupling reaction on agaroses. The activation of polysaccharides by CNBr was described by Porath's group in 1967, (Axen *et al.*, 1967; Porath *et al.*, 1967) a method which paved the way for affinity chromatography (Cuatrecasas *et al.*, 1968) and hydrophobic chromatography. The mechanism of the CNBr coupling reaction on agarose, which is more complex than on dextrans, was clarified by Kohn and Wilchek, 1981 many years after the major

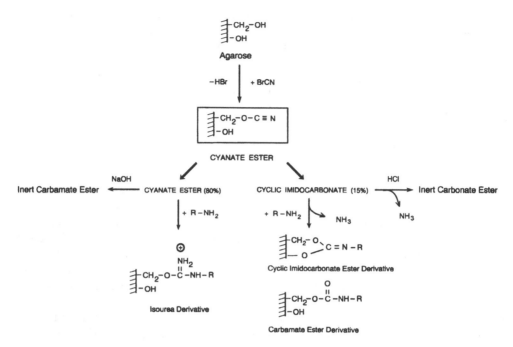

Figure 4.1 Reaction scheme for the activation of agarose by CNBr with a cyanate ester as the major stable active intermediate. The scheme is a simplified version of the one published by (Kohn and Wilchek, 1981). For further details see the text and (Kohn and Wilchek, 1981). From (Jennissen, 1995).

affinity methods had already been established. The primary stable active intermediate on CNBr-activated agarose is a cyanate ester of which ca. 15% spontaneously converts to a cyclic imidocarbonate (see simplified scheme in Fig. 4.1). The pH of the washing solution employed after activating the agarose is decisive for the amount of charges introduced since cyanate esters are selectively hydrolyzed in alkali in contrast to the imidocarbonates which are hydrolyzed in acid. If a CNBr activated gel is stabilized at low pH (Joustra and Axen, 1976) and later swollen and washed with 1 mM HCl as is the case with commercial CNBr-activated Sepharose 4B from Pharmacia (Pharmacia Fine Chemicals, 1979) only charged *isourea* coupling products are obtained e.g. when coupling primary amines or proteins. On the other hand if fresh CNBr-activated gels are washed extensively at an alkaline pH, fully uncharged *imidocarbonate/carbamate* coupling products may be obtained with primary amines (Kohn and Wilchek, 1981). Thus pure charged isourea gels, pure uncharged imidocarbonate/carbamate gels as shown in Table 4.1 or mixed gels containing different types of chemical bonds (see Fig. 4.1) can be obtained by the CNBr procedure. In general the CNBr activation procedure leads to more or less mixed gels (see also Section 1.4.2).

For simplicity apolar gels synthesized by the CNBr procedure and containing residual charges will be called "non-charge-free" hydrophobic gels (*NCF-gels*). This terminology denotes that the gels are not simple ion-exchange resins. Uncharged hydrophobic gels will be called "charge-free" hydrophobic (*CF-gels*). An excellent and easy method for

Table 4.1 Synthesis charge-containing and uncharged butyl Sepharose by the CNBr method according to (Kohn and Wilchek, 1981)

CNBr	Coupling of ^{14}C-Butylamine	
	HCL wash (isourea, charged) μmol/ml packed gel	NaOH wash (carbamate, uncharged) μmol/ml packed gel
8	24.5 ± 2.19	9.4 ± 0.12
15	30.8 ± 1.80	12.6 ± 1.01
30	80.3 ± 0.12	19.3 ± 0.67

The activation mixture contained 25 g of dry Sepharose 4B, 11 ml H_2O, 24 ml (2.5 M K_3PO_4 (pH 12), 18 ml Dioxane, 2 ml CNBr (61 g/100 ml). The mixture was incubated for 12 min at 8°C, was then sucked dry on a Büchner funnel, washed with either 750 ml 0.1 M HCl or 750 ml 0.1 M NaOH and suspended either in 100 ml HCl (0.1 M) or 100 ml NaOH (0.1 M) and stirred slowly for 30 min. The gel was sucked dry and immediately added to 2 M ^{14}C-butylamine (Höchst AG, Frankfurt; specific radioactivity 1.5 × 10^5 cpm/ml) pH 10 and stirred slowly for 3 h at 5°C. The butylamine solution was separated from the gel by suction and then the gel was washed with 200 ml each of 10 mM NaOH, 10 mM HCl and H_2O and finally suspended in 10 mM sodium β-glycerophospate, 0.01 mg/ml sodium azide, pH 7.0. The pH of the butylamine solution changed insignificantly (0.5–1%) after addition of the gel. The solubilized samples (Jennissen and Heilmeyer-Jr, 1975) were counted in triplicate and are given as mean values ± S.D. For further details see (Jennissen and Heilmeyer-Jr, 1975; Kohn and Wilchek, 1981).

obtaining purely uncharged carbamate linked alkyl agaroses is the carbonyldiimidazole method (Bethell *et al.*, 1979; Zumbrink *et al.*, 1995) which is also employed below (see also (Wilchek *et al.*, 1984) for an alternative method via chloroformates). For other methods of immobilizing chemical compounds of various types for the synthesis of hydrophobic and affinity matrices see (Hermanson *et al.*, 1992) and for novel aspects of the tresyl chloride method see (Demiroglou and Jennissen, 1990; Demiroglou *et al.*, 1994, Zumbrink *et al.*, 1995).

Discovery and development of hydrophobic interaction chromatography

The chromatographic separation of proteins by way of hydrophobic interactions was reported independently by two groups in 1972 (Er-el *et al.*, 1972; Yon, 1972) and by three additional groups in 1973 (Hofstee, 1973a; Hjerten, 1973; Porath *et al.*, 1973). Historically the method then evolved in two distinct branches. The first branch was developed by Shaltiel, Hofstee and Yon (Er-el *et al.*, 1972; Hofstee, 1973a; Yon, 1972) and centered on hydrophobic gels synthesized by the CNBr procedure (containing some charges) and on procedures run at *low ionic strength.* The second branch developed by Porath and Hjerten (Hjerten *et al.*, 1974; Porath *et al.*, 1973) focused on gels synthesized by chemical methods which did not introduce charges and which were run at *high ionic strength.* In the first branch the name *"hydrophobic chromatography"* (Shaltiel and Er-el, 1973) was coined, the dominant term for many years, whereas in the second the name *"hydrophobic interaction chromatography"* (Hjerten, 1973) predominated. The development of this novel separation method based on hydrophobic interactions taking place along these two branches was controversial for many years. Today these controversies have been resolved and in this review it will be attempted to depict the major highlights in the development of this still advancing field.

Hydrophobic non-charge-free gels (NCF-gels)

In 1972 Yon (Yon, 1972) reported that *lipophilic proteins* such as albumin or aspartate transcarbamoylase could be hydrophobically adsorbed on N-(3-carboxypropionyl) aminodecyl-agarose containing mixed hydrophobic and ionic groups ("hydrophobic affinity chromatography"). The proteins were adsorbed at low ionic strength at the isoelectric point and eluted at alkaline pH by charge repulsion (for review see Yon, 1977). In classical affinity chromatography it had been suggested by Steers *et al.* (Steers-Jr *et al.*, 1971) at that time, that a 1–2 nm long spacer should be inserted between the matrix and the immobilized ligand to increase the efficiency of biorecognition. Many groups were therefore applying the new technology and it was more or less by accident that Shaltiel's group (Er-el *et al.*, 1972) discovered "hydrophobic chromatography", since they had set out to purify glycogen phosphorylase by classical affinity chromatography on a glycogen-Sepharose column. The glycogen was immobilized via an alkyl spacer by the CNBr method and when the control experiment without glycogen i.e. with the alkyl spacer-Sepharose alone was run, they detected that phosphorylase was strongly adsorbed in the absence of glycogen on a hydrocarbon coated agarose alone (Er-el *et al.*, 1972). The surprising result in Shaltiel's experiments was that a very "normal" *hydrophilic enzyme*, phosphorylase *b*, could be purified on hydrocarbon coated agaroses to near homogeneity in one step, implicitly questioning the general doctrine of the time that all hydrophobic amino acids were buried in the interior of proteins. Phosphorylase was adsorbed *at low ionic strength* on immobilized butyl residues which had no resemblence to the substrates of the enzyme (thus excluding affinity chromatography) and was eluted by a "deforming buffer" reversibly unfolding the enzyme. Taken together with Shaltiel's systematic approach of grading the hydrophobicity of the gels via an immobilized *homologous hydrocarbon series* (Er-el *et al.*, 1972) (see the section on Chain-length parameter), the immediate impression was that here was a novel method applicable not only to hydrophobic or lipophilic proteins but also to hydrophilic and possibly to all proteins. A few months later Hofstee independently published a series of papers leading to similar conclusions (Hofstee, 1973a–c).

Hydrophobic charge-free gels (CF-gels)

Uncharged hydrophobic gels (CF-gels) were synthesized for the first time by Porath *et al.* (Porath *et al.*, 1973) who reacted benzyl chloride with agarose at high temperatures. In this system the synthesis of a graded homologous series of hydrocarbon coated agaroses was not easily feasible. However Porath demonstrated the inverse salt behavior of proteins adsorbed on such gels for the first time and thus termed this method "hydrophobic salting-out chromatography". In contrast to ion exchangers proteins were adsorbed at high salt concentrations and eluted by decreasing the ionic strength. Hjerten (Hjerten, 1973) in outlining "hydrophobic interaction chromatography" synthesized various hydrophobic supports including homologous alkylamines according to (Er-el *et al.*, 1972) via the CNBr procedure and combined them chromatographically with the salting-out effect of Porath (Porath *et al.*, 1973). These results demonstrated and generalized that proteins could also be adsorbed to NCF-matrices of the Shaltiel type at high salt concentrations and eluted by negative salt gradients just as on charge-free gels (see above). In 1974 Hjerten *et al.* (Hjerten *et al.*, 1974) described a novel preparation of uncharged hydrophobic gels by coupling alkyl and aryl groups via the glycidyl ether method which allowed the preparation of uncharged homologous series of alkyl agaroses (see also Sections on *The adsorption threshold and critical hydrophobicity of gels and on Multivalence*).

Charge containing (NCF) versus charge-free (CF) hydrophobic gels

In retrospect, although there is no doubt that uncharged hydrophobic gels are by virtue of displaying a single (pure) type of non-covalent interaction superior to the NCF-gels (see (Porath *et al.*, 1973)), it appears that all groups involved in the development of this new method observed the binding and fractionation of proteins by hydrophobic interactions. In those cases of hydrophobic NCF-gels where the CNBr activated gels had been washed by the original procedure of (Porath *et al.*, 1967) with 0.1 M NaHCO$_3$ (pH 7–8) or with 0.2 M Na$_2$CO$_3$ (pH 9–10 (Jennissen, 1976a,b)) prior to coupling with alkyl amines a large proportion of the cyanate esters was destroyed favoring uncharged coupling products. Finally it was shown by Shaltiel in a careful study that in fact very similar results are obtained on hydrophobic CF-gels as on the original NCF-gels synthesized by the CNBr method (for review see (Halperin *et al.*, 1981)). In addition it was shown by various groups (Hjerten, 1973; Hofstee and Otillio, 1978; Jennissen, 1976a,b) that the charges introduced by the CNBr method were effectively quenched by salt in the range of 0.3–3.0 M so that the NCF-supports matched their uncharged counterparts in many of their hydrophobic properties.

Nomenclature

The two major terms that finally came to use "hydrophobic chromatography" (Er-el *et al.*, 1972; Shaltiel, 1984) and "hydrophobic interaction chromatography" (Hjerten, 1973, 1981) have now been used interchangeably side by side for nearly 30 years. There is no reason why one of these terms should be more or less of a misnomer (Hjerten, 1976) than the generally accepted term "affinity chromatography". New names are coined to accommodate new scientific contexts not so much for their inner logic. The term "hydrophobic interaction chromatography" is used exclusively in this review for purely editorial reasons.

Principles of hydrophobic interaction chromatography

The chain-length parameter

Shaltiel's group (Er-el *et al.*, 1972) introduced the principle of the *variation of the alkyl chain length* of homologous alkylamines on NCF-gels comprising a homologous series of hydrocarbon coated Sepharoses (Seph-C$_n$ (Shaltiel, 1974, 1984)). They found that on a homologous series Seph-C$_1$ to Seph-C$_6$ the enzyme phosphorylase was excluded by Seph-C$_1$ and Seph-C$_2$, retarded by Seph-C$_3$ and retained by Seph-C$_4$ to Seph-C$_6$. The major conclusion of these experimental results was that an increase in the chain length by $-CH_2-$ units concomitantly increased the strength of protein binding from retardation to reversible binding to very tight binding ("irreversible" binding). In addition to this variation in affinity with the chain length the gels also changed in specificity for the adsorbed protein as was shown in later work (see (Shaltiel, 1984)). However the enzyme could only be eluted through reversible denaturation by a deforming buffer followed by renaturation to the active form. The experiments of Shaltiels group demonstrated the decisive influence of a "gradable" hydrophobic interaction between the matrix and a protein. Simultaneously the optimization of the gels allowed the purification phosphorylase from a crude extract in one step. The principle applicability of these findings was confirmed on NCF-type hydrophobic alkyl gels by various groups (Hofstee, 1973c; Jakubowski and Pawelkiewicz, 1973; Jennissen and Heilmeyer, 1975; Jost et al., 1974; Raibaud et al., 1975) and also on neutral CF-type hydrophobic alkyl gels (Rosengren et al., 1975).

The surface concentration parameter

The adsorption threshold and critical hydrophobicity of gels

In 1975 however it could first be shown that a second parameter is of equal if not greater importance for the binding of proteins to alkyl substituted gels. If, instead of the chain length, the *surface concentration of immobilized alkyl groups* (i.e. density) is varied on Seph-C_1–Seph-C_4 protein adsorption is characteristically a sigmoidal function of the surface concentration of immobilized alkyl residues (Fig. 4.2) (*surface concentration series*). In such a concentration series the strength of binding also increases from retardation to very tight binding as in the homologous series of Shaltiel. Figure 4.2 illustrates the combined effect of chain elongation and surface concentration increase on the adsorption of the enzyme phosphorylase kinase to alkyl agaroses. Chain-elongation in a homologous series leads to a leftward shift of the sigmoidal curves of the concentration series and to a loss of sigmoidicity. Thus in the concentration series of alkyl agaroses a second general parameter for the variation of the gel hydrophobicity had been discovered which was equal to or more crucial for the binding of proteins than an increase in chain length alone (Jennissen and Heilmeyer, 1975). Another important finding in this work was that a threshold value of the alkyl surface concentration, a "critical hydrophobicity can be defined at which a protein is adsorbed (Jennissen and Heilmeyer, 1975). With a ratio of alkyl residues: positive charges in the gels of ca. 10 : 1 (Jennissen and Heilmeyer, 1975) the predominance of hydrophobic interactions as the basis for adsorption was convincing. Sigmoidal adsorption curves and critical surface concentrations were also obtained from binding data in the presence of 1.1 M ammonium sulfate (see Fig. 4.3) i.e. under charge quenching (Jennissen, 1978a) and a similar behavior has also been demonstrated on charge-free hydrophobic gels at low ionic strength (Jennissen and Demirolgou, 1992). A sigmoidal binding of phosphorylase *a* to methyl-Sepharoses of increasing degree of substitution was also published several years later by Shaltiel's group (Shaltiel, 1978). Also later Rosengren et al. (Rosengren et al., 1975) showed the dependence of phycoerythrin adsorption on the density of immobilized alkyl groups in a series of uncharged Seph-C_5–Seph-C_{12} alkyl agaroses at high salt concentrations. Probably, due to the salting-out conditions and the long chain-length of the immobilized alkyl groups ($\geq C_5$), neither a pronounced sigmoidicity of binding nor a critical hydrophobicity were described. A very similar approach to the generation of graded hydrophobicity surfaces as in the concentration series (Fig. 4.2) of alkyl agaroses has been attempted in the synthesis of so-called "hydrophobicity gradients" on glass

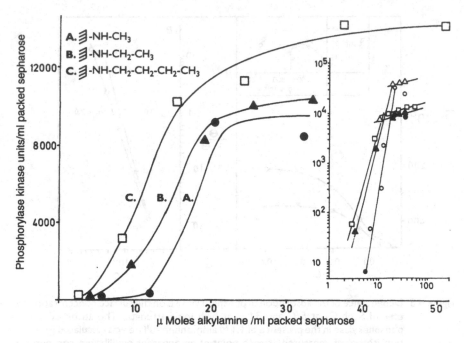

Figure 4.2 Dependence of the adsorption of phosphorylase kinase on the chain-length and surface concentration parameters of a homologous series of alkyl-Sepharoses a low ionic strength. The amount of adsorbed enzyme activity per ml packed Sepharose was calculated from the difference between the total amount of applied units and the amount excluded from the gel. The crude extract was applied to columns containing ca. 10 ml packed gel. Insert: Double logarithmic plots of adsorbed phosphorylase kinase as a function of the degree of substitution. Experiments with purified phosphorylase kinase are included. The gels were prepared by the CNBr procedure. For further details see the text. From (Jennissen and Heilmeyer, 1975). Seph-C_1: (●) crude extract; (○) purified phosphorylase kinase, Seph-C_2: (▲) crude extract; (△) purified phosphorylase kinase, Seph-C_4: (□) crude extract.

(Elwing *et al.*, 1988). However these latter gradients also contain a counter-gradient of charges which significantly influences the hydrophilicity/hydrophobicity balance in the adsorption of proteins so that such surfaces do not constitute true hydrophobicity gradients unless the charge gradient is effectively quenched.

Multivalence

The interpretation of the sigmoidal curves (Figs. 4.2–4.3) became possible when the concepts of multivalence and cooperativity of protein adsorption were developed (Jennissen, 1976b). This work was based on quantitative protein adsorption studies (for recent treatise (see (Hlady *et al.*, 1999)). It became clear that the sigmoidicity and the "critical hydrophobicity" were due to the multivalence of the interaction (i.e. the necessity for a simultaneous interaction of more than one alkyl residue or more than one separate local surface site with the protein moiety) (Jennissen, 1976b,c, 1978a; Jennissen and Botzet, 1979). The conclusion of multivalence and of protein binding on a binding-site lattice was not biased by putatively interspersed charges but could

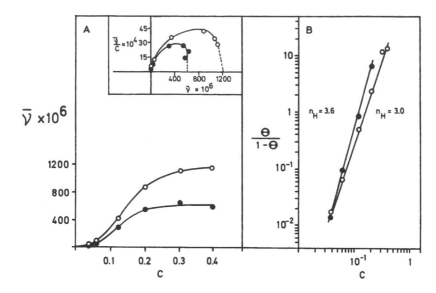

Figure 4.3 Dependence of the adsorption of phosphorylase b on the surface concentration parameter of Seph-C$_4$ at 5°C and 34°C at high ionic strength. The adsorbed amount of phosphorylase in the presence of 1.1 M ammonium sulfate was calculated from adsorption isotherms measured at each point at an apparent equilibrium concentration of free bulk protein of 0.07 mg/ml. The adsorbed amount of enzyme ($\bar{v}$) is expressed in relation to the anhydrodisaccharide content of agarose in mol/mol anhydrodisaccharide. Similarly C indicates the immobilized butyl residue concentration in relation to the anhydrodisaccharide content of agarose in mol alkylresidue/mol anhydrodisaccharide. A monomer molecular mass of 10^5 was employed for phosphorylase b. The alkyl agaroses were synthesized by the CNBr method. A. Adsorption isotherms ("lattice site binding function" (Jennissen, 1988)) of phosphorylase b in Cartesian coordinates. Insert: Scatchard plots of the sigmoidal binding curves with extrapolation of fractional saturation of 610 (5°) and 1220 (34°) μmol enzyme/mol anhydrodisaccharide (corresponding to 6.2 and 13.4 mg/ml packed gel respectively). The broken lines indicate the mode of extrapolation. (●) 5°C; (○) 34°C. B. Hill plots of the sigmoidal binding curves. (Θ) the fractional saturation was calculated from the extrapolated saturation values of the Scatchard plot (A). The Hill coefficients n$_H$ are given in the graph. The apparent dissociation constants of half-maximal saturation (K'$_{D,0.5}$) are 0.137 and 0.167 mol butylresidue/mol anhydrodisaccharide at 5° and 34° respectively (which corresponds to 14.0 and 17.0 μmol butylresidues/ml packed gel respectively). (●) 5°C; (○) 34°C. For further details see the text (Jennissen, 1978a, 1981, 1988; Jennissen and Botzet, 1993). From (Jennissen, 1978a).

be generalized from a homologous (alkyl residues alone) and to a heterologous (alkyl residues + charges) lattice which should principally not behave differently in generating sigmoidal protein binding curves in a concentration series of alkyl agaroses. In addition, it could be expected that the heterologous lattice would become "functionally" homologous by quenching the charges in the presence of 1.1 M ammonium sulfate (Jennissen, 1978a). As expected, the sigmoidal binding curves were not eliminated by high salt concentrations and on the Seph-C$_4$ concentration series protein binding now displayed a positive temperature coefficient as is characteristic for hydrophobic interactions (see Fig. 4.3) (Jennissen, 1976b, 1978a). Later a mathematical model was developed (Jennissen, 1976c, 1978a, 1981) allowing an estimation of the minimum number of alkyl residues (see Fig. 4.3B) interacting with the protein. The model of multivalence was also confirmed from a different perspective by equilibrium binding studies of phosphorylase b (~ 1 mM) with ^{14}C-hexylamine (~ 1 mM) in solution at a salt concentration of 1.1 M ammonium sulfate. In this experiment (Jennissen et al., 1982) the addition of ~ 1 mM phosphorylase b did not alter the free bulk concentration of ^{14}C-hexylamine indicating that phosphorylase b did not bind hexylamine under these conditions. This allowed the estimation of a maximal binding affinity for hexyl amine protein binding to $K_{0.5} \sim 10$–$100\,M^{-1}$ (Jennissen et al., 1982). Since in binding studies with immobilized butyl residues (Seph-C$_4$) binding constants of 9–16 $\times$ 10$^4\,M^{-1}$ for phosphorylase b had been obtained (Jennissen, 1976b; Jennissen and Botzet, 1979) this binding experiment clearly demonstrated that not even the long C$_6$ residue, when immobilized, would be capable of adsorbing a molecule of phosphorylase in a monovalent manner (i.e. on a single immobilized residue). On a gel surface only the cooperative interaction of a critical number of such immobilized residues could lead to adsorption. Since the multivalent mechanism of protein adsorption appeared to be the common denominator of most types of adsorption chromatography (hydrophobic and ion exchange) the term "multivalent interaction chromatography" was suggested (Jennissen, 1978a) but did not come to general use. Later the concept of multivalence was also applied to reversed phase chromatography (Pearson et al., 1982). The possibility of a "multi-point" or "multiple contacts" type of binding in hydrophobic protein adsorption was also envisaged in lieu of direct evidence by Hofstee and Hjerten (Hofstee, 1973b; Hjerten et al., 1974). However the concept and term of multivalence are to be preferred to terms such as "multiple contacts" since the latter term does not differentiate between the binding of a protein to separate alkyl residues (separate local surface sites) or just to different segments of one and the same alkyl residue.

Protein adsorption hysteresis

Cooperative multivalent protein binding on alkyl substituted surfaces can lead to protein adsorption hysteresis (Jennissen, 1978b, 1985, 1988; Jennissen and Botzet, 1979). In protein adsorption hysteresis, the adsorption isotherm is not retraced by the desorption isotherm, due to an increase in binding affinity after the protein is adsorbed. This indicates that protein adsorption to multivalent surfaces is thermodynamically irreversible ($\Delta_i S > 0$) and that a true equilibrium has not been reached. The binding affinity increase can be attributed to an increase in multivalence (Jennissen and Botzet, 1979) which is either due to a reorientation of the protein on the surface or to a conformational change in which buried hydrophobic contact sites (valences) are exposed by the binding strain on the adsorbed protein (Jennissen, 1985; Jennissen and Botzet, 1979). In the case of the adsorption of phosphorylase b to butyl agarose there was no evidence that an irreversible conformational change was taking place (Jennissen and Botzet, 1979), since the fully active enzyme can be desorbed from such gels by "deforming buffer" (Er-el et al., 1972) (see above). The danger of a protein undergoing an irreversible conformational change and even a denaturation after adsorption has however been shown for other proteins binding to hydrophobic matrices (Ingraham et al., 1985; Wu et al., 1986) as well as to non-hydrophobic affinity supports (Jost et al., 1974).

Adsorption hysteresis has decisive effects on the chromatographic behavior of proteins during hydrophobic interaction chromatography leading to non-linearity and skewed elution peaks in zonal chromatography and to false "irreversibility", i.e. extremely high affinity, in adsorption chromatography (Jennissen, 1981, 1986). Hysteresis can be reduced by a decrease in the surface concentration of immobilized residues which reduces multivalence (Jennissen, 1981).

The salt-parameter

Salting-out on unsubstituted hydrophilic gels

Reversible salting-out adsorption of proteins by neutral salts below their precipitation points on solid supports (silica gel, filterpaper) goes back to Arne Tiselius (Tiselius, 1948). In a column chromatography system this technique was reported by Porath (Porath, 1962) as a "zone precipitation" of serum proteins on cross-linked *dextran* (Sephadex G-100). Although in that paper no distinction is made between an actual precipitation of the proteins on the gel and an adsorptive mechanism, both factors were probably involved. The same phenomenon has also been observed on other *crosslinked* hydrogels such as Sephacryl (Ashton and Anderson, 1981) and Sepharose CL-6B (Sawatzki *et al.*, 1981). From adsorption studies of cyclohexane and 1-pentanol on highly crosslinked dextran (Sephadex G-15), which show positive temperature coefficients, anhydroglucose itself has been implicated as exhibiting nonpolarity (Mardsen, 1977). However since the nonpolar adsorption of the organic solutes also correlated with the crosslinking density of the dextran (Mardsen, 1977), which could not be differentiated from the effect attributed to glucose, the matter remains unclear. On the other hand it has been reported (Janado and Nishada, 1981) that the sugars glucose and mannose possess negative as well as positive cosolvent effects in respect to hydrophobic solutes e.g. octanol. The positive cosolvent effect is enhanced by oligomerization of the sugar (maltose, dextran) and by increasing the temperature or the salt concentration (2 M NaCl), which strongly indicates nonpolar interactions of the sugar moiety. In the case of galactose a significant positive cosolvent effect was not shown (Janado and Nishada, 1981).

The salting-out of proteins on *non-crosslinked* and non-substituted *agarose* (Sepharose 4B) was reported independently by two groups (Mevarech *et al.*, 1976; Von der Haar, 1976). At high ammonium sulfate concentrations (2–3 M), but below the precipitation point of proteins, agarose is capable of adsorbing large amounts of proteins (for review see (Von der Haar, 1979)). The proteins can be eluted by a negative ammonium sulfate concentration gradient and purified. Characteristically this adsorption is only elicited by strongly salting-out ions like sulfate, phosphate and citrate (Von der Haar, 1979) at high concentrations. No examples with other salts like NaCl have been reported. Non-crosslinked cellulose also appears to exhibit a similar behavior as an adsorbent for salted-out proteins (Ashton and Anderson, 1981; Tiselius, 1948).

The mechanism of this latter type of salting-out chromatography remains unclear, since no thermodynamic studies have been made. It may very well be that protein adsorption in these cases displays a negative temperature coefficient similar to the adsorption of phosphorylase b in the presence of 1.1 M ammonium sulfate on Seph-C_1 (see also Fig. 4.6) (Jennissen, 1976b, 1978a). Since this behavior suggests that the free energy of binding is primarily enthalpic and not hydrophobic it has been termed "exothermic" salting-out chromatography (Jennissen, 1978a). This interpretation is supported by results obtained with nucleic acids. Nucleic acids (tRNA) can also be salted-out on Sepharose 4B and various other neutral polysaccharides in the presence of 2 M ammonium sulfate as shown by Morris (Morris, 1978). Morris also found a negative temperature coefficient for the retention volumes of individual zones (fractions) of tRNA and the distance between them and concluded an enthalpic, non-hydrophobic adsorption mechanism. Surprisingly deviations in the expected temperature dependence were also observed in reversed-phase liquid chromatography with acetonitrile/water phases indicating non-hydrophobic interactions (Cole et al., 1992) even on these very hydrophobic surfaces. Therefore, as a rule the temperature dependence of the adsorption reaction can be taken to be a more sensitive parameter than a salt effect per se (e.g. salting-out) in gaining information on the actual adsorption mechanism involved (see Jennissen, 1978a).

As to the predominant non-covalent interaction responsible for the binding of proteins and nucleic acids to neutral carbohydrates under salting-out conditions a likely candidate is hydrogen bonding (C. J. O. R. Morris, personal communication, 1977). However more basic work in this area is required before final conclusions can be reached (Morris, 1978).

Another major conclusion from the above observations is that in all salting-out experiments with proteins on chemically modified hydrophilic gels (especially with high concentrations of ammonium sulfate) it is essential to run controls on the corresponding unsubstituted matrices.

Salting-out and salting-in on hydrophobic gels

Porath (Porath et al., 1973) showed that the hydrophobic adsorption of trypsin inhibitor can be enhanced by high concentrations of salts on uncharged benzyl ether agarose. Trypsin inhibitor could be purified 25-fold after being adsorbed at 3 M NaCl followed by elution in buffer without salt. These results were confirmed by Hjerten (Hjerten, 1973) on NCF-gels containing aliphatic residues by the adsorption of serum proteins at 4 M NaCl and elution by lowering the ionic strength 400-fold. A similar chromatographic technique was described by Rimerman and Hatfield (Rimerman and Hatfield, 1973) who salted out *Escherichia coli* proteins on an alanine-Sepharose with 1 M potassium phosphate and eluted with a decreasing salt concentration gradient. Application of a cell free *E. coli* extract to the column and development with a negative concentration gradient led to the elution of *E. coli* proteins in relation to their solubility in concentrated ammonium sulfate (Rimerman and Hatfield, 1973). Similarly alkaline phosphatase could be adsorbed on phenylalanine-Sepharose in the presence of 1.25 M ammonium sulfate and eluted by a negative salt gradient (Doellgast and Fishmann, 1974).

Subsequently it could be shown that the effect of salts on the adsorption and elution of proteins on alkyl agaroses indeed followed the Hofmeister series of salts (Jennissen and Heilmeyer, 1975; Raibaud et al., 1975). We could show that phosphorylase kinase is eluted ("salted-in") from a Seph-C_2-column by increasing salt gradients (Jennissen and Heilmeyer-Jr, 1975). In a series of experiments the ionic strength of the peak fractions eluted, was inversely related to the *salting-in power* of the anions ions in the gradient in agreement with the Hofmeister series of salts (see Fig. 4.4). Raibaud *et al.* (Raibaud *et al.*, 1975) reported that the concentration of salts necessary for the inhibition of β-galactosidase adsorption on a Seph-C_3-column shows a similar inverse relationship to the salting-in power of the anions employed. These experiments clearly indicated that the action of the ions was not due to a pure electrostatic but to a lyotropic effect. It could be argued that this effect is again due to the interspersed charges in the NCF-gels. However, proteins could also be eluted (salted-in) from uncharged CF-gels (octyl-Sepharose) by an increasing salt gradient as shown by (Raymond *et al.*, 1981): after adsorption of proteins at high ionic strength a first major fraction of proteins was eluted by a decreasing salt gradient followed by the elution of a second fraction by an increasing $MgCl_2$ gradient. In other experiments it could be shown that haemoglobin, serum albumin

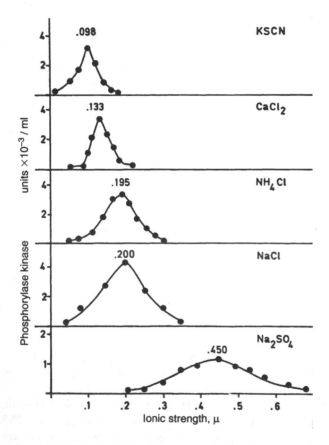

Figure 4.4 Influence of the salt parameter on the desorption of purified phosphorylase kinase from Seph-C_2 (25 μmol/ml packed gel) with salt gradients of different ionic composition. Each column with 5 ml of the above gel (CNBr method) was loaded with ca. 11 mg of the enzyme. The gradients were produced from 100 ml low ionic strength adsorption buffer and 100 ml salt containing buffer. The number at the maximum of the elution profiles indicates the ionic strength of the peak fraction. For further details see the text and legend to Fig. 4.1 and (Jennissen and Heilmeyer, 1975). (From Jennissen and Heilmeyer, 1975.)

(Memoli and Doellgast, 1975) and phosphorylase b (Jennissen, 1976a,b) were salted-out by ammnoium sulfate on NCF-alkyl Sepahroses, in column (Jennissen, 1976a) (see Fig. 4.5) and in batch experiments (Jennissen, 1976b) under conditions, where unsubstituted Sepharose showed no adsorption. Finally Pahlman *et al.* (Pahlman *et al.*, 1977) showed that the *salting-out power* of anions, for the adsorption of HSA on uncharged Seph-C_5, followed the order of the Hofmeister series of salts. In sum, these experiments again demonstrate the similar properties of the hydrophobic matrices containing some residual charges (NCF-gels) and the uncharged hydrophobic gels (CF-gels) in respect to the lyotropic action of salts on protein adsorption.

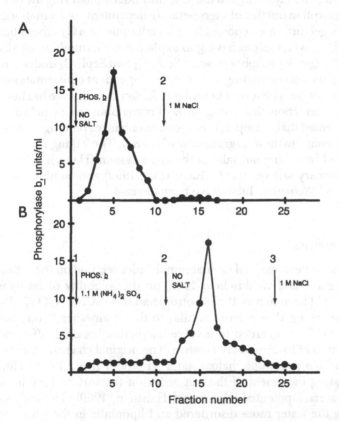

Figure 4.5 Application of the salt parameter by utilizing the inverse salt dependence for the chromatography of purified phosphorylase b on Seph-C_1 (30 μmol/ml packed gel). In this form of salting-out chromatography the equilibration buffer contained 10 mM sodium β-glycerophosphate, 20 mM mercaptoethanol, 2 mM EDTA, 20% sucrose, 0.5 μM PMSF, pH 7.0 (buffer A) to which either 1.1 M ammonium sulfate or NaCl was added. 6 mg/3 ml phosphorylase b was added to 20 ml Seph-C1 in a 2 cm i.d. × 17 cm column. Fractions of 6.5 ml were collected. The gel was prepared by the CNBr procedure. A. Application of enzyme to a column equilibrated with buffer without $(NH_4)_2SO_4$ or NaCl: (1) Application of phosphorylase b in buffer A; (2) Elution with buffer A + 1 M NaCl. B. Application of enzyme to a column equilibrated with buffer with $(NH_4)_2SO_4$: (1) Application of phosphorylase b in buffer A + 1.1 M ammonium sulfate; (2) Elution with buffer A; (3) Elution with buffer A + NaCl. For further details see the text and (Jennissen, 1976a). From (Jennissen, 1976a).

The mechanism of protein binding was further analyzed at different temperatures under equilibrium binding conditions on NCF-gels (Jennissen, 1976b; Jennissen and Botzet, 1979). At very low ionic strength (10 mM Tris/HCl, pH 7.0) the adsorption of phosphorylase b exhibited a negative temperature coefficient on Seph-C1 as well as on Seph-C4 (Jennissen, 1976b). At high ionic strength (1.1 M ammonium sulfate) Seph-C1 retained its negative coefficient but Seph-C4 now exhibited a positive temperature (see Fig. 4.3) coefficient (Jennissen, 1976b; Jennissen and Botzet, 1979) demonstrating that thermodynamically two forms of salting-out adsorption on hydrophobic gels can be distinguished as exothermic and endothermic salting-out chromatography respectively (see above) (Jennissen, 1978a). It may be argued that one may not be observing the temperature dependence of adsorption but that of a temperature dependent conformational change of the protein on the gel surface as reported for α-lactalbumin on a C_2-ether silica column (Wu et $al.$, 1986). However, besides having to explain two thermodynamically different conformational changes of phosphorylase on Seph-C1 and Seph-C4 under otherwise identical conditions, the corresponding temperature-dependent conformational changes of the protein have not been observed in solution. In fact the opposite has been shown in the hydrophobic interaction chromatography of myoglobin and cytochrome c. In this case it was documented that a temperature increase enhances binding without a major change in protein conformation (Ingraham et $al.$, 1985). The salting-in action of salts can be counteracted by salting-out salts in the same system (Hanstein, 1979). Thus various binary and ternary salt systems (el-Rassi et $al.$, 1990) and combinations with detergents (Buckley and Wetlaufer, 1990) have been devised.

Theories of salt actions on proteins

An early approach on the salt effects exerted on macromolecules is based on the action of chaotropic ions (Hamaguchi and Geiduschek, 1962) on the solubility of proteins (Hatefi and Hanstein, 1969). The action of the chaotropic anions (SCN^-, CLO_4^-, I^-, NO_3^-, Br^-), which can be arranged in a series similar to the Hofmeister (lyotropic) series (Hofmeister, 1887, 1888), is regarded to involve a structure-breaking effect on water since the ionic entropies of hydration are positive. The original chaotropic series was later supplemented by the chaotropic haloacetates (Hanstein et $al.$, 1971). Thus one can observe a decreasing increment of the salt series on the surface tension of water and an increase in surface potential (Hatefi and Hanstein, 1969). The authors conclude that "by making the water more disordered and lipophilic in the presence of the appropriate ions, it should be possible to weaken the hydrophobic bonds of membranes and multicomponent enzymes and increase the water solubility (salting-in) of particulated proteins and nonelectrolytes" (Hatefi and Hanstein, 1969). This interpretation is supported by the solvent isotope effects observed in D_2O vs H_2O (Hanstein et $al.$, 1974). The opposite effect can be observed with so-called antichaotropic salts (SO_4^{2-}, HPO_4^{2-}, F^-) which reverse the resolution of hydrophobic interactions by stabilizing the water structure (salting-out) (Davis and Hatefi, 1972) and which generally have negative values of the ionic entropy of hydration (Hanstein et $al.$, 1971). For a quantitative description of the effect of salt concentrations on the solubility of the model solute 2-methylnaphthoquinone an extended Setschenow equation has been utilized (Hanstein, 1979; Hanstein et $al.$, 1971). The general conclusion of this work, with consideration of electrostatic and dispersion forces, is that chaotropes interact indirectly with solutes (e.g. proteins) mainly through their effect on water structure (Hanstein, 1979).

The solvophobic theory of Melander and Horvath, 1977 allows the description of reversed-phase retention for a wide variety of conditions including organic solvents and neutral salts. Salting-in and salting-out is explained on the basis of the respective surface-tension-decreasing/-increasing effect of the salt which is applicable to reversed-phase chromatography as well as to hydrophobic interaction chromatography (Melander and Horvath, 1977; Melander *et al.*, 1984). Specifically in respect to retention in hydrophobic interaction chromatography it has been suggested that water plays a central role as displacing agent (Geng *et al.*, 1990). In addition to the dependence of retention on the non-polar molecular area of the protein and the interfacial tension in the aqueous salt solution there also appear to be specific salt effects (divalent cations) resulting from a direct binding to protein e.g. of $MgCl_2$ (Arakawa and Timasheff, 1984; Szepesy and Horvath, 1988). In the paper of Arakawa and Narhi (Arakawa and Narhi, 1991) this approach, that salts do not act by influencing the surface tension but by directly binding to the protein, is extended. The action of thiocyanates is therefore interpreted as due to a preferential binding to proteins followed by a destabilization of the hydrophobic interactions.

Irrespective of the mechanism, the applicability of the Hofmeister (lyotropic) series of salts, expanded by the chaotropic series, to hydrophobic interaction chromatography has been verified by many groups and these salts are important tools in controlling the adsorption and elution of proteins on these resins. The individuality of each protein in its quantitative interactions in such a system especially when the native state should be conserved, however, remains a very important factor in determining the behavior of each individual chromatographic system.

Optimization of alkyl agaroses for hydrophobic interaction chromatography

Introduction

Even now nearly 30 years after the introduction of hydrophobic interaction chromatography the method has failed to gain the same foothold in the methodological repertoire of protein chemistry as has affinity chromatography, although a large number of proteins has been successfully purified by this method (Eriksson, 1989; Hjerten, 1981; Hofstee and Otillio, 1978; Mohr and Pommerening, 1986; Ochoa, 1978; Shaltiel, 1984; Yon, 1977). In fact, a recent paper comes to the conclusion that certain "classical" commercial hydrophobic adsorbents are inadequate for an ideal downstream processing because of their high hydrophobicity (Oscarsson *et al.*, 1995). The criticism of these authors is essentially correct. The major problem encountered on such hydrophobic gels is that proteins can be very effectively adsorbed but an elution in a native state is often practically impossible. The problem therefore is to find a hydrophobic matrix with such a low hydrophobicity as to allow a binding and an elution of the intact protein. This problem is not new. The possibility of synthesizing low hydrophobicity gels has been present from the very beginning of hydrophobic interaction chromatography (Jennissen, 1976a). In fact, such a "weak-hydrophobic chromatography system" in which the protein (phosphorylase *b*) eluted as a retarded peak on Seph-C_4 at a high salt concentration was demonstrated many years ago (Jennissen, 1981). The question is therefore: Can a generally applicable method be devised for the synthesis of gels with an optimal low hydrophobicity for each protein? As will be shown below we think that such a method is conceivable.

The homologous series procedure

The synthesis of controlled hydrophobicity gels via the *homologous series* of hydrocarbon-coated Sepharoses (variation of alkyl chain length (Er-el *et al.*, 1972; Halperin *et al.*, 1981; Shaltiel, 1984)) was soon commercialized by introduction of the so-called *exploratory kit* for choosing the most appropriate column and for optimizing resolution (Shaltiel, 1974). This analytical kit, which was commercially available for some years, contained a homologous series of small columns from Seph-C_1 to Seph-C_{10} with two control columns (Shaltiel, 1974). The principle was to determine – *at low ionic strength* – the lowest member of the homologous series capable of retaining the desired enzyme or protein. This column was then selected for the purification of the desired protein. In a second step it was attempted to increase resolution by optimizing the elution procedure which ranged from mild salting-in procedures to reversible denaturation steps.

It had been shown by Hjerténs group (Hjertén, 1973; Hjertén *et al.*, 1974; Rosengren *et al.*, 1975) that proteins could also be adsorbed to homologous series of hydrophobic agaroses at high salt concentrations to be subsequently eluted by an inverse salt gradient. This was shown for the uncharged and the charge-containing gels. The optimization strategy was similar to that of Shaltiel only that elution was facilitated by an inverse salt gradient. Uncharged alkyl agaroses optimized and eluted according to the procedure outlined by Hjertén were also widely utilized and commercialized. However similar to the Shaltiel type of gels the main problem encountered in the high salt concentration approach of Hjertén was that again the proteins could often not be eluted (Oscarsson *et al.*, 1995) in the native form by the inverse salt gradient. Nevertheless this procedure or variants thereof are still the method of choice for most groups today.

The critical-hydrophobicity procedure

The importance of the second of the two procedures, i.e. optimization via the surface concentration series, has been underestimated. Although the decisive importance of the immobilized alkyl residue concentration for the hydrophobic adsorption of proteins (critical hydrophobicity) was stressed for many years (Jennissen and Heilmeyer, 1975; Jennissen, 1976b, 1978a, 1979; Jennissen and Demirolgou, 1992) no hydrophobicity gradient gel series has ever been produced commercially. Against the above background of the problems reported in hydrophobic interaction chromatography a novel rational basis for the design of a hydrophobic chromatography systems was recently introduced (Jennissen, 2000). It has been called critical hydrophobicity hydrophobic interaction chromatography (critical hydrophobicity HIC).

This concept is based on a very simple idea. High yields in hydrophobic interaction chromatography can only be obtained if the protein to be purified is fully excluded from the gel under as physiological elution conditions as possible i.e. at low ionic strength.

This means that the gel should be fully non-adsorbing under these conditions. On the other hand, since a purification is only possible if the protein is adsorbed to the gel, the matrix should be constructed in a way, that adsorption can be easily induced by other means without denaturing the protein. According to this concept, working at or near (juxtacritical) the critical hydrophobicity point should solve both problems. At critical or juxtacritical hydrophobicity of the matrix no protein is adsorbed at low ionic strength but adsorption can be induced by a finite high salt concentration with the possibility of utilizing either (a) elution chromatography by a negative salt gradient ("irreversible" adsorption conditions) or (b) a linear zonal chromatography (reversible adsorption conditions) (Jennissen, 1981). If the selected gel is significantly below the critical hydrophobicity protein adsorption may not be inducible by salt and if the gel is significantly above the critical hydrophobicity a complete elution of the protein will not be possible.

The aim of this new procedure is, therefore, to synthesize uncharged alkyl-Sepharose supports very close to the "critical hydrophobicity" of the protein under physiological conditions. Although essentially any type of molecule displaying hydrophobic properties could be coupled to the matrix, even proteins (Jennissen and Botzet, 1993), the immobilized residues should be restricted to alkane derivatives, to insure a "purity" of hydrophobic interactions. This restriction, in the first instance, also excludes pi- or d-electron containing molecules e.g. phenyl residues or sulfur atoms which should be avoided, because they may introduce additional charge-transfer interactions (Porath, 1978, 1989, Jennissen, 1995). Strongly salting-out ions should also be avoided, since they may induce nonspecific protein adsorption on the carbohydrate support itself (see discussion above). NaCl centrally located in the Hofmeister series appears to be an ideal salt to employ from the biochemical as well as the physical chemical view point. The critical hydrophobicity procedure thus involves 3 basic steps under standard conditions:

1   Selection of an *appropriate alkyl chain length* from a homologous series which is capable of adsorbing a selected protein under semiphysiological low ionic strength conditions.
2   Determination of the *critical hydrophobicity* at the predefined low ionic strength on the gel selected from the homologous series under point 1.
3   Determination of the minimal *salt concentration* (NaCl) necessary for a complete adsorption of a specified amount of the selected protein (e.g. 0.5 mg/ml packed gel) on the critical hydrophobicity support (point 2).

The three parameters can be determined by a simplified version of quantitative hydrophobic interaction chromatography (Jennissen and Demiroglou, 1992) aimed primarily at the high affinity adsorption sites. In distinction to the previously employed quantitative chromatographic method (Jennissen and Heilmeyer, 1975) the selected protein in this case is not applied to the column until equilibration is complete as determined from an identical concentration of protein or catalytic activity in the run-through and sample. Instead, a constant amount of enzyme activity or a protein (in this case fibrinogen) at an intermediate bed load is applied, followed by a wash with protein-free buffer until no more protein (enzyme activity) is detected in the run-through (see Methods). In single protein systems the adsorbed protein can then be eluted by urea or SDS to gain additional information on the adsorption state.

SELECTION OF THE APPROPRIATE ALKYL CHAIN LENGTH

The appropriate alkyl chain length is selected from test runs on Seph-C_4–Seph-C_6 similar to the homologous series method of Shaltiel at low ionic strength (see Jennissen, 2000). The surface concentration is set to ca. 20 μmol/ml packed gel. In general a constant amount of protein (ca. 0.5 mg/ml packed gel, which can be 100% adsorbed on the column of highest hydrophobicity) is applied at low or physiological salt concentration (0.15 M NaCl) to each column (1–2 ml packed gel). Then the gel in the homologous series is determined which adsorbs ca. 50% of the applied protein at a medium surface alkyl concentration of ca. 20–30 μmol/ml packed gel. In the case of the example below, ca. 50% of the applied fibrinogen was adsorbed on an uncharged Seph-C_5 gel containing 22 μmol/ml packed gel, so that Seph-C_5 was chosen for an expanded concentration series to determine the exact critical hydrophobicity point. For more information on the various methods of measuring protein adsorption in batch, column and surface spectroscopy systems (see Hlady *et al.*, 1999).

DETERMINATION OF THE CRITICAL HYDROPHOBICITY

As previously defined the critical hydrophobicity is that degree of substitution where the adsorption of a protein begins (Jennissen and Heilmeyer, 1975). As shown in Fig. 4.6 a strongly sigmoidal adsorption curve is obtained on the uncharged Seph-C_5 at a physiological NaCl concentration for the adsorption of fibrinogen as a function of the degree of substitution. The aim is to get as close as possible to the critical hydrophobicity without a significant adsorption of the protein. Since there was no measurable adsorption of fibrinogen at 12 μmol/ml packed gel and only ca. 2% was adsorbed at 13.6 μmol/ml packed gel (critical hydrophobicity, Fig. 4.6), the ideal juxtacritical hydrophobicity range was taken as 12–14 μmol/ml packed gel.

THE MINIMAL SALT CONCENTRATION FOR ADSORPTION

The non-adsorbing critical hydrophobicity gel above (13.6 μmol/ml packed gel) can now be transformed into an adsorbing gel by the addition of salt. In the case of fibrinogen this can be achieved by adding 1.5 M NaCl to the adsorbing buffer (see (Jennissen, 2000)). At lower salt concentrations the full load of fibrinogen is not adsorbed. Since the amount of fibrinogen adsorbed to the critical hydrophobicity pentyl Sepharose (13.6 μmol/ml packed gel) at low ionic strength (i.e. 0.15 M) was negligible (i.e. only 2% of applied amount), it is clear that a complete recovery of fibrinogen adsorbed at high ionic strength (1.5 M NaCl) should now be possible by simply decreasing the salt concentration to the original concentration of 0.15 M. This is indeed the case.

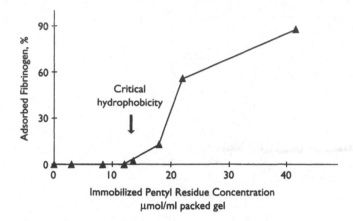

Figure 4.6 Adsorption of fibrinogen as a function of the immobilized pentyl residue concentration as derived from quantitative hydrophobic chromatography. Fibrinogen (1 mg) was applied in 1 ml to a column (0.9 cm i.d.×12 cm) containing 2 ml packed gel in 50 mM Tris/HCl, 150 mM NaCl, 1 mM EGTA, pH 7.4. Fractions of 1.5 ml were collected. The column was washed with 15 ml buffer followed by elution with 7.5 M urea. The arrow denotes the critical hydrophobicity. The uncharged gels were synthesized by the carbonyldiimidazole method. 100% equals 1 mg fibrinogen adsorbed to 2 ml packed gel of Seph-C_5. The total amount of adsorbed fibrinogen, corrected for the amount adsorbed to unsubstituted control Sepharose 4B, is shown. For further details see methods, the text and (Jennissen, 2000). From (Jennissen, 2000).

One-step purification of native fibrinogen from human blood plasma

Employing Seph-C_5 of critical hydrophobicity it is now possible to purify fibrinogen from human plasma in a single step (Fig. 4.7). The hydrophobicity of the column even suffices to purify fibrinogen from plasma not equilibrated with 1.5 M NaCl, allowing a direct application of human plasma without any preparatory steps (Fig. 4.7A). This leads to a temporary decrease in NaCl concentration (fractions 5–9), however, without any significant loss of fibrinogen. After extensive washing with 1.5 M NaCl pure fibrinogen (clottablity 93–99%, Fig. 4.7B) can be eluted at a NaCl concentration of 150 mM. In this case the total yield was 25%, which is not due to residual fibrinogen on the column but to errors inherent in the use of clottability for the calculations and losses in the run-through. Maximal yields of fibrinogen of 60% have been obtained. If blood plasma equilibrated with 1.5 M NaCl is applied to the gel and eluted by a negative salt gradient a maximal clottability of 80% is obtained (not shown).

Conclusions

Hydrophobic interaction chromatography is one of the very basic separation methods in classical biochemistry. However a simple optimization method for the purification of proteins on low hydrophobicity gels is still lacking. In the chapter it has been outlined that the successful hydrophobic interaction chromatography of proteins on

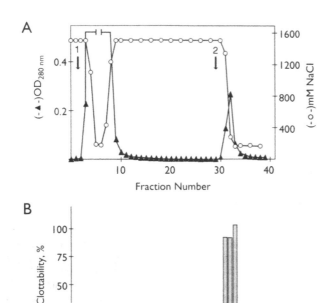

Figure 4.7 Isolation of electrophoretically pure, biologically active fibrinogen from human blood plasma in one step by hydrophobic interaction chromatography on critical hydrophobicity Seph-C₅. (A) 19 ml fresh unclotted human blood plasma (20 mM sodium citrate) was applied (arrow 1) to 20 ml packed Seph-C₅ (13.6 μmol/ml packed gel in a column 1.4 cm i.d. × 13 cm) equilibrated with 50 mM Tris/HCl, 1.5 M NaCl, pH 7.4 at a flow rate of 70 ml/h and a fraction volume of 6 ml. The non-adsorbed protein was washed out with 200 ml equilibration buffer. Elution (arrow 2) was facilitated by equilibration buffer containing a tenfold lower salt concentration of 150 mM NaCl. (B) The fractions 30–32 contain pure fibrinogen with a clottability of 93–100% with a total yield of 25%. From (Jennissen, 2000).

alkyl-matrices under standard conditions depends *on three basic parameters*: (i) the chain-length parameter, (ii) the surface-concentration parameter and (iii) the salt parameter. Only if these three parameters are optimized in an integrated manner can a successful implementation of hydrophobic interaction chromatography in protein purification be expected. The presented data strongly suggest that the *critical hydrophobicity method* for the optimization of hydrophobic supports poses a general, successful and rational approach to the purification of proteins by hydrophobic interaction chromatography. The only drawback is that hydrophobic concentration-series gel kits are not commercially available so that the application of the critical hydrophobicity method necessitates experience in the synthesis of alkyl agaroses and the quantification of the immobilized residues.

Acknowledgments

The support by the Deutsche Forschungsgemeinschaft (Je 84/9-2) and the Ministerium für Schule und Weiterbildung, Wissenschaft und Forschung NRW (Az.: IV A 6-214 005 97) is gratefully acknowledged.

References

Arakawa, T. and Narhi, L. O. (1991) Solvent Modulation in Hydrophobic Interaction Chromatography. *Biotechnol. Appl. Biochem.*, **13**, 151–172.

Arakawa, T. and Timasheff, S. N. (1984) Mechanism of Protein Salting In and Salting Out by Divalent Cation Salts: Balance Between Hydration and Salt Binding. *Biochemistry*, **23**, 5912–5923.

Ashton, A. R. and Anderson, L. E. (1981) Purification of Multiple Pea Ferredoxins at High Ionic strength on Unsubstituted Sepharose 4B. *Biochim. Biophys. Acta.*, **667**, 452–456.

Axen, R., Porath, J. and Ernback, S. (1967) Chemical Coupling of Peptides and Proteins to Polysacharides by Means of Cyanogen Halides. *Nature*, **214**, 1302–1304.

Ben-Naim, A., Wilf, J. and Yaacobi, M. (1973) *J. Phys. Chem.*, **77**, 95–102.

Bethell, G. S., Ayers, S., Hancock, W. S. and Hearn, M. T. W. (1979) A Novel Method of Activation of Cross-linked Agaroses with 1,1'-carbonyldiimidazole Which gives a Matrix for Affinity Chromatography Devoid of Additional Charged Groups. *J. Biol. Chem.*, **254**, 2572–2574.

Buckley, J. J. and Wetlaufer, D. B. (1990) Surfactant-mediated Hydrophobic Interaction Chromatography of Proteins: Gradient Elution. *J. Chromatogr.*, 99–110.

Cole, L. A., Dorsey, J. G. and Dill, K. A. (1992) Temperature Dependence of Retention in Reversed-phase Liquid Chromatography. 2. Mobile-phase Considerations. *Anal. Chem.*, **64**, 1324–1327.

Cuatrecasas, P., Wilchek, M., Anfinsen, C. B. (1968) Selective enzyme purification by affinity chromatography. *Proc. Natl. Acad. Sci. USA*, **61**, 636–643.

Davis, K. H. and Hatefi, Y. (1972) Resolution and Reconstitution of Complex II (Succinate-Ubiquinone Reductase) by Salts. *Arch. Biochem. Biophys.*, **149**, 505–512.

Demiroglou, A., Bandel-Schlesselmann, C. and Jennissen, H. P. (1994) A Novel Reaction Sequence for the Coupling of Nucleophiles to Agarose with 2,2,2-Trifluoroethanesulfonyl Chloride. *Angew. Chem. Int. Ed. Engl.*, **33**, 120–123.

Demiroglou, A. and Jennissen, H. P. (1990) Synthesis and Protein-binding Properties of Spacer-free Thioalkyl Agaroses. *J. Chromatogr.*, **521**, 1–17.

Dill, K. A. (1990) The Meaning of Hydrophobicity. *Science*, **250**, 297–298.

Doellgast, G. J. and Fishmann, W. H. (1974) Purification of Human Placental Alkaline Phosphatase. *Biochem. J.*, **141**, 103–112.

el-Rassi, Z., De-Ocampo, L. F. and Bacolod, M. D. (1990) Binary and Ternary Salt Gradients in Hydrophobic-interaction Chromatography of Proteins. *J. Chromatogr.*, **499**, 141–152.

Elwing, H., Nilsson, B., Svensson, K.-E., Askendahl, A., Nilsson, U. R. and Lundström, I. (1988) *J. Colloid Interface Sci.*, **125**, 139–145.

Er-el, Z., Zaidenzaig, Y. and Shaltiel, S. (1972) Hydrocarbon-coated Sepharoses. Use in the Purification of Glycogen Phosphorylase. *Biochem. Biophys. Res. Commun.*, **49**, 383–390.

Eriksson, K.-O. (1989) Hydrophobic Interaction Chromatography. In: Janson, J. C. and Rydén, L. (eds) *Protein Purification: Principles, High Resolution Methods and Applications*, VHC Verlagsgesellschaft mbH, Weinheim, pp. 207–226.

Fausnaugh, J. L., Kennedy, L. A. and Regnier, F. E. (1984) Comparison of Hydrophobic-Interaction and Reversed-Phase Chromatography of Proteins. *J. Chromatogr.*, **317**, 141–155.

Geng, X., Guo, L. and Chang, J. (1990) Study of the Retention Mechanism of Proteins in Hydrophobic Interaction Chromatography. *J. Chromatogr.*, **507**, 1–23.

Halperin, G., Breitenbach, M., Tauber-Finkelstein, M. and Shaltiel, S. (1981) Hydrophobic Chromatography on Homologous Series of Alkylagaroses. A Comparison of Charged and Electrically Neutral Column Materials. *J. Chromatogr.*, **215**, 211–228.

Hamaguchi, K. and Geiduschek, E. P. (1962) The Effect of Electrolytes on the Stability of the Desoxyribonucleate Helix. *J. Amer. Chem. Soc.*, **84**, 1329–1338.

Hanstein, W. G. (1979) Chaotropic Ions and their Interactions with Proteins. *J. Solid-Phase Biochem.*, **4**, 189–206.

Hanstein, W. G., Davis, K. A. and Hatefi, Y. (1971) Water Structure and the Chaotropic Properties of Haloacetates1. *Arch. Biochem. Biophys.*, **147**, 534–544.

Hanstein, W. G., Davis, K. A. and Hatefi, Y. (1974) Solvent Isotope Effects on the Structure and Function of Mitochondrial Membranes in Aqueous Media. *Arch. Biochem. Biophys.*, **163**, 482–490.

Hatefi, Y. and Hanstein, W. G. (1969) Solubilization of Particulate Proteins and Nonelectolytes by Chaotropic Agents. *Biochemistry*, **62**, 1129–1136.

Hermanson, G. T. Mallia, A. K. and Smith, P. K. (1992) Activation Methods. In: *Immobilized Affinity Ligand Techniques*, Academic Press, New York, pp. 51–135.

Hjerten, S. (1973) Some General Aspects of Hydrophobic Interaction Chromatography. *J. Chromatogr.*, **87**, 325–331.

Hjerten, S. (1976) Hydrophobic Interaction Chromatography of Proteins on Neutral Adsorbents. *Methods of Protein Separation*, **2**, 233–243.

Hjerten, S. (1981) Hydrophobic Interaction Chromatography of Proteins, Nucleic Acids, Viruses, and Cells on Noncharged Amphiphilic Gels. *Methods Biochem. Analyses*, **27**, 89–108.

Hjerten, S., Rosengren, J. and Pahlman, S. (1974) Hydrophobic Interaction Chromatography – The Synthesis and the Use of Some Alkyl and Aryl Derivatives of Agarose. *J. Chromatogr.*, **101**, 281–288.

Hlady, V., Buijs, J. and Jennissen, H. P. (1999) Methods for Studying Protein Adsorption. *Methods Enzymol*, **309**, 402–429.

Hofmeister, F. (1887) 11. Zur Lehre von der Wirkung der Salze (Über Regelmässigkeiten in der eiweissfällenden Wirkung der Salze und ihre Beziehung zum physiologischen Verhalten derselben). *Arch. Exp. Pathol. Pharmakol.*, **24**, 247–260.

Hofmeister, F. (1888) 12. Zur Lehre von der Wirkung der Salze (Über die wasserentziehende Wirkung der Salze). *Arch. Exp. Pathol. Pharmakol.*, **25**, 1–30.

Hofstee, B. H. J. (1973a) A Hydrophobic Affinity Chromatography of Proteins. *Anal. Biochem.*, **52**, 430–448.

Hofstee, B. H. J. (1973b) Immobilization of Enzymes through Non-covalent Binding to Substituted Agaroses. *Biochem. Biophys. Res. Commun.*, **53**, 1137–1145.

Hofstee, B. H. J. (1973c) Protein Binding by Agarose Carrying Hydrophobic Groups in Conjunction with Charges. *Biochem. Biophys. Res. Commun.*, **50**, 751–757.

Hofstee, B. H. J. and Otillio, N. F. (1978) Non-ionic Adsorption Chromatography of Proteins. *J. Chromatogr.*, **159**, 57–69.

Howard, G. A. and Martin, A. J. P. (1950) The Separation of C12-C18 Fatty Acids by Reversed Phase Partition Chromatography. *Biochem. J.*, **46**, 532–538.

Hubert, P. and Dellacherie, E. (1993) Molecular Interactions in Hydrophobic Chromatography. In: Ngo, T. T. (ed.) *Molecular Interactions in Bioseparations*, Plenum Press, New York, pp. 333–359.

Ingraham, R. H., Lau, S. Z. M., Taneja, A. K. and Hodges, R. S. (1985) Denaturation and the Effects of Temperature on Hydrophobic-interaction and Reversed-phase High-performance Liquid Chromatography of Proteins – Bio Gel TSK-Phenyl-5PW Column. *J. Chromatogr.*, **327**, 77–92.

Israelachvili, J. N. (1985) *Intermolecular and Surface Forces.* Academic Press, London, New York, pp. 105, 207.

Israelachvili, J. N. and Pashley, R. M. (1984) Measurement of the Hydrophobic Interaction Between Two Hydrophobic Surfaces in Aqueous Electrolyte Solutions. *J. Colloid Interface Sci.*, 98, 500–514.

Jakubowski, H. and Pawelkiewicz, J. (1973) Chromatography of Plant Aminoacyl-tRNA Synthetases on ω-aminoalkyl Sepharose Columns. *FEBS Letters*, 34, 150–154.

Janado, M. and Nishada, T. (1981) Effect of Sugars on the Solubility of Hydrophobic Solutes in Water. *J. Solution Chem.*, 10, 489–500.

Jennissen, H. P. (1976a) Basic Properties of Hydrophobic Agaroses. *Protides Biol. Fluids Proc. Colloq.*, 23, 675–679.

Jennissen, H. P. (1976b) Evidence for Negative Cooperativity in the Adsorption of Phosphorylase b on Hydrophobic Agaroses. *Biochemistry*, 15, 5683–5692.

Jennissen, H. P. (1976c) Multivalent Adsorption of Proteins on Hydrophobic Agaroses. *Hoppe-Seyler's Z. Physiol. Chem.*, 357, 1201–1203.

Jennissen, H. P. (1978a) Multivalent Interaction Chromatography as Exemplified by the Adsorption and the Desorption of Skeletal Muscle Enzymes on Hydrophobic Alkyl-agaroses. *J. Chromatogr.*, 159, 71–83.

Jennissen, H. P. (1978b) Off-rates of Phosphorylase b Bound to Hydrophobic Agaroses. *Hoppe-Seyler's Z. Physiol. Chem.*, 359, 281–282.

Jennissen, H. P. (1979) Multivalent Adsorption Mechanisms in Hydrophobic Chromatography. *J. Solid-Phase Biochem.*, 4, 151–165.

Jennissen, H. P. (1981) Immobilization of Residues on Agarose Gels: Effects on Protein Adsorption Isotherms and Chromatographic Parameters. *J. Chromatogr.*, 215, 73–85.

Jennissen, H. P. (1985) Protein Adsorption Hysteresis. In: *Surface and Interfacial Aspects of Biomedical Polymers vol. 2, Protein Adsorption*, pp. 295–320.

Jennissen, H. P. (1986) Protein Binding to Two-dimensional Hydrophobic Binding-site Lattices: Sorption Kinetics of Phosphorylase b on Immobilized Butyl residues. *J. Colloid Interface Sci.*, 111, 570–586.

Jennissen, H. P. (1988) General Aspects of Protein Adsorption. *Makromol. Chem., Macromol. Symp.*, 17, 111–134.

Jennissen, H. P. (1995) Cyanogen Bromide and Tresyl Chloride Chemistry Revisited: The Special Reactivity of Agarose as a Chromatographic and Biomaterial Support for Immobilizing Novel Chemical Groups. *J. Mol. Recogn.*, 8, 116–124.

Jennissen, H. P. (2000) Hydrophobic Interaction Chromatography: The Critical Hydrophobicity Approach. *Int. J. Bio-Chromatography*, 5, 131–163.

Jennissen, H. P. (2001) Ultra-hydrophilic Metallic Biomaterials. *Biomaterial*, 2, 45–53.

Jennissen, H. P. and Botzet, G. (1979) Protein Binding to Two-dimensional Hydrophobic Binding-site Lattices: Adsorption Hysteresis on Immobilized Butyl-residues. *Int. J. Biol. Macromol.*, 1, 171–179.

Jennissen, H. P. and Botzet, G. (1993) The Binding of Phosphorylase Kinase to Immobilized Calmodulin. *J. Mol. Recogn.*, 6, 117–130.

Jennissen, H. P., and Demiroglou, A. (1994). Verfahren zur Gewinnung von molekular einheitlichem, nativem, biologisch vollaktivem Fibrinogen aus Blut. *Ger. Offen. DE P 42 40 119 A1*, pp. 1–6, German Patent Office, Munich.

Jennissen, H. P., Demiroglou, A., and Logemann, E. (1982). Studies on the Mechanism of Protein Adsorption on Hydrophobic Agaroses. In: Gribnau, T. C. J., Visser, J. and Nivard, R. J. F. (eds) *Affinity Chromatography and Related Techniques, Analytical Chemistry Symposia Series*, vol. 9, pp. 39–49.

Jennissen, H. P. and Demirolgou, A. (1992) Base-atom Recognition in Protein Adsorption to Alkyl Agaroses. *J. Chromatogr.*, 597, 93–100.

Jennissen, H. P. and Heilmeyer-Jr, L. M. G. (1975) General Aspects of Hydrophobic Chromatography. Adsorption and Elution Characteristics of Some Skeletal Muscle Enzymes. *Biochemistry*, 14, 754–760.

Jost, R., Miron, T. and Wilchek, M. (1974) The Mode of Adsorption of Proteins to Aliphatic and Aromatic Amines Coupled to Cyanogen Bromide-activated Agarose. *Biochim. Biophys. Acta*, 362, 75–82.

Joustra, M. and Axen, R. (1976) Stability of the Binding Groups Generated by CNBr activation of Agarose. *Protides Biol. Fluids Proc. Colloq.*, 23, 525–529.

Kauzmann, W. (1959) Some Factors in the Interpretation of Protein Denaturation. *Adv. Protein Chem.*, 14, 1–63.

Kohn, J. and Wilchek, M. (1981) Procedures for the Analysis of Cyanogen Bromide-activated Sepharose or Sephadex by Quantitative Determination of Cyanate Esters and Imidocarbonates. *Anal. Biochem.*, 115, 375–382.

Lewin, S. (1974) *Displacement of Water and its Control of Biochemical Reactions*, Academic Press, New York, pp. 85, 91, 260.

Liautard, J. P. (1992) Behavior of Large Nucleic Acids in Reversed-phase High Performance Liquid Chromatography. *J. Chromatogr.*, 584, 135–139.

Mardsen, N. V. B. (1977) Similarity Between Nonionic Micelle Formation and Nonpolar Adsorption to Sephadex G-15. *Naturwissenschaften*, 64, 148–149.

Melander, W. and Horvath, C. (1977) Salt Effects on Hydrophobic Interactions in Precipitation and Chromatography of Proteins: An interpretation of the Lyotropic Series. *Arch. Biochem. Biophys.*, 183, 200–215.

Melander, W. R., Corradini, D. and Horvarth, C. (1984) Salt-mediated Retention of Proteins in Hydrophobic Interaction Chromatography – Application of Solvophobic Theory. *J. Chromatogr.*, 317, 67–85.

Memoli, V. A. and Doellgast, G. J. (1975) Heamoglobin and Serum Albumin: Salt-mediated Hydrophobic Chromatography. *Biochem. Biophys. Res. Commun.*, 66, 1011–1016.

Mevarech, M., Leicht, W. and Werber, M. M. (1976) Hydrophobic Chromatography and Fractionation of Enzymes from Extremely Halophilic Bacteria Using Decreasing Concentration Gradients of Ammonium Sulfate. *Biochemistry*, 15, 2383–2386.

Mohr, P., and Pommerening, K. (1986) Hydrophobic Interaction Chromatography. In: Mohr, P. and Pommerening, K. (eds) *Affinity Chromatography, Chromatographic Science Series*, vol. 33, Marcel Dekker Inc., New York, Basel, pp. 225–241.

Morris, C. (1978) Fractionation of Transfer Ribonucleic Acids by Chromatography on Neutral Polysaccharide Media in Reverse Salt Gradients. *J. Chromatogr.*, 159, 33–46.

Ochoa, J. L. (1978) Hydrophobic (Interaction) Chromatography. *Biochimie.*, 60, 1–15.

Oscarsson, S. (1997) Factors Effecting Protein Interaction at Sorbent Interfaces. *J. Chromatogr. B.*, 699, 117-131.

Oscarsson, S., Angulo-Tatis, D., Chaga, G. and Porath, J. (1995) Amphiphilic Agarose/Based Adsorbents for Chromatography. Comparative Study of Adsorption Capacities and Desorption Efficiencies. *J. Chromatogr. A.*, 689, 3–12.

Pahlman, S., Rosengren, J. and Hjerten, S. (1977) Hydrophobic Interaction Chromatography on Uncharged Sepharose Derivatives. *J. Chromatogr.*, 131, 99–108.

Pearson, J. D., Lin, N. T. and Regnier, F. E. (1982) The Importance of Silica Type for Reverse-phase Protein Separations. *Anal. Biochem.*, 124, 217–230.

Pharmacia Fine Chemicals (1979) Affinity Chromatography (Principles and Methods), pp. 12–18, Ljungföretagen AB, Örebro.

Porath, J. (1962) Zone Precipitation. *Nature*, 196, 47–48.

Porath, J. (1978) Explorations into the Field of Charge-transfer Adsorption. *J. Chromatogr.*, 159, 13–24.

Porath, J. (1989) Electron-Donor-Acceptor Chromatography (EDAC) for Biomolecules in Aqueous Solutions. In: Hutchens, T. W., (ed.) *Protein Recognition of Immobilized Ligands' UCLA Symposia on Mol. & Cell. Biology*, New Series, vol. 80, Alan R. Liss, Inc. New York, pp. 101–122.

Porath, J., Axen, R. and Ernback, S. (1967) Chemical Coupling of Proteins to Agarose. *Nature*, 215, 1491–1492.

Porath, J., Sundberg, L., Fornstedt, N. and Olsson, I. (1973) Salting-out in Amphiphilic Gels as a New Approach to Hydrophobic Adsorption. *Nature*, 245, 465–466.

Raibaud, O., Hoegberg-Raibaud, A. and Goldberg, M. E. (1975) Purification of *E. coli* Enzymes by Chromatography on Amphiphilic Gels. *FEBS Lett.*, 50, 130–134.

Raymond, J., Ayanya, J. L. and Fotso, M. (1981) Hydrophobic Interaction Chromatography: A New Method for Sunflower Protein Fractionation. *J. Chromatogr.*, 212, 199–209.

Rimerman, R. A. and Hatfield, G. W. (1973) Phosphate-induced Protein Chromatography. *Science*, 182, 1268–1270.

Rosengren, J., Pahlman, S., Glad, M. and Hjerten, S. (1975) Hydrophobic Interaction Chromatography on Noncharged Sepharose Derivatives. Binding of a Model Protein, Related to Ionic Strength, Hydrophobicity of Substituent, and Degree of Substitution (Determined by NMR). *Biochim. Biophys. Acta*, 412, 52–61.

Sawatzki, G., Anselstetter, V. and Kubanek, B. (1981) Isolation of Mouse Transferrin Using Salting-out Chromatography. *Biochim. Biophys. Acta*, 667, 132–138.

Shaltiel, S. (1974) Hydrophobic Chromatography. *Methods Enzymol.*, 34, 126–140.

Shaltiel, S. (1978) Hydrophobic Chromatography. In: Epton, R. (ed.) *Chromatography of Synthetic and Biological Polymers*, vol. 2, Ellis Horwood Ltd., Chichester, pp. 13–41.

Shaltiel, S. (1984) Hydrophobic Chromatography. *Methods Enzymol*, 104, 69–96.

Steers-Jr, E., Cuatrecasas, P. and Pollard, H. B. (1971) The Purification of beta-Galactosidase from *Escherichia Coli* by Affinity Chromatography. *J. Biol. Chem.*, 246, 196–200.

Szepesy, L. and Horvath, C. (1988) Specific Salt Effects in Hydrophobic Interaction Chromatography of Proteins. *Chromatographia*, 26, 13–18.

Tanford, C. (1973) *The Hydrophobic Effect: Formation of Micelles and Biological Membranes.* John Wiley & Sons, New York.

Tiselius, (1948) Adsorption Separation by Salting Out. *Arkiv. foer. Kemi., Mineralogi. och. Geologi.*, 26B, 1–5.

Von der Haar, F. (1976) Purification of Proteins by Fractional Interfacial, Salting Out on Unsubstituted Agarose Gels. *Biochem. Biophys. Res. Commun.*, 70, 1009–1013.

Von der Haar, F. (1979) Purification of Proteins by Reversible Salting Out on Unsubstituted Agarose Gels: General Methodology and Use of Variables. *J. Solid-Phase Biochem.*, 4, 207–220.

Wilchek, M. Miron, T. and Kohn, J. (1984) Affinity Chromatography. *Methods Enzymol* 104, 3–55.

Wu, S. L., Figueroa, A. and Karger, B. (1986) Protein Conformational Effects in Hydrophobic Interaction Chromatography. *J. Chromatogr.*, 371, 3–27.

Yon, R. J. (1972) Chromatography of Lipophilic Proteins on Adsorbents Containing Mixed Hydrophobic and Ionic Groups. *Biochem. J.*, 126, 765–767.

Yon, R. J. (1977) Recent Developments in Protein Chromatography Involving Hydrophobic Interactions. *Int. J. Biochem.*, 9, 373–379.

Zumbrink, T., Demiroglou, A. and Jennissen, H. P. (1995) Analysis of Affinity Supports by ^{13}C-CP/MAS-NMR Spectroscopy: Application to Carbonyldiimidazole- and Novel Tresyl Chloride-Synthesized Agarose and Silica Gels. *J. Mol. Recogn.*, 8, 363–373.

Chapter 5

Conformational behaviour of polypeptides and proteins in reversed phase and lipophilic environments

Milton T. W. Hearn

Introduction

With the development of high resolution biochromatography, reversed-phase high-performance liquid chromatography (RP-HPLC) has found wide analytical and laboratory scale preparative application in peptide and protein chemistry. The success of RP-HPLC procedures with porous *n*-alkylsilicas for the process scale purification of synthetic organic compounds and other substances of pharmaceutical interest, has been similarly matched over the past decade in the process manufacture of peptides and small polypeptides with molecular weights up to 7 000. Generally this success has not, however, been replicated with larger polypeptides (MW > 10 000) and globular proteins, although numerous examples of the isolation of functional proteins at the micro- and ultramicro-preparative level by RP-HPLC procedures can be found in the scientific literature (Hearn, 1998a; Aguilar *et al.*, 1996). Practitioners have often been discouraged from using RP-HPLC methods for the large scale purification of proteins because of their concerns about the combined influences of the acidic elution conditions that traditionally have been used with RP-HPLC procedures and the hydrophobicity *per se* of the *n*-alkylsilica sorbents. In this context, under the influence of the perturbing low pH aquo-organic solvent conditions used during the RP-HPLC separation process, *n*-alkyl ligand- or solvent-induced unfolding processes have frequently been implicated on an anecdotal basis of the loss of biological activity or the formation of multiple peak zones with samples of high compositional purity, as well as for the reduction in mass yields with proteins. Whilst these features may detract from the use of RP-HPLC as the technique of choice in large scale preparative purification protocols with proteins, these same characteristics provide a unique opportunity to study the folding/unfolding processes and conformational stability of polypeptides and proteins in aquo-organic solvents and hydrophobic environments. As a consequence, RP-HPLC can not only be used as a versatile separation technique *par excellence* for the high resolution separation and quantitation of complex mixtures of peptides and proteins, but this powerful separation method also can be employed to provide insight into the hierarchal structural features of these biosolutes. In particular, the interactive behaviour of polypeptides and proteins in hydrophobic environments associated with reversed phase chromatographic (RPC) procedures provides an opportunity to examine the conformational properties and other secondary equilibria, which these biomolecules undergo at non-polar liquid–solid interfaces.

In this chapter, different aspects of this solute–ligand interaction have been examined from the points of view of the influence of the contribution of amino acid sequence of the bioanalyte, and the nature of the changes in the secondary and tertiary structures of polypeptides and small globular proteins that occur in response to variations in the controlling chromatographic parameters. The co-utilisation of RP-HPLC procedures with different spectroscopic tools (Round *et al.*, 1994; Hearn, 1998a; Higgins *et al.*, 1997; Chao *et al.*, 1998), such as differential scanning UV/VIS spectroscopy, derivative UV or intrinsic fluorescence spectroscopy, diode array (DAD) spectroscopy with/without peak tracking algorithmic routines, circular dichroism (CD) spectroscopy and solid state ^{1}H/^{13}C nuclear magnetic resonance (solid state NMR) spectroscopy provide additional dimensions which enable the study of the role of immobilised non-polar *n*-alkyl ligands under solvated conditions to be explored. Accordingly, in this chapter specific polypeptide examples have been used to illustrate a range of case studies, whereby the selective use has been employed of amino acid replacements or deletions, or the use of single or multiple L-α- $\rightarrow$ D-α-substitutions to unravel the physicochemical basis of the changes in the α-helical or β-sheet conformational propensity of polypeptides and their synthetic analogues or homologues in different solvent and non-polar sorbent environments. Similar extension of these RP-HPLC procedures to evaluate the ligand-induced stabilisation of coiled-coil (Lau *et al.*, 1984; Hodges *et al.*, 1988; Zhou *et al.*, 1990) and amphipathic α-helical peptides (Aguilar *et al.*, 1985, 1986; Blondelle *et al.*, 1992; Purcell *et al.*, 1993, 1995; Krause *et al.*, 1995; Lazoura *et al.*, 1997) has also been examined as well as the behaviour of several globular proteins in similar RPC milieus. Although various reports in the scientific literature exists about the aberrant behaviour of globular, membrane and fibrous proteins in RP-HPLC systems, compared to studies with peptides, much less detailed, systematic work has, however, been described on the conformational behaviour of these higher molecular weight biosolutes in non-polar chromatographic sorbents with aquo-organic solvent environments. As a consequence, the physicochemical basis of the solvent- and/or ligand-induced denaturation noted with growth hormone (Hearn *et al.*, 1988; Oroszlan *et al.*, 1992), cytochrome C (Richards *et al.*, 1994a,b), lysozyme (Lu *et al.*, 1986), ribonuclease A (Cohen *et al.*, 1985), α- and β-lactalbumin (Benedek, 1988; Grinberg *et al.*, 1989; Oroszlan, 1990), trypsin (Hearn *et al.*, 1985) and soybean trypsin inhibitor (Cohen *et al.*, 1984) has yet to be fully enunciated at a detailed molecular or atomic level. This incomplete knowledge, in part, has arisen because most earlier studies have typically examined the retention and peak shape behaviour of biosolutes at only a single temperature. Determination of the combined effects of temperature and the column residency time (Hearn, 1983; Hearn *et al.*, 1985; Hearn, 1998a) on the chromatographic properties of proteins under different isocratic and gradient elution RP-HPLC conditions thus remains an important challenge, yet to be finalised, in protein biophysics.

Facilitating these practical developments has been the emergence of several sophisticated empirical, extra-thermodynamic or thermodynamic treatments. These descriptive models permit changes in retention time or peakwidth observed when polypeptides or proteins undergo secondary or tertiary structural changes to be theoretically elaborated. Over the past decade, several models, in particular, of considerable utilitarian advantage have been developed to describe the interaction between peptidic or protein solutes and the hydrocarbonaceous stationary-phase ligands in RP-HPLC (Horvath *et al.*, 1976; Snyder, 1980; Hearn, 1983; Hearn and Aguilar, 1988; Aguilar and Hearn,

1991; Hearn, 1998a). These theoretical models provide a framework for selecting appropriate chromatographic parameters to achieve enhanced resolution, as well as to aid the interpretation of the retention process *per se*.

Increasingly, the same theoretical approaches have been found appropriate to facilitate the characterisation of conformational changes which polypeptides and proteins can undergo under different experimental conditions. It is now known (Hearn, 1983; Cohen *et al.*, 1984, 1985; Aguilar *et al.*, 1985, 1986; Hearn *et al.*, 1985, 1986; Lu *et al.*, 1986; Benedek, 1988; Hearn and Aguilar, 1988; Grinberg *et al.*, 1989; Oroszlan *et al.*, 1990; Aguilar and Hearn, 1991; Oroszlan *et al.*, 1992; Purcell *et al.*, 1993; Richards *et al.*, 1994a; Round *et al.*, 1994; Krause *et al.*, 1995; Lazoura *et al.*, 1997; Hearn, 1998a) that marked variations in logarithmic capacity factor, log k, as a function of temperature (T) can be used to monitor secondary equilibrium processes with low molecular weight compounds and analogous approaches can be used to asses the conformational changes of polypeptides or proteins during the RP-HPLC chromatographic process. Consequently, analysis of the corresponding van't Hoff plot data provides (Hearn, 1983; Hearn and Aguilar, 1988; Aguilar and Hearn, 1991; Purcell, 1992; Vailaya and Horvath, 1996a,b; Hearn, 1998a) an approach to evaluate the relative flexibility and extent of solvation of these biosolute in the adsorbed and the free states as revealed from the respective changes in the entropic and enthalpic contributions to the Gibbs free energy of association and interconversion for the chromatographic interaction process.

Because of their structural complexity and size, as well as the nature of the dependency of the capacity factor k on the elutropic strength ε_m of the mobile phase, polypeptide and polypeptide separations and associated chromatographic measurements with RP-HPLC procedures have been conventionally conducted under gradient rather than isocratic elution conditions. Under gradient elution conditions, a complication is however introduced in biophysical interpretation of the experimental data due to the fact that the interaction between the polypeptide or protein and the hydrocarbonaceous ligand in the presence of aquo-organic solvent eluents is not being measured under strictly thermodynamic near-equilibrium binding conditions. Recent scientific literature (Vailaya and Horvath, 1996a,b; Boysen *et al.*, 1999, 2002; Hearn and Zhao, 1999; Purcell *et al.*, 1999; Zhao *et al.*, 1999) has provided a variety of supporting data that the relationships between the retention parameters reflecting changes in the hydrophobic contact area and the affinity of interaction of polypeptides and proteins with n-alkylsilica and other types of lipid-like sorbents may not follow linear free energy (LFERs) relationships in such dynamic (bio)solute-ligand interactive systems. The most obvious of these divergencies from ideal LFER behaviour is the well known (Hearn, 1983; Guo *et al.*, 1986; Parket *et al.*, 1986; Aguilar and Hearn, 1991; Rothemund *et al.*, 1995; Hearn, 1998a) loss of correlation between the observed and predicted retention times of polypeptides as the size of the amino acid sequence increases.

These differences become particularly manifest with polypeptides and proteins as significant changes in the nature of the secondary structural transitions associated with variations in the magnitude of the hydrophobic binding domain(s) and the interaction affinity constant(s) of these biosolutes over the temperature range between 4°C and 65°C when experiments are carried out under isocratic rather than gradient elution conditions. With this latter caveat in mind, when operated under gradient conditions RP-HPLC procedures can nevertheless offer a valuable adjunct to other experimental methods in investigations into the nature of the induction of stabilised secondary structures of polypeptides. However, to precisely follow the conformational transitions that polypeptides undergo upon their interaction with solvated hydrophobic surfaces isocratic conditions must be employed. Analogous isocratic and gradient elution procedures can also be used to evaluate the relative conformational stability of α-helical coil or coil-coil polypeptides, β-sheet polypeptides as well as globular proteins. In order for these process to be qualitatively and quantitatively assessed, the need thus arises to determine the retention and zone broadening dependencies of polypeptides and proteins under different RP-HPLC operating conditions and to relate these observation to a corresponding theoretical structure-retention relationship framework.

Retention relationships

The retention time, usually expressed in the isocratic elution mode as the dimensionless capacity factor, k, or in the case of the linear gradient elution mode as the dimensionless median capacity factor, $\bar{k}$, can be related to the change in Gibbs free energy ($\Delta\,G^0_{assoc}$)for the association of the polypeptide or protein with the non-polar ligands (and hence to the affinity of the interaction) as well as to the interactive hydrophobic surface area (ΔA_h) of the polypeptide or protein in contact with the ligand surface for a defined elution condition and temperature. In the linear gradient elution mode, the mathematical treatment known as the linear solvent strength (LSS) model has been found (Snyder, 1980; Hearn, 1983; Stadailus et al., 1984; Hearn and Aguilar, 1988; Purcell et al., 1989; Aguilar and Hearn, 1991; Purcell et al., 1993; Hearn, 1998a) to be useful for the selection of optimal elution conditions in terms of the gradient slope and duration and can be used to provide useful information about the physico-chemical and molecular properties of these biosolutes (Hearn, 1983; Melander et al., 1984; Hearn and Aguilar, 1988; Purcell et al., 1989; Aguilar and Hearn, 1991; Purcell et al., 1993, 1995; Lazoura et al., 1997; Purcell et al., 1999). The experimental derivation of k or $\bar{k}$ thus represents the starting point for all biophysical investigations which are intended to explore the consequences of conformational changes with polypeptides and proteins in RP-HPLC systems. The manner that k or $\bar{k}$ can be varied in response to adjustments in the experimental conditions, such as the isocratic or median gradient mole fraction of organic solvent modifier, ψ or $\bar{\psi}$, or the temperature, then provides essential data which can be used to evaluate the physico-chemical basis of these conformational events.

Dependence of $\log k$ on ψ and $\log \bar{k}$ on $\bar{\psi}$

Amphipathic α-helical and β-sheet structures are known to play important roles in many surface mediated biorecognition phenomena involving polypeptides and proteins. As noted above, over the past few years, RP-HPLC has emerged as a particularly powerful technique to study the influence of very subtle differences in the secondary structure of amphipathic polypeptide upon interaction with hydrophobic ligands (Aguilar et al., 1985; Hodges et al., 1988; Zhou et al., 1990; Blondelle et al., 1992; Aguilar et al., 1993; Purcell et al., 1993; Mant et al., 1993; Hodges et al., 1994; Blondelle et al., 1995; Krause et al., 1995; Purcell et al., 1995; Rothemund et al., 1995; Lazoura et al., 1997; Boysen et al., 1999, 2002; Chao et al., 1998; Hearn and Zhao, 1999; Purcell et al., 1999; Zhao et al., 1999), as well as to characterise the folding/unfolding transitions of proteins at hydrophobic surfaces (Cohen *et al.*, 1984, 1985; Hearn *et al.*, 1985; Lu *et al.*, 1986; Benedek, 1988; Hodges *et al.*, 1988; Grinberg *et al.*, 1989; Oroszlan *et al.*, 1990, 1992; Richards *et al.*, 1994a,b; Boysen *et al.*, 1999, 2002; Purcell *et al.*, 1999). This valuable feature of RP-HPLC methods complements the powerful, and widely exploited ability of the technique to resolve peptides/polypeptides differing in terms of their primary structure, diastereomeric characteristics or amino acid composition.

A variety of experimental conditions and approaches have been employed to affect changes in the reversed phase retention behaviour of amphipathic peptide/polypeptides and globular proteins, with the near-equilibrium isocratic retention model or the linear solvent strength (LSS) gradient retention model frequently employed to help the interpretation of the experimental data, and to provide information associated with the interactive properties of the polypeptide and protein solutes when isocratic and linear gradient elution conditions are used. For convenience, the dependency between the logarithm of the capacity factor, k, and the mole fraction of the organic solvent modifier, ψ, is frequently represented for isocratic data as a linear relationship. Analogous relationships can be employed to accommodate gradient retention data such that the plots of the logarithm of the median capacity factor, $\log \bar{k}$, vs the median mole fraction of organic solvent, $\bar{\psi}$, required to desorb the polypeptide or globular protein from the immobilised hydrophobic n-alkyl ligands are assumed to also follow linear dependencies. The form of the theoretical expressions governing elution relationships have thus been often represented for an isocratic elution system as:

$$\log k' = \log k_0 - S\psi \tag{1}$$

and for the corresponding linear gradient elution system as:

$$\log \bar{k} = \log k_0 - S\bar{\psi} \tag{2}$$

where, S is the slope and $\log k_0$ the Y-intercept at $\psi = 0$ or $\bar{\psi} = 0$ respectively. The parameter S is believed (Horvath *et al.*, 1976; Snyder, 1980; Hearn, 1983; Hearn and Aguilar, 1988; Aguilar and Hearn, 1991) to be related to the magnitude of the contact surface area, ΔA_h established between the solute and the hydrocarbonaceous ligand in RP-HPLC, whilst $\log k_0$ represents the affinity of the solute for the stationary surface under a defined set of mobile phase condition, such as 20% aqueous acetonitrile containing 0.1% trifluoroacetic acid (TFA).

Compared to simple organic compounds, the S and $\log k_0$ values of a polypeptide or protein at a defined temperature and solvent composition in a RP-HPLC system are relatively large (Grego and Hearn, 1978; Hearn, 1983; Cohen *et al.*, 1984; Hearn *et al.*, 1985; Hearn and Aguilar, 1986, 1988; Aguilar and Hearn, 1991; Richards *et al.*, 1994a,b; Hearn 1998a). This property has been attributed to multi-site interactions between the biosolute and the non-polar solvated ligand, which are a common feature of the retention behaviour of most polypeptides or proteins with n-alkylsilica sorbents. Determination of the resolution, R_S, of a polypeptide or protein pair, P_1 and P_2, in a RP-HPLC system with capacity factors given by k_1 and k_2 respectively, can be achieved from Equation 3, as follows:

$$R_S = \left[\frac{1}{4}\right]\left[\frac{k'_2}{k'_1}\right]\sqrt{N}\left[\frac{k'_1}{1 + k'_1}\right] \tag{3}$$

where N is the separation efficiency, and the ratio of the capacity factors (k_2/k_1) represents the selectivity, α, of the particular RP-HPLC system such that

$$\log \alpha = \log \frac{k'_2}{k'_1} = \log \frac{k'_{0,2}}{k'_{0,1}} - \psi(S_2 - S_1) \tag{4}$$

As a consequence of the dependency of k, and hence α, on the Gibbs free energy for the interaction, ΔG^0_{assoc} (see Equation 10), it is possible to inter-relate the retention behaviour of a defined set of polypeptides to the associated qualitative linear free energy relationships (QLFERs). When no secondary equilibria occur, for example when no conformational equilibria are manifested, this inter-dependency takes the form of conventional structure-selectivity maps (SSMs), which can be described in terms of logarithmic selectivity increments ($\log \alpha_{srr}$s) using control substance, such as polyglycine, as the base point for the comparison and the set of polypeptides or proteins under examination, i.e. from equations of the form

$$\log \alpha_{srr} = \tau_{srr} = f(K_{srr}) \tag{5}$$

where K_{srr} is a summated structure-retention free energy parameter which characterises the differences between two polypeptides or proteins under investigation. Such approaches have been used to compare, for example, the retention behaviour of different species variants of cytochrome C (Richards et al., 1994a) and myoglobin (Purcell et al., 1999) under different RP-HPLC conditions with n-alkyl sorbents of different chain lengths. For smaller polypeptides, advantage can be taken of the relationship implicit to Equations 4 and 5 through the use (Guo et al., 1986; Parker et al., 1986; Houghten and DeGraw, 1987; Mant and Hodges, 1991; Wilce et al., 1991, 1992, 1995) of the so-called amino acid group retention coefficients (GRCs) (or the corresponding fragmental hydrophobicity parameters hydr of the individual amino acid residues which constitute the primary structure), allowing the retention times of the polypeptides to be predicted with reasonable accuracy under a defined set of RP-HPLC chromatographic conditions. When the objective is to compare the 'native' state to an 'unfolded' state of the same polypeptide, the same approach can be employed to follow transitions in retention behaviour, but in this situation the governing dependency can be represented by

$$\log \alpha_{conf} = \tau_{conf} = f(K_{conf}) \tag{6}$$

where α_{conf} represents the relative selectivity between the 'native' and the 'unfolded' state, whilst K_{conf} represents a summated structure-conformation free energy parameter which characterises the particular conformational change that the polypeptide or protein under examination has undergone in the RP-HPLC environment.

In light of the inter-relationships which have been foreshadowed by Equations 1, 4 and 6, it is thus not surprising that empirical relationships linking the magnitude of the S-value and the molecular weight (MW) or alternatively to the accessible surface area (ΔA_{total}), as measured with water as the probe (Connolly, 1983) or the accessible hydrophobic surface area (Richards, 1977; Rose et al., 1985; Makhatadze et al., 1990; Aguilar et al., 1994) (ΔA_{hsa}) of a polypeptide or protein. Although several procedures for the evaluation of the accessible hydrophobic surface area, ΔA_{hsa}, can be employed, the most commonly used method involves adaptation of the Rose-Privalov calculations.

As a consequence, these empirical relationships linking S and ΔA_{hsa} are typically represented in the form (Snyder, 1980; Hearn, 1983; Hearn and Aguilar, 1988; Aguilar and Hearn, 1991; Richards *et al.*, 1994b; Purcell, 1995; Hearn, 1998a) of

$$S = a(\text{MW})^b = a(\Delta A_{\text{total}})^b = a(\Delta A_{\text{hsa}})^b \tag{7}$$

where a, a, a, b, b and b are coefficient which vary according to the properties of the polypeptide or protein as well as the chromatographic conditions.

Solvophobic theory has been used to derive a relationship between $\log k$ (or $\log \bar{k}$) and a number of physicochemical properties (Horvath, 1976; Grego and Hearn, 1978; Snyder, 1980; Hearn and Grego, 1981; Melander *et al.*, 1984; Purcell *et al.*, 1992; Aguilar *et al.*, 1993; Vailaya and Horvath, 1996a,b; Boysen *et al.*, 1999, 2002; Hearn, 1998a; Hearn and Zhao, 1999; Purcell *et al.*, 1999; Zhao *et al.*, 1999) as follows:

$$\log k' = \log k_0 - (N\Delta A_h + 4.836\, N^{1/3}(k^e - 1)V^{2/3})/RT \tag{8}$$

where A_h is the relative hydrophobic contact area, N is Avogadro's number, V is the mean molar volume of the solvent, R is the gas constant, T is the absolute temperature (in K) and e is the ratio of the energy required for the formation of a cavity with the surface area equal to the solute surface area and the energy required to extend the planar surface of the liquid by the same area. Rearrangement of Equations 1 and 8 yields the following relationship between S and the solvophobic parameters for a defined temperature and range of ψ or $\bar{\psi}$:

$$S = a\Delta A_h + b\kappa^e - c \tag{9}$$

where a, b and c are constants defined by the particular RP-HPLC system for a specified polypeptide or protein. The implication of this Equation 9 is that the S value can thus be indirectly related to the interactive hydrophobic contact area (ΔA_h,) as derived from the solvophobic theory, whilst the $\log k_0$ value can be related to the affinity of interaction of the biosolute for the non-polar ligands. The values of ΔA_h and the corresponding ΔA_{total} or ΔA_{hsa} values for a polypeptide or protein may be the same or different depending on whether additional changes in the secondary structure are induced on adsorption of the biosolute to the non-polar stationary phase compared to the secondary and tertiary structural changes that occur in the bulk mobile phase. Consequently, ΔA_h often exhibits a fractional relationship to ΔA_{total} (or ΔA_{hsa}) with $\Delta A_h/\Delta A_{\text{total}}$ 1. Since the magnitudes of ΔA_{total} and ΔA_h are expected to be dependent on temperature, the codicil arises that the S-value should also be temperature dependent. The S-value should thus satisfy an extra-thermodynamic relationship defined by the derivative $(S/T)_{jj+1}$ where j and $j + 1$ represent two different states of the polypeptide or protein. Changes in the magnitude of the S and $\log k_0$ parameters as a function of temperature therefore represent important probes for the change in the secondary structure of polypeptides or proteins that arise during their interaction with hydrophobic surfaces of RP-HPLC sorbents.

Although first order dependencies of the kind represented as Equations 1–8 provide useful approximations of the influence of ψ or $\bar{\psi}$ on $\log k$ or $\log \bar{k}$, it is worth recalling that over the complete range of mole fractions of the organic solvent modifier from

0 ψ 1.0, much more complex bimodal solvophobic-silanophilic retention dependencies (Horvath *et al.*, 1976; Schoenmakers *et al.*, 1979; Bij *et al.*, 1981; Hearn and Grego, 1981; Hearn, 1993, 1998a) occur with *n*-alkylsilica sorbents in RP-HPLC and analogous bimodal dependencies are evident with polymer-based reversed phase sorbents as well. Figure 5.1 illustrates the characteristics of this bimodal dependency with polypeptides and proteins, whereby the log k values show a curvilinear dependency with decreasing values over a defined ψ-range (typically up to 60% acetonitrile with most *n*-alkylsilicas) but which manifest increasing values at higher ψ-ranges. As has been extensively documented (Grego and Hearn, 1978; Schoenmakers *et al.*, 1979; Bij *et al.*, 1981; Hearn and Grego, 1981a,b; Hearn, 1983; Hearn and Aguilar, 1988; Hearn, 1998a; Aguilar and Hearn, 1991; Hearn and Zhao, 1999; Zhao *et al.*, 1999) the shape and position of these bimodal dependencies of log k on ψ are determined by the solvational properties of the organic solvent modifier. Hydrogen donor solvents thus exhibit different log k vs ψ dependencies to those found for solvents with hydrogen acceptor characteristics. When linear gradient elution conditions are employed with such solvent systems, it is thus not surprising that some of the biophysical information on the characteristics of the log k vs ψ dependencies are averaged as the corresponding log $\bar{k}$ vs $\bar{\psi}$ plots, which can take on a more linear appearance. For this reason, it is desirable for the chromatographic measurements to be carried out under isocratic conditions. Although this may not always initially appear feasible due to the physical or chemical properties of the polypeptide or protein, recent studies (Boysen and Hearn *et al.*, 2001a; Hearn and Zhao, 1999) with a range of wild-type and recombinant proteins, including the transcription factors *fos* and *jun*, have indicated that in practice a window of suitable isocratic elution conditions can be selected which allow these measurement to be made. In practice, this window of isocratic conditions can be achieved by utilising the derived gradient elution $\bar{\psi}$ values as a 'spotter' values around which the range of isocratic ψ-values are then selected.

Dependence of log k and log $\bar{k}$ on temperature at fixed values of ψ or $\bar{\psi}$

Temperature plays a profound effect on the retention and peak width behaviour of polypeptides and proteins in all chromatographic systems. Because of the nature of the hydrophobic effect, the influence of temperature is particularly noticeable in RP-HPLC with these biomolecules. The relationship of the capacity factor, as log k (or log $\bar{k}$), on temperature (T) for a chromatographic system of phase ratio, Φ, can be expressed through its dependency on the standard free energy change, ΔG^0_{assoc}, namely

$$\log k = -\Delta G^0_{assoc}/RT + \log \qquad (10)$$

and

$$\Delta G^0_{assoc} = \Delta H^0_{assoc} - T\Delta S^0_{assoc} \qquad (11)$$

For a thermodynamically favourable retention process, the values of ΔG^0_{assoc} for different polypeptide and protein solutes are anticipated to be negative.

According to the van't Hoff equation

$$\log k' = -\frac{\Delta H^0_{assoc}}{RT} + \frac{\Delta S^0_{assoc}}{R} + \log \Phi \qquad (12)$$

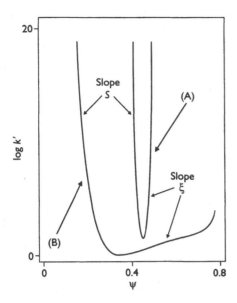

Figure 5.1 Schematic representation of the retention dependencies of polypeptides and proteins chromatographed on a reversed phase sorbent exhibiting solvophobic (hydrophobic adsorption) and lipophobic (polar adsorption) characteristics. The figure illustrates two case histories (A and B) for the dependency of the isocratic logarithmic capacity factor $\log k'$ vs the mole fraction of the organic solvent modifier, ψ, (or the linear gradient logarithmic median capacity factor $\log \bar{k}'$ vs the median mole fraction of the organic solvent, $\bar{\psi}$). As the contact hydrophobic area, ΔA_h, of the biosolute-non-polar ligand increases, the slope, S, of the solvophobic aspect of the plot increases, whilst the slope, ξ, of the lipophobic aspect of the plot may either increase or decrease according to the molecular properties and surface anisotropy of the biosolute. Shown in this figure is the case (A) where the $\log k'$ value of polypeptide or protein exhibits a strong dependence on ψ for both the hydrophobic and lipophobic/silanophilic aspects of the interaction, with the retention dependency characterised as a narrow window of solvent compositions over which elution can be achieved. Typically, when a retro-elution approach is attempted in case A utilising the lipophobic aspect of the dependency from higher ψ-values and exploiting the decreasing $\log \bar{k}'$ values as the ψ-value becomes smaller, the polypeptide or protein is often recovered in a denatured/unfolded state. As a consequence, the use of this aspect of the $\log \bar{k}'$ vs ψ dependency is better suited to the analytical recovery of chemically modified polypeptides or proteins, i.e. after reduction and alkylation, cyanogen bromide cleavage, etc., as part of the characterisation of the primary structure and to remove guanidine hydrochloride, salts or other low molecular weight contaminants. However, when the solvophobic aspect of the $\log \bar{k}'$ vs ψ dependency is exploited in the usual manner by employing mobile phase compositions of increasing solvent content to achieve a smaller $\log \bar{k}'$ value, then recovery of the polypeptide or protein in near native state can be achieved, taking into account the influence of column residency or temperature. Also shown in this figure is the situation (B) which prevails with some polypeptides and proteins that show a shallow lipophobic/silanophilic dependency on the ψ-value. This situation has been noted when hydrogen donor solvents have been employed, such as iso-propanol as the organic solvent modifier. In this case, the solvophobic component of the dependencies may also show a shallower slope, i.e. smaller S-value, which in the case of complex mixtures of polypeptides or proteins leads to some loss of resolution since a unique elution window may not occur for the polypeptide or protein of interest.

where ΔH_{assoc}^0 and ΔS_{assoc}^0 are the enthalpy and entropy changes associated with the chromatographic migration process, respectively, R is the universal gas constant, T is the absolute temperature and is the phase ratio of the chromatographic system.

For some structurally simple organic molecules, such as benzene derivatives, linear relationships in the van't Hoff plots have been observed (Gilpin and Sisco, 1980; Gilpin and Squires, 1981), suggesting that for these compounds the values of ΔH_{assoc}^0 and ΔS_{assoc}^0 remain essentially unchanged over the experimentally investigated temperature range. However, the situation with n-alkylsilica sorbents with many organic compounds as well as polypeptides and proteins is more complicated than would appear from such observations. Various authors have pointed out that phase transitions in the bonded n-alkyl stationary-phase ligands may cause non-linear relationship in the van't Hoff plots (Gilpin and Sisco, 1980; Gilpin and Squires, 1981; Vailaya and Horvath, 1996a,b; Boysen et al., 1999, 2002; Hearn and Zhao, 1999) Gilpin et al. (1980) have, for example, found that transition temperatures for n-octyl (C_8), n-nonyl (C_9) and n-decyl (C_{10}) ligands immobilised to porous silica, initially pre-treated with equal volumes of acetonitrile and water, were 40.7, 0.7°C; 51.8, 2.1°C and 60.1, 1.0°C respectively, when pure water was used as the eluent. These differences correspond to an increase in the transition temperature of approximately 10°C per each additional methylene unit in the bonded n-alkyl chain. Based on this empirical rule, the predicted transition temperatures for n-butyl- (C_4) and n-octadecyl- (C_{18}) ligands would be outside the temperature range of most RP-HPLC separations carried out with polypeptides and proteins. Several studies, including molecular dynamics simulation investigations (Yarovsky et al., 1994; Klatte and Beck, 1995; Yarovsky et al., 1995a, 1997) of n-alkylsilica surfaces have confirmed that the C_4-ligand has reduced flexibility compared to the C_8- or C_{18}-ligand in terms of the respective gauche-trans disposition of the methylene units. The n-butyl chains thus exhibit a 'picket-fence'-like appearance to the docking polypeptide of protein on its approach and adsorption to the RP-HPLC sorbent, whereas the n-octyl and n-octadecyl chains assume the appearance of collapsed lipid-like droplets in water-rich eluents and only become extensively extended when the mole fraction of the organic solvent, ψ, reaches a significant value. As a consequence, differences in the slope of the van't Hoff plots can be anticipated to arise with polypeptides and proteins if a C_4-, C_8- or C_{18}-sorbent is employed.

In addition, it should be noted that the carbon number in the bonded n-alkyl chain is not the only factor affecting the linearity of van't Hoff plots. According to the observations of Cole et al. (1992a,b), linear van't Hoff plots were found for benzene on a n-octadecylsilica adsorbent with a bonded ligand density lower than 2.84 $\mu mol/m^2$ were linear over a wide temperature range (-5 to 80°C). In the case where the bonded ligand density was higher than 3.06 $\mu mol/m^2$, however, non-linear relationships were observed. Thus, the ligand density of the n-alkyl sorbent as well as the chain length must be considered as further variables in the chromatographic behaviour of polypeptides and proteins in RP-HPLC systems. Moreover, ineffective coverage of the silica matrix, irrespective of whether a type A or a type B silica is employed, will lead to additional modes of selectivity associated with silanophilic effects. For these reasons, the use of shielded or hindered n-alkyl ligands of shorter chain length have attracted considerable attention as a compromise between the intrinsic hydrophobicity of the sorbent surface, adequacy of ligand coverage and chemical or thermal stability (Lockmuller and Wilder,

1979; Hearn, 1983; O'Hare *et al.*, 1983; Glajch *et al.*, 1987; Hearn and Aguilar, 1988; Lork *et al.*, 1989; Aguilar and Hearn, 1991; Chloupek *et al.*, 1994; Hancock *et al.*, 1994; Hearn, 1998a). Finally, as noted previously the kind of organic modifier added to the aqueous mobile phase in these RP-HPLC systems can also be expected to affect the shape of van't Hoff plot.

Dependence of $\log k$ and $\log \bar{k}$ on temperature at different values of ψ or $\bar{\psi}$

For small peptides and some polypeptides of intermediate size, the changes in the enthalpic and entropic terms with variation of the organic solvent composition and temperature offer interesting insight into the processes of interaction with RP-HPLC systems. For example, it has been noted in several studies (Boysen *et al.*, 1999, 2001; Hearn and Zhao, 1999; Purcell *et al.*, 1999; Zhao *et al.*, 1999) that both the ΔH^0_{assoc} and ΔS^0_{assoc} values for different polypeptides incrementally change with increasing modifier concentration in the mobile phase at a defined temperature. Illustrative of these dependencies of ΔH^0_{assoc} and ΔS^0_{assoc} on the concentration of the organic solvent modifier in the mobile phase and temperature are the plots (Boysen and Hearn, 2001a) of $\log k$ vs $1/T$ for the hormonal polypeptide insulin over the range of $\psi = 0.25–0.29$ respectively (Fig. 5.2). Although overall, non-linear van't Hoff dependencies are observed (the basis of which is discussed subsequently in this chapter) within a narrow temperature range at a defined modifier concentration, the plots shown in these figures can be approximated as linear dependencies. Based on such results, the virial coefficients of enthalpy and entropy changes with respect to the modifier concentration at a constant temperature

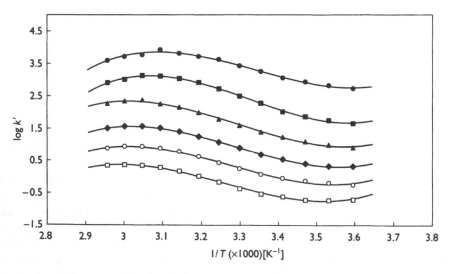

Figure 5.2 van't Hoff plots for bovine insulin determined at different isocratic organic solvent modifier concentrations with a *n*-butyl-(C₄)-silica Bakerbond sorbent using acetonitrile-water mobile phases containing 0.1% trifluoroacetic acid. The organic solvent modifier volume fractions were: ●, 26%; ▼, 27%; ■, 28%; ▲, 29%; ○, 30% and □, 31% respectively. Data selected from Boysen *et al.*, 1999.

can be defined (Hearn & Zhao, 1999) namely

$$\zeta = \frac{\partial \left(\Delta H^0_{assoc} \right)_T}{\partial \psi} \tag{13}$$

and

$$\theta = \frac{\partial \left(\Delta S^0_{assoc} \right)_T}{\partial \psi} \tag{14}$$

Data (Hearn and Zhao, 1999) for the virial coefficients parameters ζ and θ for glucagon, β-endorphin and bombesin are listed in Table 5.1. It can be seen that at the low temperature range (5–35°C), the $\partial \left(\Delta H^0_{assoc} \right)_T / \partial \psi$ values, ζ, for these three polypeptides are positive, but at higher temperatures (i.e. in the range 55–85°C), however, slightly positive or negative values of $\partial \left(\Delta H^0_{assoc} \right)_T / \partial \psi$ values, ζ, are observed, depending on the particular peptide. As to the dependency of $\partial \left(\Delta S^0_{assoc} \right)_T / \partial \psi = \theta$, over the lower temperature range (5–35°C) these virial coefficients are also positive, but become negative over the higher temperature range (55–85°C). Such behaviour is typical of non-classical enthalpy-entropy compensation phenomena. Enthalpy-entropy compensation effects are a manifestation of another type of extra-thermodynamic relationship that polypeptides and proteins can undergo in RP-HPLC environments. In these cases, the molecular interactions between the polypeptide or protein and the immobilised hydrocarbonaceous ligands generally involve significant enthalpy changes and a more restricted conformation of the biosolute when in the bound state, which is concomitantly associated (Everett, 1983) with a large change in the entropy.

What is the basis of these changes in the virial coefficients of enthalpy and entropy as the mole fraction of organic solvent in the mobile phase changes? From the available experimental results obtained with a range of polypeptides, it is clear that these changes are usually not associated with polypeptide degradation within the chromatographic system. For example, electrospray mass spectrometric (ES-MS) studies have confirmed that many polypeptide and small globular proteins can be recovered from the RP-HPLC systems operated at these elevated temperatures without any compositional modification, although in other cases some chemical modifications, such as deamidation or α- $\to$ β-aspartic acid rearrangement via α-aminosuccinimido-intermediates, have

Table 5.1 Virial coefficient parameters for enthalpic, ζ, and entropic, θ, changes with respect to organic solvent modifier concentration, ψ, for bombesin, β-endorphin and glucagon for the chromatographic interaction process, using a n-butyl (C4)-silica sorbent and acetonitrile-water mobile phases

Peptide	$\zeta = \dfrac{\partial \left(\Delta H^0_{assoc} \right)_T}{\partial \psi}$ (kJ · mol^{-1}) · (1%)$^{-1}$			$\theta = \dfrac{\partial \left(\Delta S^0_{assoc} \right)_T}{\partial \psi}$ (J · mol^{-1}K^{-1}) · (1%)$^{-1}$		
	$T = 5$–35 °C	$T = 35$–55 °C	$T = 55$–85 °C	$T = 5$–35 °C	$T = 35$–55 °C	$T = 55$–85 °C
Glucagon	2.2	−0.3	−0.6	2.9	−5.2	−6.1
β-Endorphin	2.8	1.4	−0.9	4.1	−0.7	−7.5
Bombesin	1.2	1.1	3.1×10^{-3}	0.7	0.3	−2.9

been noted. Generally, the results thus provide further confirmation that the variations observed in these virial coefficients is a function of changes in the conformational status of the biosolute(s) under the particular chromatographic conditions.

From kinetic arguments, at lower temperatures, polypeptide and protein biosolutes can be expected to adopt more constrained conformations. It has been previously shown that peptides such as bombesin, β-endorphin or neuropeptide Y (*loc cit*) exist in a partial α-helical conformation in the presence of some organic solvents, including acetonitrile (Aguilar *et al.*, 1985; Purcell *et al.*, 1992, 1993; Mant *et al.*, 1993; Vailaya and Horvath, 1996a; Higgins *et al.*, 1997; Lazoura *et al.*, 1997; Boysen and Hearn, 2001a). As a consequence, when a hydrogen bond acceptor solvent is employed, an increasing organic modifier concentration may be stabilising the secondary structure of the polypeptide in the bulk as well as the bound states, resulting in a less negative value of ΔS^0_{assoc} for the chromatographic migration process and a positive value of $\partial(\Delta S^0_{assoc})_T/\partial\psi$. In contrast, at higher temperatures, the conformation of most polypeptides and proteins becomes more extended and flexible in the less viscous solvent environment of the mobile phase at these higher temperatures, i.e. under these unfolding conditions, negative values of $\partial(\Delta S^0_{assoc})_T/\partial\psi$ will be observed. As foreshadowed above, the chromatographic migration process with polypeptides and proteins will involve a series of solvation-desolation steps that affect both the hydrocarbonaceous ligands as well as the polypeptide/protein itself. Organic solvents, e.g. acetonitrile, that tend to stabilise the secondary structures of polypeptides, and which minimise the exposure of the hydrophobic core of the protein if it has a globular tertiary structure, can thus be expected (Grego and Hearn, 1978; Hearn and Grego, 1981a,b; Hearn, 1983; Creighton, 1984; Hearn *et al.*, 1985; Hearn and Aguilar, 1988; Aguilar and Hearn, 1991; Hearn, 1998a; Hearn and Zhao, 1999) to lead to a less complex RP-HPLC chromatographic peak profiles and higher mass recovery of the native form(s) of the protein. On the other hand, organic solvents that destabilise the secondary or tertiary structure of a polypeptide or protein will in many cases generate (Hearn and Grego, 1981a; Aguilar and Hearn, 1991; Hearn, 1998a; Hearn and Zhao, 1999; Purcell *et al.*, 1999; Hearn and Zhao, 1999) denatured forms of the biosolute, often accompanied by significantly decreased recoveries of mass and bioactivity.

When LFERs prevail, then the overall change in enthalpy (or entropy) can be represented by the sum of the incremental changes in enthalpy (or entropy) such that if two components (the polypeptide or protein, P, and the hydrocarbonaceous ligand, L) are involved

$$\Delta H^0_{assoc,overall} = \Delta H^0_{assoc,p} + \Delta H^0_{assoc,l} \tag{15}$$

and

$$\Delta S^0_{assoc,overall} = \Delta S^0_{assoc,p} + \Delta S^0_{assoc,l} \tag{16}$$

where $\Delta H^0_{assoc,p}$ and $\Delta S^0_{assoc,p}$ refer to the enthalpy and entropy changes for the transfer of the biosolute, P, from the mobile phase to the stationary-phase surface, including desolvation of the solute and interaction in the bulk phase of the solvent molecules released from the desolvation of P on binding to the hydrocarbonaceous surface. Similarly, $\Delta H^0_{assoc,l}$ and $\Delta S^0_{assoc,l}$ represents the enthalpy and entropy change in the hydrocarbonaceous ligands, L, arising from the adsorption of the biosolute onto the stationary-phase surface, including removal of the mobile phase molecules from the stationary-phase surface to allow solute access, and the reorganisation of these ligand molecules leading to the formation of a cavity in the stationary liquid phase for the partially accommodation of the biosolute and the close contact interaction of the solute with the stationary-phase ligand. Thus

$$\frac{\partial \left(\Delta H^0_{\text{assoc, overall}} \right)_T}{\partial \psi} = \frac{\partial \left(\Delta H^0_{\text{assoc},p} \right)_T}{\partial \psi} + \frac{\partial \left(\Delta H^0_{\text{assoc},l} \right)_T}{\partial \psi} \tag{17}$$

and

$$\frac{\partial \left(\Delta S^0_{\text{assoc, overall}} \right)_T}{\partial \psi} = \frac{\partial \left(\Delta S^0_{\text{assoc},p} \right)_T}{\partial \psi} + \frac{\partial \left(\Delta S^0_{\text{assoc},l} \right)_T}{\partial \psi} \tag{18}$$

Elsewhere, Hearn and Zhao (Hearn and Zhao, 1999) have provided a comprehensive elaboration of the effect of temperature on $\partial(\Delta H^0_{\text{assoc, overall}})_T/\partial \psi$ and its physicochemical significance. Since the $\partial(\Delta H^0_{\text{assoc, overall}})_T/\partial \psi$ values for polypeptides with preferred secondary structures can markedly change over different temperature ranges, it can be concluded that the number and type of amino acid side chain and backbone functional groups within structured polypeptides that are exposed for interaction with solvent molecules in the mobile phase at lower temperature ranges (i.e. 10°C) when a polypeptide is adsorbed to the non-polar stationary-phase ligands are different to those presented by the same polypeptide when bound to the hydrocarbonaceous ligands at the higher temperature range (i.e. 25°C) due to conformational changes of the polypeptide. Similar considerations also apply to globular proteins. Experimental results discussed subsequently (*loc cit*) with low molecular weight compounds such as toluene, nitrobenzene and phenol, or small peptides which lack any secondary structure, support this conclusion. Whether this 'low temperature' behaviour involves the so-called hydrophobic compression effect (Arakawa and Timasheff, 1984; Jensen *et al.*, 1997) evident with globular proteins in bulk solutions at low temperatures requires further investigation. However, the RP-HPLC results are consistent with the general consensus on the influence of the hydrophobic effect, with the exposure of the 'hydrophobic core' of a polypeptide or protein minimised in polar solvent environments through the intermediacy of conformational stabilisation effects.

Recent molecular dynamics and molecular modelling simulation studies (Yarovsky *et al.*, 1994, 1995, 1997; Klatte and Beck, 1995) have shown that upon docking of the polypeptide onto the solvated *n*-alkyl ligand such conformational changes are energetically favoured. Figure 5.3 illustrates a situation that may prevail in the case of bombesin (Yarovsky *et al.*, 1997) prior to, and following, docking of this polypeptide onto a C_8-ligand system, as determined by such computational molecular simulation procedures. It is well known that many biologically active polypeptides interact with their specific receptors *via* hydrophobic forces. Several avenues of independent investigation have provided support for the possibility that the receptor bound conformations of a polypeptide are similar to that observed at a lipid-water interfaces (Galactionov *et al.*, 1988; Nikiforovich *et al.*, 1991; Galaktionov and Marshall, 1993). Similar molecular mechanics procedures to those employed (Yarovsky *et al.*, 1997) with bombesin can be adapted to enable the calculation of relatively stable molecular conformations for polypeptides in the presence of water-lipophilic phases in general. As a consequence, the nature of the orientations of the amino acid side chains of the polypeptide or protein in these lipid rich environments can be evaluated, in terms of either partition or solvophobic models of penetration and cavity capture of the biomolecule by the lipophilic phase. Importantly, such computational approaches enable the relevance of 'retention/conformational structure' molecular relationships to be tested and support for this attractive hypothesis evaluated. Clearly, strong parallels exist between the use of molecular mechanics and dynamics procedures for the computational assessment of the 'interactive conformation' of a polypeptide or protein in the lipophilic environment of RP-HPLC systems and the 'bioactive conformation' of these molecules in the presence of their membrane-associated receptor. In this, and other contexts, RP-HPLC procedures are thus acting as experimental probes for biomembrane mimetic systems, fulfilling an analytical role as a novel form of 'molecular recognition chromatography'.

Exploiting this analogy, Pidgeon et al. (Pidgeon et al., 1994; Rhee et al., 1994; Yin et al., 1998) as well as Bayerl et al. (Murphy and Gill, 1990; Reinl and

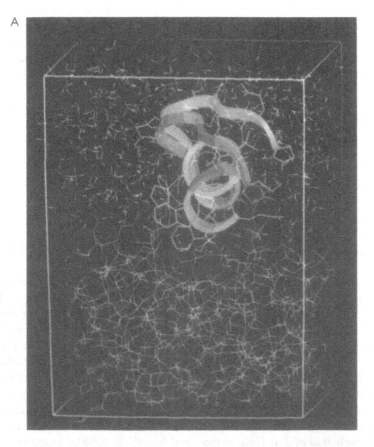

Figure 5.3 (Continued)

B

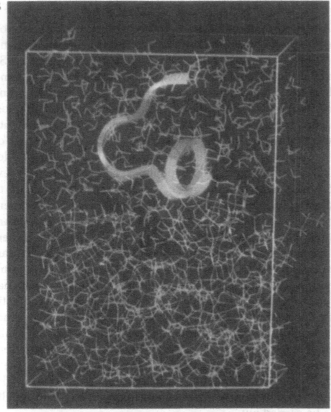

Figure 5.3 Molecular modelling simulation of the conformations of the polypeptide bombesin, prior to and following docking to n-octadecyl ligands immobilised onto a silica surface. The figure illustrates a typical structure of the bombesin – RP-HPLC sorbent – water complex obtained by the constant temperature/constant volume molecular dynamics procedures with the relative surface accessibility of the bombesin amino acid residues in a typical conformation adopted upon binding to the RP-HPLC sorbent. Data taken from Yarovsky et al., 1995b, 1997. In panel (A) is shown the orientation of bombesin with the lowest van der Waals interaction energy chosen as the starting geometry of the peptide-sorbent complex, In panel (B) is shown the bombesin-sorbent system configuration following exploration of the full Cartesian space using molecular dynamics and simulated annealing methods. For this purpose, all silica atoms except for the surface hydroxyl groups were kept immobilised, whilst the surface hydroxyl groups, the n-butyl chains, the peptide and the solvent were free to move. The peptide torsional bonds were restrained to 180°. Initial energy minimisation by means of the steepest descent followed by the conjugate gradient method was used to relax the system. The system was then equilibrated at 300 K and then 'heated' by standard computational methods to 1000 K in 25 K increments every 1 ps. The configurational space was then sampled for 25 ps. Slow cooling of the system was then performed by decreasing the temperature by 25 K every 2 ps until the temperature reached 300 K. The time development of the system was simulated for 200 ps in total, with 100 ps for the equilibration stage and 100 ps for the data collection. The energy of the system reached 36 kcal/mol at this stage.

Bayerl, 1994; Hetzer *et al.*, 1998) have prepared immobilised artificial membranes by immobilising various lipophilic compounds, such as phosphatidylcholine (PC), dipalmitoyl phosphatidylcholine (DPPC) phosphatidylglycerol (PG), phosphatidylserine (PS), phosphatidylethanolamine (PE) and related ether derivatives, onto porous silica and other support materials. Phase transitions at specific temperature values corresponding to those found with liposomes can be observed with such immobilised lipids and phospholipids. Because of the surface heterogeneity of these ligates when incorporated into silica-based sorbents following immobilisation *via* the standard aminopropyl-(AP-) or thiocyanatopropyl-(NCS-) chemistries, these systems however generate bizarre profiles in terms of their $\log k$ vs $1/T$ dependencies with polypeptides. Despite claims by several subsequent investigators that such systems provide 'new and sensitive methods' to monitor the conformational properties of polypeptides and proteins in an environment that more closely reflecting a biological membrane, this optimism has yet to be substantiated. There are several underlying reasons for this caution. Firstly, most researchers in the field hold the view that such studies are more efficiently and reproducibly carried our on biosensor chips or as two-phase liposome systems. Secondly, the aberrant retention and thermodynamic behaviour observed with these lipophilic sorbents has its origins in several important factors, including lack of reproducibility in synthetic procedures, variability in quality control of these immobilised lipophilic sorbents and, finally, their unavailability for rigorous evaluation and replication of the claimed results by the scientific community. These deficiencies, which do not occur with the current generations of n-alkyl ligate sorbent systems, continue to constrain progress in these areas. As a consequence, detailed, systematic and encompassing investigations into the thermodynamic characteristics of polypeptide-ligate interactions with such lipophilic sorbent systems have yet to be carried out.

Dependence of S and $\log k_0$ values on temperature and ψ or $\overline{\psi}$

From the above discussion, it is apparent that with different classes of polypeptides and proteins significant transitions in the magnitude of the S and $\log k_0$ values can occur with increasing temperatures, as a result of perturbation of the secondary or tertiary structure of these biosolutes. Under ideal linear elution chromatographic conditions with a completely aqueous mobile phase the relationship between the capacity factor and the Gibbs free energy change for the interaction can be given by:

$$\log k_0 = \frac{-\Delta G^0_{0/w}}{RT} + \log \Phi \tag{19}$$

where $\Delta G^0_{0/w}$ is the standard free energy change for the process of adsorbing the solute from a pure water mobile phase onto the non-polar stationary-phase surface.

Equation 19 suggests that $\log k_0$ value is a measure for $\Delta G^0_{0/w}$, reflecting the affinity of the solute for the hydrocarbonaceous ligands in neat water. In ideal cases with conformationally rigid solutes, plots of $\log k_0$ vs $1/T$ should thus generate straight lines. If the biosolute undergoes a conformational change with a half life ($t_{1/2}$) comparable to the overall time (t_R) of the mass transport phenomenon associated with the biosolute-ligand interaction, then marked deviation from linearity would be observed.

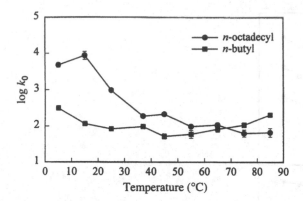

Figure 5.4 Plots of the log k_0 vs $1/T$ dependencies for the linear polypeptide bombesin generated from the experimental data obtained with n-octadecyl silica (●) and n-butylsilica (■) Bakerbond wide pore sorbents and 0.1% trifluoroacetic acid acetonitrile-water mobile phase conditions. Data selected from Purcell et al., 1992.

Figures 5.4 and 5.5 illustrate the plots of $\log k_0$ vs $1/T$ for the conformationally flexible polypeptide bombesin and several low molecular weight control solutes (N-acetyl-L-α-phenylalanine ethyl ester, N-acetyl-L-α-tryptophanamide and penta-L-α-phenylalanine). It can be seen that the $\log k_0$ vs $1/T$ plots for the small solutes are nearly linear. The corresponding plot for bombesin follows a non-linear relationship. Other hormonal polypeptides, such as β-endorphin, neuropeptide Y, insulin-related peptides or glucagon, similarly show (Cohen *et al.*, 1984; Purcell *et al.*, 1992; Aguilar *et al.*, 1993; Hearn and Zhao, 1999) non-linear $\log k_0$ vs $1/T$ plots with C$_4$-, C$_8$- or C$_{18}$-sorbents. From data of this kind, the conclusion has been drawn (Hearn and Zhao, 1999) that extrapolation of $\log k$ vs ψ plots, and particularly the $\log k$ vs ψ plots, to derive the notional affinity constants, $K_{assoc,0}$, for the interaction of a polypeptide or protein with a RP-HPLC sorbent in the presence of a completely aqueous mobile phase has to be treated with considerable caution in cases where deviations from van't Hoff plot linearity are found.

Moreover from Equations 1, 10 and 19, an expression linking the S-value with the free energy parameters can be obtained in the following manner. Since

$$\Delta G^0_{assoc} = -RT(\log k) + RT \log \Phi \qquad (20)$$

by differentiating Equations 1 and 20 with respect to ψ, we have

$$\frac{\partial (\log k')_T}{\partial \psi} = -S \qquad (21)$$

and

$$\frac{\partial (\Delta G^0_{assoc})_T}{\partial \psi} = -RT \frac{\partial (\log k')_T}{\partial \psi} \qquad (22)$$

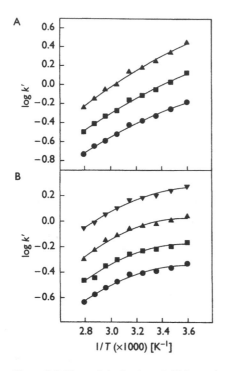

Figure 5.5 Plots of the log k_0 vs $1/T$ dependencies for the low molecular weight control solutes, N-acetyltryptophanamide (A) and N-acetylphenylalanine ethyl ester (B) generated from the experimental data obtained with a *n*-butylsilica Bakerbond sorbent and 0.1% tri-fluoroacetic acid acetonitrile-water mobile phase conditions. Data taken from Purcell *et al.*, 1992; Hearn and Zhao, 1999. The legend code for the mobile phase ψ-value conditions is : (a) ●, 10%; ▼, 15%; ■, 20%; and for (b) ●, 25%; ▲, 30%; ■, 35%; ▼, 40% respectively.

Substitution of Equation 21 into Equation 22 yields

$$\frac{\partial \left(\Delta G_{assoc}^0 \right)_T}{\partial \psi} = RTS \tag{23}$$

In an analogous fashion, differentiation of Equation 11 with regard to ψ, we have

$$\frac{\partial \left(\Delta G_{assoc}^0 \right)_T}{\partial \psi} = \frac{\partial \left(\Delta H_{assoc}^0 \right)_T}{\partial \psi} - T \frac{\partial \left(\Delta S_{assoc}^0 \right)_T}{\partial \psi} \tag{24}$$

Based on the above equations, the relationship between the slope term, S, derived from the plot of log k vs ψ (or the corresponding plot of log k vs ψ) and thermodynamic parameters can be expressed as

$$S = \frac{1}{RT} \frac{\partial \left(\Delta H_{assoc}^0 \right)_T}{\partial \psi} - \frac{1}{R} \frac{\partial \left(\Delta S_{assoc}^0 \right)_T}{\partial \psi} \tag{25}$$

Substitutions of Equation 25 in terms of the virial coefficients, given as Equations 13 and 14, permits S to be represented by Equation 26 as follows:

$$S = \frac{\zeta}{RT} + \frac{\theta}{R} \qquad (26)$$

Transitions associated with conformational behaviour of polypeptides and proteins can thus be revealed when the experimentally obtained values of the virial enthalpic coefficient, ζ, i.e. $\partial(\Delta H^0_{assoc})_T / \partial \psi$, and the virial entropic coefficient, i.e. $\partial(\Delta S^0_{assoc})_T / \partial \psi$ are compared with the predicted S values of the same polypeptides and proteins, assuming that linear elution behaviour occurred with no secondary equilibrium process participating for the purposes of the calculation, i.e. the retention process could be physically described according to Equation 1. Illustrative of this experimental approach are the examples of the plots of S vs T for β-endorphin, glucagon and bombesin shown in Fig. 5.6 with the predicted (solid lines) and experiment data points (filled points) determined under isocratic conditions, whilst the corresponding ζ and data are listed in Table 5.1. As can be seen from Fig. 5.6, for β-endorphin the S vs T plot shows two transition temperatures (ca. 35°C and ca. 55°C), but for glucagon and bombesin, only one transition temperature in each case was observed (near 35°C or 55°C respectively). Because the S parameter of a polypeptide or protein is composed of two physicochemical terms, ΔA_h and k^e (see Equation 9), with possible compensation of the so-called entropy-enthalpy compensation effect (Hearn, 1983; Hearn and Aguilar, 1988; Murphy and Gill, 1990; Oroszlan, 1990; Lee, 1991; Hearn, 1998a) also involved in the solute-ligate interaction, the determination of the changes in the magnitude of the S parameter directly from the retention dependencies of log k on ψ may in some cases with polypeptide and protein not be as sensitive a discriminator as the measurement of the corresponding changes in the derived free energy parameters, ΔG^0_{assoc}, ΔH^0_{assoc} or ΔS^0_{assoc}, calculated from van't Hoff plot analysis. In terms of monitoring conformational changes of polypeptide and protein solutes in RP-HPLC environments, use of thermodynamic rather than empirical parameter values are thus preferred.

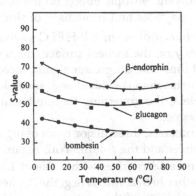

Figure 5.6 Plots of the S-value vs T for the polypeptides β-endorphin, glucagon and bombesin, separated on a n-butylsilica Bakerbond sorbent with acetonitrile-water mobile phase conditions. The solid lines represent the calculated values of S at different T-values calculated according to Equation 25, whilst the code for the experimental data points, acquired from Hearn and Zhao, 1999, is as follows: ▼, β-endorphin; ■, glucagon; ●, bombesin respectively.

Behaviour of polypeptides with preferred secondary structures: general comments

The interactive structure of polypeptides and proteins are influenced by many factors including those mediated by coulombic, hydrogen bonding, van der Waals and hydrophobic phenomena. Although the hydrophobic effect was first discussed (Kauzmann, 1959; Tanford, 1973) in terms of the stabilisation of the secondary and tertiary structure of polypeptides and proteins over 40 years ago comprehensive physicochemical descriptions of the nature of the underlying forces involved in hydrophobic phenomena, and how they are manifested in reversed phase chromatographic systems, still remain elusive. In terms of the chromatographic interactions involved in the RP-HPLC of polypeptides and proteins, the solvophobic model (Horvath *et al.*, 1976; Grego and Hearn, 1978; Hearn, 1983; Hearn and Aguilar, 1988; Aguilar and Hearn, 1991; Vailaya and Horvath, 1996a,b; Hearn, 1998a) has proved to be the most robust theoretical treatment currently available. Other models (Hearn, 1982, 1984; Dill, 1987; Dorsey and Dill, 1989), based on partition or adsorption considerations, have also gained some popularity. From a physical perspective, the interface between an aqueous milieu and an immobilised lipid-like moiety represents a very significant environment for the interaction of most types of biological molecules, and polypeptides and proteins are no exception. When these latter types of biomacromolecules have a high propensity to interact with lipid-like moieties, their surface structures are invariably composed of clusters of non-polar amino acid residues which are brought into close proximity as a result of the secondary and tertiary structural constraints arising from folding processes.

When favourable polypeptide or protein folding occurs, the free energy change associated with folding, $\Delta G^0_{folding}$, is negative, despite the significant increase in order of the system. This favourable $\Delta G^0_{folding}$ outcome is a direct consequence of an increase in the intra-chain (amide backbone and side chain) hydrogen bonding effects and hydrophobic associations of non-polar functional groups on the one hand, and a decrease in the solute-solvent hydrogen bonding and solute-solvent entropic effects on the other. Surprisingly, the value of $\Delta G^0_{folding}$ for many polypeptides and proteins is of similar magnitude to the value of ΔG^0_{assoc} for an interactive process in RP-HPLC systems. The choice of organic solvent, the time of residency on the sorbent surface, the temperature and other chromatographic variables all thus take on greater significance in the RP-HPLC separation of polypeptides and proteins than is evident with small, low molecular weight organic compounds. Nevertheless, the governing thermodynamic and extra-thermodynamic considerations are the same.

In terms of polypeptide or protein secondary structures, three major types of organisation have been documented, the helix, the β-sheet and the β-turn. With regard to helical secondary structures, the α-helix (3.6 amino acid residues with a rise of 1.5 Å per turn) represents the dominant type, although other helical motifs (e.g. the 3_{10}-helix and the π-helix) are known depending on the periodicity of the participating amino acid residues. Similarly, β-sheet structures exist as parallel and antiparallel strands with periodic rise of 3.2 Å and 3.4 Å per unit and 2 amino acid residues per unit. In the case of the β-sheet structures, hydrogen bonding occurs between polypeptide chains, whilst in the case of the helical motifs, between 10 and 16 atoms contribute intra-turn to the generation of each hydrogen bonding unit. Similarly, the balance between the hydrogen bonding and hydrophobic phenomena on the one hand, and the coulombic and van der Waals effects on the other, determine the tertiary structural organisation which characterises a folded protein. Conformational changes with polypeptides and proteins will thus involve *inter alia* changes in the hydrogen bonding characteristics as well as the hydrophobic interaction features of the molecule. The former process will be largely reflected in changes in the enthalpy of the polypeptide or protein, whilst that latter process is often associated with entropically driven phenomena. Although in a RP-HPLC environment the enthalpic, entropic and heat capacity characteristics cannot be independently manipulated, with the availability of sufficient experimental data, the impact of changes in the chromatographic conditions on these thermodynamic parameters can be qualitatively and quantitatively characterised. The polypeptide and protein examples detailed in the following three sections illustrate the generality of these conclusion.

Behaviour of β-endorphin and neuropeptide Y: prototype examples of the retention behaviour of α-helical polypeptides

Illustrative of the behaviour of polypeptides and polypeptides that can assume α-helical conformations in bulk solution as well as at hydrophobic surfaces are the characteristic transitions in the retention and peak width behaviour of β-endorphin, a 31-residue polypeptide first recognised for its analgesic properties and isolated from brain/pituitary/hypothalamic tissue (Smyth and Zacharian, 1980) and neuropeptide Y, a 36 amino acid carboxy terminally amidated peptide, first isolated from porcine brain (Taylor and Kaiser, 1986). The chromatographic behaviour of these two polypeptides have been used in this section to illustrate the typical changes that can occur with amphipathic α-helical polypeptides as the relevant RP-HPLC experimental conditions, such as temperature, residence time or *n*-alkyl ligand chain length, are varied. Additionally, these variations in retention and peak width behaviour provide a platform to examine the molecular basis of the inter-relationships linking structure-function and structure-retention dependencies. For this reason, it is useful to summarise here in a concise manner, several relevant aspect of the biological and structural properties of these examples, since they provide interesting case studies that are relevant to most other bioactive polypeptides and illustrate the potential of exploring conjointly these structure-function and structure-retention dependencies.

β-endorphin

The endogenous opoid activity of the neuropeptide β-endorphin and its synthetic analogues has been extensively investigated with the objective to delineate the role of this 31-mer in the regulation of the pain response. In common with a number of other neuroendocrine peptide hormones, β-endorphin is derived from pro-opiocorticotropin (POMC) by proteolytic cleavage from this precursor protein. Within its primary structure β-endorphin contains the pentapeptide motif Tyr-Gly-Gly-Phe-Met associated with a enkephaloidic peptide functional response typified by this class of endogenous analgesics. The interaction of this pentapeptide unit of β-endorphin with opoid receptors is believed to be mediated by the ability of the C-terminal 19-mer segment to assume an amphipathic α-helix in the presence of the hydrophobic environment of the receptor(s) (Wu *et al.*, 1981; Tatemoto, 1982).

As noted above, the relative propensity of a particular polypeptide to assume a preferred secondary structure under a selected set of RP-HPLC conditions can be ascertained for a range of different solvent conditions, either off-line or on-line by CD spectrometry, utilising the wavelength dependence of the mean molar ellipticity, $[\theta]$ (deg.cm^2.dmol^{-1}), calculated from $[\theta] = (\text{MRW} \cdot \theta)/C \cdot l$, where MRW is the mean amino acid residue molecular weight, C is the concentration (g.cm^{-3}), l is the pathlength (cm) and Θ is the ellipticity (deg), with comparison of the derived spectra to reference spectra representing pure α-helix, β-sheet, β-turn and random structures in order to determine the contribution of each structure to the overall CD spectra. Although in aqueous phosphate buffered solutions β-endorphin does not assume any significant secondary structure as revealed from CD measurements, in the presence of methanol, acetonitrile or trifluoroethanol the secondary structure of this polypeptide becomes more stabilised taking on a α-helical content of up to ca. 30%. As evident from Fig. 5.7, the individual log k vs ψ plots (Purcell *et al.*, 1992) of β-endorphin at different temperatures with aqueous acetonitrile gradient conditions show a high linear correlation, although it is apparent from these plots that the S-values are not constant over the temperature range examined. As evident from the work of Hearn and Zhao (1999), when similar data were acquired for β-endorphin under isocratic rather than gradient conditions, it was found that the slope dependencies obtained from the log k vs ψ measurements were different to those derived from the corresponding log k vs ψ measurements. Moreover, when shorter N- or C-terminal truncated variants of β-endorphin were subjected to similar types of analysis, greater convergence of the results between the isocratic and gradient measurements resulted.

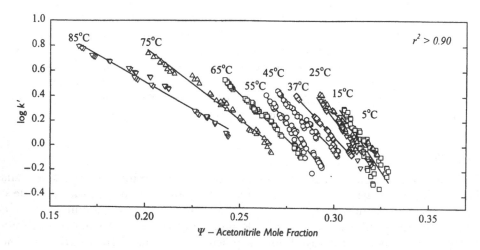

Figure 5.7 Plots of log k' versus the median mole fraction of the organic solvent, ψ, for β-endorphin separated on a *n*-butylsilica Bakerbond sorbent with acetonitrile-water mobile phase conditions at different temperatures over the range 5°C through 85°C. The experimental data from these linear gradient elution experiments was selected from Purcell *et al.*, 1992.

What then is the origin of these divergencies between the isocratic and the gradient data and retention data obtained at different temperatures and solvent compositions with RP-HPLC sorbents? With β-endorphin and its synthetic analogues of similar size, one indicator that secondary equilibrium processes must be occurring is the observation that the S-values for these polypeptides are dependent on the n-alkyl chain length of the hydrocarbonaceous sorbent. Results from the work of Purcell et al. (1992, 1993) with β-endorphin cogently illustrate that this behaviour is associated with the participation of dynamic polypeptide species, the structure(s) of which is(are) dependent on subtle differences in the solvent composition, time of residence on the n-alkyl sorbent or changes in temperature. As revealed from CD investigations using acetonitrile concentrations approximating the solvent percentages at which the polypeptide can be eluted from a C_4 or a C_{18} sorbent, β-endorphin has been found to assume about a 30% α-helical content from a previously β-sheet and random coil population of conformers in completely aqueous buffers.

Although the favourable adsorption of a polypeptide onto a reversed phase sorbent will be associated with a negative value of the ΔG^0_{assoc}, the greater ordering of the conformation of a polypeptide in the presence of the n-alkyl ligand will result in a (large) negative change in the entropy of association ($\Delta S^0_{assoc} \ll 0$) of the chromatographic system, whilst disordering of the polypeptide solute on the surface of the RP-HPLC sorbent will be characterised by a positive value of ΔS^0_{assoc}. Moreover, if the system does not involve any secondary equilibrium processes or temperature dependencies of the enthalpic or entropic components of the system, then according to Equation 7 linearity in the plots of $\log k$ vs $1/T$ would be expected. As evident from the data shown in Fig. 5.8, for the isocratic elution measurements (Hearn and Zhao, 1999), curvilinear van't Hoff plots are observed for β-endorphin, consistent with a transition from one state to another, with the transition midpoint(s) characterised by a critical temperature value(s). These data with β-endorphin can also be compared to similar curvilinear $\log k$

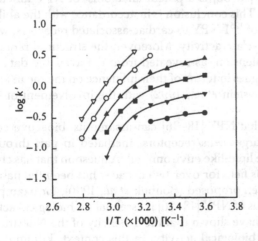

Figure 5.8 Plots of the $\log k'$ vs $1/T$ for the isocratic elution of β-endorphin at different organic modifier concentrations on a n-butylsilica Bakerbond sorbent using acetonitrile-water mobile phases. Data was selected from Hearn and Zhao, 1999. The code for the different mobile phase compositions is as follows: $\triangledown$, 25%; $\circ$, 26%, $\blacktriangle$, 27%; $\blacksquare$, 28%; $\blacktriangledown$, 29%; and $\bullet$, 30% respectively.

vs $1/T$ plots obtained with bovine insulin (Fig. 5.2). Such results imply that the ΔH^0_{assoc} and ΔS^0_{assoc} terms are dependent on both the temperature and the solvent composition. For example, for temperatures up to 45°C the derived ΔS^0_{assoc} values for β-endorphin with a C_{18}-sorbent were found to be negative, but of relatively similar value, indicating a slight induction of order of the system had occurred as the mole fraction of the organic solvent modifier was increase over the range $0 < \psi < 0.4$. In contrast, at temperatures higher than 45°C but over the same range $0 < \psi < 0.4$, the derived ΔS^0_{assoc} values of β-endorphin with the same C_{18}-sorbent were positive, and only became negative at a ψ-value of ca. 0.2. Moreover, in such circumstances, the virial coefficients ζ and θ (which represent the slope of the plots of ΔH^0_{assoc} vs ψ and ΔS^0_{assoc} vs ψ respectively) will be negative and the plot of these dependencies will pass through the value of $\Delta H^0_{assoc} = 0$ and $\Delta S^0_{assoc} = 0$ at critical values of ψ. When increasingly negative values of ΔS^0_{assoc} are observed, such behaviour implies that as the mole fraction of the organic solvent modifier, ψ, is increased, then greater stabilisation of the preferred conformation(s) of the polypeptide occur(s) on adsorption to the solvated non-polar ligand, up to and including the ψ-value required to desorb the polypeptide. For this process to occur, a significant change in the solvational status of the solute within the binding cavity of the associated non-polar ligand must occur, i.e. ΔH^0_{assoc} must also become large and negative in order for the value of ΔG^0_{assoc} to reach a small, but negative value.

Neuropeptide Y

The biological properties of neuropeptide Y (NPY) analogues have been extensively investigated in various structure-function studies over the past 10 years, documenting the ability of the C-terminal fragment encompassing the sequence from amino acid residues 18–36, i.e. NPY-[18–36], to elicit a hypotensive response slower in onset and longer in duration than the hypertensive effect observed (Boublik et al., 1989) with NPY-[1–36] and suggesting that NPY-[18–36] is a potent antagonist of NPY function (Balasubramaniam and Sheriff, 1990). This conclusion is in accordance with the ability of NPY-[18–36] to inhibit the binding of ^{125}I-NPY to cardiac-associated receptors, with no effect itself on cardiac adenylate cyclase activity. Moreover, the structural requirements for NPY-[18–36]-induced hypotension, as revealed from the available data on the structure-function of various analogues in terms of their influence on the mean arterial pressure (MAP), is consistent (Feinstein et al., 1992) with the involvement of the N-terminus of NPY-[18–36].

Collectively, these results suggest that NPY-[18–36] can assume its 'bioactive conformation(s)' in the presence of its target cells/receptors, mediated in part through interaction with the plasma membrane lipid-like environment. A question that has challenged peptide chemist working in this field for over two decades has been the nature of these conformations. It has also been proposed (Boublik et al., 1990), for example, that an α-helical motif in the C-terminus of NPY-[18–36] is essential for biological activity. Other studies (Spicer et al., 1990) have shown that the α-helicity of the N-terminal region is not a strict requirement for biological activity. In this context, Edmundson helical wheel analysis (Aguilar et al., 1993) has revealed that NPY-[18–36] can assume a strongly amphipathic helical structure. Consequently, it is likely that NPY-[18–36] adopt this helical conformation upon reaching lipid rich receptor environments, be they the receptor pocket or the non-polar cavity of a reversed phase ligand surface. Induction of an amphipathic helical structure within NPY-[18–36] as the polypeptide interacts with lipid surfaces may therefore play an important role in both its receptor recognition as well as in the chromatographic retention and peakwidth processes. The ability to monitor the surface-induced stabilisation of the secondary structure of NPY-[18–36] analogues with analogous hydrophobic surfaces thus represents an important approach in the characterisation of the structure-function and structure-retention relationships of NPY-[18–36].

In order to ascertain whether NPY-related polypeptides can assume a preferred secondary structure under the conditions that are widely employed in RP-HPLC separations, the availability of independently derived spectroscopic data is particularly useful. As discussed in previous sections of this chapter, circular dichroism measurements offer a versatile approach to achieve this outcome. With the NPY-[18–36]-related polypeptides (the same approach can be employed as a general strategy with most other polypeptides), the propensity of the L → D substituted NPY-[18–36] analogues to adopt α-helical structures in hydrophobic environments can be measured by CD methods, variations in α-helical content correlated with the reversed phase retention behaviour, and insight gained into the interactive conformation of these polypeptides in this nonpolar environment. Such CD studies performed (Boublik *et al.*, 1989; Spicer *et al.*, 1990) in 30% trifluoroethanol (TFE) in aqueous buffer confirmed that NPY-[18–36] adopts an α-helical structure, whilst [1]H-nuclear magnetic resonance analysis of NPY-[18–36] in TFE/H_2O (9:1) has also revealed (Mierke *et al.*, 1992) that NPY-[19–34] can adopt an α-helical structure.

Generally, in exploring the conformational behaviour of polypeptides with RP-HPLC in conjunction with other spectroscopic procedures, it is however prudent to utilise a range of different solvent conditions other than the standard 90% TFE condition, since the extent of secondary structure stabilisation can be very dependent on the solvent composition. Thus, as shown (Lazoura *et al.*, 1997) in a recent study, NPY-[18–36] does not adopt any helical structure in phosphate (P_i) buffer. However, the α-helical content increased to ca. 35% in 40% aqueous acetonitrile-P_i buffer and to ca. 75% in 90% TFE-P_i buffer (Fig. 5.9). Thus, the degree by which the 40% aqueous acetonitrile-P_i buffer (a solvent composition corresponding to the RP-HPLC elution conditions) or the 90% TFE-P_i buffer enhanced the intramolecular interactions within the polypeptide and stabilise the α-helical structure adopted by NPY-[18–36] differed significantly when compared to a totally aqueous environment. Although the mechanism by which organic solvents induce secondary structure formation with peptides remains ill-defined, it is thought to involve interaction of the peptide dipoles in specific preferred conformations with the solvent molecules, thus leading to the stabilisation of particular conformations over others through the participation of intramolecular hydrogen bonds and solvent – amide hydrogen bonding (Stores *et al.*, 1992; Hodges *et al.*, 1998). As commented elsewhere in this chapter, the selection of hydrogen-donor vs hydrogen-acceptor solvents thus becomes an important consideration when the physicochemical basis of the chromatographic behaviour and conformational vagaries of polypeptides and proteins are examined by RP-HPLC techniques.

Moreover, as revealed by CD measurements (Lazoura *et al.*, 1997), the α-helical content of NPY-[18–36] varied considerably when different single D-α-amino acid substitutions were carried out, irrespective of whether an aqueous phosphate (P_i) buffer,

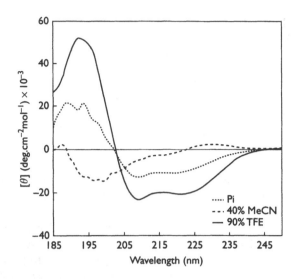

Figure 5.9 Circular dichroism results for the polypeptide neuropeptide Y-[18–36] (NPY-[18–36]) in 15 mM sodium phosphate, pH 2.2, buffer, (····); in 40% acetonitrile-15 mM sodium phosphate, pH 2.2, buffer (- - - -); and in 90% trifluoroethanol-15 mM sodium phosphate, pH 2.2, buffer (—)-at 25°C. Data taken from Lazoura *et al.*, 1997.

a 40% acetonitrile-phosphate buffer or a 90% trifluoroethanol-phosphate buffer system was employed, as illustrated in Fig. 5.10. In the aqueous P_i buffer all of the D-α-substituted peptides exhibit essentially extended structures, but in 40% aqueous acetonitrile-P_i and 90% TFE-P_i all of the D-α-NPY-[18–36] peptide analogues appeared to adopt a significant degree of α-helical structure in the presence of these organic solvent conditions. In 40% aqueous acetonitrile, the α-helical content of analogues with D-α-substitutions in the central region of NPY-[18–36] (i.e. residues His^{26}–Thr^{32}) appear to be particularly affected, indicating that residues encompassing this region are critical for maintenance of the preferred secondary structure. In contrast, the α-helical content of the [D-Asn]^{29}-NPY-[18–36] was not significantly reduced compared to the corresponding all L-analogue, indicating that the D-α-isomeric substitution at this position does not significantly disrupt the overall α-helical conformation, i.e. the chiral substitution of this residue is not a critical determinant for the maintenance of the amphipathic α-helix. In 90% TFE, the reduced α-helical content, exhibited by the analogues [D-Ala]^{23}- to [D-Arg]^{35}-NPY-[18–36] suggests that these residues are also located within the α-helical domain of NPY-[18–36]. Under these conditions, [D-Tyr]^{27}-NPY-[18–36] has the highest α-helical content indicating that the L → D substitution at Tyr^{27} can enhance intra-helical hydrogen-bonding in the hydrophobic environment provided by 90% TFE, and analogous processes may occur in the hydrophobic environment of the reversed phase ligand.

These conclusions are also consistent with Edmundson helical wheel representation of NPY-[18–36], shown in Fig. 5.11, which clearly illustrates (Lazoura *et al.*, 1997) the propensity of this polypeptide to adopt an amphipathic α-helical structure. According to the value of the hydrophobic moments (Eisenberg *et al.*, 1982) calculated for

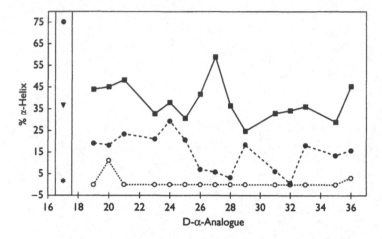

Figure 5.10 Circular dichroism results for the polypeptide neuropeptide Y-[18–36] (NPY-[18–36]), and the NPY-[18-36] analogues systematically substituted at each amino acid residue by the D-α-enantiomer, in 15 mM sodium phosphate, pH 2.2, buffer, (· · · ·); in 40% acetonitrile-15 mM sodium phosphate, pH 2.2, buffer (- - - -); and in 90% trifluoroethanol-15 mM sodium phosphate, pH 2.2, buffer (—) at 25°C. Data taken from Lazoura *et al.*, 1997. Also shown in this figure are the results for the L-α-NPY-[18–36] polypeptide in 15 mM sodium phosphate, pH 2.2, buffer, (○); in 40% acetonitrile-15 mM sodium phosphate, pH 2.2, buffer (●); and in 90% trifluoroethanol-15 mM sodium phosphate, pH 2.2, buffer (■) at 25°C.

NPY-[18–36] (H.M. = 0.72) and for NPY-[19–34] (H.M. = 0.97) the amphipathic nature of NPY-[18–36] is predominantly associated with the central region of the molecule. This amphipathic feature of NPY-[18–36] is illustrated in the lateral presentation shown in Fig. 5.11 where the hydrophobic moment is orientated downwards. The amino acid residues (indicated by the filled circles), located in the lower face of the α-helix could thus constitute a hydrophobic binding domain when NPY-[18–36] adopts this conformation.

Irrespective of whether the polypeptide either partitions into, or alternatively adsorbs to, a hydrophobic cavity on the non-polar surface of the sorbent, as a general observation, the increased degree of secondary structure observed with many polypeptides in the presence of RP-HPLC ligands may be attributed to enhanced intra-molecular and inter-molecular interactions, stabilising either a preferred α-helical or β-sheet structure adopted by the polypeptides in these non-polar environments. Both hydrogen bonding (and thus largely solvation and enthalpically dependent processes) and hydrophobic interactions (and thus largely entropically driven processes) can occur to different extents, depending on the amino acid sequence of the polypeptide or protein. Again, the potential of utilising data derived from analysis of the virial coefficients ζ and θ can be mentioned. It can be noted with the NPY-related polypeptides that in 40% aqueous acetonitrile-P_i or 90% aqueous TFE-P_i (solvent conditions that simulate the mobile phase elutropicities for the elution (Lazoura *et al.*, 1997) of these D-α-peptides from RP-HPLC sorbents), the polypeptides assumed a significant α-helical content, with the α-helical structure predominantly favoured in the central region of the NPY-[18–36] molecule.

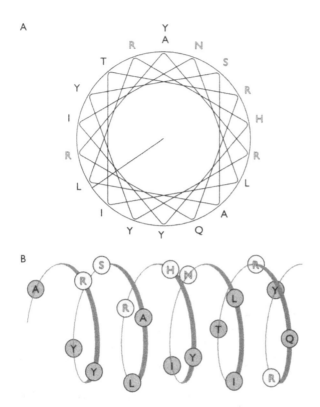

Figure 5.11 Edmundsen wheel representation of neuropeptide Y-[18–36] (NPY-[18–36]) in the annular and lateral projections. The hydrophobic amino acid residues which form the putative amphipathic sites of this polypeptide are highlighted Lazoura *et al.*, 1997 as either black letters (annular projection) or black circles (lateral projection), using the one letter code for the amino acids.

Thus, when RP-HPLC procedures were employed (Aguilar *et al.*, 1993; Lazoura *et al.*, 1997) with *n*-butyl (C_4)-, *n*-octyl (C_8)- and *n*-octadecylsilica (C_{18})–silica sorbents and acetonitrile or *i*-propanol as the organic modifier with the same series of NPY-[18–36] analogues with single D-α-substitutions, significant changes in the chromatographic parameters related to the contact area and affinity of interaction were observed. These findings demonstrate that the D-α-substitutions at residues Tyr^{27}–Thr^{32} severely disrupt the secondary structure of NPY-[18–36]. In the experiments with the NPY-[18–36] analogues shown as Fig. 5.12, the retention measurements were obtained on a C_{18}-silica at 25°C with gradient times of 30, 45, 60, 90 and 120 min respectively, at a flow rate of 1 ml/min, temperatures of 4°C, 25°C, 37°C, 60°C and 80°C, and linear elution gradients from water containing 0.1% TFA to water-acetonitrile (50 : 50) containing 0.09% TFA. The retention behaviour of the NPY-[18–36] analogues, shown in Fig. 5.12, indicates that significant selectivity and resolution differences can be achieved between a number of these D-α-substituted analogues, as has been recognised previously with other peptide diastereomers involving L $\rightarrow$ D or LL $\rightarrow$ DD substitutions (Hearn, 1982, 1983, 1984, 1998a; Blevins *et al.*, 1984; Hearn and Aguilar, 1988; Kirby *et al.*, 1993;

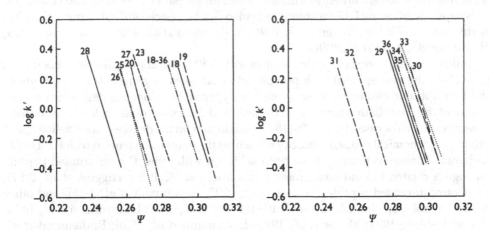

Figure 5.12 Plots of the log k' vs the median mole fraction of the organic solvent, ψ, for the polypeptide neuropeptide Y-[18–36] (NPY-[18–36]), systematically substituted at each amino acid residue by the D-α-enantiomer. In this figure, the experimental data Lazoura et al., 1997 were obtained using a C_{18}-silica Bakerbond wide pore sorbent and the elution conditions of 0.1% trifluoroacetic acid in water to 0.09% trifluoroacetic acid in acetonitrile-water (50:50) over gradient times of 30, 45, 60, 90 and 120 min at a flow rate of 1 ml/min at 25°C were used. The numbers refer to the position of the L-α- → D-α-substitution.

Krause *et al.*, 1995; Beyermann *et al.*, 1996; Rothemund *et al.*, 1996; Keah *et al.*, 1998). If all of the NPY-[18–36] analogues interacted with the immobilised C_{18} ligands without any preferred orientation or conformation and the relative selectivity was only dependent on the composition and not the chirality of the sequence, then each D-α-substitution should exert the same relative influence on the retention times and the retention plots of log $\bar{k}$ vs $\bar{\psi}$ for all analogues should be super-imposable. The fact that this was not observed, however, demonstrates that the interactive behaviour of the different peptides is particularly sensitive to the position of the D-amino acid substitutions.

It is noteworthy that the analogues with D-substitutions in the N- and C-terminal regions (e.g. residues Ala[18], Arg[19] and Arg[33]–Tyr[36]) were characterised by longer retention times than the all L-NPY-[18–36] peptide indicating that the hydrophobic contact region has increased. In addition, [D-Asn][29]- and [D-Leu][30]-NPY-[18–36] exhibited similar retention times to the L-α-NPY-[18–36] suggesting that the hydrophobic contact region of these peptides were unaffected by D-α-substitutions at these positions. However, D-α-substitution of the central region amino acid residues (Tyr[20]–Ile[28] and Ile[31]–Thr[32]) significantly affected the peptide-ligand interaction and resulted in earlier elution times. For example, [D-Ile][28]-NPY-[18–36] exhibited the smallest retention time of all the analogues indicating that the chromatographic contact region of this peptide had been significantly affected as a result of this chiral substitution. Overall, the retention data for the NPY-[18–36] analogues demonstrate that single D-amino acid substitutions within a polypeptide sequence can result in changes in retention time as a consequence of the variation in the size, orientation and composition of the hydrophobic contact region established between the peptide and the immobilised hydrophobic *n*-alkyl ligands. Recent investigations with other amphipathic hormonal and coiled-coil polypeptides following L D-substitutions lead to similar conclusions (Blevins *et al.*, 1984; Kirby *et al.*, 1993; Beyermann *et al.*, 1996; Rothemund *et al.*, 1996; Chao *et al.*, 1998; Hearn, 1998a; Keah *et al.*, 1998).

In this chapter, various reported studies with NPY-related peptides have been used to explore the concept that with polypeptide analogues in general the magnitude of the hydrophobic binding domain of each polypeptide analogue is dependent on the nature of the contributing amino acid residues and the extent of its preferred secondary structure, i.e. in the case of the NPY-[18–36] analogues on the degree of its α-helicity, and this physicochemical property directly influences the extent of retention with RP-HPLC sorbents. Analogous findings have been achieved with other D-α-substituted peptide analogues related to viral coat proteins (Eisenberg *et al.*, 1982; Higgins *et al.*, 1997), corticotropin-related peptides (Krause *et al.*, 1995; Beyermann *et al.*, 1996) and other hormonal polypeptides (Blevins *et al.*, 1984; Kirby *et al.*, 1993; Landenheim *et al.*, 1994; Li and Debber, 1994; Meyer *et al.*, 1995; Beyermann *et al.*, 1996; Rothemund *et al.*, 1996; Sanchez *et al.*, 1996; Hodges *et al.*, 1998; Keah *et al.*, 1998). A relationship should exist between the propensity of individual amino acid residues in their L-α- or D-α-chiral configurations, in terms of their ability to induce preferred secondary structures in polypeptides (reflected in the case of α-helical polypeptides as the percentage α-helicity, or in the case of β-sheet peptides the percentage of β-sheet content, as determined from CD measurements or other independent techniques) and the variations in RP-HPLC retention time for different D-α-substituted analogues.

In the case of the NPY-[18–36] analogues this trend is clearly evident (Lazoura *et al.*, 1997). Similar observations with L-α-amino acid residues substituted with D-α- or non-natural amino acids can be found in the literature with other classes of polypeptides, i.e. with β-endorphin-related polypeptides (Wu *et al.*, 1981; Tatemoto *et al.*, 1982) and coil-coil related polypeptides (Hodges *et al.*, 1998; Kohn *et al.*, 1998). Fig. 5.13 shows the dependence of percentage helicity in 40% acetonitrile and 90% trifluoroethanol, for each NPY analogue as a function of retention time (Aguilar *et al.*, 1993; Lazoura *et al.*, 1997) with a 120 min. gradient elution RP-HPLC system at 25°C. As evident from Fig. 5.13, the α-helical content of the NPY-[18–36] D-α-substitution analogues determined in 40% acetonitrile correlates with the relative retention times (but not the *S*-values) of the corresponding analogues determined with a C_{18}-sorbent, with a correlation value of $r^2 = 0.60$. In contrast, no correlation was observed between the α-helical content in 90% trifluoroethanol and the relative retention times of these D-α-substituted NPY-[18–36] analogues chromatographed on the C_{18}-silica. This result is consistent with different modes of stabilisation by trifluoroethanol and acetonitrile of the polypeptide secondary structure, as a result of the different hydrogen bonding properties of these two organic solvents. Whilst the CD data analysis of the secondary structures of the NPY-[18–36] analogues in bulk solvents provides insight into their conformations in solution, the CD data *per se* do not take into consideration the induction of secondary structure(s) upon interaction with the C_{18} ligands under the RP-HPLC conditions. This latter feature can be directly assessed in an on-line manner with CD spectrometers through the use of quartz cuvettes, surface modified *in situ* with *n*-alkyl ligands (Blondelle *et al.*, 1992). Moreover, temperature-programming studies with CD spectrometric measurements is a commonly used procedure to follow the conformational changes of polypeptides

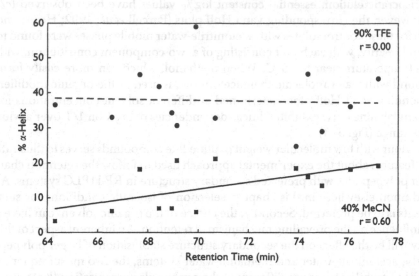

Figure 5.13 Dependence of the percentage α-helicity as determined from circular dichroism measurements in 40% acetonitrile-15 mM sodium phosphate, pH 2.2, buffer (■); and in 90% trifluoroethanol-15 mM sodium phosphate, pH 2.2, buffer (•) at 25°C and the retention time of the polypeptide neuropeptide Y-[18-36] (NPY-[18-36]), and its systematically substituted L-α → D-α-amino acid analogues. In these experiments, the retention time of the NPY-[18-36] and its D-α-analogues were determined with a 120 min linear gradient from 0.1% trifluoroacetic acid in water to 0.09% trifluoroacetic acid in acetonitrile-water (50 : 50) at a flow rate of 1 ml/min, using a n-octadecylsilica Bakerbond wide pore sorbent.

and proteins and similar procedures can be employed also in this simulated RP-HPLC environment.

As discussed above in this chapter, advantage can be taken of the temperature dependencies of the retention parameters, with the experimental results related to changes in polypeptide secondary structure. This outcome can be illustrated utilising the case of the NPY-[18–36] analogues through the dependencies of S- and log k_0-values over the range from 4–80°C with a C_{18} sorbent. In order to eliminate effects arising from the phase transition of the ligands immobilised onto the sorbent and to accommodate the behaviour of peptidic solutes which lack any secondary structure, low molecular weight control compounds such as N-acetyl-L-phenylalanine ethyl ester, N-acetyl-L-tryptophanamide or even small peptides, e.g. angiotensin-I, -II or -II, can be included in the analysis as control solutes under the same experimental conditions. Compounds such as N-acetyltryptophanamide and N-acetylphenylalanine ethyl ester, in particular, represent useful control solutes for thermo-dynamic studies with n-alkylsilica adsorbents and aquo-organic solvent eluents since they are small, highly diffusible molecules with no secondary structure and hence do not manifest any conformational changes under the different chromatographic conditions.

With such control substances essentially constant S-values and uniform decreases in log k_0-values are usually observed with increasing temperature when gradient elution procedures are employed, consistent with the known averaging of the thermodynamic behaviour for the interaction of these control solutes with n-alkyl ligands. However, in the case of isocratic elution, essential constant log k_0 values have been observed (c/f Fig. 5.5). However, the corresponding van't Hoff plots (Purcell *et al.*, 1992; Hearn and Zhao, 1999) for these control solutes with acetonitrile-water mobile phases were found to deviate from linearity, with each plot consisting of a two-component contribution, with a transition temperature near to 45°C. When methanol, which can more easily form hydrogen bond with water molecule than acetonitrile, is used as the organic modifier, the corresponding van't Hoff plots determined at different solvent concentrations for N-acetylphenylalanine ethyl exhibited linear dependencies of log k on 1/T over a wide temperature range (Fig. 5.14).

This behaviour with low molecular weight peptide-like compounds serves to illustrate several key features about the experimental approach used to follow the retention characteristics of polypeptides with preferred secondary structure in RP-HPLC systems. As commented upon elsewhere in this chapter, selection of isocratic conditions for such measurements is to be preferred. Secondly, the choice of the organic solvent can have a significant influence on the prevailing mechanism of retention. An inherent aspect of this dependency will be the effect on the secondary structure stabilisation of larger polypeptides. Clearly, acetonitrile-water and methanol-water systems, the two most frequently used RP-HPLC mobile phases are different in their molecular organisation (Katz *et al.*, 1986), as noted by various investigators. The characteristics of methanol-water solution chemistry is apparently controlled by competitive hydrogen bonding (Johnson *et al.*, 1986; Katz *et al.*, 1989), whilst acetonitrile is a poorer former of hydrogen bonds (Johnson *et al.*, 1986) and is organised in aggregates or loosely defined clusters in aqueous solution (Katz *et al.*, 1986; Meyer *et al.*, 1995; Kohn *et al.*, 1998). These differences in solution properties thus cause significant difference in the retention and selectivity behaviour with polypeptides as well as other biomacromolecules in RP-HPLC (Horvath *et al.*, 1976; Hearn, 1982, 1984; Aguilar and Hearn, 1991; Hearn, 1998a; Mant and Hodges, 1991). The deviations from linearity observed with acetonitrile based eluents

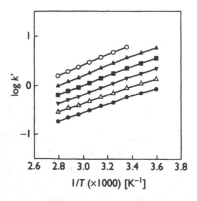

Figure 5.14 Plots of the log k' vs 1/T dependencies for the low molecular weight control solute, N-acetylphenylalanine ethyl ester, generated from the isocratic experimental data obtained with a n-butylsilica Bakerbond sorbent and 0.1% trifluoroacetic acid methanol-water mobile phase conditions. Data selected from Purcell *et al.*, 1992; Hearn and Zhao, 1999. The legend code for the mobile phase ψ-value conditions is: ○, 25%; ▲, 30%; ■, 35%; ▼, 40%; △, 45%; ●, 50% respectively.

with these low molecular weight compounds may be due to changes in orientation of the organic compound moieties on interaction with the stationary phase as well as in the re-organisation of acetonitrile and water molecules in the mobile phase induced by the elevated temperature. Such behaviour is, however, also reminiscent of the enthalpy-entropy compensated phenomena observed (Lowensehuss and Yellin, 1975; Jino et al., 1988; Rowlen and Harris, 1991) when both enthalpy and entropy show a temperature dependence. The relevance of such temperature-dependent processes in the RP-HPLC of polypeptides and proteins will be described subsequently.

The observed dependence (Aguilar et al., 1993; Lazoura et al., 1997) of the S and log k_0 values on temperature for the L-α-NPY-[18–36] and its analogues in the presence of a C_{18} sorbent is illustrated in Fig. 5.15 with a transition in retention behaviour evident between 25°C and 37°C. These changes in the S and log k_0 values can be contrasted to the relatively constant values observed for control compounds such as the amino acid derivatives and the angiotensin II/III peptides. Collectively, these results suggest that the interactive nature of the hydrophobic binding region of L-α-NPY-[18–36], localised on one face of the proposed amphipathic helix (Fig. 5.11), is disrupted at temperatures between 25°C and 37°C. Similar large changes in the S and log k_0 values of these NPY-[18–36] peptides with temperature have also been observed (Aguilar et al., 1993) using the C_4- and C_8- ligands, indicating that the behaviour evident with such polypeptides is a generic event. However, the shape and position of the S and log k_0 transitions for NPY-[18–36] and its D-α-substituted analogues depends on the chain length and densities (in μ mol/m^2) of the n-alkyl ligands, a finding illustrating the influence of the orientation, conformation and surface coverage (density) as well as the net hydrophobicity of the immobilised non-polar ligand on the induction of polypeptide conformation.

Inherent to the dependencies of the S and log k_0 values on temperature for the NPY-[18–36] D-α-substituted analogues shown in Fig. 5.16 is additional information on

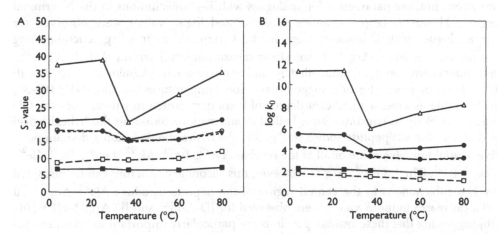

Figure 5.15 Plots of the S- and log k_0-values vs temperature, T, for the polypeptide neuropeptide Y-[18–36] (NPY-[18–36]), with each L-α-amino acid systematically substituted by the D-α-enantiomer, determined (Lazoura et al., 1997) with a n-octadecylsilica Bakerbond wide pore sorbent and acetonitrile-water-0.1% trifluoroacetic acid mobile phases over the temperature range of 5°C through 85°C. □, standard 2 [N-acetyl-L-tryptophanamide]; ■, standard 1 [N-acetyl-L-phenylalanine ethyl ester]; ●, angiotensin I; ○, angiotensin II; ◆, angiotensin III; △, NPY [18–36].

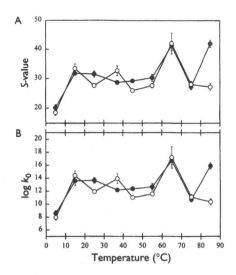

Figure 5.16 The dependence of the (A) *S*-values and the (B) log k_0-values of sperm whale myo-globin (○ = SMyo) and *apo*-myoglobin (● = *apo*-SMyo) on temperature, *T*, with a *n*-octadecylsilica Bakerbond sorbent. In these experiments (Purcell *et al.*, 1999), the elution conditions of a linear gradient of between 30 min and 90 min were employed using as the eluent a linear gradient of water-0.1% trifluoroacetic acid to acetonitrile-water-(1 : 1)-0.1% trifluoroacetic acid, pH 2.1, at temperatures ranging from 5°C through to 85°C respectively.

the relative conformational stability of each analogue. At 4°C, there were only small variations in these parameters for analogues with D-α-substitutions in the N-terminal region. However, large variations in the *S* and log k_0 values were observed for the analogues with D-α-substitutions in the C-terminal region (e.g. encompassing amino residues Ala^{23}–Arg^{33}). Results from measurements (Lazoura *et al.*, 1997) in the *n*-octadecyl environment, parallelled by similar observations (Aguilar *et al.*, 1993) with the *n*-butyl or *n*-octyl ligands, suggest that at low temperatures the all L–NPY-[18–36] polypeptide assumes a significant degree of secondary structure which, from the CD studies, is likely to constitute an α-helical conformation. Based on the helical wheel projections for this peptide shown in Fig. 5.11 the hydrophobic binding domain puta-tively would involve some or all of the residues Tyr^{20}, Tyr^{21}, Ala^{23}, Leu^{24}, Tyr^{27}, Ile^{28}, Leu^{30}, Ile^{31}, Thr^{32}, Gln^{34}, Arg^{35}. However, this secondary structure can be disrupted by D-α-substitutions in the central region of the peptide (residues Ala^{23}–Arg^{33}). At 4°C, decreases in the *S* values were observed for [D-Asn]^{29} and [D-Arg]^{33}–NPY-[18–36] suggesting that these residue positions are particularly important for maintenance of the conformation adopted by NPY-[18–36] at this temperature. At 25°C, large vari-ations in the *S* values were observed for NPY analogues containing D-α-substitutions between residues Ala^{23}–Ile^{28} with smaller changes apparent for the N- and C-terminally substituted analogues. Since CD studies indicate that a partial a α-helical structure is maintained in the central region with D-α-substitutions between residues Ala^{23}–Ile^{28}, perturbation of this structure will cause large variations in the *S* and log k_0 values of these analogues as the temperature is increased. As noted above, in the case of the D-α-substituted NPY-[18–36] analogues, no correlation was evident between the % helix observed in 40% aqueous acetonitrile or 90% aqueous trifluoroethanol and the S-values at 4°C (r = 0.48 and 0.38 respectively). This lack of correlation indicates that the S-value is a measure of the surface-bound contact area, i.e. the ΔA_h, and as such reflects the surface area of the trapped 'interactive conformation' species encompassing polypeptide secondary structures with an extent of helical content(s) that can differ from that found for the polypeptide in the bulk mobile phase milieu, either through induced stabilisation or destabilisation effects upon binding of the polypeptide to the hydrophobic surface. Finally, the results with NPY-related polypeptides also suggest that the secondary structure(s) which exist(s) at 4°C became destabilised at 25°C. This transition in the S and log k_0 values became even more evident near 37°C, as the interactive structure of each analogue assumed a more random coil structure.

In summary, in the general context of other linear, structurally unconstrained polypeptides which can adopt preferred α-helical secondary structures at a water-lipid interface, these observations with β-endorphin- and NPY[18–36]-related polypeptides serve to demonstrate the type of consequences which can be anticipated for the interactive behaviour of these polypeptides with n-alkyl ligands in RP-HPLC systems. This behaviour will be manifested as temperature-dependent and condition-dependent phenomena that will vary in the magnitude and scope for polypeptides of different sequence or amino acid chirality. This discriminatory power of RP-HPLC, enabling the orientational contribution of the amino acid residues which constitute the hydrophobic binding domain to be assessed at each temperature thus represents, from a physicochemical perspective, one of the major attributes of RP-HPLC techniques with polypeptides.

Behaviour of gramicidin analogues: prototype examples of the behaviour of β-sheet polypeptides

Relatively little similar work on the conformational stability work of β-sheet polypeptides in RP-HPLC systems has been reported in the scientific literature, partly a reflection of the propensity of polypeptides of this type to aggregate in solution. A large number of synthetic β-sheet polypeptides have, however, been purified using reversed phase procedures, including polypeptides related to the activin $\beta_A\beta_A$–$\beta_E\beta_E$ loop polypeptides, β-amyloid[1–43] (Vyas and Duffy, 1995), the cysteine-knot gonadotropin protein hormones, follitropin (FSH) (Cattini-Schultz, 1995) and thyrotropin (TSH) (Gomme et al., 1998), and other β-sheet polypeptides (Narita and Kojima, 1989; Al-Obeidi et al., 1995; Krause et al., 1996). The recent investigations of Kondejewski et al. (1998) with gramicidin S related analogues provide a clear demonstration of the potential that similar RP-HPLC procedures can offer for the characterisation of the conformational vagaries of β-sheet polypeptides in structure-function studies. Other work with synthetic peptides believed to have a high propensity for β-sheet structures are however less convincing (Steer et al., 1998) with inconclusive biophysical results, presumably due to the use of uncharacterised model peptides and gradient elution conditions rather than the more rigorous application of isocratic procedures for such measurements.

Gramicidin S is a well-known membrane active cyclic decapeptide with an amphipathic nature and antiparallel β-sheet structure. In several investigations (Jelokhami-Niaraki et al., 1998; Kondejewski et al., 1998a,b), systematic substitution of each amino acid residue with its enantiomer has been employed as the vehicle to permit elucidation of the lipid-binding propensities of different gramicidin S analogues, exploiting the unique selectivity dependencies of this class of polypeptide in RP-HPLC systems. The β-sheet structures of different gramicidin S analogues were found to be disrupted to varying extents, depending on whether the substitution occurred in H-bonding or non-H-bonding sites within the β-strands, or whether these replacements occurred in positions associated with β-turn residues. The changes in the anti-microbial and haemolytic activities of these D-α-gramicidin S analogues was found (Jelokhami-Niaraki et al., 1998; Kondejewski et al., 1998a) to correlate with the extent of conformational perturbation of each analogue as assessed by RP-HPLC investigations. Interestingly, the extent of gramicidin S-induced formation of lipid nonlamellar phases and the gramicidin S-induced increase in liposome permeability also appeared (Kondejewski et al., 1998) to be correlated with the changes in the RP-HPLC retention behaviour. Based on these and other investigations with β-sheet polypeptides, e.g. activin $\beta_A\beta_A$ loop polypeptides, it is apparent that the application of similar RP-HPLC methodologies will increase in popularity for the analysis of the interactive behaviour of β-sheet polypeptides provided attention is given to the proper use of isocratic procedures.

The effect of temperature on the RP-HPLC behaviour of intermediate molecular weight globular proteins: myoglobin, hen egg white lysozyme and cytochrome c

As discussed above, for small peptides without any secondary structure, the S-values, derived from linear regression of the plots of the k vs ψ or $\bar{k}$ vs $\bar{\psi}$, can be directly related to the hydrophobic contact areas, ΔA_hs, of the peptides in contact with the non-polar ligands, whilst the log k_0-values are a measure of the affinities of the peptides for the reversed phase ligands. With larger polypeptides and globular proteins, on the other hand the hydrocarbonaceous surfaces can promote significant conformational changes, although not necessarily leading to completely denatured, random coil structures. These changes in conformation will affect the magnitude of the ΔA_h term. With ribonuclease (Cohen et al., 1985) or trypsin (Hearn et al., 1985; Hearn, 1998a), for example, comparison of the conformational properties of the 'surface-unfolded' molecules with the urea-unfolded structures of these proteins indicated that the 'surface-unfolded' molecules still retained a significant amount of secondary structure under some RP-HPLC conditions, although partial denaturation of these proteins had clearly occurred. Analysis of the S, log k_0 and bandbroadening (as $4\sigma_v$) dependencies of globular proteins and folded polypeptides on temperature under conditions of increasing residency times can thus be used to provide insight into the macroscopic characteristics of the interaction.

Sperm whale myoglobin (SMyo) is an oxygen carrying protein of 153 amino acid residues found in the muscle of this cetacean. In the crystalline state, the native protein forms a compact globular structure of dimensions $45 \times 35 \times 25$ Å (Kendrew et al., 1960; Takano et al., 1977), with the polypeptide backbone folded predominantly as a helical ($\sim$75%) molecule, with 8 major helical segments designated as helices A to H. The prosthetic haem group is located in a crevice near the surface of the SMyo with the haem iron directly associated with the proximal His[93] residue located in the F helix. Under acidic conditions in bulk solution, the haem moiety reversibly dissociates from the polypeptide chain (Ragone et al., 1987), accompanied by a loss in the helical content of the molecule (apo-SMyo is ~ 60% helix). This low pH unfolding process is characterised by the loss of structure around the haem binding site (Wodak and Janin, 1981; Bismuto et al., 1989) and is facilitated by a hinge-like motion (Sternlicht and Wilson, 1967) between the two domains of Myo which exist between amino acid residues 1–79 and 80–153. The RP-HPLC behaviour of the protein in phosphate-buffered or TFA-based aquo-organic solvent elution systems at pH values <7.0 with n-alkyl sorbents reflects this event, with the elution profile consistent with the presence of apo-SMyo and the free prosthetic haem group. Thus, proteins containing co-factors or prosthetic groups that can be reversibly displaced by pH- or solvent-mediated effects can be anticipated to generally show similar behaviour, under analogous RP-HPLC conditions. Typical of this type of circumstance, the retention behaviour of Myo under most RP-HPLC conditions, is essentially indistinguishable from that of apo-SMyo. Illustrative of this behaviour is the temperature dependence of the S- and log k_0-values for Myo and apo-SMyo chromatographed (Purcell et al., 1999) on a C_{18} sorbent shown in Fig. 5.16. These findings are consistent with the progressive inter-conversion of native SMyo to partially unfolded apo-SMyo species, and finally to more extended (random coil) apo-SMyo species under the RP-HPLC chromatographic conditions, involving the generation of similar ensembles of conformational intermediates for both proteins.

The tertiary structure of hen egg white lysozyme (HEWL), a 129 amino acid polypeptide with a molecular mass of 14.6 kDa, has been extensively characterised by X-ray crystallographic and NMR techniques (McDonald and Phillips, 1967; Redfield and Dobson, 1988), confirming that the tertiary structure of this protein involves two ordered domains or lobes joined by a hinge-region which contains the catalytic cleft of the enzyme. The first domain (or the A-domain) contains 4 short α-helices and a 3_{10}-helix, whilst the B-domain consists of a 3 stranded antiparallel β-sheet, a short 3_{10}-helix and a long loop region. The high thermal and pH stability of HEWL has been attributed to the 4 intra-chain disulphides which confer a compact ($45 \times 30 \times 30$ Å), roughly ellipsoid structure to this protein. Reduction of these disulphide bonds, followed by alkylation to prevent reformation of the cystine bonds, disrupts the tertiary structure of HEWL (Pfeil and Privalov, 1976).

Consequently, it can be anticipated that the RP-HPLC behaviour of HEWL and the fully reduced and alkylated HEWL should be significantly different and, in fact, this is what is observed in the presence of the n-alkyl ligands as the temperature is increased. For example, distinctly different RP-HPLC retention behaviour has been documented (Purcell et al., 1999) for HEWL and the fully reduced and alkylated HEWL when these proteins were chromatographed in the presence of a C_4 sorbent (Fig. 5.17) with native HEWL demonstrating essentially constant S- and log k_0-values as the temperature was increased from 5°C to 55°C, whilst the corresponding parameters for the fully reduced and alkylated HEWL showed considerable variations with temperature. These observations indicate that similar ensembles of interactive structures were involved for HEWL over the entire temperature range investigated with the C_4 sorbent, consistent with the relative stability of the native protein under these conditions. In contrast, the fully reduced and alkylated HEWL in the presence of the C_4 ligand demonstrated two pronounced transitions in both the S- and log k_0-values

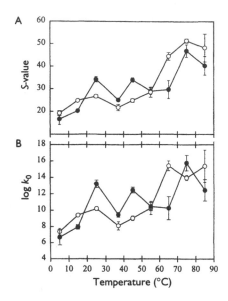

Figure 5.17 The dependence of the (A) S-values and the (B) log k_0-values of hen egg white lysozyme (○ = HEWL) and carboxymethylated hen egg white lysozyme (● = cm-HEWL) on temperature, T, with a n-octadecylsilica Bakerbond sorbent. In these experiments (Purcell et al., 1999), the elution conditions of a linear gradient of between 30 min and 90 min were employed using as the eluent a linear gradient of water-0.1% trifluoroacetic acid to acetonitrile-water-(1 : 1)-0.1% trifluoroacetic acid, pH 2.1, at temperatures ranging from 5°C through to 85°C respectively.

around 25°C and 65°C, consistent with large increases in the interactive contact area of the fully reduced and alkylated HEWL. Such observations serve to demonstrate that HEWL and carboxymethylated-HEWL can adopt different interactive structures at hydrocarbonaceous surfaces of different n-alkyl chain length.

The above studies with SMyo and HEWL indicate the features which can be expected for other globular proteins which have a relatively high level of conformational stability in their native state. In particular, such studies with model proteins, including SMyo, HEWL, α- and β-lactoglobin, ribonuclease A, or soya bean trypsin inhibitor, provide useful tests of the versatility of the experimental and theoretical approach to reliably gauge the influences of the magnitude of the residency time, the temperature optimum and the n-alkylsilica type, and adaptation to other types of polypeptides or proteins is relatively straightforward. For example, data available (Purcell et al., 1999)on the retention behaviour of HEWL in the presence of a C_{18} sorbent reveal a transition in the S and log k_0 parameters near to 55°C which is not evident with the C_4 sorbent. This information was then exploited in subsequent studies (Boysen and Hearn, 2001a) in this laboratory on the unfolding behaviour of the transcription factors, *fos* and *jun*, in the presence of similar n-alkylsilica sorbents. Observations of this kind are consistent with the conclusion that the ligand characteristics of the hydrocarbonaceous sorbent can significantly affect the chromatographic behaviour (and the interactive structure) of HEWL and other globular proteins. Molecular dynamics studies

(Yarovsky *et al.*, 1994, 1995, 1997; Klatte and Beck, 1995) have shown that at the same ligand density, the C_4 ligand is more constrained than the C_{18} ligand when immobilised onto an equivalent type of silica surface. Involvement of the head groups of this more rigid C_4 'picket fence' structure compared to the more flexible C_{18} headgroups in the interaction with HEWL may thus account for these changes in the retention parameters.

A further way that the retention dependencies of globular proteins can be investigated involves the use of species or genetically engineered protein variants. Illustrative of this approach are the observations reported (Richards *et al.*, 1994) for cytochrome c variants. Cytochrome c is a mitochondrial protein of ca. 104 amino acid residues, which folds to form a tertiary structure (Dickerson *et al.*, 1971; Gao *et al.*, 1990) with five α-helices, a small section of two stranded anti-parallel β-sheets, four type II β-turns, 2 type III β-turns and an intertwining regions of random coil structure. In all prokaryotic and eukaryotic cytochrome c, the haem iron is axially coordinated by thio-ether sulphur atom from Met[80], the imidazole nitrogen atom of His[18] and by the atoms of two other amino acid side chains. Because the haem group is covalently bonded to the main chain structure of the protein through 2 thio-ether linkages via Cys[14] and Cys[17], in RP-HPLC systems dissociation of the haem group does not occur. Various investigations (Ridge *et al.*, 1981; Nall *et al.*, 1988) on the folding of cytochrome c have confirmed that formation of transient intermediates represents crucial steps in the formation of native cytochrome c. The effects of substitution of surface accessible amino acid residue as well as other residues more buried within the internal architecture of the protein have been extensively investigated with both species variants as well as with protein variants produced by recombinant DNA techniques.

Illustrative of the approach which can be employed to examine the thermal stability of the *holo*-forms of globular proteins containing a chemically immobilised prosthetic group are the S and log k_0 results (Richards *et al.*, 1994) shown as Fig. 5.18 for equine, tuna, canine and bovine cytochrome c's chromatographed on a C_{18} sorbent. The increases noted in the S- and log k_0-values as T was increased are consistent with a progressive unfolding of both the *holo*- and *apo*-forms of this protein, with the relative differences indicative of contact area differences between the *holo*- and *apo*-cytochrome c's. Over the range of temperatures from 5–85°C, the log k vs $1/T$ plots for the equine cytochrome c at two notionally different solvent compositions were essentially linear. In contrast, other cytochrome c's, e.g. canine cytochrome c, showed more divergent, curvi-linear van't Hoff dependencies consistent with lower thermal stability. Moreover, significant differences in the S- and log k_0 values were observed between cytochrome c variants, despite a high degree of amino acid sequence homology. Examination of the 3-dimensional structures of these protein variants, provides, however, an explanation for these RP-HPLC characteristics. These molecular modelling studies suggested that specific amino acid residues are directly involved in the chromatographic contact region of the cytochrome c's when they are associated with the immobilised non-polar *n*-alkyl ligands. *In situ* limited proteolysis studies, as well a comparative data with cytochrome c's in which the distribution of the key amino residues was selectively modified, lead to similar conclusions (Boysen and Hearn, 2001a). Similar observations on the non-linear behaviour of van't Hoff dependencies have been made with insulin variants, transcription factors and polypeptide hormones such as β-endorphin, glucagon and activin-β_A (Aguilar *et al.*, 1991; Hearn, 1998a, 2000).

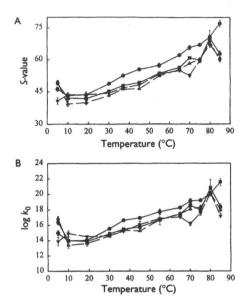

Figure 5.18 The dependence of the (A) S-values and the (B) log k_0-values of the *holo*-form of
equine (●), tuna (■), canine (▲) and bovine (▼) cytochrome c's and on temperature,
T, with a *n*-octadecylsilica Bakerbond sorbent. In these experiments (Richards *et al.*,
1994a), the elution conditions of a linear gradient of between 30 min and 120 min
were employed using as the eluent a gradient of water-0.1% trifluoroacetic acid to
50% acetonitrile-water-0.09% trifluoroacetic acid, pH 2.1, at temperatures ranging
from 5°C through to 85°C respectively.

As a general consideration, evident from the polypeptide and protein case studies
described above, non-linear van't Hoff plots of polypeptides and proteins in RP-HPLC
systems represent a relatively common occurrence. Such non-linear dependencies of
log k on $1/T$ are, from a thermodynamic perspective, usually associated with significant changes in the heat capacity of the solute-ligate complex, with the associated
changes in the enthalpy and entropy positive at low temperatures and becoming negative at high temperatures. Implicit to such behaviour is also the involvement of
extra-thermodynamic relationships, such as molecular surface area dependencies and
enthalpy-entropy compensation effects. For these reasons, experimental approaches
to extrapolated thermodynamic and molecular descriptor data based on isocratic measurements offers considerable potential. In order to place the retention behaviour which
polypeptides and proteins can manifest in RP-HPLC environments into this thermodynamic framework, the next section of this chapter thus examines in greater detail, the
origin of the non-linear van't Hoff plots with these biomacromolecules in the presence
of immobilised non-polar ligands.

Observations on the origin of the non-linear van't Hoff behaviour of
polypeptides and proteins in hydrophobic RP-HPLC environments

As discussed above, in adsorption chromatographic procedures, such as RP-HPLC, the
study of the dependencies of the retention parameters upon the experimental conditions

provides important insights into the nature of the physicochemical factors and the molecular descriptors that are associated with the interactive process(es) established between a polypeptide or protein and the immobilised chromatographic ligands. These dependencies have in the past been evaluated in terms of extra-thermodynamic or empirical relationships, frequently, as the linearised plots of the logarithmic retention factor, $\log k$, of a polypeptide or protein, P, vs the concentration, c_i, of the displacing solvent or other chemical species. The slopes of these dependencies, when linearised, are referred to as the S-value in the case of the reversed phase mode (the H-value in the case of the hydrophobic interaction mode (Hearn, 1998a, 2000, 2001) or the Z-value in the case of the ion exchange mode (Aguilar et al., 1991; Hearn 1998a, 2000) whilst the extrapolated intercept of these linearised plots as c_i 0, i.e. the corresponding $\log k_0$ values, can then be analysed in terms of relative affinity constants or linear free energy relationship terms, such as steri-molar descriptors that characterise the chromatographic properties of these biosolutes.

With n-alkylsilica-based RP-HPLC investigations with low molecular weight organic compounds and various biomacromolecules, linear elution development, i.e. near-equilibrium, chromatographic behaviour, has generally been assumed. In such cases, the influence of changes in the secondary equilibrium manifested by these solutes under the influence of the perturbing, solvated n-alkyl ligand has usually not been incorporated. Where such secondary equilibria, i.e. ionisation events or ion-pairing processes, do occur and become significant, then steps are usually taken by the investigator to ensure that only one chromatographic species is present by adjusting the mobile phase composition. In these simpler cases, the changes in the thermodynamic parameters of the separation process for a solute, i, can be depicted in terms of criteria specified by the Gibbs–Helmholtz relationship, namely:

$$\Delta G^0_{assoc,i} = \Delta H^0_{assoc,i} - T\Delta S^0_{assoc,i} \tag{11}$$

Under 'ideal' conditions, the properties of the solute, the mobile phase and the chromatographic surface are all assumed to be invariant with regard to the temperature, T. Hence, the contributions from the corresponding changes in enthalpy, $\Delta H^0_{assoc,i}$, or entropy, $\Delta S^0_{assoc,i}$, to the overall Gibbs free energy change, $\Delta G^0_{assoc,i}$, associated with the interaction of the solute i with the sorbent, as well as the phase ratio of the system, Φ, will also be independent of temperature. When such conditions prevail, the dependency of $\log k'_i$ on $1/T$ takes the form of the well known linear van't Hoff plot that have been observed experimentally with small peptides (Hearn and Grego, 1981; Hearn, 1983; Aguilar et al., 1986; Hearn and Aguilar, 1987a; Purcell et al., 1989, 1992; Lee et al., 1997; Hearn, 1998a, 2000; Hearn and Zhao, 1999). In a large number of investigations with polypeptides and proteins separated under similar RP-HPLC conditions divergencies from this ideal behaviour have, however, been detected, with the retention behaviour of these polypeptides and proteins indicative of dependencies of ΔH^0_{assoc}, ΔS^0_{assoc} and the heat capacity, C^0_p, of the system on temperature.

From Equations 10 and 11, under conditions of linear elution chromatography when the enthalpic (ΔH^0_{assoc}) and entropic (ΔS^0_{assoc}) changes associated with the retention process are independent of temperature, then $\log k'_i$, of a polypeptide and protein, P_i, can be related from fundamental thermodynamic considerations to the temperature, T, through Equation 12 As noted above, for a chromatographic system where the phase ratio, Φ, and the enthalpic or the entropic properties of the solute and the heterogeneous hydrophobic surface of the sorbent are invariant with temperature, the values of ΔH^0_{assoc} and ΔS^0_{assoc} associated with the interaction of P_i with the immobilised non-polar ligands can be derived as classical van't Hoff plots from the slope and intercept values respectively by linear regression analysis of the log k vs $1/T$ data. In the case of RP-HPLC separations with polypeptides and proteins, the extent of fit of the experimental data to the linearised form of the van't Hoff dependency thus can be used to provide insight into whether linear elution conditions prevail or whether additional factors are involved in the polypeptide (or protein) interaction with the non-polar ligand, i.e. whether, for example, destabilisation of the secondary or tertiary structure of P_i occurs under the perturbing conditions of the investigation. Moreover, detailed analysis of the log k vs $1/T$ dependencies has the potential to provide insight into whether the mechanism of the interaction of P_i with the hydrophobic surface involves the participation of additional secondary equilibrium processes which are dependent on temperature. Three situations can be contemplated for the interaction of polypeptides or proteins with an immobilised hydro-carbonaceous ligand, whereby the heat capacity, C^0_p, of the system is (i) also invariant with regard to temperature (the *isothermic* scenario); (ii) dependent on temperature, but with the constraint that the dependency of heat capacity on temperature is first order (the *homothermic* scenario); or (iii) non-linearly dependent on temperature (the *heterothermic* scenario).

In the bulk state, the heat capacity C^0_p of a substance is usually defined as the quantity of heat necessary to raise the temperature of a unit mass of the substance by one degree Kelvin. Analogous considerations can be applied to ligate-ligand systems, such as a polypeptide interacting with a n-alkyl ligand, provided the state characteristics of the complex can be defined. Under these conditions, when a unit mass of the ligate-ligand complex initially in a state defined by P, V and T undergoes a small change defined by P, V and T then a change in a particular parameter or quantity, U, associated with the ligate-ligand interaction may be represented by the equations of state as a function of P, V and T such that

$$\Delta U = \frac{\partial U}{\partial P}\Delta P + \frac{\partial U}{\partial V}\Delta V + \frac{\partial U}{\partial T}\Delta T \tag{27}$$

where P is the pressure (in Pascal units), V is the molar volume and T is the absolute temperature in degree Kelvin.

Accordingly, the change in the internal energy, E, of the system can be written in terms of the change in entropy, S, by the perfect differential

$$dE = TdS - PdV \tag{28}$$

where

$$\left(\frac{\partial E}{\partial S}\right)_V = T \tag{29}$$

$$\left(\frac{\partial E}{\partial V}\right)_S = -P \tag{30}$$

and

$$\left(\frac{\partial T}{\partial V}\right)_S = -\left(\frac{\partial P}{\partial S}\right)_V \tag{31}$$

Similarly, the enthalpy, H, of the system can be defined in terms of the internal energy, E, such that

$$H = E + PV \tag{32}$$

or

$$dH = TdS + VdP \tag{33}$$

and hence

$$\left(\frac{\partial T}{\partial P}\right)_S = \left(\frac{\partial V}{\partial S}\right)_P \tag{34}$$

The heat capacity, C_p^0, for a polypeptide-non-polar ligand system can be expressed according to the Kirchoff's relationships as:

$$C_{p,i}^0 = T\partial S_{assoc,i}^0/\partial T \tag{35}$$

where

$$\Delta S_{assoc}^0 = \int \frac{\Delta C_p^0}{T} dT \tag{36}$$

and

$$C_p^0 = \partial H_{assoc}^0/\partial T \tag{37}$$

where

$$\Delta H_{assoc}^0 = \int \Delta C_p^0 dT \tag{38}$$

and

$$C_p^0 \partial T = \partial E + P\partial V - \mu\partial\mu \tag{39}$$

where E represents the incremental difference in the internal energy of the system. According to Equation 39, C_p^0 is related to the change in the standard enthalpy and the standard pressure-volume product (PV) terms, whilst the term μ takes into account contributions from processes not defined by the criteria of Stefan–Boltzman–Maxwell laws. If the interaction of the polypeptide or protein, P_i, with the immobilised ligands satisfies these criteria, i.e. no effects other than standard changes in P, V and T are involved, then Equation 39 becomes

$$C_p^0 \partial T = \partial E + P\partial V \tag{40}$$

and hence

$$C_p^0 \partial T = \partial H_{assoc}^0 - \partial(PV) + P\partial V \tag{41}$$

or

$$C_p^0 \partial T = \partial H_{assoc}^0 - V\partial P \tag{42}$$

Evaluations of the interaction of P_i with the immobilised hydrocarbonaceous ligands in terms of Equations 35–42, however, do not represent complete descriptions of the binding process, because the condition(s) under which the thermal energy of the system is increased has not been specified. If the heat capacity of the system is increased under the conditions of constant pressure, P, then. Equation 42 can be simplified and the specific heat capacity at constant pressure can be defined in terms of Equation 43 as follows:

$$C_p^0 \partial T = (\partial H_{assoc})_p \qquad (43)$$

or

$$C_p^0 = (\partial H_{assoc}/\partial T)_p \qquad (44)$$

In addition, the equilibrium association constant, K_{assoc}, for the interaction of P_i with the hydrophobic surface of the sorbent is a function of temperature, with the dependency represented in the form:

$$K_{assoc} = e^{-\Delta G_{assoc}^0/RT} \qquad (45)$$

where the value of the Gibbs free energy change for the interaction, ΔG_{assoc}^0 is a function of temperature only. By substituting and rearranging the relevant terms of Equation 45, the following dependency can be derived:

$$\partial \left(\log K_{assoc}\right) = -1/R \; x \left(\left(T \; x \; \partial G_{assoc}^0/\partial T\right)/T^2\right) \qquad (46)$$

Following substitution with Equation 11, Equation 46 can be arranged such that

$$\partial \log K_{assoc}/\partial T = H_{assoc}^0/RT^2 \qquad (47)$$

Since the equilibrium association constant, K_{assoc}, for the interaction of a polypeptide, P_i, with a solvated hydrocarbonaceous n-alkyl ligand is related to the capacity factor through the relationship:

$$K_{assoc} = \Phi \; x \; k' \qquad (48)$$

thence

$$\partial \log k'/\partial T = H_{assoc}^0/RT^2 \qquad (49)$$

In adsorption situations in which ΔH_{assoc}^0 is invariant with temperature, i.e. under binding conditions whereby over a range of temperatures the value of ΔH_{assoc}^0 does not vary appreciably, then the following expression is obtained:

$$\log k' = -\Delta H_{assoc}^0/RT + I \qquad (50)$$

with the term I incorporating contributions from both the entropic and the phase ratio terms in the form $I = \Delta S_{assoc}^0 + \log \Phi$. If changes in phase ratio and entropy are also assumed (or found) to be independent of temperature, then the plots of $\log k$ vs $1/T$ will generate a straight line, typical of classical van't Hoff plots. In all other cases where a temperature dependency exists, non-linear plots of $\log k$ vs $1/T$ will occur. As evident from the data shown in Fig. 5.2 for bovine insulin, a 51-mer polypeptide, as well as for the examples of β-endorphin, neuropeptide Y, and even the relatively small polypeptides such as bombesin or glucagon discussed elsewhere in this chapter, such non-classical behaviour occurs with polypeptides, whereby ΔH^0_{assoc}, ΔS^0_{assoc} and log Φ are dependent on temperature, and the plots of log k vs $1/T$ do not follow linear dependencies. According to Kirchoff's relationships, if the heat capacity is invariant with temperature, then the dependency of the ΔH^0_{assoc} and ΔS^0_{assoc} contributions on temperature can be expressed as

$$\Delta H^0_{assoc} = \Delta C^0_p (T - T_H) \tag{51}$$

and

$$\Delta S^0_{assoc} = \Delta C^0_p \log (T/T_s) \tag{52}$$

where the T_H and T_S refer to the temperatures at which ΔH^0_{assoc} 0 and ΔS^0_{assoc} 0 respectively. When such temperature invariant heat capacity conditions occur, then the dependency of log k on temperature can be approximated by the logarithmic expression,

$$\log k' = \frac{\Delta C^0_p}{R} \left(\frac{T_H}{T} - \log \frac{T_s}{T} - 1 \right) + \log \Phi \tag{53}$$

On the other hand, when temperature-dependent heat capacity conditions prevail, then the dependency of log k on temperature can be more appropriately approximated (Vailaya and Horvath, 1996a,b) by a polynomial expression as represented by Equation 54, i.e.

$$\log k' = a + b(1/T) + c(1/T)^2 + d(1/T)^3 + \ldots + \log \Phi \tag{54}$$

Hence,

$$\partial \log k'/\partial T = (\partial \log k'/\partial(1/T)) x (\partial(1/T)/\partial T) \tag{55}$$

and thus

$$\log k_i/T = -(1/T)^2 x \left(b + 2c(1/T) + 3d(1/T)^2 + \ldots \right) \tag{56}$$

In these homothermic and the heterothermic scenarios, the change in enthalpy can be thus represented by

$$\Delta H^0_{assoc} = -R x \left(b + 2c(1/T) + 3d(1/T)^2 + \ldots \right) \tag{57}$$

whilst the change in heat capacity can be represented as

$$\Delta C^0_p = \partial \Delta H^0_{assoc}/\partial T \tag{58}$$

$$= m/(T)^2 + n/(T)^3 + \ldots \tag{59}$$

where $m = 2Rc$ and $n = 6Rd$, etc.

As noted by Vailaya and Horvath (1996a,b) for low molecular weight compounds, such as dansyl amino acids, when non-linear plots of log k vs $1/T$ are observed, then

$\log k$ will reach a maximal value at the temperature corresponding to T_H since the slope of the plots of $\log k_i$ vs $1/T$ at any temperature is proportional to the ΔH^0_{assoc} value at that temperature. Analogous situations appear to prevail with polypeptides and proteins in RP-HPLC systems. Given that the slope of the plot of ΔG^0_{assoc} vs T at a given temperature is determined by the ΔS^0_{assoc} value at that temperature, then in the homothermic and the heterothermic situations ΔG^0_{assoc} is also predicted to reach a maximal value at T_S. From Equations 50–58, the parameters ΔC^0_p, T_H and T_S corresponding to isothermic, homothermic and heterothermic interaction processes for polypeptides and proteins in the presence of lipophilic ligands can in principle be evaluated from the non-linear van't Hoff plots using non-linear least squares regression and associated curve fitting procedures.

Illustrative of the above considerations are the plots of $\log k$ vs ψ (acetonitrile) for bovine insulin shown in Fig. 5.20. These data were determined (Boysen *et al.*, 1999) from isocratic measurements obtained over the ψ-range of $0.26 < \psi < 0.31$ and with temperatures from 5°C to 65°C in 5°C increments respectively. In Figs 5.19 and 5.20 are shown the corresponding three-dimensional grid plots for the S- and $\log k_0$-values for bovine insulin, as the temperature and the ψ-values were varied. Again, the trend expected for a prevailing retention mechanism based on hydrophobic interactions for the polypeptide binding to the immobilised non-polar ligand was evident with the $\log k$ values decreasing as the ψ-values were increased.

The curvilinear behaviour evident in the van't Hoff plot analysis of bovine insulin Fig. 5.20 can be contrasted with the retention data for the polypeptide

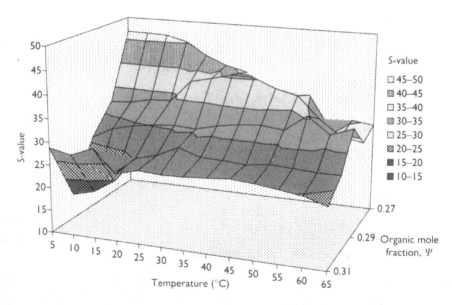

Figure 5.19 The dependence of the S-values of bovine insulin on temperature, T, and the mole fraction of organic modifier, ψ, determined with a n-octadecylsilica Bakerbond sorbent. In these experiments (Boysen et al., 2002), isocratic elution conditions were employed encompassing the range of ψ-values from $0.3 < \psi < 0.40$ using water-0.1% trifluoroacetic acid eluents adjusted to the correct ψ-value with acetonitrile.

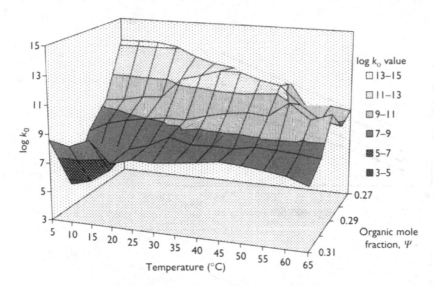

Figure 5.20 The dependence of the log k_0-values of bovine insulin on temperature, T, and the mole fraction of organic modifier, ψ, determined with a n-octadecylsilica Bakerbond sorbent. In these experiments (Boysen *et al.*, 2001), isocratic elution conditions were employed encompassing the range of ψ-values from $0.3 < \psi < 0.40$ using water-0.1% trifluoroacetic acid eluents adjusted to the correct ψ-value with acetonitrile.

pair, L-α-DDALYDDKNWDRAPQRCYYQ (A) and its retro-all D-α-QYYC-RQPARDWNKDDYLADD isomer (B) also determined as a function of temperature and organic solvent content under similar RP-HPLC conditions (Fig. 5.21, where in the case of these two 20-mer polypeptides essentially linear van't Hoff plot features were evident. Although these two polypeptides are composed of the same amino acid residues, polypeptide B involves a reversal of the direction of the amino acid sequence, but an inversion of the chirality at the α-carbon atom of each residue. Polypeptide B can thus assume a similar topological shape in solution as polypeptide A, although polypeptide A and B exhibit mirror image CD spectra (Boysten *et al.*, 2001). As confirmed by molecular modelling, CD and 2D-nuclear magnetic resonance investigations (Higgins *et al.*, 1997; Boysen *et al.*, 2001), polypeptides A and B exhibit similar α-helicity in these lipophilic environments, but readily generate random coil structures at relatively low temperatures. Compared to the RP-HPLC retention behaviour of these two 20-mer peptides, the variations in the log k values of bovine insulin b-chain were much less regular as the temperature was increased. This behaviour was manifested as cross-over transitions in the log k vs ψ plots, suggesting that the mechanism of the polypeptide-sorbent interaction was not conserved at different temperatures.

Support for this conclusion with insulin related polypeptides was reinforced following determination of the extra-thermodynamic parameters, S- and log k_0. Significant changes were found to occur (Boysen *et al.*, 1999; Hearn *et al.*, 1998) with both the S- and log k_0-values for bovine insulin b-chain and the intact bovine insulin molecule, as the temperature was varied from 5°C to 65°C, with these changes not proceeding in a monotonously regular fashion. Moreover, as the organic solvent content, ψ, was

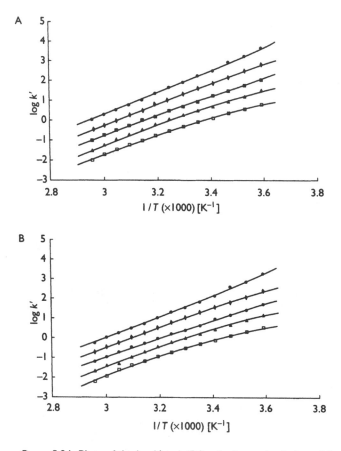

Figure 5.21 Plots of the log k' vs $1/T$ for the isocratic elution of the 20-mer polypeptide pair, L-α-DDALYDDKNWDRAPQRCYYQ (A) and D-α-QYYCRQPARDWNKDDYLADD (B), at different organic modifier concentrations on a *n*-butylsilica Bakerbond wide pore sorbent using acetonitrile-water-0.1% trifluoroacetic acid mobile phase conditions. Data was taken from Boysen *et al.*, 1999, 2001; Boysen and Hearn, 2001b. The code for the different mobile phase compositions used in this investigation is as follows: ●, 17%; ▼, 18%; ■, 19%; ▲, 20%; □, 21% respectively.

increased, decreases in the S- and log k_0-values for these polypeptides also occurred. At the lower temperatures, minimum values for the S- and log k_0-values were reached at specific acetonitrile concentrations, ψ_{min}s, with the value of ψ_{min} depending on the temperature. Studies with other insulin-related polypeptides eluted at different temperatures from similar RP-HPLC sorbents under linear gradient conditions with eluents of similar composition to those employed in these isocratic investigations have also lead to similar observations of temperature-dependent changes in the derived S- and log k_0-values (Purcell *et al.*, 1992; Hearn *et al.*, 1999; Sitaram *et al.*, 1999; Wang *et al.*, 1998), although the magnitudes of these changes in the isocratic investigations were found to be considerably larger. Presumably, these variations in the S vs T and log k_0 vs T dependencies of polypeptides, as revealed by bovine insulin b-chain, are reflecting fundamental differences between the adsorption and desorption processes which

Table 5.2 Correlation coefficient, r^2

ψ ACN	Regression order 2				Regression order 3				
	a	b	c	r^2	a	b	c	d	r^2
0.31	15.4	7.46	0.82	0.9502	−523.27	488.26	−150.91	15.45	0.9966
0.30	6.35	1.45	−0.12	0.9527	−534.44	496.22	−152.44	15.51	0.9953
0.29	0.84	2.43	−0.73	0.9583	−554.95	513.90	−157.28	15.94	0.9985
0.28	1.39	2.79	−0.82	0.9654	−543.88	504.58	−154.41	15.64	0.9972
0.27	−23.12	18.27	−3.18	0.9432	−753.74	690.64	−208.98	20.95	0.9986
0.26	−28.60	21.44	−3.55	0.9258	−627.86	572.92	−172.35	17.18	0.9939

Data for the degree of fit of the isocratically derived experimental data for bovine insulin to the isothermic, homothermic and heterothermic models for the retention of this polypetide to a n-octadecylisilica sorbent, determined at different ψ-values over the range of $0.26 < \psi < 0.31$ respectively. The coefficients of the homothermic and heterothermic relationships implicit to Equations 50–59 for the $\log k'$ vs $1/T$ dependencies of bovine insulin were as follows: 1st order: $\log k' = b(1/T) + a$; 2nd order: $\log k' = c(1/T)^2 + b(1/T) + a$, 3rd order: $\log k' = d(1/T)^3 + c(1/T)^2 + b(1/T) + a$. The corresponding correlation coefficients, r^2, for the 1st order isothermic relationship were: for $\psi = 0.31$: 0.9457, for $\psi = 0.30$: 0.9526, for $\psi = 0.29$: 0.9554, for $\psi = 0.28$: 0.9624, for $\psi = 0.27$: 0.8993, and for $\psi = 0.26$: 0.8257 respectively.

occur with this polypeptide, as well as other polypeptides and proteins, which also show non-linear van't Hoff plot relationships, under the isocratic and gradient elution modes.

The pronounced curvilinear nature of the plots of $\log k$ vs $1/T$ for bovine insulin (Fig. 5.20), determined from the isocratically derived data at different ψ-values, is particularly evident with the profiles reaching maxima that were dependent on both temperature and solvent composition. The extent of correlation of the experimental data to a second order and third order model, characteristic of the homothermic and heterothermic models (Boysen and Hearn, 2001a) is shown in Table 5.2. Also shown in Table 5.2 is the degree of fit of the data to the logarithmic form of the $\log k$ vs $1/T$ dependency, i.e. the degree of fit of the experimental data in terms of Equations 50–58. The characteristic shapes of these van't Hoff plots for bovine insulin (as well as other polypeptides or proteins which exhibit similar non-linear van't Hoff dependencies) can thus be interpreted in terms of Kirchoff's relationships, and the values of the respective coefficients a, b, c, d, ... of Equation 54 derived. Representative values for these coefficients bovine insulin are also given in Table 5.2.

The conclusion can be reached from comparison of the fitted parameters derived from Equations 52 and 53 that both expressions correlate well with the experimental data for bovine insulin under these specific chromatographic conditions. It can also be noted that Equation 52 yields the average value of ΔC_p^0 and Equation 53 yields the mean value of ΔC_p^0 vs $1/T$ at different solvent compositions. From the ΔG_{assoc}^0 vs T plots, ΔG_{assoc}^0 reaches a maximal value at the temperature corresponding to T_S, thus permitting this key transition temperature for the change in the binding structure of bovine insulin in these different solvent compositions to be derived. Based on these considerations, plots of ΔC_p^0 vs T can be generated for polypeptides and proteins in these RP-HPLC systems. In the case of bovine insulin non-linear dependencies were observed (Boysen et al., 1999; Hearn et al., 1999; Wang et al., 1998) between ΔC_p^0 and T, consistent with the participation of a heterothermic process for the interaction of this polypeptide with the n-octylsilica in the different aquo-acetonitrile environments. It is also interesting to note that these heat capacity changes were negative, as was also found to be the case for the changes in free energy, the latter observation consistent with a thermodynamically favourable process for the interaction of the polypeptide with the sorbent. Furthermore, these data clearly indicated that both the enthalpy and entropy of the interaction for polypeptides with non-polar sorbents under different iso-cratic elution conditions can have a strong temperature dependency. For example, at low temperatures both the enthalpy and entropy changes for bovine insulin are posi-tive, decrease with increasing temperature and at high temperatures become negative. Dansyl amino acids have also been found (Vailaya and Horvath, 1996a) to exhibit a similar pattern of dependencies.

The consequences of the types of thermodynamic behaviour that is manifested by the 20-mer polypeptides, A and B, or by the insulin-related polypeptides, (as well as the other examples discussed in this chapter) are clearly very important, since such manifestations underpin the so-called enthalpy-entropy compensation effect (Lumry and Rajender, 1970; Krug et al., 1976; Melander et al., 1978; Everett, 1983). Moreover, such observations have an important bearing on the interpretation of the molecular pro-cesses associated with the surface-induced conformational changes that can be readily observed experimentally in RP-HPLC systems, but which have only previously been empirically enunciated in extra-thermodynamic terms with polypeptides and globular proteins in the perturbing environment of the reversed phase sorbent. Importantly, the approach described above provides both a theoretical and an experimental framework to explore the role of molecular descriptors and conformational effects in reversed phase systems with biomacro-molecules and thus to gain greater insight into the nature of the hydrophobic effect itself.

Bandwidth dependencies and the participation of interconverting intermediates of polypeptides and proteins in dynamic RP-HPLC systems

When a polypeptide or protein undergoes conformational changes in a RP-HPLC envi-ronment, several fundamental processes or considerations must arise. Firstly, for the conformers to be resolvable and become evident as broadened, asymmetric or discrete peak shapes, the interconversion rate constants (i.e. the $t_{1/2}s$ must be slower or of a similar time scale as the mass transport events (i.e. t_Rs) associated with the chromato-graphic migration and the detector time constant. Secondly, when such conformational equilibria are manifested, it is obvious that the peak capacities (PCs) of the RP-HPLC system will be very responsive to changes in flow rate, particle size of the non-polar sor-bent, relative retention, time of residency of the polypeptide or protein on the sorbent, and particularly the surface interaction kinetics ($k_{int}s$) associated with the binding and desorption of the interconverting species from the hydrocarbonaceous sorbent. These dependencies can be descriptively expressed through the relationships:

$$PC = \Delta t_R / 4\sigma_V \tag{60}$$

$$PC = \frac{\log 10}{4} \left[\frac{S\Delta\psi k^{0.25}}{Fd_p} \right] \left[\frac{D_m t_0}{C} \right]^{0.5} \tag{61}$$

where Δt_R is the difference in separation time, $4\sigma_V$ is the peak width, F is the flow rate, d_p is the particle size of the sorbent, D_m is the diffusion coefficient of the biosolute, t_0

is the void volume of the packed chromatographic column, assuming that the extra-column dead volume is negligible, and C is the Knox parameter which accommodates the resistance to mass transfer at the stationary phase surface and is directly relate to k_{int}s.

When no secondary equilibria occur, Equation 61 predicts that the plots of PC vs $[k]^{0.25}/[C]^{0.5}$ should be linear for a specific chromatographic system of known F, d_p and t_0. In contrast, when the contact area of the biosolute changes, i.e. when the S-values are not constant, and/or when the k_{int}s for the biosolute-ligand interaction do not involve a first order rate equation, then curvilinear dependencies of PC on $[k]^{0.25}/[C]^{0.5}$ are predicted. Studies with myosin related peptide (Hearn and Aguilar, 1987a), β-endorphin analogues (Aguilar et al., 1985, 1996) and other proteins, e.g. fos and jun (Boysen and Hearn, 2001a), have confirmed these predictions. Illustrative of the changes in peak capacity which can arise under such RP-HPLC conditions are the data for β-endorphin shown in Fig. 5.22. Thus, the presence or absence of bandwidth changes, as revealed from changes in the peakwidth at $4\sigma_V$ or peak capacity PC, provides a very useful measure of the constancy of the molecular shape as the polypeptide or protein migrates

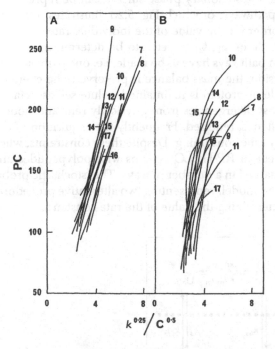

Figure 5.22 Plot (A) shows the peak capacity (PC) vs $[k]^{0.25}/[C]^{0.5}$ determined according to Equation 60 for a series of β-endorphin related polypeptides (7–17), and in plot (B) the corresponding PC dependency on $[\bar{k}']^{0.25}/[C]^{0.5}$ determined from gradient retention data with a n-octadecylsilica sorbent. Data selected from Hearn and Aguilar, 1987a. The elution conditions involved gradients from 20 min through 120 min using a water-0.1% trifluoroacetic acid to 50% acetonitrile-water-0.1% trifluoroacetic acid mobile phases at 20°C. The amino acid sequences of these peptides/polypeptides were as follows: 7, GGFM; 8, GGFMT; 9, GGFMTS; 10, GGFMTSE; 11, GGFMTSEK; 12, GGFMTSEKSQ; 13, GGFMTSEKSQTP; 14, GGFMTSEKSQTPLVT; 15, GGFMTSEKSQTPLVTL; 16, GGFMTSEKSQTPLVTLF; 17, GGFMTSEKSQTPLVTLFK.

down a RP-HPLC chromatographic bed. In this context, RP-HPLC procedures are more discriminatory than high performance size exclusion chromatography (HPSEC) for the recognition of conformational transitions with polypeptides or proteins, although the latter procedure has been employed in a number of investigations for this purpose (Corbett and Roche, 1984; Shalongo *et al.*, 1989). Moreover, the changes in $4\sigma_V$ and *PC*, which become evident when conformational changes ensue in a RP-HPLC system, provide a basis to examine the resultant changes in the diffusion coefficients (Snyder, 1980; Hearn and Aguilar, 1986) for the 'native' as well as the 'unfolded' species within these non-polar environments.

The simplest scenario that can be envisaged when a polypeptide or protein unfolds within the lipophilic environment of an immobilised *n*-alkylsilica sorbent involves the participation of a native state, *N*, and an unfolded state, *U*, with the intermediacy of a number of transition states, $I_1, I_2, \ldots$ etc., which may or may not correspond to the same molten globule intermediate(s) as observed in the bulk solvent. Similar scenarios can be written for the case whereby a polypeptide or protein becomes more stabilised in terms of its conformation when it binds to a non-polar stationary phase. These inter-conversions within the mobile and at the stationary phase surface can be represented in terms of a variety of descriptive pathways, of which Fig. 5.23. illustrates one case. It is important to recognise that in order for the value of the individual rate constants to be measured, e.g. for the magnitude of $k_{12}, k_{21}, \ldots$ etc., to be determined, certain assumptions inherent to the retention pathways have to be made, i.e. one pathway represents the rate limiting interconversion, the mass balance is preserved, the chemical structural integrity of the polypeptide or protein is maintained, solute self-association does not occur, etc. To minimise gross divergencies from physically relevant models, complementary data may be, and often is, required. Frequently the acquisition of this independent information can be very time consuming. Despite these constraints, when conformational interconversions occur in RP-HPLC systems with polypeptides and proteins, these processes can be formalised in a number of ways. The 'stochastic probability model' and the 'chemical reactor' model, representing two alternative procedures to achieve analytical solutions for determining the value of the rate constants.

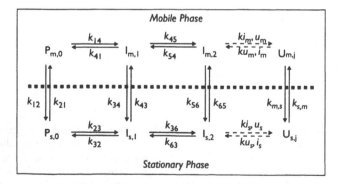

Figure 5.23 Schematic for the interconversion of a polypeptide or protein, P, in a native state (*N*), an unfolded state (*U*) or in partial folded states ($I_1, I_2, I_3, \ldots, I_n$) in the presence of a polar mobile phase and a non-polar stationary phase. The individual forward and reverse rate constants for the interconversion between the free and the bound species are shown as k_{ij} and k_{ji} respectively.

In the case of the stochastic model (Keller and Giddings, 1960; Hearn *et al.*, 1985; Hearn, 1986) the fraction of the time that each species, N, U or I_1, I_2, ..., spends in one form can be represented by a time increment, t, with the probability that this species exists in the range $t + \Delta t$ given by $P(t)$. Thus, if the polypeptide or protein molecular starts in the state $P_{N,m'}$, the probability that after one cycle of interconversions it can still be found in the state $P_{N,m}$ can be represented for a four state system by:

$$P_{N,m}^1 dt = [r_1 r_2 (1 - t)/t] \exp[-r_1(1 - t) - r_2 t] I [4r_1 r_2 (1 - t)]^{0.5} t \qquad (62)$$

where

$$r_1 = (\Phi k_{12} k_{23} + k_{14} k_{21}) tR/k_{21} \qquad (63)$$

$$r_2 = (\Phi k_{32} k_{43} + k_{34} k_{41}) tR/k_{34} \qquad (64)$$

$$I = \frac{\exp 2[r_1 r_2 (1 - t)]^{1/2}}{4\pi^{1/2} [r_1 r_2 (1 - t)]^{3/4}} \qquad (65)$$

and t is the separation time.

At a separation time of $t = 0$, a mixture of conformers corresponding to the polypeptide or protein in its native state, $P_{N,0}$, its fully unfolded state, $P_{U,0}$, and its partially folded state, $P_{I,0}$, will be introduced into the chromatographic system. Overall, the ratio of $P_{N,0}$ and $P_{U,0}$ will then change according to whether destabilisation or stabilisation of the conformation ensues until the separation time is finalised, i.e. until a point in the normalised time is reached where $t = 1$. Under conditions of relatively rapid interconversion between $P_{N,0}$ and $P_{U,0}$, i.e. where conditions of relatively rapid adsorption/desorption kinetics and high mass recovery prevail, the overall concentration profile for the migration of the conformer mixture can be represented as the sum of the probability functions, properly weighted for the fraction a and b of $P_{N,0}$ and $P_{U,0}$ present in the mixture at time $t = 0$, i.e.

$$P(t) = a \left[P_1^1(t) + P_1^4(t) \right] + b \left[P_4^1(t) + P_4^4(t) \right] \qquad (66)$$

$$P(t = 0) = a \exp(-r_1) \qquad (67)$$

$$P(t = 1) = b \exp(-r_2) \qquad (68)$$

If it is assumed that the species P_N and P_U migrate as Gaussian peak zones, and their diffusion constants D_ms) are the same or very similar, then the concentration profiles for the polypeptide or protein species can be derived since both $P(t = 0)$ and $P(t = 1)$ become discrete functions, and the peaks are separated by the incremental time Δt. Experimental data for the changes in bandshape as a function of flow rate and residency time of several globular proteins, e.g. bovine trypsin or α-lactoglobin, show good correlation to the predictions (Hearn *et al.*, 1985) derived from this stochastic model when relatively simply interconversion pathways are involved. In more complex cases, such as when cooperative or non-cooperative inter-conversions occur as part of a multi-step conformational process, the current procedural difficulties in either measuring the individual rate constants of the accompanying non-Gaussian peakshapes, or the sparsity of sufficient experimental data to enable reliable curve fitting routines to be employed, can result in a number of conceptual and computational challenges with the application of the stochastic probability model which limit its usefulness.

The 'chemical reactor' model addresses some of these limitations by treating the process of conformational interconversion as a reversible 'chemical reaction'. Expressions can then be derived (Jacobsen et al., 1984; Melander et al., 1984; Henderson and Horvath, 1986; Hearn, 2001) which enable the first and second moments of the elution profile to be obtained. Illustrative of this approach, is the expression shown as Equation 69 for the resolution of the species P_N and P_U reversibly migrating along a reversed phase column, whereby:

$$R_S = \frac{t_0 \Phi (k_{12}/k_{21} - k_{43}/k_{34})(1 - eD_a)}{4(\sigma_1 + \sigma_2)} \tag{69}$$

and

$$D_a = \frac{L(\Phi k_{12} k_{23} + k_{14} k_{21})(k_{14} + k_{41})}{(k_{14} k_{21}) u_0} \tag{70}$$

where Φ is the phase ratio, k_{ij} are the respective rate constants for adsorption, desorption and interconversion, σ_i is the peak widths of the component i, L is the column length, u_0 is the linear velocity of the mobile phase and D_a, the so-called Damkohler parameter, represents the ratio of the time taken for the polypeptide or protein species to migrate along the column in the mobile phase to the relaxation time for the conformational interconversions in the same chromatographic RP-HPLC system. When the Damkohler parameter is very large or very small, i.e. when $D_a > 1000$ or $D_a < 0.001$, only a single peak zone will be in evidence, corresponding either to the native or to the unfolded species respectively. However, in the intermediate range of $0.1 \leq D_a \leq 10$, the elution profile will assume a much more complex appearance, with asymmetric or badly skewed peak zones, multiple peak envelops or even fully base-line resolved peaks of the same notional molecular composition but different conformational status and retention time. The extent that this latter scenario occurs will be conditional on the nature of the equilibrium distribution of the various conformational species of the polypeptide or protein, the chromatographic efficiency of the system, the temperature of the separation and the characteristics of the other chromatographic parameters selected. As noted below, appropriate presentation and analysis of the experimental data can provide very useful and comparative insights into the relative conformational stability of different polypeptides and proteins in various RP-HPLC environments or the propensity of various polypeptides to assume a preferred conformation in the presence of non-polar ligands.

A codicil which arises from the use of the stochastic as well as the 'chemical reactor' models, is that the interconversion of a native form of a polypeptide or protein to an unfolded form will involve the participation of one or more transition state intermediates (cf Fig. 5.23). As a consequence, a modified form of the Eyring transition state model (Laidler, 1978; Jensen et al., 1997) can be applied to evaluate the conformational kinetics for this interconversion at a specific temperature when the various ensembles of conformers form discernible chromatographic peaks. Thus, at each temperature, the rate of interconversion of species P to species I or from species I to species U can be determined from the relationship

$$\log \left[A_0/A_t \right] = k_i t \tag{71}$$

where A_0 and A_t are the peak areas of the polypeptide or protein species in state $N, I_1, I_2, \ldots$, or U at time $t = 0$ and $t = t + \Delta t$, and k_i is the pseudo-first order rate constant for the overall interconversion. According to the Eyring transition state model (Jensen et al., 1997; Laidler, 1978; Hearn and Zhao, 1999), the slope of the plot of $\log k_i$ vs $1/T$ is related to the standard enthalpy of activation, $\Delta H_{int}^{\ddagger}$, for the interconversion, i.e.

$$\partial (\log k_i)/\partial (1/T) = - \left(\Delta H_{int}^{\ddagger} + RT \right)/R \tag{72}$$

whilst the standard free energy change of activation, $\Delta G_{int}^{\ddagger}$ and the standard entropy of activation $\Delta S_{int}^{\ddagger}$ for the interconversion of the polypeptide or protein between different conformational states can be calculated from the relationships:

$$\Delta G_{int}^{\ddagger} = -RT \log \left(\bar{h} ki/k_B T \right) \tag{73}$$

$$\Delta G_{int}^{\ddagger} = \Delta H_{int}^{\ddagger} - T \Delta S_{int}^{\ddagger} \tag{74}$$

where R is the Gas constant, h is Planck's constant and k_B is the Boltzmann constant. As a consequence, determination of the gradient of the plots of the logarithmic fractional area of individual conformer species versus the residency time, and the slope of the plots of $\log k_i$ vs $1/T$ permits the kinetic basis of the multi-zoning events to be quantitatively evaluated.

Multizoning behaviour of the type described above has previously been documented for bovine insulin (Hearn, 1998a; Sitaram et al., 1999), trypsin (Hearn et al., 1985), small peptides and several other intermediate molecular weight polypeptides and proteins (Cohen et al., 1984a,b, 1985; Aguilar et al., 1985, 1986; Hearn et al., 1985; Lu et al., 1986; Hearn and Aguilar, 1987a; Benedek, 1988; Hearn et al., 1988; Grinberg et al.,1989; Lin and Karger, 1990; Oroszlan et al., 1990, 1992; Purcell et al., 1993; Richards et al., 1994; Boysen et al., 2001, 2002; Hearn et al., 1999; Purcell et al., 1999; Sitaram et al., 1999; Wang et al., 1998) at 25°C under certain RP-HPLC conditions. The following examples on the changes in peakwidth behaviour for β-endorphin, sperm wahale myoglobin (SMyo)/apomyoglobin (apo-SMyo)and hen egg white lysozyme (HEWL) in RP-HPLC systems as the temperature and residency time are varied further illustrate (Aguilar et al., 1985, 1986; Purcell et al., 1992, 1993, 1999; Hearn and Zhao, 1999) the above kinetic considerations. The polypeptide, β-endorphin, can be again used to provide (Aguilar et al., 1985, 1986; Purcell et al., 1993) an interesting example of the pronounced dependencies which amphipathic polypeptides can manifest in terms of their bandbroadening behaviour in the presence of n-alkyl ligands of different chain length. In Figs 5.24a and b show the dependence of the experimental bandwidth on temperature and residence time for β-endorphin chromatographed on two different RP-HPLC sorbents (C_{18} and C_4 respectively) of similar n-alkyl ligand density. In the case of the C_{18} sorbent, β-endorphin exhibited a relatively planar temperature dependency over

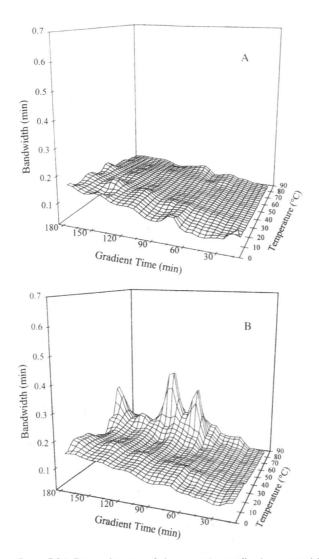

Figure 5.24 Dependencies of the experimentally determined bandbroadening for β-endorphin on temperature, *T*, and residency time, t_T, when chromatographed on a n-octadecyl Bakerbond sorbent (A) or a n-butyl Bakerbond sorbent (B). Data taken from Purcell *et al.*, 1993.

the range of residency times examined. In contrast with the C_4 sorbent, β-endorphin showed a much more complex profile in terms of bandbroadening changes as the temperature and residency time were systematically varied. As noted above, β-endorphin is known to assume an amphipathic α-helical structure in the presence of non-polar ligands, with β-endorphin analogues with intact C-terminal sequences displaying a greater propensity for assuming this secondary structure than shorter peptides such as α-endorphin. This secondary structure propensities is illustrated in the helix probability profile (Mattice *et al.*, 1981) and the Edmundsen wheel projections shown as Figs 5.25 and 5.26.

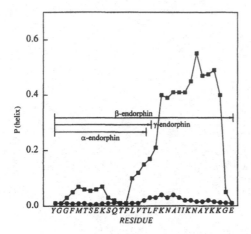

Based on these results, associated experimental data on the receptor specificities (Dill, 1987; Dorsey and Dill, 1989), and spectroscopic studies demonstrating that β-endorphin exists largely as a random coil structure in aqueous buffers, but assumes a defined helical structure in the presence of acetonitrile, methanol or lipid-like compounds such as dode-cylsulphate, the conclusion has been drawn by a number of investigators (Mattice and Robinson, 1981; Wu *et al.*, 1981; Janssen *et al.*, 1984; Aguilar *et al.*, 1985, 1986; Taylor and Kaiser, 1986; Purcell *et al.*, 1992) that β-endorphin undergoes surface-associated conformational changes in the presence of the *n*-alkyl and other non-polar ligands. Because the bandbroadening behaviour of β-endorphin in the presence of the C_{18} lig-and remained largely invariant over the temperature range of 5–85°C, yet showed (Purcell *et al.*, 1993) substantial changes in the presence of the C_4 ligand under the same chromatographic conditions, these differences again highlight the effects that can be achieved when a collapsed droplet-like non-polar stationary phase surface (character-istic of the C_{18}-type of RP-HPLC sorbents) versus a picket-fence non-polar stationary phase surface (characteristic of the C_4-type of RP-HPLC sorbents) is employed. By utilising two or more *n*-alkyl ligand sorbents of similar ligand densities and support material characteristics, insight into these dynamic capabilities of polypeptides can then be uniquely assessed.

Similar types of complex multizoning behaviour to that described for amphipathic polypeptides has also been noted for small globular proteins, such as sperm whale myo-globin (SMyo). For example, immediately following injection into a column packed with a non-polar RP-HPLC sorbent, at a specified temperature and mobile phase composi-tion, a defined population of conformational ensembles of SMyo and *apo*-SMyo will be adsorbed onto the *n*-alkylsilica. However, as the residency time or the temperature is increased, new ensembles of conformers can emerge depending on their activation

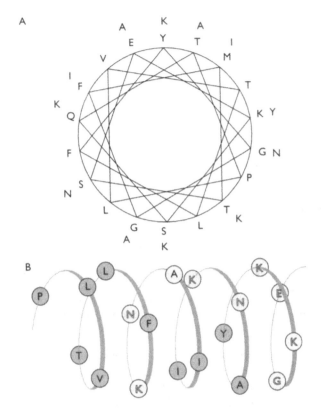

Figure 5.26 Edmundsen wheel representation of β-endorphin in the annular projection (A), whilst in the panel (B) the lateral projection of the amino acid residues which form the putative amphipathic α-helix of the C-terminal region of this polypeptide are highlighted.

energies and the selected conditions. As described above, analysis of the experimental bandwidths of SMyo/*apo*-SMyo (or for that matter other proteins) under these RP-HPLC conditions will, according to Equations 62–70, thus yield information related to the kinetics of these secondary equilibrium phenomena, including the dissociation of the prosthetic groups and conformational interconversions that may occur on the chromatographic timescale (Melander, 1984; Hearn, 1986; Benedek, 1988; Purcell *et al.*, 1993; Hearn, 1998a). Illustrative of this approach are the RP-HPLC results reported (Purcell *et al.*, 1999) for the bandbroadening behaviour of a sprem whale myoglobin (SMyo) sample (which *in situ* generates various *apo*-SMyo species) and a previously isolated *apo*-SMyo preparation as a function of temperature and time of residency at the hydrophobic surface of the adsorbent and depicted as 3-D mesh surfaces for the C_4 and C_{18} sorbents in Fig. 5.27 respectively.

As evident from these Figures, generally the overall trends in the bandbroadening were similar for both the SMyo *in situ* generated *apo*Myo species and the pre-isolated *apo*-SMyo species particularly at temperatures above 15°C when these proteins were chromatographed on a C_4 or C_{18} sorbent. This behaviour is consistent with the initial dissociation of the prosthetic haem group from SMyo, yielding *in situ* generated chromatographic species that resemble the ensembles of *apo*-SMyo species which were conformationally similar, if not identical, to those present in the pre-isolated *apo*-SMyo preparation. Closer inspection of the experimental data for the SMyo *in situ* generated *apo*Myo species and the pre-isolated *apo*-SMyo species with the C_{18} sorbent revealed some subtle differences in the degree of bandbroadening over limited temperature ranges. These observations also paralleled similar trends observed (Purcell *et al.*, 1999) for the changes in S-values of these molecules. For example, in the temperature range between 5–15°C, larger bandbroadening changes were evident for SMyo *in situ* generated *apo*Myo species than for the pre-isolated *apo*-SMyo species in the presence of the C_{18} ligands as the time of surface incubation was increased. This bandbroadening behaviour suggests the possibility that the conformational species present in the SMyo *in situ* generated *apo*Myo species had not reached the same stage of unfolding on the reversed phase surface as had occurred with the pre-isolated *apo*-SMyo sample under similar conditions of low (< 15°C) temperature and short residency times. Much less prominent difference in bandbroadening were observed for SMyo *in situ* generated *apo*-SMyo species and the pre-isolated *apo*-SMyo species with the C_4 sorbent as the residency time or temperature was varied.

As shown in Fig. 5.27, over the entire temperature range investigated with the C_4 sorbent, the pre-isolated *apo*-SMyo sample exhibited relatively constant bandwidths, suggesting that this pre-isolated *apo*-SMyo sample was slightly less structured than the transient SMyo *in situ* generated *apo*-SMyo species which was formed under the C_4 and C_{18} sorbent conditions. Consistent with this conclusion on the bandbroadening behaviour of the SMyo *in situ* generated *apo*-SMyo species are the observation into the stability of the *apo*-SMyo structure (Griko *et al.*, 1988; Goto *et al.*, 1990) in solution at low pH, which have shown that *apo*-SMyo is less structured and has more rapid denaturation kinetics than SMyo. The unfolding of SMyo in solution has also been shown to be a multi-state process with the equilibrium between the native, the fully unfolded and various molten globule conformational states responsive to changes in pH, temperature, or the concentrations of dissociants, such as urea or Gd-HCl (Griko *et al.*, 1988; Goto *et al.*, 1990a,b) Under conditions of low ionic strength, *apo*-SMyo is maximally unfolded (Griko *et al.*, 1988) at pH 2.0, but a further decrease of pH causes the protein to refold to the so-called A-state with properties similar to those of the molten globule state which exists (Hagihara *et al.*, 1993) in 1 M guanidium chloride at 20°C. In the perturbing RP-HPLC environment of the aquo-acetonitrile-0.1% trifluroacetic acid eluent at pH 2.1, analogous conformational intermediates may also arise, assuming that the observed bandbroadening differences reflect transiently trapped protein intermediates on this unfolding trajectory. As such, the peakwidth features of SMyo represent one type of multi-zoning behaviour in the RP-HPLC of polypeptides and proteins, in which the loss of a prosthetic group is an inherent part of the unfolding process.

The peakwidth behaviour of native hen egg white lysozyme (HEWL) and carboxymethylated HEWL illustrates a second type of complex interconversion process. In this case, complex multi-zoning separations of different HEWL (or carboxymethylated HEWL) chromatographically generated species have been observed by a number of investigators (Oroszlan *et al.*, 1990; Richards *et al.*, 1994; Purcell *et al.*, 1999) when these proteins were chromatographed with either the C_4 and C_{18} sorbents under

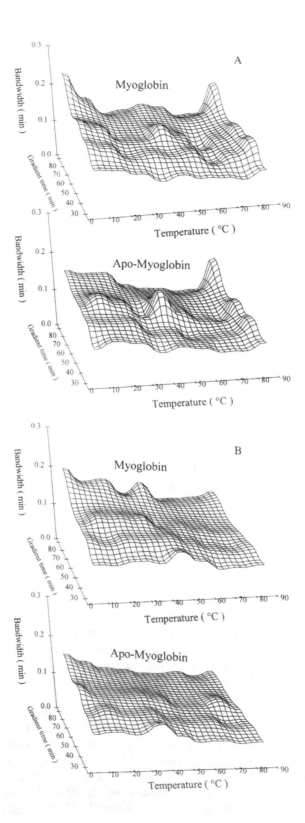

Table 5.3 Interaction rate constants, k_{int}, for hen egg white lysozyme (HEWL), α-lactoglobin (α-LAC) and carboxymethylated hen egg white lysozyme (cm-HEWL) on different non-polar sorbents. In these experiments the interaction rate constants were determined according to Equation 71 respectively

Protein	Sorbent	Rate constant, $k_{int}(min^{-1})$	Ref
HEWL	C18	1.6×10^{-3}	38
HEWL	C4	4.5×10^{-3}	38
α-LAC	C2-ether	7.42×10^{-3}	22
α-LAC	C1-ether	1.75×10^{-3}	22
cm-HEWL	C18	1.6×10^{-3}	38
cm-HEWL	C4	1.0×10^{-3}	38

various solvent conditions and over an extended temperature range of 5–85°C. Typically, in RP-HPLC systems, the elution profiles of HEWL or carboxymethylated HEWL at temperatures between 5–65°C can be characterised as generating relatively symmetrical peaks which either progressively broaden as the temperature is lowered or generate two or more peaks as the temperature is increased. The appearance of multiple peaks for HEWL represents an extreme case of the multi-zoning effect (Hearn, 1986), whereby changes in the interactive structures of slowly interconverting species are sufficiently large to permit these molecules to be resolved and thus to form distinct components in the elution profile. Under such conditions, ensembles of the more unfolded intermediates will be retained if larger hydrophobic contact areas are generated.

Table 5.3 lists the apparent rate constants, k_{int}s, for the interconversion of the HEWL, carboxymethylated HEWL and α-lactoglobin in RP-HPLC and analogous HIC environments, with the k_{int} values derived on the basis that this process can be described according to the pseudo-first order kinetics of Equations 71–73. Although the apparent rate constants for the interconversion of native HEWL to partially or fully unfolded species on the C_{18} and C_4 sorbent were of similar magnitude, the peak broadening behaviour of HEWL with the C_{18} sorbent has been found (Purcell *et al.*, 1999) to be more complex, in terms of larger variations in the respective S-values and affinities for the C_{18} sorbent over the temperature ranges investigated. Collectively, these data suggest that the interaction of HEWL with the C_{18} sorbent leads to a greater extent of unfolding than occurs with the C_4 sorbent, an observation consistent with literature precedents with other polypeptides and proteins with C_{18} and C_4 sorbents (Connolly, 1983; Cohen *et al.*, 1984b, 1985; Hearn and Aguilar, 1987; Benedek, 1988; Lin and Karger, 1990; Makhatadze *et al.*, 1990; Oroszlan *et al.*, 1990; Boysen *et al.*, 1999). This

Figure 5.27 The dependence of experimental bandwidth on the gradient time and column temperature for sperm whale myoglobin (SMyo) and *apo*myoglobin (*apo*-SMyo) on temperature, *T*, with a *n*-octadecylsilica Bakerbond wide pore sorbent (A) and a *n*-butylsilica Bakerbond wide pore sorbent (B). In these experiments (Purcell *et al.*, 1999), the elution conditions employed were a linear gradient of between 30 min and 90 min from water-0.1% trifluoroacetic acid to acetonitrile-water-(1 : 1)-0.1% trifluoroacetic acid, pH 2.1, at temperatures ranging from 5°C through to 85°C respectively.

temperature-induced process thus appears to involve the progressive exposure of more of the hydrophobic 'core' of HEWL to the solvated n-octadecyl ligands of the RP-HPLC sorbent and a slightly faster rate of denaturation leading to the formation of less compact structures. The conclusion can thus be drawn about the chromatographic behaviour of native and carboxymethylated lysozyme that slowly interconverting species were generated during the thermal denaturation in the presence of reversed phase sorbents. Stopped flow CD measurements (Miranker *et al.*, 1991) and hydrogen exchange experiments (Kuwajima *et al.*, 1991) have indicated that in solution the bending motion of the domain structures of HEWL occurs in a time frame of approximately 10 μs, whereas changes in the tertiary structure occur within the timeframe of seconds (Kuwajima, 1989). Chromatographic mass transfer events also occur within this time frame, and thus this technique has the potential ability to trap conformational intermediates during the chromatographic process. Whether the RP-HPLC environment with n-alkylsilicas provides a suitable tool for characterisation of conformational intermediates that are identical to those detected in bulk solvents or whether this technique monitors unrelated ensembles of conformational intermediates travelling on different folding/unfolding trajectories requires further experimentation. The application of appropriate on-line or *in situ* detection methods will help to resolve this conundrum and enable, in part, the informational content of solution-based studies to be correlated with analogous data obtained with surface-based procedures. Recent studies with *in situ* time resolved fluorescence measurements (Oroszlan *et al.*, 1990) and *in situ* CD spectroscopic detection (Blondelle *et al.*, 1992; Yarovsky *et al.*, 1995b) have indicated that such measurements are now feasible, whilst techniques such as solid state NMR, ESR or FT-IR potentially may also find application. Finally, the integration of microcalorimetric methods with surface based procedures inherent to RP-HPLC measurements can also more be realised.

Conclusions

Over the past two decades, high performance liquid chromatography (HPLC), and reversed phase HPLC (RP-HPLC) in particular, have become indispensable methods for the analysis of peptides and proteins as part of biochemical and biological research investigations. Furthermore, as documented in this chapter it is now feasible with RP-HPLC procedures to explore the characteristic transitions associated with the interconversions of the secondary and tertiary structures that polypeptides and proteins can undergo when they interact with immobilised n-alkyl ligands or other hydrophobic ligands in the presence of aquo-organic solvent environments. As such, RP-HPLC procedures have the potential to provide very useful experimental avenues to explore the role of the hydrophobic effect in the stabilisation of the conformation of polypeptides and proteins in heterogeneous, dynamic systems. Because of this potential, RP-HPLC procedures, as well as the other interactive modes of HPLC such as high performance ion exchange chromatography (HPIEX) and high performance hydrophobic interaction chromatography (HPHIC), represent more than just powerful separation tools, but also versatile experimental opportunities to derive information on the biophysical behaviour of biomacromolecules at solvated chemical surfaces.

Acknowledgments

The funding support of the Australian Research Council and the National Health and Medical Research Council of Australia is gratefully acknowledged.

Glossary of terms and symbols

α	ratio of the capacity factors (k_2'/k_1') representing the separation selectivity,
α_{conf}	relative selectivity between the 'native' and the 'unfolded' state,
C	Knox parameter which accommodates the resistance to mass transfer at the stationary phase surface and is directly relate to k_{int},
c_i	concentration of the displacing solvent,
C_p^0	heat capacity of the interactive solute-ligate system,
D_a	Damkohler parameter, represents the ratio of the time taken for the polypeptide or protein species to migrate along the column in the mobile phase to the relaxation time for the conformational interconversions between the N and U states of the polypeptide or protein in the same chromatographic system.
D_m	diffusion coefficient of the biosolute,
d_p	is the particle size of the sorbent,
ΔA_h	interactive hydrophobic surface area,
ΔA_{total}	total accessible surface area,
ΔG_{assoc}^0	Gibbs standard free energy for the association of the polypeptide or protein with the non-polar ligands,
$\Delta G_{o/w}^0$	Gibbs standard free energy change for the process of adsorbing the solute from a pure water mobile phase onto the non-polar stationary-phase surface,
$\Delta G_{int}^{\ddagger}$	change in the standard free energy of activation for the interconversion of the polypeptide or protein between different conformational states,
ΔH_{assoc}^0	enthalpy changes associated with the chromatographic process,
$\Delta H_{int}^{\ddagger}$	standard enthalpy of activation for the interconversion of a polypeptide or protein between different conformational states,
ΔS_{assoc}^0	entropy change associated with the chromatographic process,
$\Delta S_{int}^{\ddagger}$	change in the standard entropy of activation for the interconversion of a polypeptide or protein between different conformational states,
Δt_R	difference in separation time,
F	flow rate (ml/min),
Φ	phase ratio of the chromatographic system,
f_{hydr}	fragmental hydrophobicity parameters,
$\bar{h}$	Planck's constant,
K_{assoc}	equilibrium association constant,
k_B	Boltzmann constant.
κ^e	ratio of the energy required for the formation of a cavity with the surface area equal to the solute surface area and the energy required to extend the planar surface of the liquid by the same area,
k'	dimensionless capacity factor $(= (t_e - t_0/t_0)$,
$\bar{k}$	dimensionless median capacity factor in the linear gradient elution mode,
K_{conf}	summated structure-conformation free energy parameter,

k_{ij}	respective rate constants for adsorption, desorption and interconversion, K_{int} surface interaction kinetics associated with the binding and desorption of interconverting species,
k_{srr}	summated structure-retention free energy parameter,
L	column length,
$\log \alpha$	logarithmic selectivity increment,
$\log k'$	logarithm of the capacity factor, k',
$\log \bar{k}$	logarithm of the median capacity factor, $\bar{k}$,
$\log k_0$	Y-intercept of the plot of $\log k'$ vs ψ or the plot of $\log \bar{k}$ vs $\bar{\psi}$ at $\psi \rightarrow 0$ or $\bar{\psi} \rightarrow 0$ respectively,
N	separation efficiency expressed as theoretical number of plates,
PC	peak capacities of the polypeptides or proteins in the RP-HPLC system.
Θ	virial coefficient for the entropy change with mole fraction of the organic solvent $\partial \left(\Delta S^0_{assoc} \right)_T / \partial \psi = \theta$,
R	Gas constant,
R_s	resolution of the chromatographic separation,
S	slope of the plot of $\log K'$ vs ψ,
$\bar{S}$	slope of the plot of $\log \bar{k}$ vs $\bar{\psi}$,
σ_v	peak width of the eluted polypeptide,
t_0	void time of a packed chromatographic column, assuming that the extra-column dead volume is negligible,
t_{srr}	summated structure retention coefficients,
T	absolute temperature (in K),
u_0	linear velocity of the mobile phase (cm/min),
V	mean molar volume of the solvent,
ψ	isocratic mole fraction of organic solvent modifier,
$\bar{\psi}$	median gradient mole fraction of organic solvent modifier,
ζ	virial coefficient for the enthalpy change with mole fraction of the organic solvent, $\partial \left(\Delta H^0_{assoc} \right)_T / \partial \psi$.

References

Aguilar, M. I., Hodder, A. N. and Hearn, M. T. W. (1985) *J. Chromatogr.*, **327**, 115–138.

Aguilar, M. I., Hodder, A. N. and Hearn, M. T. W. (1986) *J. Chromatogr.*, **352**, 52–66.

Aguilar, M. I. and Hearn, M. T. W. (1991) In: *HPLC of Proteins, Peptides and Polynucleotides, Contemporary Topics and Applications* (ed. M. T. W. Hearn); VCH Publishers, New York, pp. 247–275.

Aguilar, M. I., Hodder, A. N. and Hearn, M. T. W. (1991) In: *HPLC of Proteins, Peptides and Polynucleotides, Contemporary Topics and Applications* (ed. M. T. W. Hearn); VCH Publishers, New York, pp. 199–245.

Aguilar, M. I., Mougos, S., Boublik, J., Rivier, J. and Hearn, M. T. W. (1991) *J. Chromatogr.*, **646**, 53–65.

Aguilar, M. I., Richards, K. L., Round, A. J. R. and Hearn, M. T. W. (1994) *Pept. Res.*, **7**, 207–217.

Aguilar, M. I. and Hearn, M. T. W. (1996) *Meth. Enzymol.*, **270**, 1–25.

Al-Obeidi, F. A., Hadley, M. E., Pettit, B. M. and Hruby, V. J., (1995) *J. Am. Chem. Soc.*, **111**, 3413–3416.

Arakawa, T. and Timasheff, S. N. (1984) *Biochemistry*, **23**, 5924–5929.

Balasubramaniam, A. and Sheriff, S. (1990) *J. Biol. Chem.*, **265**, 14724–14727.

Benedek, K. (1988) *J. Chromatogr.*, **458**, 93–104.

Beyermann, M., Fechner, K., Furkert, J., Krause, E. and Bienert, M. (1996) *J. Med. Chem.*, **39**, 3324–3330.

Bij, K. E., Horvath, Cs., Melander, W. R. and Nahun, A. (1981) *J. Chromatogr.*, **203**, 65–72.

Bismuto, E., Irace, G. and Gratton, E., (1989) *Biochemistry*, **28**, 1508–1512.

Blevins, D. D., Burke, M. F. and Hruby, V. J., In: *Handbook of HPLC for the Separation of Amino Acids, Peptides and Proteins.* CRC Press, Boca Raton, FL, (1984) **2**, pp. 137–143.

Blondelle, S. E., Buttner, K. and Houghten, R. A. (1992) *J. Chromatogr.*, **625**, 199–206.

Blondelle, S. E., Ostresh, J. M. Houghten, R. A. and Pérez-Payá, E. (1995) *Biophys. J.*, **68**, 351–359.

Boublik, J., Scott, N., Taulane, J., Goodman, M., Brown, M., and Rivier, J. (1989) *Int. J. Pept. Prot. Res.*, **33**, 11–15.

Boublik, J. H., Spicer, M. A., Scott, N. A., Brown, M. R. and Rivier, J. E. (1990) *Ann. N. Y. Acad. Sci.*, **611**, 27–34.

Boysen, R. and Hearn, M. T. W. (2001a) *J. Pept. Res.*, **57**, 1–10.

Boysen, R. and Hearn, M. T. W. (2001b) In: *Current Protocols in Protein Science* (ed. J. E. Colligan, B. M. Dunn, H. L. Ploegh, D. W. Speicher and P. J. Wingfield) John Wiley and Sons, New York, **8**, 1–40.

Boysen, R. I., Wang, Y., Keah, H. H. and Hearn, M. T. W. (1999) *J. Biophys. Chem.*, **77**, 79–97.

Boysen, R. I., Jong, A. and Hearn, M. T. W. (2001) *Biophys. J.*, in press.

Boysen, R. I., Jong, A. J. O., Wilce, J. A., King, G. and Hearn, M. T. W. (2002) *J. Biol. Chem.*, **277**, 23–31.

Cattini-Schultz, S. V., Stanton, P. G., Robertson, D. M. and Hearn, M. T. W. (1995) *Pept. Res.*, **8**, 214–226.

Chao, H., Bautista, D. L., Litowski, J., Irwin, R. T. and Hodges, R. S. (1998) *J. Chromatogr.*, in press.

Chloupek, R. C., Hancock, W. S., Marchylo, B. A., Kirkland, J. J., Boyes, B. E. and Snyder, L. R. (1994) *J. Chromatogr.*, **686**, 45–59.

Cohen, K. A., Schellenberg, K., Karger, B. L., Grego, B. and Hearn, M. T. W. (1984a) *Anal. Biochem.*, **140**, 223–235.

Cohen, S. A., Benedek, K., Dong, S., Tapuhi, Y. and Karger, B. L. (1984b) *Anal. Chem.*, **56**, 217–221.

Cohen, S. A., Benedek, K., Tapuhi, Y., Ford, J. C. and Karger, B. L. (1985) *Anal. Biochem.*, **144**, 275–284.

Cole, A. and Dorsey, J. G. (1992a) *Anal. Chem.*, **64**, 1317–1323.

Cole, A. and Dorsey, J. G. (1992b) *Anal. Chem.*, **64**, 1324–1331.

Connolly, M. L. (1983) *J. Appl. Cryst.*, **16**, 548–558.

Corbett, R. J. T. and Roche, R. S. (1984) *Biochemistry*, **23**, 1888–1993.

Creighton, T. E., In: *Proteins: structure and molecular properties.* W. H. Freeman & Co., New York, pp. 286–304.

Dickerson, R. E., Takano, T., Eisenberg, D., Kallai, O. B., Samson, L., Cooper, A. and Margoliash, E. (1984) (1971) *J. Biol. Chem.*, **246**, 1511–1535.

Dill, K. A. (1987) *J. Phys. Chem.*, **91**, 1980–1986.

Dorsey, J. G. and Dill, K. A. (1989) *Chem. Rev.*, **89**, 331–346.

Eisenberg, D., Weiss, R. M. and Terwilliger, T. C., (1982) *Nature*, **299**, 371–374.

Everett, D. H., In: *Adsorption from Solution* (eds R. H. Ottewill, C. H. Rochester and A. L. Smith) Academic Press, New York, pp. 1–45.

Feinstein, R. D., Boublik, J. H., Kirby, D., Spicer, M. A., Craig, A. G., Malewicz, K., Scott, N. A., Brown, M. R. and Rivier, J. E. (1983) (1992) *J. Med. Chem.*, 35: 2836–2843.

Galaktionov, S. G., Tseytin, V. M. and Vakser, I. A., (1988) *Biophysics*, **33**, 595–603.

Galaktionov, S. G. and Marshall, G. R. (1993) *Biophys. J.*, **65**, 608–615.

Gao, Y., Boyd, J., Williams, R. J. and Pielak, G. J., (1990) *Biochemistry*, **30**, 6994–7003.

Gilpin, K. and Sisco, W. R. (1980) *J. Chromatogr.*, **194**, 265–284.

Gilpin, K. and Squires, J. A. (1981) *J. Chromatogr. Sci.*, **19**, 195–210.

Glajch, J. L., Kirkland, J. J. and Kohler, J. (1987) *J. Chromatogr.*, **384**, 81–88.

Gomme, P. T., Thompson, P. T., Stanton, P. G. and Hearn, M. T. W., (1998) *J. Pept. Res.*, in press.

Goto, Y. L., Calciano, L. J. and Fink, A. L., (1990a) *Proc. Natl. Acad. Sci. USA.*, **87**, 573–577.

Goto, Y., Takahashi, N. and Fink, A. L., (1990b) *Biochemistry*, **29**, 3480–3488.

Grego, B. and Hearn, M. T. W. (1978) *J. Chromatogr.*, **317**, 67–80.

Griko, Yu. V., Privalov, P. L., Venyaminov, S. Yu., Kutyshenko, V. P. (1988) *J. Mol. Biol.*, **202**, 127–138.

Grinberg, N., Blanco, R., Yarmush, D. M. and Karger, B. L., (1989) *Anal. Chem.*, **61**, 514–520.

Guo, D., Mant, C. T., Taneja, A. K., Parker, J. M. R. and Hodges, R. S. (1986) *J. Chromatogr.*, **359**, 499–531.

Hagihara, Y., Aimoto, S., Fink, A. L. and Goto, Y. (1993) *J. Mol. Biol.*, **231**, 180–184.

Hancock, W. S., Chloupek, R. C., Kirkland, J. J. and Snyder, L. R. (1994) *J. Chromatogr.*, **686**, 31–43.

Hearn, M. T. W. and Grego, B. (1981a) *Chromatographia*, **14**, 589–592.

Hearn, M. T. W. and Grego, B. (1981b) *J. Chromatogr.*, **218**, 497–507.

Hearn, M. T. W. and Grego, B. (1981c) *J. Chromatogr.*, **203**, 349–363.

Hearn, M. T. W. and Grego, B. (1981d) *J. Chromatogr.*, **218**, 497–515.

Hearn, M. T. W., In: *Advances in Chromatography*, (eds J. C. Giddings, P. Brown and J. Cazes) Marcel Dekker, Inc., New York, **20**, pp. 1–82.

Hearn, M. T. W. (1982) In: *HPLC: Advances and Perspectives* (ed. Cs. Horvath), Academic Press, New York, **3**, pp. 87–155.

Hearn, M. T. W. (1983) *Meth. Enzymol.*, textbf1984, **104**, 190–212.

Hearn, M. T. W., Hodder, A. N. and Aguilar, M. I. (1985) *J. Chromatogr.*, **327**, 47–66.

Hearn, M. T. W. (1986) In: *Chemical Separations: Science and Technology*, (eds J. D. Navratil, C. J. King, Litarvan Press, Arvada, CO, pp. 77–98.

Hearn, M. T. W. and Aguilar, M. I. (1986a) *J. Chromatogr.*, **359**, 31–54.

Hearn, M. T. W. and Aguilar, M. I. (1986b) *J. Chromatogr.*, **352**, 35–66.

Hearn, M. T. W. and Aguilar, M. I. (1987a) *J. Chromatogr.*, **392**, 33–49.

Hearn, M. T. W. and Aguilar, M. I. (1987b) *J. Chromatogr.*, **397**, 47–70.

Hearn, M. T. W. and Aguilar, M. I. (1988) In: *Modern Physical Methods in Biochemistry*, (eds A. Neuberger and L. L. M. Van Deenen), Elsevier Publ., Amsterdam, pp. 107–142.

Hearn, M. T. W., Aguilar, M. I., Nguyen, T. and Fridman, M. (1988) *J. Chromatogr.*, **435**, 271–284.

Hearn, M. T. W. (1998a) In *Protein Purification, Principles, High Resolution Methods, and Applications*, (eds J. C. Janson and L. Ryden), VCH Publ., New York, pp. 239–282.

Hearn, M. T. W. (2000) In: *Handbook of Bioseparations*, (ed. S. Ahuja), Academic Press, New York, 72–235.

Hearn, M. T. W. (2001) In: *HPLC of Biopolymers* (eds K. Gooding and F. E. Regnier) Marcel Dekker, Inc., New York, N.Y., 99–245.

Hearn, M. T. W., Boysen, R., Wang, Y. and Muraledaram, S. (1999) In: *Peptide Science – Present and Future* (ed. Y. Shimonishi) Kluwer Academic Publishers b.v., 246–250.

Hearn, M. T. W. and Zhao, G. L. (1999) *Anal. Chem.*, **71**, 4874–4885.

Henderson, D. E. and Horvath, Cs. (1986) *J. Chromatogr.*, **368**, 203–213.

Hetzer, M., Heinz, S., Grage, S. and Bayerl, T. M., (1998) *Langmuir*, **14**, 982–984.

Higgins, K. A., Bicknell, W., Keah, H. H. and Hearn, M. T. W. (1997) *J. Pept. Res.*, **50**, 421–435.

Hodges, R. S., Semchuk, P. D., Taneja, A. K., Kay, C. M., Parker, J. M. R., Mant, C. T. (1988) *Peptide Res.*, **1**, 19–30.

Hodges, R. S., Zhu, B.-Y., Zhou, N. E. and Mant, C. T., (1994) *J. Chromatogr.*, **676**, 3–15.

Hodges, R. S., Tripet, B. and Wagschal, K., In: *Peptides: Structure, Function and Comformation* (ed. J. Tam) Mayflower Press, Mayflower Sci. Press, Kingswinford, in press.

Horváth, Cs., Melander, W. and Molnár, I., (1998) (1976) *J. Chromatogr.*, **125**, 129–156.

Houghten, R. and DeGraw, S. T. (1987) *J. Chromatogr.*, **386**, 223–228.

Jacobsen, J., Melander, W. R., Vaisnys, G. and Horvath, Cs., (1984) *J. Phys. Chem.*, **88**, 4536–4542.

Janssen, P. S., van Nispen, J. W., Hamelinck, R. L., Melgers, P. A. and Goverde, B. C. (1984) *J. Chromatogr. Sci.*, **22**, 234–238.

Jelokhami-Niaraki, M., Kondejewski, L. H., Farmer, S. W., Hancock, R. E., Kay, C. M. and Hodges, R. S., In: *Peptides: Structure, Function and Conformation* (ed. J. Tam) Mayflower Press, Mayflower Sci. Press, Kingswinford, in press.

Jensen, W. A., Armstrong, J.McD., diGiorgio, J. and Hearn, M. T. W. (1998) (1997) *Biochim. Biophys. Acta*, **1338**, 186–198.

Jino, K., Nagosh, T. and Tanaka, N. (1988) *J. Chromatogr.*, **346**, 1–10.

Johnson, B. P., Khaledi, M. G. and Dorsey, J. G. (1986) *Anal. Chem.*, **58**, 2354–2362.

Katz, E. D., Ogan, K. and Scott, R. P. W. (1986) *Anal. Chem.*, **352**, 67–73.

Katz, E. D., Lochmuller C. H. and Scott, R. P. W. (1989) *Anal. Chem.*, **61**, 349–362.

Kauzmann, W. (1959) *Adv. Prot. Chem.*, **14**, 1–87.

Keah, H. H., Kecorius, E. and Hearn, M. T. W. (1998) *J. Pept. Res.*, **51**, 2–11.

Keller, R. A. and Giddings, J. C. (1960) *J. Chromatogr.*, **3**, 205–210.

Kendrew, J. C., Dickerson, R. E., Strandberg, B. E., Hart, R. G., Davis, D. R., Phillips, D. C. and Shore, V. C. (1960) *Nature*, **185**, 422–427.

Kirby, D. A., Miller, C. L. and Rivier, J. E. (1993) *J. Chromatogr.*, **648**, 257–265.

Klatte, S. J. and Beck, T. L. (1995) *J. Phys. Chem.*, **99**, 16024–16029.

Kohn, W. D., Kay, C. M. and Hodges, R. S., In: *Peptides: Structure, Function and Conformation* (ed. J. Tam) Mayflower Press, Mayflower Sci. Press, Kingswinford, in press.

Kondejewski, L. H., Jelokhami-Niaraki, M., Hancock, R. E. and Hodges, R. S. (1998a) In: *Peptides: Structure, Function and Conformation* (ed. J. Tam) Mayflower Press, Mayflower Sci. Press, Kingswinford, in press.

Kondejewski, L. H., Semchuk, P. D., Daniels, L., Wilson, I. and Hodges, R. S. (1998b) In: *Peptides: Structure, Function and Conformation* (ed. J. Tam) Mayflower Press, Mayflower Sci. Press, Kingswinford, in press.

Krause, E., Beyermann, M., Dathe, M., Rothemund, S. and Biernet, M. (1995) *Anal. Chem.*, **67**, 252–258.

Krause, E., Beyermann, M., Fabian, H., Dathe, M., Rothemund, S. and Bienert, M. (1996) *Int. J. Pept. Prot. Res.*, **48**, 559–568.

Krug, R. R., Hunter, W. G. and Grieger, R. A. (1976) *J. Phys. Chem.*, **80**, 2335–2340.

Kurosu, Y., Sasaki, T., Takakura, T., Sakayanagi, N., Hibi, K. and Senda, M. (1990) *J. Chromatogr.*, **515**, 407–414.

Kuwajima, K. (1989) *Proteins*, **6**, 87–103.

Kuwajima, K., Garvey, E. P., Finn, B. E., Mathews, C. R. and Sugai, S. (1991) *Biochemistry*, **30**, 7693–7703.

Laidler, K. J. (1978) In: *Physical Chemistry with Biological Applications*, Benjamin Cummings, Menlo Park, NC, pp. 365–426.

Landenheim, E. E., Taylor, J. E., Coy, D. H. and Moran, T. H., (1994) *Eur. J. Pharmacol.*, **271**, 7–9.

Lau, S. Y. M., Taneja, A. K. and Hodges, R. S. (1984) *J. Chromatogr.*, **317**, 129–140.

Lazoura, E., Maidonis, I., Bayer, E., Hearn, M. T. W. and Aguilar, M. I. (1997) *Biophys. J.*, **72**, 238–246.

Lee, B. (1991) *Proc. Natl. Acad. Sci. U.S.A.*, **88**, 5154–5158.

Lee, T.-H., Thompson, P. E., Aguilar, M. I. and Hearn, M. T. W. (1997) *Int. J. Pept. Prot. Res.*, **48**, 93–102.

Li, S. and Debber, C. M. (1994) *Nature Struct. Biol.*, **1**, 368–370.

Lin, S. and Karger, B. L. (1990) *J. Chromatogr.*, **499**, 89–102.

Lockmuller, C. H. and Wilder, D. R. J. (1979) *J. Chromatogr. Sci.*, **17**, 574–579.

Lork, K. D., Unger, K. K., Bruckner, H. and Hearn, M. T. W., (1989) *J. Chromatogr.*, **476**, 135–143.

Lowensehuss, A. and Yellin, N. (1975) *Spectrochim. Acta*, **31**, 207–215.

Lu, X. M., K. Benedek, K. and Karger, B. L. (1986) *J. Chromatogr.*, **359**, 19–29.

Lumry, R. and Rajender, S. (1970) *Biopolymers*, **9**, 1125–1132.

Makhatadze, G. I., Medvedkin, V. N. and Privalov, P. L., (1990) *Biopolymers*, **30**, 1001–1010.

Mant, C. T. and Hodges, R.S. (1993) In: *High Performance Liquid Chromatography of Peptides and Proteins: Separation, Analysis and Conformation*. CRC Press, Boica Raton, Fl, pp. 589–658.

Mant, C. T., Zhou, N. E. and Hodges, R. S. (1993) In: *The Amphipathic Helix* (ed. R. M. Epand) CRC Press, Roca, FL, pp. 39–45.

Mattice, W. L. and Robinson, R. M. (1981) *Biochem. Biophys. Res. Comm.*, **101**, 1311–1317.

McDonald, C. C. and Phillips, D. C. (1967) *J. Am. Chem. Soc.*, **89**, 6332–6341.

Melander, W. R., Campbell, D. E. and Horvath, Cs. (1978) *J. Chromatogr.*, **158**, 215–230.

Melander, W. R., Corradini, D. and Hovath, Cs. (1984) *J. Chromatogr.*, **317**, 67–80.

Melander, W. R., Lin, H. J., Jacobsen, J. and Horvath, Cs, (1984) *J. Phys. Chem.*, **88**, 4527–4536.

Meyer, J. P., Davis, P., Lee, K. B., Porreca, F. and Hruby, V. J. (1995) *J. Med. Chem.*, **38**, 3462–3470.

Mierke, D. F., Dürr, H., Kessler, H. and Jung, G., (1992) *Eur. J. Biochem.*, **206**, 39–48.

Miranker, A., Radford, S. E., Karplus, M. and Dobson, C. M., (1991) *Nature*, **349**, 633–636.

Murphy, K. P. and Gill, S. J. (1990) *J. Thermochim. Acta*, **172**, 11–19.

Nall, B. T., Osterhout, J. J. and Ramdas, L., (1988) *Biochemistry*, **27**, 7310–7314.

Narita, M. and Kojima, Y. (1989) *Bull. Chem. Soc. Jpn.*, **62**, 3572–3578.

Nikiforovich, G. V., Hruby, V. J., Prakash, O. and Gehrig, C. A. (1991) *Biopolymers*, **31**, 941–955.

O'Hare, M. J., Capp, M. W., Nice, E. C., Cooke, N. H. C. and Archer, B. G. (1983) In: *High Performance Liquid Chromatography of Peptides and Proteins*, (eds M. T. W. Hearn, F. E. Regnier and C. T. Wehr) Academic Press, New York, pp. 161–172.

Oroszlan, P., Blanco, R., Lu, X.-M., Yarmush, D. M. and Karger, B. L. (1990) *J. Chromatogr.*, **500**, 481–502.

Oroszlan, P., Wicar, S., Wu, S.-L., Hancock, W. S. and Karger, B. L. (1992) *Anal. Chem.*, **64**, 1623–1631.

Parker, J. M. R., Guo, D. and Hodges, R. S., (1986) *Biochemistry*, **25**, 5425–5432.

Pfeil, W. and Privalov, P. L. (1976) *Biophys. Chem.*, **4**, 41–50.

Pidgeon, C., Ong, S., Choi, H. S. and Liu, H. I. (1994) *Anal. Chem.*, **66**, 2701–2709.

Purcell, A. W., Aguilar, M. I. and Hearn, M. T. W. (1989) *J. Chromatogr.*, **476**, 125–133.

Purcell, A. W., Aguilar, M. I. and Hearn, M. T. W. (1992) *J. Chromatogr.*, **593**, 103–110.

Purcell, A. W., Aguilar, M. I. and Hearn, M. T. W. (1993) *Anal. Chem.*, **65**, 3038–3047.

Purcell, A. W., Aguilar, M. I., Wettenhall, R. E. H. and Hearn, M. T. W. (1995) *Peptide Res.*, **8**, 160–170.

Purcell, A. W., Aguilar, M. I. and Hearn, M. T. W. (1999) *Anal Chem.*, **71**, 2440–2451.

Ragone, R., Colonna, G., Bismuto, E. and Irace, G., (1987) *Biochemistry*, **26**, 2130–2134.

Redfield, C. and Dobson, C. M. (1988) *Biochemistry*, **27**, 122–136.

Reinl, H. M. and Bayerl, T. M. (1994) *Biochemistry*, **33**, 140791–14099.

Rhee, D., Markovich, R., Chac, W. G., Qiu, A. X. and Pidgeon, C. (1994) *Anal. Chim. Acta*, **297**, 377–386.

Richards, F. M. (1977) *Ann. Rev. Biophys. Bioeng.*, **6**, 151–176.

Richards, K. L., Aguilar, M. I. and Hearn, M. T. W. (1994a) *J. Chromatogr.*, **676**, 17–31.

Richards, K. L., Aguilar, M. I. and Hearn, M. T. W. (1994b) *J. Chromatogr.*, **676**, 33–41.

Ridge, J. A., Baldwin, R. L. and Labhardt, A. M., (1981) *Biochemistry*, **20**, 1622–1630.

Rose, G. D., Geselowitz, A. R., Lesser, G. J., Lee, R. H. and Zehfus, M. H. (1985) *Science*, **229**, 834–838.

Rothemund, S., Krause, E., Beyermann, M., Dathe, M., Engelhardt, H. and Bienert, M. (1995) *J. Chromatogr.*, **689**, 219–226.

Rothemund, S., Krause, E., Beyermann, M., Bienert, M., Sykes, B. D. and Sonnichsen, F. D. (1996) *Biopolymers*, **39**, 207–219.

Round, A. J., Aguilar, M. I. and Hearn, M. T. W. (1994) *J. Chromatogr.*, **661**, 61–75.

Rowlen, K. L. and Harris, J. M. (1991) *Anal. Chem.*, **63**, 964–973.

Sanchez, Y. M., Haack, T., Gonzalez, M. J., Ludevid, D., and Giralt, E. (1996) In: *Peptides: Chemistry, Structure and Biology*, (eds P. T. P. Kauyama and R. S. Hodges) Mayflower Sci. Press, Kingswinford, pp. 558–560.

Schoenmakers, P. J., Billiet, H. A. H. and de Galan, L. D., (1979) *J. Chromatogr.*, **185**, 179–190.

Shalongo, W., Jagannadham, M. V., Flynn, C. and Stellwagen, E. (1989) *Biochemistry*, **28**, 4820–4826.

Sitaram, B. R., Keah, H. H. and Hearn, M. T. W. (1999) *J. Chromatogr. A*, **857**, 263–273.

Smyth, D. G. and Zacharian, S. (1980) *Nature*, **288**, 613–615.

Snyder, L. R. (1980) In: *HPLC – advances and perspectives* (ed. Cs. Horváth) Academic Press, New York, pp. 207–316.

Spicer, M. A., Boublik, J. H., Feinstein, R. D., Goodman, M., Brown, M. and Rivier, J. (1990) *Ann. N. Y. Acad. Sci.*, **611**, 359–361.

Stadalius, M. A., Gold, H. S. and Snyder, L. R. (1984) *J. Chromatogr.*, **296**, 31–59.

Steer, D. L., Thompson, P. E., Blondelle, S. E., Houghten, R. A. and Aguilar, M. I. (1998) *Int. J. Pept. Res.*, **51**, 401–412.

Sternlicht, H. and Wilson, D. (1967) *Biochemistry*, **6**, 2881–2892.

Storrs, R. W., Truckses, D. and Wemmer, D. E., (1992) *Biopolymers*, **32**, 1695–1702.

Takano, T. (1977) *J. Mol. Biol.*, **110**, 537–568.

Tanford, C. (1973) In: *The Hydrophobic Effect*, John Wiley & Sons, New York, pp. 1–220.

Tatemoto, K. (1982) *Proc. Natl. Acad. Sci. USA*, **79**, 5485–5489.

Taylor, J. W. and Kaiser, E. T. (1986) *Pharmacol. Rev.*, **38**, 291–319.

Vailaya, A. and Horvath, Cs. (1996a) *Biophys. Chem.*, **62**, 81–90.

Vailaya, A. and Horvath, Cs. (1996b) *Indust. Eng. Chem. Res.*, **35**, 2964–2982.

Vyas, S. B. and Duffy, L. K. (1995) *Biochem. Biophys. Res. Comm.*, **206**, 718–722. B-amyloid.

Wang, Y., Guo, Z, Boysen, R. I. and Hearn, M. T. W. (1998) *J. Pept. Res.*, in press.

Wilce, M. C., Aguilar, M. I. and Hearn, M. T. W. (1991) *J. Chromatogr.*, **548**, 105–116.

Wilce, M. C., Aguilar, M. I. and Hearn, M. T. W. (1992) *J. Chromatogr.*, **632**, 11–18.

Wilce, M. C., Aguilar, M. I. and Hearn, M. T. W. (1995) *Anal Chem.*, **34**, 1210–1219.

Wodak, S. J. and Janin, J. (1981) *Biochemistry*, **20**, 6544–6552.

Wu, C. S., Lee, N., Ling, N., Chang, J. K., Loh, H. and Yang, J. T. (1981) *Mol. Pharmacol.*, **189**, 302–306.

Yarovsky, I., Aguilar, M. I. and Hearn, M. T. W. (1994) *J. Chromatogr.*, **660**, 75–84.

Yarovsky, I., Aguilar, M. I. and Hearn, M. T. W. (1995a) *Anal. Chem.*, **67**, 2145–2153.

Yarovsky, I., Aguilar, M. I. and Hearn, M. T. W. (1995b) *Proc. Lorne Protein Conf.*, 203–204.

Yarovsky, I., Aguilar, M. I. and Hearn, M. T. W. (1997) *J. Phys. Chem.*, **101**, 10962–10971.

Yin, J. M., Liu, H. L. and Pidgeon, C. (1998) *Biorg. Med. Chem. Letts.*, **8**, 179–182.

Zhao, L. X., Purcell, A. W., Aguilar, M. I. and Hearn, M. T. W., (1999) *J. Chromatogr.*, **853**, 263–274.

Zhou, N. E., Mant, C. T. and Hodges, R. S. (1990) *Peptide Res.*, **3**, 8–20.

Chapter 6

Affinity chromatography

Jaroslava Turková

Introduction

In principle, affinity chromatography is a form of adsorption chromatography, which is based on the exceptional ability of biological molecules to form specifically and reversibly complexes with complementary substances immobilized on a solid matrix. These are generally called ligands, affinity ligands or affinants. The complexes of enzymes with their inhibitors, substrates, cofactors, effectors, antibodies with their antigens or haptens, lectins with glycoproteins or polysaccharides, complexes of nucleic acids, hormones and toxins with receptors, transport proteins with vitamins or sugars, etc., may be mentioned as examples (Lowe and Dean, 1974; Jakoby and Wilchek, 1974; Scouten, 1981; Mohr and Pommerening, 1985; Turková, 1978, 1993; Hermanson *et al.*, 1992; Schott, 1984; Wilchek and Bayer, 1990). The complexes of biologically active compounds with dyes are described in dye ligand affinity chromatography (Vijayalakshmi and Bertrand, 1989), with metal ions in metal chelate affinity chromatography (Porath, 1975), etc. These different approaches are grouped under the generic name "Pseudobio specific ligand affinity chromatography" was discussed in details in a review by M. A. Vijayalakhsmi (1989). If one of the components of the complex is immobilized, a specific sorbent is formed for the second component assuming that the conditions necessary for the formation of this complex exist. The binding sites of the immobilized substances must be sterically accesible after their binding to the solid support, and they must not be deformed by immobilization.

A solid support with a covalently bound affinant is used as the stationary phase in a chromatographic column. A diagrammatic representation of the process of affinity chromatography is shown in Fig. 6.1. When a crude mixture containing the biologically active products is passed through the column of affinity adsorbent, all the compounds which, under given experimental conditions, have no complementary binding site for the immobilized affinity ligand will pass through, unretarded. By contrast, products showing an affinity for the insoluble affinant are adsorbed on the column. They can be released by elution with a solution of a soluble affinity ligand or by changing the solvent composition by so-called deforming buffers (e.g. by a change in pH, ionic strength, temperature, etc.).

New applications of affinity chromatography resulting from a change-over from soft gel supports to small rigid particles used in high-performance affinity chromatography (HPLAC) have been reviewed by Ohlson *et al.* (1989). A comparison of HPLAC wih soft gel affinity chromatography (AC) is shown in Fig. 6.2. Mechanically stable, rigid particles, with small and uniform sizes, provide high flow rates with good mass

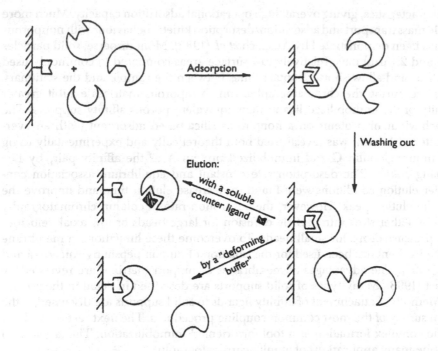

Figure 6.1 Diagrammatic representation of the process of bioaffinity chromatography.

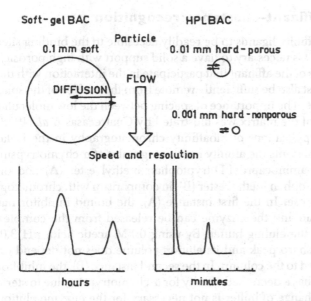

Figure 6.2 A comparison of affinity chromatography using soft gel or porous and nonporous small hard particles.

transfer characteristics, giving overall high operational adsorption capacity. Much more favourable mass transport and adsorption/desorption kinetic behaviour with nonporous support has been demonstrated by Anspach et al. (1989). Monodisperse, solid particles (0.7-, 1.5- and 2.1-μm) have relatively low surface areas compared to commonly used porous silicas and allow shorter contact times between the sample and the stationary phase surface during the chromatographic run. Nonporous matrices exhibit greater accessibility of the immobilized ligand than equivalent porous affinity supports. The elution behaviour of proteins on a nonporous silica-based adsorbent (with an average diameter of 1.4 μm) was investigated both theoretically and experimentally using human immunoglobulin G and immobilized protein A as the affinity pair, by Lee and Chuang (1996). The desorption rate constant and equilibrium association constant under elution conditions were found to decrease elution time and improve the shape of the elution peak. However, the adsorption rate in column chromatography is limited by either slow intraparticle diffusion for large beads or low axial velocities and high pressure drops for small beads. To overcome these limitations, a membrane based bioadsorbent has been used for the isolation of human pepsin by Kučerová and Turková (1997). The advantages of membranes as support matrixes are reviewed by Charcosset (1998). Many types of solid supports are described in detail in the second section. Methods of attachment of affinity ligands to solid supports are discussed in the section on survey of the most common coupling procedures. The next section is about biospecific complex formation as a tool for oriented immobilization. The last section will describe many applications of affinity chromatography.

General principles of affinant–substance recognition

In order for the immobilized affinity ligands to be readily accesible to the binding sites of biological macromolecules, it is necessary to have a solid support with high porosity. Moreover, the chemical groups of the affinant that participate in the interaction with the macromolecular substance must also be sufficiently remote from the surface of the solid matrix to avoid steric hindrance. The importance of spacing between the low molecular weight ligand and the surface of the matrix was illustrated by Cuatrecasas et al. (1968) in one of the first successful applications of bioaffinity chromatography in the isolation of enzymes. Figure 6.3 represents the affinity chromatography of α-chymotrypsin, on Sepharose coupled with ε-aminocaproyl-D-tryptophan methyl ester (A) and on Sepharose coupled with D-tryptophan methyl ester (B), in comparison with chromatography on unsubstituted Sepharose. In the first instance (A), the bound inhibitor has high affinity for α-chymotrypsin and the enzyme can be released from the complex only by decreasing the pH of the eluting buffer. By using 0.1 M acetic acid, pH 3.0, α-chymotrypsin is eluted in a sharp peak and its elution volume does not depend on the volume of the sample applied to the column. In the second instance (B), the inhibitor coupled directly on Sepharose has a decreased affinity for α-chymotrypsin, due to steric hindrance. In this instance a change of buffer is not necessary for the enzyme elution and, as it can be seen from the graph, the enzyme is eluted in a much larger volume following the inactive material. In order to verify that nonspecific adsorption on the carrier did not take place, chromatography of α-chymotrypsin on an unsubstituted carrier was carried out (C) as well.

Studies on the conformation of model peptides in membrane-mimetic environments (Gierasch et al., 1982) lead us to expect that steric accessibility of the reactive groups

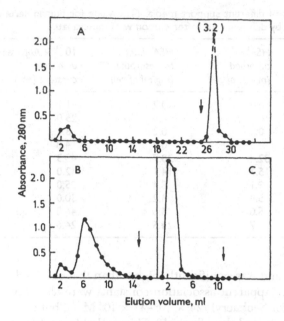

Figure 6.3 Affinity chromatography of (α-chymotrypsin on inhibitor Sepharose columns. The columns (50 × 5 mm) were equilibrated and run with 0.05 M Tris-hydrochloric acid buffer of pH 8.0. Each sample (2.5 mg) was applied in 0.5 ml of the same buffer. The columns were run at room temperature with a flow-rate about 40 ml/h and fractions, I ml, were collected. The arrows indicate a change of elution buffer (0.1 M acetic acid, pH 3.0). (A) Sepharose coupled with (ε-aminocaproyl-D-tryptophan methyl ester, (B) Sepharose coupled with D-tryptophan methyl ester, (C) unsubstituted Sepharose. The first peaks in A and B were devoid of enzyme activity. Reproduced with permission from P. Cuatrecasas *et al.* (1968) *Proc. Natl. Acad. Sci. U.S.A.*, **61**, 634–643.

of the affinity ligand will not only be determined by their distance from the surface of the solid support but will also depend on the interfacial water region, which does not stabilize the same conformation as does bulk water. The arrangement of the solvent layers on the surface of the solid support will also obviously be one of the main factors affecting the penetration of the bound molecules to the surface of the support. As a logical consequence the mode of immobilization has a greater effect on the interaction of the substances with low molecular weight ligands than with high molecular ones.

Angal and Dean (1977) studied the effect of matrix on the binding of human serum albumin to the sulphonated aromatic dye Cibacron Blue immobilized on ten solid supports. Cibacron Blue was attached to cellulose (Whatman Biochemicals, Maidstone, Kent, U.K.), acrylamide-cross linked dextran Sephacryl (Pharmacia, Uppsala, Sweden), co-polymerized polyacrylamide-agarose mixed gels Ultrogels Ac A54 and Ac A44 (LKB Instruments, Croydon, Surrey, U.K.), agaroses Sepharose 6B, 4B and 2B (Pharmacia G.B. Ltd., London, U.K.) and to epichlorohydrin-crosslinked Sepharose CL6B, CL4B and CL2B. Bioaffinity column supports were compared by frontal analysis. These results are summarized in Table 6.1. A 16-fold range in ligand concentration was observed between matrices despite the similarity of the coupling conditions used. The molar effectiveness of the agarose adsorbents ranged between 0.064 and 0.157 mol of

Table 6.1 Comparison of the properties of different support media. (The value for human serum
albumin adsorbed is calculated by difference and after elution with thiocyanate)

Support material	Ligand concn. (μg/ml of gel)	HSA[1] adsorbed (mg/ml of gel)	HSA eluted by desorption (mg/ml of gel)	$10^{-3} \times$ Apparent association constant (M^1)
Cellulose	3.2	0.8	0.2	1.1
Sephacryl	1.9	10.7	8.4	25.0
Ultrogel AcA54	0.3	0.2	0.2	3.1
Ultrogel AcA44	0.4	0.3	0.2	4.8
Sepharose 6B	2.3	32.4	20.7	45.3
Sepharose 4B	1.5	15.7	14.1	42.0
Sepharose 2B	0.9	9.1	8.4	35.0
Sepharose CL6B	0.7	5.4	4.2	30.0
Sepharose CL4B	0.4	5.0	4.6	46.8
Sepharose CL2B	0.2	1.7	24.6	24.6

1 Human serum albumin.

human serum albumin/mol of dye and was significantly higher than that obtained for
cellulose and the various Ultrogels. Apparent association constants were also similar
for all substituted Sepharoses and for Sephacryl (24×10^3–47×10^3 M^{-1}), but were at
least a factor of 10 lower for cellulose and the Ultrogels. This probably explains the
observed lower working capacities of these adsorbents.

The main principle governing the specific interactions of biological macromolecules
is the complementarity of the binding sites. For example, the high binding affinity of
specific substrates results from the perfect fit of configurationally and conformationally
oriented groups of the substrate with the complementarily located groups or sites on
the enzyme. This is true not only with respect to their spatial arrangement, but also
with regard to the nature of the complementary parts of the molecules. However, the
means by which an affinity ligand can be bound to a solid support is restricted because
the ligand must be coupled by that part of the molecule which does not participate
in the biospecific binding. In addition, the immobilization of the affinant should not
cause a change in its conformation nor should it affect the nature of its binding sites.
The overall effectiveness of an affinity adsorbent depends on the extent to which this
is achieved.

The importance of the mode of attachment of nucleotides to a solid support in relationship to the efficiency of the affinity chromatography of kinases and dehydrogenases
has been demonstrated by Harvey *et al.* (1974). The adsorbent N[6]-(6-aminohexyl)-
AMP-Sepharose contains AMP bound to Sepharose via of the N[6] of adenine moiety:

while in the sorbent P^1-(6-aminohexyl)-P^2-(5'-adenosine) pyrophosphate-Sepharose, AMP is linked *via* 5'-phosphate:

The affinity of various dehydrogenases and kinases for these two adsorbents is shown[*] in Table 6.2. Glucose-6-phosphate dehydrogenase, D-glyceraldehyde 3-phosphate dehydrogenase and myokinase adsorbed only to P^1-(6-aminohexyl)-P^2-(5'-adenosine) pyrophosphate-Sepharose, while alcohol dehydrogenase and glycerokinase were bound only to N^6-(6-aminohexyl)-5'-AMP-Sepharose. Lactate dehydrogenase, malate dehydrogenase, 3-phosphoglycerate kinase and pyruvate kinase adsorbed to both sorbents, while hexokinase and creatine kinase were bound to neither of them. These results reflect the nature of the enzyme-nucleotide interactions and it can be concluded that while the free 5'-phosphate group is essential for the binding, for example, to alcohol dehydrogenase or glycerokinase, it has a completely different role in the interaction of glyceraldehyde 3-phosphate dehydrogenase. In this instance the decisive role is played by the adenosine moiety of the affinant. The much stricter binding requirements with hexokinase and creatine kinase evidently result in these enzymes not being bound to either of the adsorbents. However, hexokinase from yeast extracts was isolated by use of ATP complexed with immobilized boronic acid (Matrex Gel phenylboronate from Amicon, Lexington, Mass., U.S.A.) by Bouriotis *et al.* (1981).

Table 6.2 Comparison of the binding of various enzymes to N^6-(6-aminohexyl)-5'-AMP-Sepharose (I) and P^1-(6-aminohexyl)-P^2-(5'-adenosine)-pyrophosphate-Sepharose (II)

Enzyme Code number	Name	Binding (β)[*]	
		I	*II*
E.C.1.1.1.27	Lactate dehydrogenase	>1000[**]	>1000[**]
E.C.1.1.1.49	Glucose 6-phosphate dehydrogenase	0	170
E.C.1.1.1.37	Malate dehydrogenase	65	490
E.C.1.1.1.1	Alcohol dehydrogenase	400	0
E.C.1.2.1.12	D-Glyceraldehyde 3-phosphate dehydrogenase	0	>1000[**]
E.C.2.7.2.3	3-Phosphoglycerate kinase	70	260
E.C.2.7.1.40	Pyruvate kinase	100	110
E.C.2.7.1.1	Hexokinase	0	0
E.C.2.7.4.3	Myokinase	0	380
E.C.2.7.1.30	Glycerokinase	122	0

[*] Binding (β) is the KCl concentration (mM) at the centre of the enzyme peak when the enzyme is eluted with a linear gradient of KCl.
[**] Elution was effected by a 200-μl-pulse of 5 mM NADH.

High molecular weight affinity ligands usually offer more possibilities for the preparation of affinity adsorbents. A series of very active affinity adsorbents has been prepared by direct attachment of various proteins to a solid support. Survey of the most common coupling procedures, and several examples are given in the section, Application of affinity chromatography, Tables 6.11 and 6.12. However, a very important condition in this instance is that the attachment to the solid support should not cause a change in the native conformation of the ligand. To protect the binding site of the lectin, Clemetson *et al.* (1977) coupled the lectins to Sepharose 4B after CNBr-activation in the presence of 2% of the appropriate sugar.

A solution that may overcome both a low stability and capacity of biospecific sorbents for some glycoproteins may lie in their immobilization through their carbohydrate moieties. Because the active sites of enzymes and antibodies reside in their protein moieties, immobilization of these glycoproteins through their carbohydrate moieties is useful not only for the stabilization of the protein conformation, but it may also confer a greater accessibility to their active sites. By the way of illustration, Bílková *et al.* (1997) recently described the attachment of anti-chymotrypsin antibodies to hydrazide-derivatized bead cellulose. The molar ratio of biospecifically adsorbed chymotrypsin molecules to immobilized antibody was 2 : 1, the value predicted for the enzyme occupancy on each of the antigen binding sites of immunoglobulin G.

Increased accessibility and stability of the active sites of the antibodies can be achieved also by oriented immobilization using the sorption and the cross-linkage of Fc parts of antibodies to immobilized Protein A. Oriented immobilization by the use of this biospecific complex formation with additional types of different complexes is shown in the section on Biospecific Complex formation as a tool for oriented immobilization. In the past decade the interaction between biotin and avidin or streptavidin has provided the basis for the establishement of the avidin-biotin technology (Wilchek and Bayer, 1990).

In order to minimize the nonspecific binding of inert compounds to affinity sorbents their affinity ligands should be used at the lowest possible content. The importance of the low concentration of the affinity ligand and the effect of the uneven surface of the gel are illustrated in Fig. 6.4.

This figure illustrates schematically the surface of the macroreticular hydroxy-alkylmethacrylate polymer in the form of aggregated beads. After the binding of the affinity ligand via the spacer, well accessible, less accessible and sterically inaccessible molecules of the affinity ligand can be recognized. This steric hindrance may in many cases explain the low saturation of molecules of the immobilized ligand with the isolated compound and the heterogeneity in the affinity of immobilized ligands. For the preparation of a homogeneous bioaffinity sorbent it is hence necessary to select conditions for the ligand-carrier binding under which the density of the affinity ligand is low and the ligand is preferentially bound only to readily accessible sites (Fig. 6.4).

The low density of the affinity ligand is also required to prevent nonspecific binding. The bottom part of the figure illustrates the sorption of macromolecules, e.g. enzymes, which do not have a complementary binding site for the immobilized affinity ligand. This binding is caused by the high density of the immobilized affinity ligand, permitting the formation of multiple nonspecific bonds between the macromolecules in solution and the solid phase. These nonspecific bonds allow the compounds present in the mobile phase to bind to the affinity ligand, the spacer and the surface of the solid matrix.

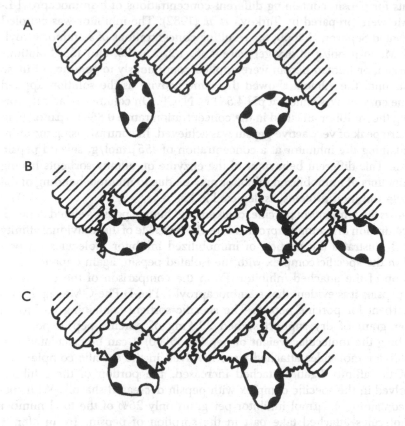

Figure 6.4 Schematic illustration of the effect of concentration of an immobilized affinity ligand
and uneven surface of a solid carrier on specific and nonspecific sorption. (A) Specific
complementary "one-to-one" bonding of isolated enzyme. (B) Nonspecific multi-point
bonding of isolated enzyme in incorrect orientation (Left), in specific multi-point bonding (middle) and in steric hindered bonding (right). (C) Nonspecific multi-point bonding
of inert protein.

These multiple nonspecific bonds may be stronger than a single complementary bond
between the isolated enzyme and immobilized complementary affinity ligand, e.g. an
inhibitor. When the nonspecific multiple bonds are involved in addition to the specific
complementary bond (middle part of the figure) they increase the strength of the binding
in the specific complex. This results in the elution of an enzyme in several fractions and
also gives rise to difficulties in enzyme elution. The multiple nonspecific bonds may
then lead to binding of the enzyme to the immobilized ligand in an incorrect orientation
(middle part of the figure left). Thus, affinity chromatography may yield good results
only on a sorbent containing a low affinity ligand concentration (top part of the figure)
where the enzyme can bind only via the complementary bond to the immobilized
affinity ligand at a ratio of 1 : 1.

In order to determine experimentally the effect of the concentration of the immobilized inhibitor on the course of affinity chromatography of proteolytic enzymes,

specific sorbents for pepsin containing different concentrations of ε-aminocaproyl-L-Phe-D-Phe-OMe were prepared by Turková *et al.* (1982). The inhibitor was coupled to epoxide-activated Separon H 1000; the resulting concentrations of ε-aminocaproyl-L-Phe-D-Phe-OMe in μmol/g of dry gel were 0.85, 1.2, 2.5, 4.5, and 155. Solutions of porcine, chicken, or human pepsin were applied continuously to columns of these affinity sorbents until the effluent showed the same activity as the solution applied (cf. Fig. 6.5). The enzyme was eluted at pH 4.5 (1 M NaCl). On columns of affinity sorbents containing the inhibitor attached in the concentration range 0.85–4.5 μmol/g, in all cases one sharp peak of very active pepsin was achieved. In contrast, using the affinity sorbent containing the inhibitor at a concentration of 155 μmol/g, several pepsin peaks were seen. This different behaviour of the enzyme on affinity sorbents having low and high amounts of immobilized inhibitor may be due to multiple bonding of the enzyme molecule and inert proteins, as depicted in Fig. 6.4.

Figure 6.6 shows the amounts of porcine, chicken, and human pepsins eluted depending on the concentration of ε-aminocaproyl-L-Phe-D-Phe-OMe of the individual affinity sorbents. Part B illustrates the portion of immobilized inhibitor molecules (in percent) involved in the specific complex with the isolated pepsin, again depending on the concentration of the attached inhibitor. From the comparison of the curves for the individual pepsins it is evident that ε-aminocaproyl-L-Phe-D-Phe-OMe-Separon is a very good sorbent for porcine pepsin. The specific sorbent containing 0.85 μmol of inhibitor per gram of dry support sorbed 29.4 mg of porcine pepsin per g of dry sorbent. Using the molecular weight of pepsin (35000) it can be calculated that 99% of the inhibitor molecules attached were involved in the specific complex. As the amount of the affinity ligand attached increased, the portion of the inhibitor molecules involved in the specific complex with pepsin decreased sharply. With specific sorbents containing 4.5 μmol inhibitor per gram only 26% of the total number of inhibitor molecules attached take part in the sorption of pepsin. In an affinity sorbent with the lowest concentration of the affinity ligand, all the molecules of the affinity ligand are fully available for the formation of the complex with the isolated enzyme.

Liu and Stellwagen (1987) used Cibacron Blue F3GA immobilized at several densities to study the different adsorptions of monomeric octopine dehydrogenase and tetrameric lactate dehydrogenase. They determined that the half-time for desorption of lactate dehydrogenase from Cibacron Blue F3GA-Sepharose CL-6B was nearly identical (27 s) to the mass transfer half-time of the protein in the matrix. The change in the visible adsorbance of Cibacron F3GA accompanying its complexation with lactate dehydrogenase was used to observe the kinetics of complexation. The results of their experiments indicated that it is chromatographic mass transfer and not the chemistry of complexation that limits zonal chromatography. This is why the effect of immobilized dye concentration on protein complexation is usualy studied using zonal chromatography.

When the sorbed substance is released from the specific sorbent, the effect of the heterogeneity of the immobilized affinity ligand should be born in mind (Amneus *et al.*, 1976). Fig. 6.7. shows the separation patterns of chymotrypsins and trypsins from mouse pancreatic homogenates on various preparations of Sepharose with coupled soybean trypsin inhibitors (STI). Assuming that the difference in elution conditions reflects differences in biological activities, the former can be used for the characterization

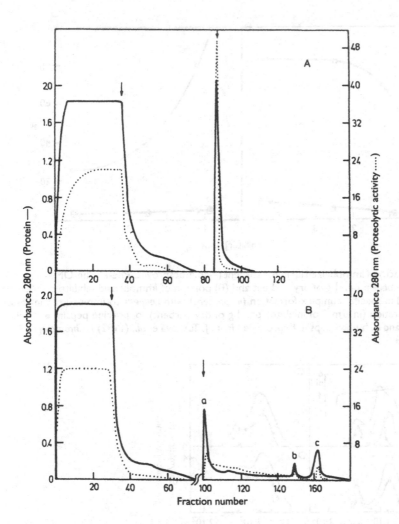

Figure 6.5 Affinity chromatography of porcine pepsin on (ε-aminocaproyl-L-Phe-D-Phe-OCH$_3$-Sepharon columns with (A) low and (B) high concentrations of the immobilized inhibitor. The solution of crude porcine pepsin was applied continuously (see text) onto the affinity columns (5 ml) equilibrated with 0.1 M sodium acetate (pH 4.5). At the position marked by the first arrow equilibrating buffer was applied to the columns to remove unbound pepsin and nonspecifically adsorbed proteins. The second arrow indicates the application of 0.1 M sodium acetate containing 1 M sodium chloride (pH 4.5). Fractions (5 ml) were taken at 4-min intervals. The inhibitor concentration of affinity sorbents were (A) 0.85 and (B) 155 μmol/g of dry support. Solid line, protein; broken line, proteolytic activity. a, b and c, fractions of pepsin of the same specific proteolytic activity. Reproduced from J. Turková *et al.* (1982) *J. Chromatogr.* **236**, 375–383.

of the molecule. The applicability of the adsorbent then depends on the functional homogeneity of the immobilized affinity ligand.

The heterogeneity of association constants of an adsorbent can be caused by (1) the heterogeneity of the biospecific ligand used for the preparation of sorbent, (2) various

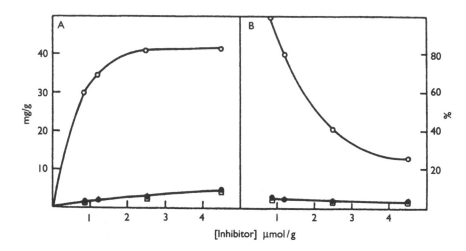

Figure 6.6 (A) Capacity of immobilized inhibitor sorbent (ε-aminocaproyl-L-Phe-D-Phe-OMe-Separon) in mg of pepsin per 1 g of dry sorbent and (B) portion of immobilized inhibitor molecules involved in specific complex formation (in percent) with respect to immobilized inhibitor concentration (in μmol of inhibitor per 1 g of dry sorbent). o, porcine pepsin; •, chicken pepsin, and α, human pepsin. Reproduced from J. Turková et al., (1982) *J. Chromatogr.*, **236**, 375–383.

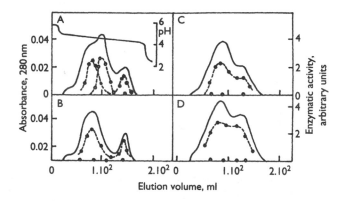

Figure 6.7 Separation patterns of mouse chymotrypsin on Sepharose 4B substituted with different preparations of soybean trypsin inhibitor [STI; STI(W) = inhibitor obtained from Worthington Biochemical Corp., STI(S) = inhibitor obtained from Sigma]. Solid line, absorbance or pH; (•), chymotryptic activity; (o), tryptic activity. (A) unmodified STI(W)-Sepharose, coupled at pH 7.2; (B) Chymotrypsin-modified STI(W)-Sepharose, coupled at pH 7.2; (C) chymotrypsin-modified STI(W)-Sepharose, coupled at pH 8.5; (D) chymotrypsin-modified STI(S)-Sepharose, coupled at pH 7.2. Reproduced with permission from H. Amneus et al. (1976) *J. Chromatogr.*, **120**, 391–397.

changes of the ligand under the effect of immobilization, and (3) various modifications of the affinity ligand caused by the sample.

(1) *Heterogeneity of the ligand before immobilization*
   High molecular weight affinity ligands of biological origin, such as proteins, nucleic acids and carbohydrates, used for the preparation of a specific sorbent, may be

genetically heterogeneous and such heterogeneity can be found in both commercial and non-commercial ligand preparations. It is evident that the presence of impurities in immobilized affinants having a similar or stronger affinity towards the isolated molecules may impair the use of a specific sorbent in gradient separations.

(2) *Alteration of the affinity ligand by immobilization*

The effective activity of the ligand can be changed in various ways by the effect of immobilization. The microenvironment formed by the matrix (charge density, steric hindrance, etc.) may affect the interaction of the immobilized ligand with the isolated molecules to a considerable extent and in a variety of ways, and it can also influence the structure of the affinity ligand itself. Immobilization also brings about changes in the chemical structure, with ensuing change in the molecular properties of the affinity ligand. Here, for example, the number of bonds between the affinity ligand and the solid support plays a considerable role. A comparison of Figs. 6.7B, C clearly shows the unfavourable effect of an increased number of bonds between the molecules of STI and Sepharose 4B, caused by the increase in pH from 7.2 to 8.5 during the coupling after cyanogen bromide activation.

(3) *Modification of the affinity ligand after immobilization*

The fractionated material can contain components that modify the function of the attached affinity ligand. These components may be similar to the compounds being isolated, although they need not be. The enzymes, for example proteases and nucleases, present in crude extracts may cleave the coupled affinants (proteins, nucleic acids) and thus reduce the capacity of the adsorbent for the binding of the specific complementary compound. In addition to this degradation of the affinity ligand, the enzymes and other chemicals present in the fractionated mixture can modify the properties of the coupled affinant specifically, giving rise to forms with retained but changed affinities. All three of the above mentioned effects can be followed in Fig. 6.7. Soybean trypsin inhibitor (Kunitz) obtained from both Worthington Biochemical Corp. [STI(W)] and Sigma [STI(S)] was bound on Sepharose activated with cyanogen bromide. The attached STI was further modified with a solution of α-chymotrypsin: the adsorbent column was washed with a solution of α-chymotrypsin at pH 8 and a flow-rate of 10 ml/h for 24 h and, after incubation, α-chymotrypsin was eluted with a buffer of pH 2.5. From Fig. 6.7A it is evident that when the unmodified STI(W)-Sepharose coupled at pH 7.2 was used, only poor resolution occurred between the two peaks with chymotryptic activity and the peak with tryptic activity. Two further peaks with tryptic activity were eluted still later, at much lower pH values. After a modification of STI(W)-Sepharose with a solution of chymotrypsin, elution of the tryptic activity simultaneously with the chymotryptic activity no longer took place. At the same time, good resolution of the two peaks with chymotryptic activities was obtained. If STI(W)-Sepharose, prepared by coupling at pH 8.5 and modified with a solution of chymotrypsin, was used for separation, the resolution of the two peaks with α-chymotryptic activities deteriorated considerably, in the same manner as when modified STI(S)-Sepharose coupled at pH 7.2 was used (Fig. 6.7D). If various amounts of activated pancreatic homogenate were fractionated on modified STI(W)-Sepharose, prepared at pH 7.2, then with increasing load of the adsorbent the two peaks with chymotryptic activities were eluted at higher pH values (see Table 6.3) and they were less well resolved. The gel had a capacity of 9 mg of α-chymotrypsin per ml. After

Table 6.3 Elution conditions for mouse chymotrypsin (CHT-I and CHT-II) of chymotrypsin-modified STI(W)-Sepharose, coupled at pH 7.2

Number of pancreas applied	CHT activity not retained (%)	pH of solution CHT-I	CHT-II
0.5	0	4.75	4.30
1	0	4.90	4.35
2	3	5.05	4.50
4	57	>5.10	4.80

the chromatography of nine pancreatic homogenates, this capacity decreased to 0.2 mg/ml.

Solid matrix supports

Required characteristic

One of the most important factors in the development of affinity chromatography and of immobilized enzymes is the development of solid supports. A correct choice of solid support and the covalent coupling between the matrix and the affinity ligand may be essential for the success of the desired affinity chromatographic separation. Solid matrix supports can also have a considerable impact on the stability of the immobilized affinity ligand and the adsorbed material. A solid support may even constitute an affinity ligand itself, e.g. polysaccharides for some lectins. An increasing number of different types of supports, their activated forms and biospecific matrices prepared from them, are now becoming commercially available as ready-to-use adsorbents. Within the scope of this chapter only rudimentary solid supports are described and briefly discussed.

An ideal matrix for a successful application in bioaffinity chromatography and for the immobilization of enzymes should possess the following properties (Porath, 1974):

1   insolubility;
2   sufficient permeability and a large specific area;
3   high rigidity and a suitable form of particles;
4   zero adsorption capacity;
5   chemical reactivity permitting the introduction of affinity ligands;
6   chemical stability under the conditions required for the attachment, adsorption, desorption and regeneration;
7   resistance to microbial and enzymatic attack;
8   hydrophilic character.

Complete insolubility is essential, not only for the prevention of losses of affinity adsorbent, but also to prevent contamination of the substance being isolated by the dissolved matrix.

Table 6.4 shows the amount of α-chymotrypsin and glycine bound to 1 ml of hydroxyalkyl methacrylate gels of various pore sizes, depending on the exclusion (molecular weights) and surface areas (Turková *et al.*, 1973). It is obvious that the amount of bound α-chymotrypsin depends directly on the surface area, which is largest for Spheron 300 and 500. The amount of bound glycine indicates that there are relatively small differences in the number of reactive groups.

Essentially the same conclusion may be drawn from the studies of Narayanan *et al.* (1990) on the influence of the physical properties of the base matrix in the preparative bioaffinity chromatography of proteins. They synthesized and characterized four silica-based high performance bioaffinity media differing in pore size and surface area. The surface characterization and coupling of concanavalin A to four silica gels treated with hydrophilic polymer to which glutaraldehyde was covalently attached is shown in Table 6.5. In order to compare the accessible surface areas of the media, in addition to Con A the binding capacities of lactoglobulin, horseradish peroxidase, glyceraldehyde-3-phosphate dehydrogenase and thyroglobulin were also determined. A large protein like thyroglobulin (molecular weight 670 000) was not coupled at all to a silica preparation with an average pore diameter of 8.8 nm while a medium sized protein like peroxidase (molecular weight 40 000) bound less to a silica preparation with an average pore diameter of 77.6 nm despite the large pore size. Con A immobilized to four silica preparations was used for bioaffinity chromatography of horseradish peroxidase. Although the Con A concentration bound to silica with mean pore diameter of 40.8 nm is comparable to that bound to a preparation with mean pore diameter 19.0 nm, the

Table 6.4 Amounts of chymotrypsin and glycine bound to hydroxyalkyl methacrylate gels (Spheron) as a function of their surface areas

Gel	Exclusion mol. wt.	Specific surface area (m^2/ml)	Amount of bound glycine (mg/ml)	Amount of bound chymotrypsin (mg/ml)	Relative proteolytic activity
Spheron 10^5	10^8	0.96	0.5	0.73	–
Spheron 10^3	10^6	5.9	3.1	7.8	44
Spheron 700	700 000	3.6	2.8	6.7	49
Spheron 500	500 000	23	2.6	17.1	37
Spheron 300	300 000	19.5	3.15	17.7	44
Spheron 200	200 000	0.6	2.3	6.9	53
Spheron 100	100 000	0.2	2.6	2.6	38

Table 6.5 Surface characterization and properties of glutaraldehyde-P preparations of 4 silica gels with coupled concanavalin A

Preparation	1	2	3	4
Property				
Pore volume (ml/g)	0.26	0.66	0.83	0.77
Pore surface area (m^2/g)	130	143	85	46
Pore diameter (median)(nm)	8.8	19.0	40.8	77.6
Carbon coverage (m^2/g)	385	424	460	280
Aldehyde $(\mu mol/m^2)$	1.3	1.8	1.53	1.3
Con A (mg/g)	80	140	104	86

Pore volume, pore surface area, and pore diameter were determined by mercury intrusion porosimetry and corrected for interparticle voids.

adsorption capacity for peroxidase on the Con A-silica with smaller pore is higher. The use of the same sorbents for bioaffinity separation of small molecules (p-nitrophenyl sugar derivatives) shows that the pore diameter is much less important for their binding.

By contrast, the bioaffinity adsorption of cells on an immobilized ligand occurs exclusively at the external surface of the support. Therefore, in this type of separation, it is best to select a support with an exclusion limit as low as possible in order to favour ligand immobilization on the external surfaces of the beads.

In order to eliminate the kinetically limited access of adsorbed material to the affinity ligand and recovery of the adsorbed material due to internal diffusion, nonporous solid supports have been increasingly used (Anspach *et al.*, 1990). The advantage of membrane-based immobilized ligand was demonstrated by Kučerová and Turková (1997).

Rigid and a suitably shaped particles are needed to obtain useful flow rate. When an affinant is prepared, it is important that it should be bound to the carrier, and the excess of the affinant that is not bound must be washed out. Similarly, when substances that form a specific and reversible complex with the bound affinant are isolated, it is important that, as far as possible, only their retention should take place on the column. This is one of the main reasons why carriers that contain ionogenic groups, such as the copolymer of ethylene with maleic anhydride, which contain free carboxyl groups after the affinant has been attached, have never been as widely applied in affinity chromatography as agarose based sorbents (no ionogenic groups present).

The support must possess a sufficient number of chemical groups that can be activated and become capable of binding affinants. Activation should take place under conditions that do not change the structure of the support. No less important are the chemical and mechanical stabilities of the carrier under the conditions of attachment of the affinant, and also at various pH values, temperatures and ionic strengths, the possible presence of denaturating agents, etc., which may be necessary for good sorption and elution of a substance. Repeated use of a specific adsorbent depends on achieving the necessary stability.

A related requirement is that the specific sorbents should not be vulnerable to the attack by microorganisms and enzymes. This requirement is best fulfilled by inorganic supports, such as silica, or by synthetic polymers, such as polyacrylamide or hydroxyalkyl methacrylate gels.

Solid support having hydrophilic character is desirable not only to minimize non-specific sorption and inactivation, but also because a hydrophobic support can decrease the stability of some affinity ligands or eluted material by denaturation analogous to that produced by organic solvents. Table 6.6 shows the characteristics required of supports as a function of the type of chromatography: low pressure (LPLAC), medium pressure (MPLAC) or high pressure liquid affinity chromatography (HPLAC).

Biopolymers

Water molecules are essential for the structure and function of biologically active compounds. Affinity chromatography is, therefore, generally performed in the aqueous phase and hydrophilic biopolymers are usually employed as solid supports, mainly natural polysaccharides, such as cellulose, dextran, agarose and, to a lesser extent,

Table 6.6 Characteristics required of an affinity support as a function of the type of chromatography

	LPLAC	MPLAC	HPLAC
Rigidity	+	+	+++
Porosity	++(+)	+	+
Hydrophilic character	+++	+++	+
Secondary interaction	−	−	−
Cost	+	+	+
Activable functional groups	+++	+++	+

starch. The derivatization with ligands necessary for the affinity chromatography to be carried out can be performed relatively simply via their OH groups.

Cellulose and its derivatives

Cellulose is formed by linear polymers of β-1,4-linked D-glucose units with an occasional 1,6-bond:

Commercially available celluloses are generally crosslinked with bifunctional reagents, such as 1-chloro-2,3-epoxypropane, and they are very stable to chemical attack. Glycosidic bonds are sensitive to acid hydrolysis, and under extreme conditions an almost quantitative decomposition to pure crystalline D-glucose may take place. On interaction with oxidative reagents, such as periodate, aldehyde and carboxyl groups are formed. Cellulose can be also destroyed by microbial cellulases.

Cellulose and its derivatives are produced by a number of firms. In addition to Whatman (Maidstone, Great Britain) and Schleicher & Schüll (Zürich, Switzerland), Serva (Heidelberg, F.G.R.), and Bio-Rad Labs. (Richmond, Calif., U.S.A.) supply p-amino-benzoylcellulose under the trade name Cellex PAB and aminoethyl-cellulose under the name Cellex AE. Miles Labs (Slough, Great Britain) produce a hydrazide derivative of CM-Cellulose (Enzite-CMC-hydrazide), bromoacetylcellulose (BAC) and m-aminobenzyl-oxymethylcellulose (AMBC).

Macroporous regenerated cellulose in regular beaded form is produced under the trade mark Perloza by Lovochemie a.s. (Lovosice, Czech Republic). Beaded cellulose and its derivatives, in comparison with other biopolymer spherical materials, show good mechanical strength and resistence to shape deformation and, therefore, provide better through-flow layers in columns. Good mechanical strength is preserved in spite of the high porosity. Due to its chemical composition it is highly hydrophilic and is well tolerated by biosystems. Its insolubility in water and a number of other

solvents allows it to be used in aqueous media. The hydrazide derivative of Perloza
was used by Bílková *et al.* (1997) to prepare an immunosorbent for oriented immobilization of α-chymotrypsin. Medium-pressure Matrex Cellufine gels supplied by
Amicon Co. (Danvers, MA, U.S.A.) are composed of spherical, beaded cellulose. They
offer low non-specific adsorption, outstanding physical strength and high pressure operating capabilities, all at a low cost. The use of Cellufine in bioaffinity chromatography
has been described by Anspach *et al.* (1990). The use of fibrous cellulose particles as
matrices for DNA-bearing supports is described by Hermanson *et al.* (1992) in their
chapter about immobilized nucleic acids. The isolation of poly-mRNA from tumor
cells by use of an oligo(dT)-cellulose slurry in an Eppendorf EVENT 4160 vacuum
filtration unit was described by Noppen *et al.* (1996). This method can be used for
mRNA determination or purification in diagnostics as well as in biological and medical
research.

To solve purification problems encountered during a scale up from laboratory to
industrial use, Hou and Mandaro (1986) have developed a radial flow chromatography method based on a cellulosic media derivatized with vinyl polymers. The method
employed for grafting the polymer onto the cellulose yields a matrix with a high charge
density and thus a very high adsorption capacity. A schematic representation of the
radial flow Zeta cartridge is shown in Fig. 6.8. The cartridge was constructed by rolling
a thin sheet matrix around a central rod with webbing between the layers of the matrix
to allow swelling of the media and to provide an even distribution of the fluid throughout the matrix. The fluid flows radially from the outside to the inside of the cartridge
through the layers of the grafted media (ion exchange or affinity), and it is then collected by the flow paths engraved on the central core, and exits through the ports

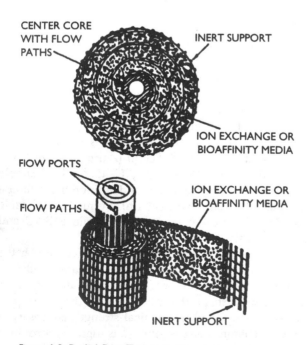

Figure 6.8 Radial flow Zeta cartridge.

located at the top of the cartridge. Zeta cartridges and several Zeta affinity products were produced by CUNO Inc. (Cergy-Pontoise, France). Mem Sep TM Chromatography Cartridges, which are ready to use and provide a microporous network of pure regenerated cellulose in a column-type housing configuration, containing several affinity membrane cartridges are produced by MILLIPORE (Bedford, MA, U.S.A.). More information about the production and application of cellulose membranes is provided in the section on Membranes and tubes.

Dextran gels

Dextran is a branched-chain glucose polysaccharide produced in solutions containing sugar by various strains of *Leuconostoc mesenteroides*. Soluble dextran, prepared by fractional precipitation with ethanol of partially hydrolysed crude dextran, contains more than 90% of α-1,6-glucosidic linkages with 1,2-, 1,3- and 1,4-glucoside branching. When crosslinked with 1-chloro-2,3-epoxypropane in alkaline solution, dextran affords a three-dimensional gel with the general structure:

$$
\begin{array}{l}
-\text{O}-\text{CH}_2 \\
\quad\quad\quad \text{O} \\
\text{OH} \quad -\text{O}-\text{CH}_2 \\
\text{HO} \quad\quad\quad\quad \text{O} \\
\quad\quad \text{O} \quad \text{OH} \quad -\text{O}- \\
\quad\quad \text{CH}_2 \quad \text{HO} \\
\quad\quad \text{CH}-\text{OH} \quad\quad \text{OH} \\
\quad\quad \text{CH}_2 \\
\quad\quad \text{O} \\
\text{HO} \\
\quad \text{OH} \quad -\text{O}- \\
\quad\quad\quad \text{O} \\
\quad -\text{O}-\text{CH}_2
\end{array}
$$

The most prominent producer of dextran gels, supplied under the trade name Sephadex, is Pharmacia Biotech. (Uppsala, Sweden). The gels are very stable against chemical attack; for example, exposure to 0.25 M sodium hydroxide solution at 60°C for 2 months has no effect. The glucosidic bond is sensitive to hydrolysis at low pH, although it is stable in 0.02 M hydrochloric acid for 6 months, or in 0.1 M hydrochloric acid or 88% formic acid for 1–2 h (Lowe and Dean, 1974). Aldehyde or carboxyl groups are formed under the action of oxidizing agents. Dextran gels can withstand heating in an autoclave at 110°C (in solution) for 40 min, or at 120°C, when dry. Drying and swelling is reversible. The gels swell to some extent even in ethanol, ethylene glycol, formamide, N,N-dimethylformamide and dimethyl sulphoxide.

A molecular sieve produced by covalent crosslinking of allyl-dextran with N,N′-methylene-bis-acrylamide, has been developed by Pharmacia Biotech. (Uppsala, Sweden) under the trade name Sephacryl. The advantage of this matrix is the good flow rate, because the support is exceptionally rigid. Unfortunately the nonspecific adsorption is increased compared to other dextran gels.

They are widely used without any modification as specific sorbents for the isolation of a series of lectins. One example is the isolation of concanavalin A from jack bean seeds (Nandedkar *et al.*, 1987). The use of dextran gels is partly restricted by their rather low porosity.

Agarose and its derivatives

Agarose is a polysaccharide present in crude agar in a polymeric mixture of agaropectin and agarose. The separation of agarose out of the polysaccharide mixture is based on differences in solubility and chemical reactivity, which is associated with the anionic character of agaropectins. Cooling aqueous agarose solutions below 50°C allows the development of agarose gels in bead, pellet, or spherical forms.

Agarose is a linear polysaccharide consisting of alternating 1,3-linked β-D-galactopyranose and 1,4-linked 3,6-anhydro-α-L-galactopyranose residues:

Arnott *et al.* (1974) postulated on the basis of X-ray studies that the polysaccharide chains form a double helix, then aggregate via hydrogen bridges and hydrophobic interactions into fibers or bundles with ordered structures. This network phase in a gel, which may contain up to 100 times more water than agarose, contains relatively large voids through which large macromolecules can diffuse. In contradistinction, a gel network comprising of a comparable concentration of crosslinked soluble polymer, such as the crosslinked dextrans, would lead to a lattice in which the mean pore size would be considerably smaller. These relationships are shown diagrammatically in Fig. 6.9 and suggest that agarose shows particularly useful special properties as a chromatographic medium. The exclusion limit may be varied within wide range because the pore size is inversely proportional to the agarose concentration (Mohr and Pommerening, 1985).

The main producers of agarose are Pharmacia Biotech. (Uppsala, Sweden), under the trade name Sepharose, Bio-Rad Labs. (Richmond, Calif., U.S.A.), under the trade name Bio-Gel A and Reactifs IBF (Villeneuve la Garenne, France) under the trade name Ultrogel A. Agarose gels under the name SAG (Ago-Gel) -10, -6, -4 and -2 with molecular weight exclusion limits of $25 \times 10^4 - 15 \times 10^7$ are supplied by Seravac Labs. (Maidenhead, Great Britain) and Mann Labs. (New York, N.Y., U.S.A.)

Supports with large beads are advantageous for the affinity chromatography of cells, since they can pass through such columns without being physically trapped. For this purpose an agarose gel has been developed with the trade name Sepharose 6MB. The macrobeads have a large diameter (250–350 μm), uniform shape, and low nonspecific adsorption of cells. The stability of an agarose matrix can be considerably increased by crosslinking with epichlorohydrin, 2,3-dibromopropanol or divinyl sulphone. In 1975, Sepharose CL(2B, 4B, 6B) was introduced, prepared from appropriate types of Sepharoses by crosslinking with 2, 3-dibromopropanol in strongly alkaline medium and desulphating the resulting gel by alkaline hydrolysis under reducing conditions. The crosslinking of Sepharose CL does not decrease the effective pore size, thus suggesting that crosslinks take place mainly between chains within a single gel fiber, probably between oxygen in position 2 of the anhydrogalactose residue (Mohr and Pommerening, 1985). The increased stability of Sepharose CL is shown in Table 6.7.

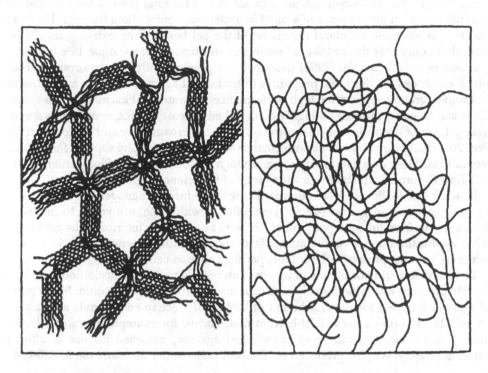

Figure 6.9 A comparison between a cross-linked dextran (Sephadex) matrix and agarose gel matrix (right), at equivalent polymer concentration. The aggregates in agarose gels may contain $10–10^4$ bundles of polysaccharide helices. Reproduced with permission from Arnott *et al.* (1974) *J. Mol. Biol.*, **90**, 269–284.

Table 6.7 Comparison of stability between normal and covalent cross-linked agarose gels

	Sepharose	*Sepharose CL*
pH	4–9	3–14
Temperature (°C)	0–40	<70
Solvents	Aqueous solutions containing high concentrations of salts, urea guanidine. HCl, detergents Dimethylformamide-H_2O (1:1) Ethyleneglycol-H_2O (1:1)	Aqueous solutions, 6 M guanidine. HCL, 8 M urea and detergents in a pH range 3–11 Organic solvents
Sterilization	No autoclaving	Autoclaving at pH 7 and 110–120°C
Chaotropic ions (KSCN)	Low stability	High stability

It is inadvisable to dry and re-swell the agarose gels. When agarose is not in use it should be stored in the wet or moist state and protected from microbial growth by means of a suitable bacteriostatic agent. A number of antimicrobial agents are commonly used: 0.02% sodium azide, 0.5% butanol, trichlorobutanol and saturated toluene. Other bacteriostatic agents should only be used if they are known to be innocuous to the structure of agarose. In general, when agarose gels are stored for long periods they should be kept below 8°C in the presence of a suitable bacteriostat but without freezing. Freezing results in irreversible structural disruption of the gel beads. Freeze-drying should be carried out only after the addition of protective substances, for example 15% lactose.

Gustavsson and Larsson (1996) described the preparation of superporous agarose which combines the desirable properties of traditional agarose supports and those of a chromatography support for high performance separations. Pharmacia Biotechnol. (Uppsala, Sweden) produces a highly cross-linked agarose matrix, resulting in a very rigid gel, under the trade name Superose 6B. Both the crosslinking and narrow particle size (20–40 μm) contribute to its performance as a chromatography support for HPLC-separations. Their new names for Sepharose high performance bioaffinity columns are "Hi Trap Columns" which have a wide range of life science applications.

Reactifs IBF (Villeneuve la Garenne, France) produces Magnogel A4R which is a support composed of agarose (4% w/v) cross-linked with epichlorohydrin. Its magnetic nature results from the incorporation of 7% (w/v) Fe_3O_4 in the interior of the gel beads. It has applications under conditions not favorable to column operation, e.g. in viscous solutions or in the presence of insoluble particles such as cell debris.

The polysaccharide backbone of agarose can readily undergo substitution reactions to yield products with a moderately high capacity for further derivatisation. Many types of agarose activated for the attachment of biologically active compounds and a variety of affinity sorbents are available from many firms, for example Sigma (St. Louis, MO, U.S.A.), etc. Derivatives of cross-linked agarose, modified for use in affinity chromatography, are also produced by Bio-Rad Labs. under the trade name Affi-Gel.

Synthetic copolymers

The advantages of high-performance liquid bioaffinity chromatography, shown in Fig. 6.2, and the usefulness of the preparation of biologically active compounds on a pilot or industrial scale, are the impetus behind the continuous development of synthetic polymers. The main appeal of solid supports for these applications is their inherent mechanical stability which provides good flow characteristics even under high pressures. They can be operated at pressures up to 100 p.s.i., and usually tolerate a wide pH range. They are suitable for affinity ligand immobilization and provide bioaffinity supports with high capacities. They are biologically inert and thus, they are not subject to enzymatic or microbial degradation. The chemical structure of these supports can be characterized by their polyethylene backbone, which creates excellent chemical and physical stability. They also contain modifiable side chains R_1, R_2, R_3, R_4:

$$\begin{array}{ccc} R_1 & & R_2 \\ | & & | \\ -\,C & - & C\,- \\ | & & | \\ R_3 & & R_4 \end{array}$$

Only a limited number of synthetic polymers will be described. However, many synthetic copolymers exist and biospecific sorbents prepared from them are produced by many firms.

Acrylamide derivatives

Polyacrylamide gels are produced by copolymerization of acrylamide with the bifunctional crosslinking agent N,N'-methylenebisacrylamide. The monomers used in this synthesis are highly toxic and thus should be handled with care.

Polyacrylamide gels are composed of a hydrocarbon skeleton onto which carboxamide groups are bound:

$$\begin{array}{c}
NH_2 \\
| \\
C=O \\
| \\
---CH_2-CH-CH_2-CH-CH_2-CH--- \\
| | \\
C=O C=O \\
| | \\
HN NH_2 \\
| \\
CH_2 \\
| \\
HN \\
| \\
C=O \\
---CH_2-CH-CH_2-CH-CH_2-CH_2--- \\
| | \\
C=O C=O \\
| | \\
HN NH_2
\end{array}$$

The main producer of polyacrylamide gels is Bio-Rad Labs (Richmond, CA, U.S.A.) under the trade name Bio-Gel P. This gel is produced with a range of pore sizes, from Bio-Gel P-2 with a molecular weight exclusion limit of 1800, to Bio-Gel P-300 with a molecular weight exclusion limit of 400 000. Gels of different porosities are available in beads with 50–100, 100–200, 200–400 and 400 mesh size. Commercial polyacrylamide beads are available in the dry state and are swollen by mixing with water or aqueous solutions for periods of 4–48 h depending on the porosity. Bio-Gel P products are stable in most eluants used in biochemical studies, including dilute solutions of salts, detergents, urea and guanidine hydrochloride, although high concentrations of these reagents may alter the exclusion limits by up to 10%. The use of media with pH values outside the range 2–10 is to be avoided since some hydrolysis of the amide side groups may occur with the consequent appearance of ion-exchange groups. The use of oxidising agents such as hydrogen peroxide is also inadvisable.

Non-specific adsorption to the matrix backbone is restricted to very acidic, very basic and aromatic compounds and is evidenced by their delayed emergence from the chromatographic bed. Ionic groups on the matrix are almost non-existent.

Polyacrylamide gels are biologically inert and refractory to attacks from microorganisms. Because the gel particles adhere strongly to clean glass surfaces, Inman and Dintzis (1969) recommend the use of siliconized glass or polyethylene laboratory vessels. They can easily be converted into solid carriers suitable for the binding of a series of affinants (Inman and Dintzis, 1969).

Non-ionic synthetic supports are obtained by copolymerization of N-acryloyl-2-amino-2-hydroxymethyl-1, 3-propane diol with hydroxylated acrylic bifunctional monomer. Hydrophilic supports under the trade name Trisacryl GF are manufactured by IBF Reactifs (Villeneuve la Garenne, France). The chemical structure of the polymer Trisacryl GF05 is:

$$
\begin{array}{cccc}
& \text{CH}_2\text{OH} & & \text{CH}_2\text{OH} \\
& | & & | \\
\text{NH}-\text{C}-\text{CH}_2\text{OH} & & \text{NH}-\text{C}-\text{CH}_2\text{OH} \\
| \quad | & & | \quad | \\
\text{CO} \quad \text{CH}_2\text{OH} & & \text{CO} \quad \text{CH}_2\text{OH} \\
| & & | \\
-\text{CH}-\text{CH}_2-\text{CH}-\text{CH}_2-\text{CH}-\text{CH}_2-\text{CH}-\text{CH}_2- \\
| \quad | & & | \quad | \\
\text{CO} \quad \text{CH}_2\text{OH} & & \text{CO} \quad \text{CH}_2\text{OH} \\
\text{NH}-\text{C}-\text{CH}_2\text{OH} & & \text{NH}-\text{C}-\text{CH}_2\text{OH} \\
| & & | \\
\text{CH}_2\text{OH} & & \text{CH}_2\text{OH}
\end{array}
$$

By strictly controlling the polymerization process, it is possible to synthesize a complete line of products, covering a wide range of molecular weight exclusion from 3000 (Trisacryl GF05) to about 20 million (Trisacryl GF 2000).

Trisacryl is characterized by a high degree of hydrophilicity, due both to the presence of primary alcohol groups and also to the secondary amide function. It can be used under pressures up to 2–3 bar and is not affected by organic solvents such as alcohols, ketones, dioxane, or chlorinated solvents. It is stable at low (−20°C) and high (121°C) temperatures. Denaturing agents have no effect on the gel because its structure involves no hydrogen bonds. It is also stable to acidic pH, but less stable to high pH because of the slow hydrolysis of the amide linkage. Oligo(dT)-substituted Trisacryl was used for the purification of polyadenylated mRNA by Sene *et al.* (1982). Bonnafous *et al.* (1983) described cell bioaffinity chromatography with using of Trisacryl and ligand immobilized through cleavable mercury-sulphur bonds.

Methacrylate supports

The copolymerization of hydroxyalkyl methacrylate with alkylene dimethacrylates gives rise to heavily crosslinked xerogel microparticles which subsequently aggregate and yield macroporous spheroids (Čoupek *et al.*, 1973). Their structure is shown in Fig. 6.10. These gels have some chemical properties in common with agarose, for example, the hydroxyl groups of the gel can be activated with cyanogen bromide (Turková *et al.*, 1973).

Hydroxyalkyl methacrylate supports have been marketed under the trade name Separon HEMA (manufactured by Tessek s.r.o., Prague, Czech Republic), or under the trade name Spheron (manufactured by Lachema, Brno, Czech Republic). These supports have good chemical and mechanical stability and are stable to heating in 1 M sodium glycolate at 150°C for 8 h or boiling in 20% hydrochloric acid for 24 h. They are biologically inert and are not attacked by microorganisms. They can be employed in organic solvents, a property which was used to advantage during the binding of peptides (Turková *et al.*, 1976). The inner structure, pore size, and distribution, specific surface, and quantity of reactive OH groups can be varied, with a molecular weight exclusion

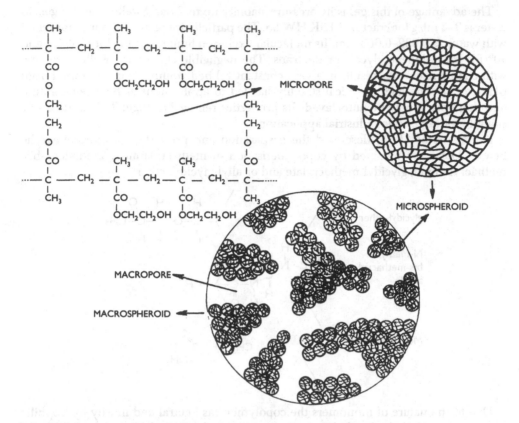

Figure 6.10 Structure of hydroxyalkyl methacrylate copolymer (Separon, Spheron).

limit ranging from 20 000 to 20 000 000. A comparison of some properties of seven types of Spherons are shown in Table 6.4. Because of its high rigidity this matrix shows excellent flow properties. High performance liquid bioaffinity chromatography (HPLBAC) of porcine pepsin on Separon H1000, modified with ε-aminocaproyl-L-phenylalanyl-D-phenylalanine methylester, has been described by Turková *et al.* (1981). The excellent stability of this matrix allows its application to large scale operations and to industrial production (Mohr and Pommerening, 1985).

Hydroxyethylmethacrylate support is also produced under the trade name Dynospheres by Dyno Particles (Lillestrom, Norway). Their monodisperse microparticles with a size range of 0.3–5 μm are promising synthetic polymers for HPLAC application.

Toyo Soda Manufacturing Co. (Tokyo, Japan) has developed a semi-rigid gel, a copolymer of oligoethyleneglycol, glycidylmethacrylate and pentaerythrol dimethacrylate under the trade name Toyopearl. The identical copolymer under the name Fractogel TSK HW Type is sold by E. Merck (Darmstadt, Germany).

Optimal conditions for the activation of free hydroxyl groups on the gel matrix by epichlorohydrin and subsequent immobilization of ligands were investigated by Matsumoto *et al.* (1982). They successfully prepared affinity adsorbents for bioaffinity chromatography of lectins and trypsin. Shimura *et al.* (1984) used Toyopearl HW-65S with attached p-aminobenzamidine for the high-performance bioaffinity chromatography of plasmin and plasminogen.

The advantage of this gel is its pressure stability up to 7 bar. Swelling of dry gels in water is 3–4 ml/g for Fractogel TSK HW-65. The particle size of this support, moistened with water, is 0.032–0.063 mm. Its molecular exclusion limit is 5×10^6 for proteins and 10^6 for polyethylene glycols or dextrans. The negligible change in swelling volume with changing eluents, results in a very constant gel bed volume. It may be used from pH 1 to 14. The high chemical stability has led to applications at high temperature and therefore it may be autoclaved. Its properties render Fractogel TSK particularly suitable for large scale industrial application.

Krämer *et al.* (1978) described the preparation and properties of oxirane acrylic beads. These are obtained by copolymerisation of methacrylamide, methylene-bis-methacrylamide, glycidyl-methacrylate and or allyl-glycidyl-ether:

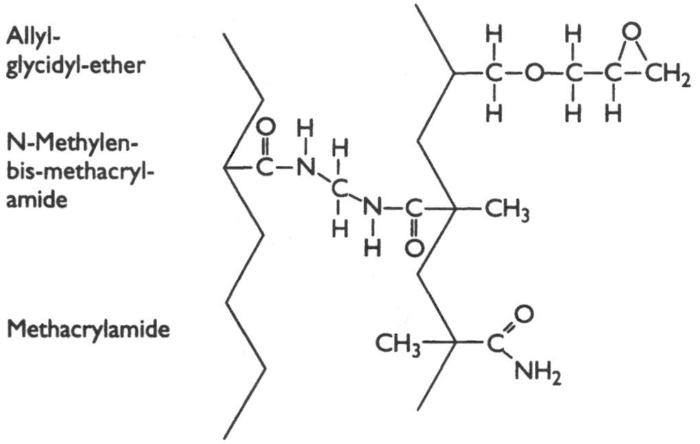

Due to the nature of monomers the copolymer has neutral and mostly hydrophilic matrix, with a slight hydrophobic component due to the methyl groups along the polymer backbone. The oxirane group content is 1000 μmol/g dry beads. The beads are macroporous and they show a water regain of 2.5 ml/g of dry beads. This water regain is independent of pH (0.5–12.5) and ionic strength. The beads are morphologically and chemically stable under these conditions, even if exposed to them for several weeks. The mechanical stability upon stirring is very good. At present, oxirane acrylic beads are produced under the trade mark Eupergit C by Röhm Pharma GMBH (Darmstadt, F.R.G.).

High-performance immunoaffinity chromatography (HPIAC) using Eupergit C beads was developed and optimized by Fleminger *et al.* (1990b). They immobilized antibodies against carboxypeptidase A onto Eupergit C beads of sizes 150 μm (standard, porous), 30 μm (C30N, porous) and 1 μm (C1Z, nonporous). Carboxypeptidase A was adsorbed to immunosorbents in cited order: more than 1000 mg/g of first solid support, more than 100 mg/g and 6.5 mg/g of 2nd and 3rd solid supports. However, antigen binding capacities of used immunosorbents were 0.75, 0.8 and 0.95 mol of carboxypeptidase A/mol of antibodies.

Polystyrene and its derivatives

Polymer-coated polystyrene/divinylbenzene beads under the name Poros matrix have been developed by PerSeptive Biosystems (Cambridge, Massachusetts, U.S.A.). The backbone of the matrix is unique in that it contains a network of large and small pores within each spherical bead (Hermanson *et al.*, 1992). The Poros matrix structure consists of large 'through pores' (600–800 nm) that allow rapid flow into the interior of the bead and a network of 'diffusive pores' (50–100 nm) that gives the support good capacity for affinity applications. The polymer coating provides active sites for futher modification and also blocks the harsh hydrophobic character of the styrene core. Depending on the particular application, PerSeptive has used cross-linked polyethyleneimine as well as a proprietary polyhydroxylic polymer to coat the particles. Since the base matrix is a stable cross-linked polystyrene, the chemical and physical nature of the support is exceptionally robust. The media is resistant to extremes in pH (1–14) and is compatible with all common buffers and solvents used in HPLC. It can also withstand 0.5 N NaOH and 1.0 N HCl for cleaning and sterilizing purposes. The physical stability of the matrix is reflected by its maximum pressure limit of 3000 psi. In particular, activation of the proprietary hydroxyl-containing polymer coating has yielded affinity supports based on the immobilization of protein A and iminodiacetic acid, as well as various specific immunoglobulins. Both reductive amination and tresyl-mediated coupling protocols have been used with success.

Saito and Nagai (1983) coupled antibody on a plastic surface using polystyrene tubes (Falcon, Div. of Becton, Dickinson and Co., Cockeysville, MD, U.S.A.) treated with 0.5% toluene 2,4-diisocyanate dissolved in carbon tetrachloride. The polystyrene tube coated with anti-rabbit γ-globulin goat serum allowed a simple separation of the free tracer in a radioimmunoassay of thyroid-stimulating hormone and prolactin.

Superparamagnetic polystyrene Dynabeads, consisting of (Fe_2O_3)-containing core covered with a polymer are produced by the firm DYNAL A.S. (Oslo, Norway).They have a smooth surface that is easily coated with antibodies or other selecting molecules. Combined with a magnet, Dynabeads make a unique tool in positive or negative separation. Monosize magnetic particles in selective cell separation were used by Ugelstad *et al.* (1988) for the successful clinical application of immunomagnetic beads for depletion of tumor cells or T lymphocytes from bone marrow. Information about cell separation and protein purification by the use of Dynabeads are in second edition of Technical Handbook (1996), which can be obtained from Dynal a.s.

Combination of biopolymers with synthetic polymers

In order to preserve the polyacrylamide porosity during activation, copolymers of agarose and polyacrylamide have been produced. This matrix combines the advantages of each individual polymer, while extending the potential range of derivatisation procedures by virtue of the availability of both amide and hydroxyl groups for activation (Doley *et al.*, 1976). Polyacrylamide-agarose gels with varying porosities are produced under the name Ultrogels AcA by IBF Reactifs (Villeneuve la Garenne, France). A schematic representation of the Ultrogel AcA matrix is shown in Fig. 6.11.

Ultrogel AcA is available in four types, each having a three-dimensional polyacrylamide lattice enclosing an interstitial agarose gel. The gels are pre-swollen and calibrated within a narrow particle size range of 60–140 µm.

During chemical reactions involving one of the polymers, certain precautions must be taken in view of both polymers properties. Thus the gel must not be exposed to strongly alkaline media, since the amide groups will be hydrolyzed to carboxylic acids. The limited heat resistance of the agarose must equally be respected: Ultrogel AcA must not be exposed to temperatures greater than about 40°C.

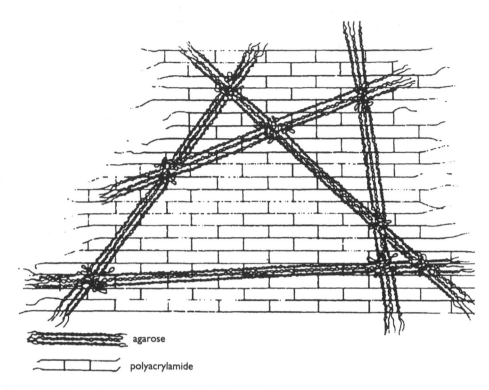

Figure 6.11 Schematic representation of the Ultrogel AcA matrix.

Immunosorbents prepared with glutaraldehyde-activated Ultrogel AcA are of special interest for the one-step purification of antibodies from whole serum (Guesdon and Avrameas, 1976). Polyacrylic hydrazido-Sepharose derivatives possess the advantages of both, agarose and acrylamide gels. At neutral pH they carry no charge and they contain a large number of modifiable groups. The preparation of polyacrylhydrazido-agarose based on periodate oxidation of Sepharose followed by reaction with poly-acrylhydrazide has been described by Miron and Wilchek (1981). These yielded matrices which were colourless and stable after reduction with sodium borohydride. Polyacrylhydrazido-agarose could be used either directly or after further modification with various reactive groups. A support having similar properties is dextran crosslinked with N,N'-methylenebisacrylamide (Belew *et al.*, 1978). This is produced by Pharmacia (Uppsala, Sweden) under the trade name Sephacryl and is discussed in more detail in paragraph about dextran.

Magnogel Ac A44 produced by IBF Reactifs (Villeneuve la Garenne, France) is a magnetized support, derived from Ultrogel Ac A44 (Guesdon and Avrameas, 1977). The polyacrylamide-agarose beads contain 7% Fe_3O_4 in the interior, thus enabling them to be separated in the magnetic field. The gel may be activated either through the agarose or polyacrylamide moieties. This gel is suitable for magnetic bioaffinity chromatography (Groman and Wilchek, 1987). This material offers advantages where easy and rapid manipulation of particles are desirable, such as when unstable materials are being isolated, when the extract is viscous or contaminated with solids, or in the separation of cell types.

Inorganic supports

Inorganic supports have been reviewed by Weetall and Lee (1989). They classified these supports into a few major categories: metals, metal oxides, ceramics, and glasses. They described the preparations, properties and applications (for the immobilization of antibodies) of porous glass, porous silica, titania, alumina and zirconia bodies, and iron and nickel oxides. These supports have an inherent advantage in their rigidity. Since inorganic particles are friable, one should not use a stirring bar when working with these materials. Particles can be separated by several convenient methods. These include: filtration, centrifugation, settling, aspiration, or magnetic separation. Several of these methods can be utilized for sizing inorganic particles, particularly when clumping has occurred or when one wants particles of only a specific size range. Particles may be sized on the basis of settling times, centrifugation speed or filter porosity. The best method for sizing can be selected by considering the size range that is desired, and by choosing the method most likely to yield the desired particle size.

Controlled pore glass

Controlled pore glass (CPG) is synthesised by heating certain borosilicate glasses to 500–800°C for prolonged periods of time. These glass mixtures separate on such heat treatment into borate- and silicate-rich phases. The borate phase can be dissolved by treatment with acid, leaving a network of extremely small tunnels with pore diameters 3–6 nm. Subsequent treatment with mild caustic soda removes silica material from the pore interiors and thus enlarges the pore diameter. Careful control of the various treatments can lead to a porous glass in the range 4,5–250 nm. Glass derivatives have outstanding mechanical stability. The rigidity of the beads permits high flow rates and facilitates fast and efficient separations. Glass beads are resistant to microbial attack and may be readily sterilised by disinfectants or autoclaving. The latter is a prime consideration in the purification of pyrogen-free enzymes destined for *in vivo* or clinical studies.

CPG has ion-exchange properties due to its silanol (−Si−OH) surface. The same silanol functions can be exploited as anchor points for coating chemistries that largely eliminate the non-specific adsorption. CPG is very resistent to acid but rapidly degrades at pH greater than 8.0. Glass will also dissolve at an appreciable rate in deionized water. Working buffers should be neutral and contain at least 0.05 M salt or, preferably, be slightly acidic.

Corning Glass Works have demonstrated that glass, when treated with γ-aminopropyltriethoxysilane, becomes a suitable support for affinity chromatography (Weetal and Filbert, 1974). The silanization process created by a reaction between the surface silanol groups and the amino-functional silane coupling agent:

$$\begin{array}{c} O \\ | \\ -O-Si-OH \\ | \\ O \\ | \end{array} + \begin{array}{c} O-CH_2CH_3 \\ | \\ CH_3CH_2-O-Si-O-(CH_2)_3-NH2 \\ | \\ O-CH_2CH_3 \\ | \end{array} \longrightarrow \begin{array}{c} O \\ | \\ -O-Si-O- \\ | \\ O \\ | \end{array} \begin{array}{c} O-CH_2CH_3 \\ | \\ Si-O-(CH_2)_3-NH_2 \\ | \\ O-CH_2CH_3 \\ | \end{array}$$

The reaction can be performed in either organic or aqueous media and the resulting alkylamino-glass can subsequently be used to immobilize affinity ligands. Commercially available porous glass packing materials are produced among others by the Bio-Rad Labs. (Richmont, Calif., U.S.A.) under the trade name Bio-Glass, by Corning Glass Works (Corning, N.Y., U.S.A.), Waters Assoc. (Milford, Mass., U.S.A.) Electro-Nucleonics, Inc. (Fairfield, N.Y., U.S.A.) and Pierce Chemical Company (Rockford, Il., U.S.A.) under the name CPG.

Glyceryl-CPG is a controlled pore glass whose surface has been chemically modified to produce a hydrophilic, non-ionic coating which shares most of the same operating characteristics as conventional CPG. The degree of adsorption of glutamate dehydrogenase on various derivatized glass surfaces was studied by Du Val et al. (1984). Glycerolpropyl glass was the weakest adsorber of the protein. Glyceryl-CPG is distributed by Electro-Nucleonics Inc. (Fairfield, N.Y., U.S.A.) Another supplier of glycophase-coated supports under the name glycophase G/CPG is the Pierce Chemical Company (Rockford, Il., U.S.A.). This company uses triethoxypropyl glycidosilane as the alkylsilane.

Ivanov et al. (1985) compared epoxy-containing porous glass, prepared with γ-glycidoxypropyltriethoxysilane, and carbonylchloride-containing matrices, prepared by grafting copolymers of N-vinylpyrrolidone and acryloylchloride onto the surface of γ-aminopropyl-silylated porous glass, for the isolation of neuraminidase from the influenza virus. A biospecific sorbent prepared from the polymer-containing glass enabled the isolation of neuraminidase with a 3–4 times higher specific activity than on the adsorbent prepared from epoxy-containing glass. In order to prevent the non-specific adsorption of proteins from human serum to wide porous glass with disaccharides bound through a polyacrylamide spacer, Rapoport et al. (1997) pretreated the column of adsorbent with 5% bovine serum albumin during 16 h and then washed it with 10 mM phosphate buffered saline.

Phillips et al. (1985) used nonporous glass beads (particle diameter < 10 μm) to eliminate the diffusional effects due to the pore. Cibacron Blue F3GA coupled to nonporous glass beads, porous silicas and soft gels was employed by Anspach et al. (1989) to investigate equilibration times for the adsorption of lysozyme on the different dye-affinity sorbents. In the batch mode, equilibration times varied from 20 s for nonporous glass beads (20–30 μm) to more than 60 min in the case of a porous sorbent with a particle diameter of 100–300 μm and 60 nm pore size.

Porous and nonporous silica

The structure of silica is amorphous and its composition can be expressed as $SiO_2 \times H_2O$. Its basic unit is tetrahedral (SiO_4) and its porosity depends on the mode of preparation. Silica gel is formed from silicic acid sols by polycondensation of orthosilicic acid. Submicroscopic elemental particles are formed which retain micelles of the starting acid in the interior. The silica is bound by siloxane Si–O–Si bonds. Every elemental particle touches the surfaces of several neighbouring particles and in this way a conglomerate is formed containing pores of various diameters. The occurence of these inner spaces is very high and after drying they contain large specific inner surface areas of hundreds of m^2/g.

The main advantage of silica is its inherent mechanical stability which provides good flow characteristics even under high pressure. The use of silica with pore sizes ranging from 6 to 400 nm, or nonporous silica in small particles 1.5–10 μm, is recommended to provide good mass transfer when performing protein separations. Silica is a commonly used support for high-performance affinity chromatography. Slightly acidic silanol groups on the silica surface act as centres for the non-specific adsorption. Under alkaline working conditions (pH > 8) the surface of silica gel exhibits a high solubility which results in the contamination of the purified product. The problems of non-specific adsorption and the solubility of silica have been largely overcome by derivatization of the silanol groups with silanes, yielding silica derivatives coated with a hydrophilic layer. The most common reagent for blocking silanol groups is 3-glycidoxypropyltrimethoxy silane. The resulting epoxy silica can be used for the direct attachment of affinity ligands or can become the starting material for the synthesis of other products. As an example can be cited the hydrazide-activated silica supports for HPLAC developed by Ruhn *et al* (1994). They prepared diol-bonded silica from Nucleosil Si-300 or 1000 (Alltech, Deerfield, Il., U.S.A.) coated with 3-glucidoxypropyltrimethoxy silane by hydrolysis with sulfuric acid. After periodate oxidation of the diol-silica, an aldehyde silica was produced and used for the optimization of hydrazide-activated silica synthesis by use of oxalic or adipic dihydrazide. After activation, remaining aldehyde groups were reduced by adding $NaBH_4$. Dihydrazide-activated silica was used to immobilize the periodate oxidized carbohydrate moieties of antibodies, horse radish peroxidase and tRNA. The long term stability of dihydrazide-activated silica was studied before and after its use in biomolecule immobilization. The activated support was stable for 2–6 weeks when stored at 5–25°C. Periodate oxidized antibodies coupled to dihydrazide-activated supports were stable for at least one month in solvents commonly used in HPLC. Nonporous monodisperse silica beads have been described by Unger *et al* (1986). Decreasing the particle diameters from 10 to 1.5 μm, or less, increases the surface area within a given column volume. From both theoretical and practical considerations, nonporous monodisperse silicas of small particle diameter should thus be very useful for rapid analytical and micropreparative affinity chromatography. Anspach *et al* (1990) describe the improvement of affinity chromatographic performance using adsorbents prepared from nonporous monodisperse silicas. The elution of proteins from nonporous silica-based adsorbents was investigated both theoretically and experimentally using human immunoglobulin G and immobilized protein A as the affinity pair by Lee and Chung (1996). Nonporous silica (average diameter of 1.4 μm) was silanized with γ-amino-propyltriethoxysilane and activated with glutaraldehyde. A comparison was made between predicted and experimental elution peaks from chromatography of IgG on immobilized protein A. The desorption rate constant and equilibrium association constant under elution conditions were found to have a substantial effect on elution time and peak shape.

Many silica gel supports are available commercially in both irregular or spherical shapes, either uncoated or glycophase coated. Among them are, for example, silica-based supports under the trademark LiChrospher Si, LiChrospher Diol, etc. (E. Merck, Darmstadt, F.R.G.), Porasil A-F (Waters Associates, Milford, MA, U.S.A.), Progel-TSK columns (SUPELCO, Bellefonte, PA, U.S.A.). Ultraaffinity-EP is one of the commercially available epoxide silicas available in prepacked columns (Beckmann Instruments, Berkeley, CA, U.S.A.). Immobilization of the ligand onto such a matrix can be performed by passing the material through the column slowly, over a predetermined time period. The use of anti-chaotropic anions such as phosphates and sulphates is recommended since they stabilize the protein during derivatization and increase their interaction with the activated support. Columns, cartridges or kits of a silica activated with epoxide functional bonded phases are sold under the name Durasphere AS by Alltech Associates, Inc. (Deerfield, Il., U.S.A.).

Iron and nickel oxides

Iron oxide core containing particles can be prepared by several methods. One method involves the use of commercially available iron oxide powders. These can be silanized directly and used for the attachment of affinity ligands (Weetall and Lee, 1989). An even dispersion of magnetic material (γFe_2O_3 and Fe_3O_4) throughout the bead is in Dynabeads which are produced by DYNAL A.S. (Oslo, Norway). This firm supplies uncoated Dynabeads, activated Dynabeads and Dynabeads precoated with specific ligands. They are the uniform, superparamagnetic, monodisperse polymer particles. Information about them is in paragraph about polystyrene and its derivatives.

Commercially available particles consisting of an iron oxide core coated with a silane polymer terminating in amine (particle size 1–2 μm), carboxyl (particle size 0.5–1 μm), or sulphydryl (particle size 1–3 μm) functional groups are supplied by Advanced Magnetics Corp. (Cambridge, MA, U.S.A.) The same firm also offers a variety of proteins including Protein A, avidin and goat anti-mouse antiserum coupled to particles (Groman and Wilchek, 1987). Magnogel, which consists of iron oxide entrapped in a polyacrylamide-agarose envelope, has been discussed in page 162. Latex particles impregnated with iron oxide are also commercially available from Seradyn Inc. (Indianapolis, IN., U.S.A.). These materials show paramagnetic properties and have been successfully used in immunoassays. Nickel oxides produced by precipitation, or directly from a chemical supply house, have been used in a manner similar to the iron oxides (Weetall and Lee, 1989).

Membranes and tubes

Membranes are in many way similar in structure to synthetic beaded polymer supports. However, synthetic membranes have advantages as support matrixes in comparison to conventional bead supports because they are not compressible and they eliminate diffusion limitations. As a result higher throughput and faster processing times are possible in membrane systems (Charcosset, 1998). Membrane formation, characterization and applications are described already in a monograph "Affinity Membranes, Their Chemistry & Performance in Adsorption Separation Processes" by Klein (1991). The chemical composition of membranes varies greatly. Sheets can be constructed from any number of primary polymers including cellulose, polyamide (nylon), polyacrylonitrile and many other materials. The most widely used membranes for proteins purification include cellulose and nylon.

Hydrophilic affinity microporous membranes composed of reactive reinforced cellulosic polymers has been introduced by Memtec Corporation (Hermanson *et al.*, 1992). This membrane posesses reactive aldehydes for covalent coupling of amino groups of proteins and other ligands. Reinforced cellulosic polymers are suitable for pleated and specially cut membranes. Similar cellulose membranes produced by Sartorius (Göttingen, Germany) have been used for selective removal of human serum amyloid

P component from rat blood by immunoaffinity in an extracorporeal circulation system (Adachi *et al.*, 1996).

Synthetic polyamides, known as nylons, are a family of condensation polymers of dicarboxylic acids and α,ω-diamines. Several types of nylon, differing only in the number of methylene groups in the repeating alkane segments, are available in a variety of physical forms, such as fibres, hollow fibres, foils, membranes, powders, and tubes.

The purification of phosphofructokinase from yeast cell homogenate using selective adsorption-desorption with Immunodyne nylon membrane has been described by Huse *et al.* (1990). Immunodyne, Biodyne A and Loprodyne nylon membranes are supplied by Pall Filtrationstechnik (Dreilich, F.R.G.). Immunodyne membranes are pre-activated nylon membranes developed for the covalent fixation of molecules via hydroxyl, carboxyl or amino groups. The reactive groups of Immunodyne membrane have the ability to selectively bind phosphofructokinase and phosphoglycerate kinase from yeast cell extract. The kinetics of phosphofructokinase binding to various nylon membranes is shown in Table 6.8. The decrease in the phosphofructokinase activity in the homogenate with the Immunodyne membrane can be explained by the action of the group used to preactivate this membrane as an affinity ligand. Elution of phosphofructokinase from the nylon sorbent by adenine nucleotides is in agreement with this interpretation. The described membrane technique is extremely simple and does not require sophisticated equipment. The membrane was cut and transferred to a polyethylene bottle. After filling the bottle with 10 mM sodium hydroxide solution the membrane adhered loosely to the wall. Figure 6.12 shows the bottle with the membrane fixed with rubber bands to a rotating shaft in a horizontal position. This arrangement allows the use of small volumes and utilization of the whole membrane area. The biospecific adsorption of protein from particle containing cell homogenates may be superior to other methods as the first step in the extraction of cell homogenates, at least on a milligram scale.

A non-interactive polymer (hydrophilic polyvinylidene difluoride) is the base material of Immobilon AV Affinity Membrane (IAV) produced by Millipore (Bedford, MA, U.S.A.). A variety of ligands containing amines or thiols can be covalently immobilized to chemically activated hydrophilic microporous membranes in a range of pH conditions (pH 4–10), ionic strengths (0.01–1.0 M) and temperatures (0–37°C). By varying

Table 6.8 Time-course of phosphofructokinase (PFK) binding to different nylon mebranes

Time of incubation (min)	PFK activity (U/ml) in the cell homogenate			
	Control	Immunodyne	Biodyne A	Loprodyne
0	15.7	–	–	–
60	14.2	7.6	14.7	15.3
120	14.9	4.8	14.2	15.8
	(0.42)	(0.46)	(0.46)	(0.42)

Aliquots of 6 ml of yeast cell homogenate were incubated with the respective nylon membranes and assayed for PFK activity at the indicated times. An incubation without a membrane was performed as a control. Values in parentant are the specific activities at the end of incubation determined in the supernatant after centrifugation at 25 000 g.

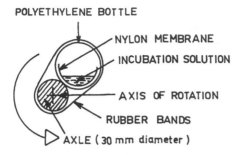

Figure 6.12 Treatment of the nylon filters with a small volume of incubation solution within a bottle fixed to a rotating shaft. Reproduced with permission from K. Huse *et al.* (1990) *J. Chromatogr.*, **502**, 71–177.

these parameters, the user can immobilize nanogram to milligram amounts of proteins ($150 \, \mu g/cm^2$ is approximately a protein monolayer). Kučerová and Turková (1997) coupled 3,5-diiodo-L-tyrosine to this membrane and used it for the isolation of pepsin from a crude extract of human gastric mucosa. The advantage of membrane-based immobilized ligand when batch-wise isolation was used was that the time for sorption and desorption of pepsin was very short.

The Affinity-15 Membrane Chromatography System is produced also by Sepracor Inc. (Marlborough, MA, U.S.A.). Affinity ligands are covalently bound to the membrane using a stable, secondary amine linkage, and therefore ligand leaching is virtually eliminated. Membrane technology for protein purification increases the speed, lowers the costs, and simplifies the protein purification.

Commercial availability of activated solid supports and biospecific adsorbents

The rapid development of many new unmodified or activated supports, biospecific sorbents in beads, columns, cartridges etc. is documented in the catalogues of many companies and in The International Product Magazine for Biotechnology (BPI, Elsevier, B. P. 214, B-1210 Brussels, Belgium). A well-equipped separations laboratory should have a variety of commercially available matrices at hand, as well as a full range of vendor catalogs and technical data sheets on file. Fortunately, a large number of reliable suppliers offers a wide range of practical and efficient matrices. An appendix of the book of Hermanson *et al.* (1992) contains the manual listing vendors of various useful support materials. Tables 6.4 and 6.5 in the book of Turková (1993) also contain examples of commercially available supports with full names and addresses of suppliers. However, many suppliers or their commercially available supports have been rapidly changing and therefore some information here may be outdated.

Survey of the most common coupling procedures

When selecting the method of attachment, the primary consideration is which groups of the affinity ligand can be used to form a linkage to a solid support without affecting the binding site. The attachment also should not introduce non-specifically adsorbing groups. From this point of view, it is often best to first couple a spacer to an affinant and then attach it to a solid support. The linkage between the surface of a solid support and an affinant should be stable during adsorption, desorption and regeneration. When choosing an appropriate method, one should bear in mind the dependence of the stability of the affinant on the reaction conditions. It should also be noted that the coupling procedure may be influenced by both the nature of the solid matrix and the substance to be attached. When bifunctional compounds are used for the coupling, complications arising from the crosslinking of both the carrier and the proteins with one another can be expected. Therefore reaction conditions, such as pH, temperature and time, should be chosen and monitored carefully during coupling.

When chemically inert solid supports are available, the preparation of biospecific adsorbents consists of two-steps (1) activation or functionalization of this chemically inert support, and (2) coupling of the ligand. The activation is dictated chiefly by the nature and the stability of the matrix itself. Thus, for example, conditions applicable to the derivatization of glass would totally destroy agarose and vice versa.

Effect of the nature of proteins and solid supports

The amount of protein to be coupled, the stability and the biological properties of immobilized biomolecules can be affected by the choice of the solid support and the method of coupling. In order to determine the effect of the nature of the support and the character of the proteins coupled, several proteins, namely, serum albumin, trypsin, chymotrypsin, papain and trypsin inhibitor antilysine were attached to glycidyl methacrylate copolymer, oxirane-acrylic beads, epoxy-activated Sepharose and 3-(2′,3′-epoxypropoxy)propyl derivatives of glass and silica (Zemanová *et al.*, 1981). Figure 6.13 (A and B) shows the difference in the coupling of proteins (in mg/g of dry support) to methacrylate copolymer and agarose. It is evident from the figures that the amount of protein attached as a function of pH is affected by both, the character of the proteins and the nature of the solid support.

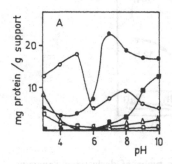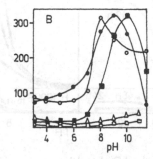

Figure 6.13 Effect of pH on the coupling of: o, serum albumin; •, papain; □, antilysin; ■, trypsin and △, chymotrypsin (A) to the glycidyl methacrylate copolymer and (B) to the epoxy-activated Sepharose 6B. Data from I. Zemanová et al. (1981) *Enzyme Microb. Technol.*, **3**, 229–232.

The effect of the solid support was much less pronounced when various proteins were immobilized using benzoquinone. The smaller effect of the solid support was seen when the effect of pH was investigated on the benzoquinone-mediated immobilization of trypsin, chymotrypsin and serum albumin, either to hydroxyalkyl methacrylate copolymer (Stambolieva and Turkovà, 1980) or agarose (Brandt *et al.*, 1975).

Support modification and affinity ligand immobilization

Epoxide-containing supports

Carrier epoxides may react with amino, carboxy, hydroxy and sulphydryl groups, with some aromatic nuclei such as indole, imidazole, etc., saccharides polynucleotides, adipic acid dihydrazide etc. The S–C, N–C and O–C bonds formed are extremely stable (Turková, 1993). The pH profiles for the coupling of glycyl-D-phenylalanine to the hydroxyethyl methacrylate copolymer, Separon HEMA, derivatized to both, high and low extents of epoxides is shown in Fig. 6.14. The coupling rate was also affected by the structure of the bound amino component. The quantity of the substance immobilized and the reaction rate increased with the increasing hydrophobicity of the compounds to be immobilized. The coupling reaction of Separon $H1000E_{max}$ with 1,6-diaminohexane was very fast, being complete after 6 h.

The same Separon was used by Smalla *et al.* (1988) for the study of the influence of salts on the coupling of different enzymes. Figure 6.15 shows the dependence of

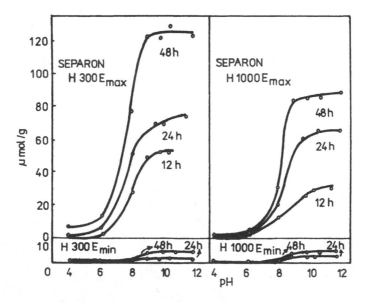

Figure 6.14 Coupling of glycyl-D-phenylalanine to various types of derivatized Separons as a function of pH and time. The content of epoxide groups: Separon $H300E_{max}$ = 1550 μmol/g of solid support, Separon $H1000E_{max}$ = 1770 μmol/g, Separon $H300E_{min}$ = 240 μmol/g, Separon $H1000E_{min}$ = 140 μmol/g. Data from J. Turková *et al.* (1981) *J. Chromatogr.*, **215**, 165–179.

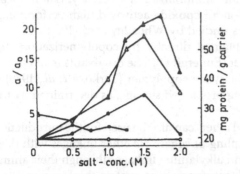

Figure 6.15 Dependence of the activity and protein binding of aminoacylase-Separon HEMA E conjugate on the salt added during the immobilization reaction. Aminoacylase (5 mg) in 2.5 ml 0.2 M phosphate buffer (pH 8.0); 50 mg Separon HEMA E, 20 h at 5°C. Salts added: ($\triangle$), $(NH_4)_2SO_4$, ($\square$), Na_2SO_4, ($\bullet$), $(NH_4)_2HPO_4$, (o) NaCl. a_0, activity of the enzyme-carrier conjugate in the absence of salts; a, activity of the enzyme-carrier conjugate in the presence of salts as indicated. ($\triangle$) $(NH_4)_2SO_4$ addition and protein binding (right axis). Aminoacylase (10 mg) in 2.5 ml phosphate buffer (pH 8.0); 50 mg Separon HEMA E, 30 h at 5°C. Data from K. Smalla et al. (1988) Biotechnol. Appl. Biochem., 10, 21–31.

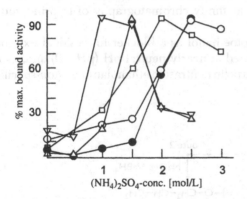

Figure 6.16 Dependence of the activity of proteinase-Separon HEMA E conjugate on the ammonium sulphate concentration in the medium during immobilization. Maximum bound activity (%) of immobilized proteinases: (∇) pepsin (5 mg) in 2.5 ml 0.1 M acetate buffer (pH 8); ($\triangle$) elastase (2.5 mg) in 2.5 ml 0.1 M phosphate buffer (pH 8); ($\square$) subtilisin (0.5 mg) in 2.5 ml 0.2 M phosphate buffer (pH 8); (o) chymotrypsin (5 mg) in 2.5 ml 0.1 M phosphate buffer (pH 8); ($\bullet$) trypsin (5 mg) in 2.5 ml 0.1 M phosphate buffer (pH 8). Coupling conditions: 50 mg Separon HEMA E, 15 h at 20°C for pepsin, chymotrypsin and trypsin, 20 h at 5°C for subtilisin and elastase. Data from K. Smalla et al. (1988) Biotechnol. Appl. Biochem., 10, 21–31.

the activity and protein binding of aminoacylase-Separon HEMA E conjugate on the salt used for the immobilization reaction. Aminoacylase-Separon H1000E$_{max}$ with the highest activity was achieved using ammonium sulphate. However, as Fig. 6.16 shows, the optimum concentration of immobilized protein depends on the concentration of this salt. The study of the effect of different concentrations of $(NH_4)_2SO_4$ on the coupling of thermitase, trypsin, chymotrypsin, pepsin, elastase, subtilisin and carboxypeptidase A showed varying effects of added salts on the immobilization efficiency. Salt-induced immobilization of deoxy-oligonucleotides on an epoxide-activated high-performance liquid chromatographic affinity support was studied by Wheatley *et al.* (1996).

Epoxide-containing supports can be obtained directly by copolymerization, for example of glycidyl methacrylate copolymer (Eupergit C). The disadvantage of biospecific sorbents prepared from glycidyl methacrylate copolymer (Turková *et al.*, 1978) is the formation of new epoxide groups during prolonged storage, as determined by the coupling of different dipeptides.

Bisoxiranes (e.g. 1,4-butanediol diglycidyl ether) can also be used for the introduction of reactive oxirane groups suitable for coupling of sugars *via* ether linkages with their hydroxyl groups. Proteins and peptides form alkylamine linkages through their amino groups. Thioether linkages are formed with substances that contain thiol groups.

Coupling of the antibiotic, novobiocin, *via* its phenolic hydroxy group to epoxy-activated Sepharose was performed and the product used for the bioaffinity chromatography of DNA gyrase by Staudenbauer and Orr (1981). Kanamori *et al.* (1986) used Sepharose 4B or Toyopearl HW-65 (Fractogel TSK) after activation with epichlorohydrin for the preparation of two formyl carriers, as shown in Fig. 6.17. A large amount of m-aminobenzamidine was efficiently immobilized on both types of carriers. Formyl groups remaining on the adsorbents were converted into hydroxymethyl groups by reduction with sodium borohydride. All of the adsorbents were successfully used for both low- and high-performance liquid bioaffinity chromatography of trypsin-family proteases.

Fleminger *et al.* (1990b) used β-mercaptoethanol as a blocker for residual oxirane groups of Eupergit C. Blocking is performed at nearly neutral pH (pH 8.0) and, as it does not form charged groups with the matrix (in contrast to ethanolamine), non-specific ionic adsorption of proteins is eliminated.

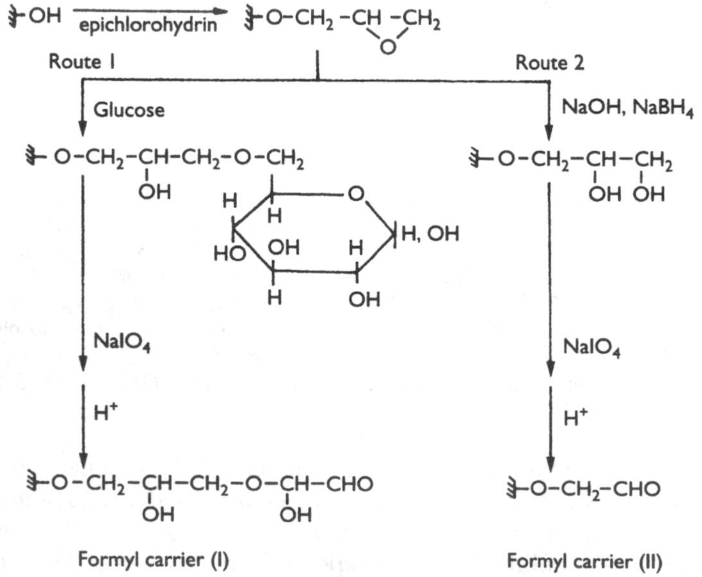

Figure 6.17 Preparation of formyl carriers.

Hydrazide derivatized solid supports

A review of hydrazido-derivatized supports in affinity chromatography has been published by O'Shannessy (1990). Under suitable mild conditions, oxidation of glycoproteins with periodate results in the generation of reactive aldehydes which can subsequently be bound with nucleophiles such as primary amines or hydrazides. Both primary amines and hydrazides react with aldehydes only when they are in the unprotonated form. The very low pK of hydrazides, usually around 2.6, in contrast to primary amines, which have pK value in the range of 9–10, allows one to significantly reduce the formation of Schiff bases between protein and oligosaccharide by performing the coupling reaction under mildly acidic conditions between pH 4.5–5.5. Under such conditions the majority of the primary amines of the protein moiety are protonated and unreactive. Secondly, the product of coupling between an aldehyde and a hydrazide is a hydrazone, which is much more stable than a Schiff base and, according to many authors, does not require reduction (Fig. 6.18). However, van Sommeren *et al.* (1993) observed ligand leakage during both storage and chromatography on immunosorbent prepared by the attachment of antibody to hydrazide-activated agarose. When such condition of poor stability occurs, the hydrazone produced can be stabilized by performing the reaction in presence of sodium cyanoborohydride (hydrazine derivative: conjugate-CH₂NHNH-support).

Lamed *et al.* (1973) have described the coupling of several nucleotide di- and triphosphates, after periodate oxidation to adipic acid dihydrazide coupled to CNBr-activated Sepharose. To 1 ml Sepharose hydrazide in 0.1 M sodium acetate (pH 5) was added

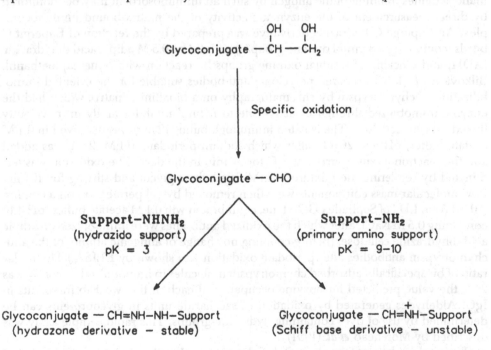

Figure 6.18 Flow diagram summarizing the chemistry involved in the site-specific immobilization of glycoconjugates *via* their carbohydrate moiety onto hydrazido-derivatized and amino-derivatized matrices.

4–5 μmole of periodate oxidized nucleotide in 2.5 ml of the same buffer. The suspension was stirred for 3 h at 4°C, after which 7.5 ml of 2 M NaCl solution was added and stirring continued for another 30 min to remove unbound nucleotide. Control reactions were carried out with unoxidized nucleotides. The absorbance of the supernatant was measured to determine the extent of binding. The amounts of bound nucleotide ranged from 3 to 4.5 μmoles per ml Sepharose with the various nucleotides. Only trace amounts (0.1–0.2 μmole/ml gel) of nonoxidized nucleotides were adsorbed on the Sepharose hydrazide. The advantages of Sepharose hydrazide over aminoethyl cellulose is that stable products are obtained without further reduction with sodium borohydride, and unreacted hydrazide groups do not impose ion-exchange properties on the resin at neutral and high pH. In the case of nucleosides, nucleotides and RNA, immobilization onto hydrazido-derivatized matrices would appear to be the method of choice.

Enzymes with carbohydrate moieties and antibodies contain their active site in the polypeptide part of the molecules. The presence of carbohydrate increases the stability of glycoproteins. The carbohydrate moiety of the protein, either after periodate or enzymatic oxidation – can readily be immobilized to supports containing hydrazide groups, giving conjugates with very good steric accessibility of their active sites and with an increased stability (Turková et al., 1997).

Fleminger et al. (1990a) described the optimization of oriented immobilization of periodate-oxidized monoclonal antibodies on hydrazide derivatives of Eupergit C. They used carboxy-peptidase A (CPA) and horseradish peroxidase (HRP) as antigens and selected monoclonal antibodies (mAbs) that did not inhibit the respective enzymatic activities. Binding of the antigen by such an immunosorbent may be monitored by direct measurement of the enzymatic activity of the matrix-bound immunocomplex. An Eupergit C-hydrazide derivative was prepared by the reaction of Eupergit C beads (containing 0.8 mmol oxirane group/g) with 0.1 or 0.5 M adipic acid dihydrazide (ADH) and blocking of residual oxirane groups by reaction with β-mercaptoethanol. Bílková et al. (1997) prepared polyclonal anti-bodies suitable for the oriented immobilization of chymotrypsin by chromatography on a bioaffinity matrix which had the enzyme immobilized through its active site to natural inhibitor antilysin, covalently linked to bead cellulose. The isolated immunoglobulin (12 mg) was dissolved in 0.1 M acetate buffer, pH 5.5 (20 ml), after which sodium periodate (0.1 M, 2 ml) was added and the reaction mixture stirred at 4°C for 30 min in the dark. The oxidation was terminated by rendering the mixture 20 mM in ethylene glycol and stirring for 10 min. Low-molecular-mass components were then removed by gel permeation on a column (10 × 1.5 cm I.D.) of Sephadex G-25 Fine, equilibrated wih 0.1 M acetate buffer (pH 4.8) containing 0.5 M NaCl, after which the oxidized antibodies were immobilized on adipic acid dihydrazide cellulose. (Before coupling no change of antigenic affinity of the anti-chymotrypsin antibodies after periodate oxidation was shown by ELISA.) The molar ratio of biospecifically adsorbed chymotrypsin molecules to immobilized antibody was 2 : 1, the value predicted for enzyme occupancy of each of the two Fab fragments in IgG. Aldehydes generated by oxidation of saccharide units in glycoproteins can be determined by use of dyes containing hydrazide groups. This rapid, simple assay was described by Morehead et al. (1991).

Chemical oxidation of the oligosaccharides may result in the oxidation of some amino acid residues (such as serine, threonine, proline and methionine), a decrease in enzymatic activity. Oxidation of sugar residues by periodate or enzymatic oxidation is shown in Fig. 6.19. Petkov *et al.* (1990) used enzymatic oxidation of D-galactose of the carbo-hydrate moiety of glucose oxidase by galactose oxidase in the presence of catalase. Galactose oxidase (0.7 ml) and catalase (0.3 ml) were added to glucose oxidase (10 mg in 3 ml of 0.1 M phosphate buffer, pH 7.0) and left to react at 20°C for 6 h. The reaction mixture was gel filtered through a Sephadex G 25 Fine column (23.0 × 1.5 cm I.D.) equilibrated with 0.1 M acetate buffer pH 4.8 containing 0.5 M NaCl. The oxidized enzyme was coupled to hydrazide derivatives of O-α-D-galactosyl Separon H1000 or Sepharose 4B. Both solid supports were modified with adipic acid dihydrazide after their activation with galactose oxidase. Each immobilized glucose oxidase possesed higher activity than could be achieved by other procedures.

Carbohydrate moieties in the Fc portion of immunoglobulin G are key structural features needed for their physiological complexation by complement. The Fc fragment

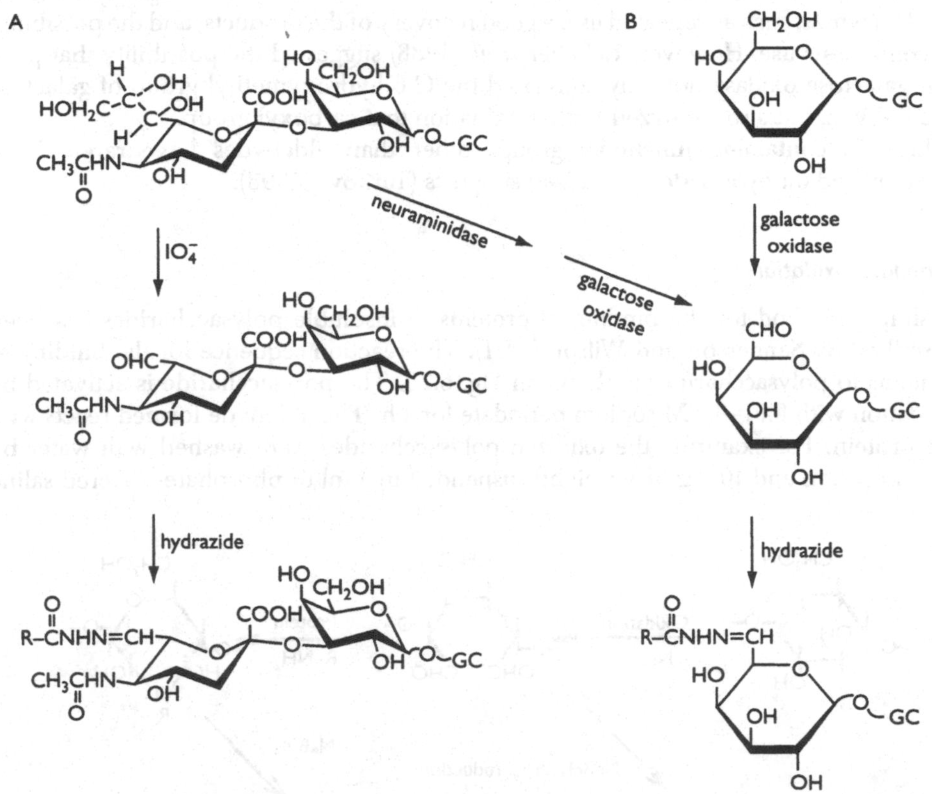

Figure 6.19 Two major reaction schemes for coupling hydrazide reagents to (oxidized) sugar residues. In (A), sialyl groups of glycoconjugates are oxidized chemically with periodate and the resultant aldehyde may be reacted with an appropriate hydrazide. In (B), galactose (or N-acetylgalactosamine) residues are oxidized enzymatically, using galactose oxidase, to the respective C-6 aldehydoderivative which undergoes subsequent interaction with an appropriate hydrazide. In cases where galactose (or N-acetylgalactosamine) residues appear penultimate to terminal sialyl residues, hydrazides may be coupled to the sialoglyco-conjugate by the combined enzymatic action of neuraminidase and galactose oxidase, as shown.

contains two carbohydrate chains with N-acetylneuraminic acid and galactose as terminal sugars. Therefore, Solomon *et al.* (1990) could use instead of periodate oxidation of carbohydrate moieties of antibodies against carboxypeptidase A and horse radish peroxidase enzymatic oxidation of these antibodies. Concomitant treatment of carbohydrate moieties of the antibodies with neuraminidase and galactose oxidase generated aldehyde groups in the oligosaccharide moieties of immunoglobulins. They showed that the co-immobilization of neuraminidase and galactose oxidase on Eupergit C-ADH beads provides an economical, efficient and selective system for the enzymic oxidation of monoclonal antibodies without impairing their immunological activity. Both enzymes are glycoproteins and therefore immobilization through their carbohydrate moieties after periodate oxidation was used. After coupling of the enzymes to the carrier, the preparations were treated with 0.2 M acetaldehyde in 0.1 M acetate buffer (pH 5.5) for 2 days to block the residual reactive hydrazide groups. Co-immobilized galactose oxidase and neuraminidase exhibits the well known advantages of immobilized enzymes, such as repeated use, a good recovery of the products, and the possibility of continuous use. However, Kelleher *et al.* (1988) suggested the possibility that purified galactose oxidase not only converted the C-6 hydroxymethyl group of galactose to aldehyde, but also catalyzed further oxidation to a carboxyl group.

Ligands containing functional groups other than aldehydes have rarely been immobilized on hydrazido-derivatized supports (Turková, 1993).

Periodate oxidation

A simple method for the binding of proteins to insoluble polysaccharides has been described by Sanderson and Wilson (1971). The reaction sequence for the binding of proteins to polysaccharides is shown in Fig. 6.20. The polysaccharide is activated by oxidation with 0.01–0.5 M sodium periodate for 1 h. The aldehyde formed reacts with the protein. For example, the oxidized polysaccharides were washed with water by centrifugation and 10 mg (dry weight) suspended in 1 ml of phosphate-buffered saline

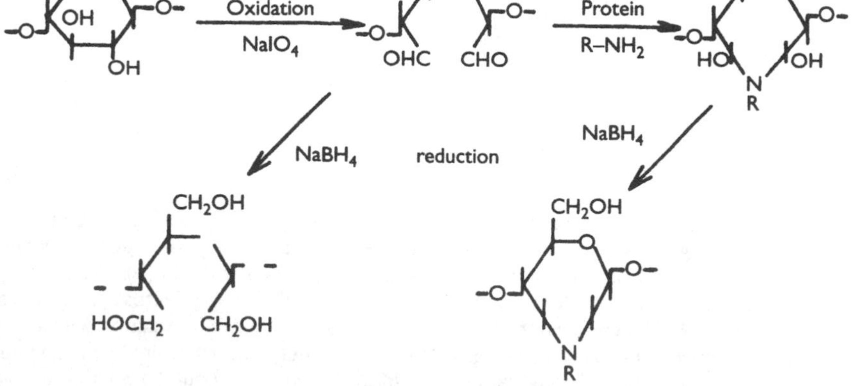

Figure 6.20 Reaction sequence for the binding of proteins to polysaccharides.

(pH 8) containing 10 mg of bovine serum albumin and agitated continuously for 20 h. Subsequent reduction with sodium borohydride (a freshly prepared 1% solution) led to the stabilization of the bonds between the protein and the polysaccharide, and to the reduction of the residual aldehyde groups.

The use of the immobilization *via* reductive alkylation for the coupling of trypsin to periodate-oxidized glucose-Separon and cellulose beads enables a comparison of the methacrylate matrix with natural polysaccharide supports (Turková, 1993). The amount of trypsin coupled onto periodate-oxidized glucose derivative Separon H1000-glc in relation to pH first increases moderately with increasing pH, but above pH 8 the increase is steep up to pH 10. The amount of the immobilized trypsin and its activity, determined by means of benzoyl-L-arginine p-nitroanilide as substrate, increases with increasing concentration of free trypsin in the reaction mixture during the coupling. Just as in the case of the preceeding gel, the rate of binding of trypsin onto cellulose in bead form increases with increasing pH. However, the solubilization of cellulose derivatives also increases with pH, due to alkaline degradation yielding soluble immobilized trypsin fractions and soluble oxidized oligosaccharides. Just as with glucose–hydroxyalkyl methacrylate gel, the amount of bound trypsin, as well as its activity, increase with increasing concentration of free trypsin in the reaction mixture during the coupling. The Schiff base-type bond between the oxidized glucose matrix and the peptide is very unstable and reduction with sodium borohydride is necessary for stabilization.

In order to compare the coupling of ligands to solid supports *via* presumed aldehyde groups we determined the amount of Gly-D,L-Phe coupled to periodate-oxidized glucose-Separon and to Separon with attached hexamethylene diamine and activated by glutaraldehyde as a function of pH (Koelsch *et al.*, 1986). From Fig. 6.21 it is evident that the two activated matrices are clearly different. Another big difference between these two types of aldehyde groups was also found in the stability of bonds with glycyl-D, L-phenylalanine. Unlike the case with oxidized glucose residues, in which the reduction with NaBH₄ is necessary, the bond between glutaraldehyde and dipeptide is very

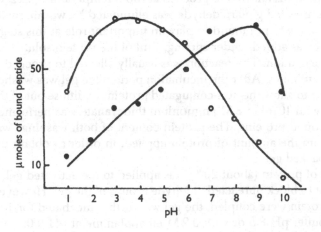

Figure 6.21 pH Dependence of the amount of Gly-D,L-Phe (μmol/g of dry support) bound to glucose-Separon H 1000 oxidized by NaIO₄ (•) and Separon H 1000-NH₂ activated by glutaraldehyde (o). Data from R. Koelsch et al. (1986) *Biotechnol. Lett.*, **8**, 283–286.

stable. There is no difference between reduced and untreated preparation. In both variants no release of nitrogen was found after 11 weeks at pH 7.0 and 24°C.

Glutaraldehyde activation technique

The glutaraldehyde activation procedure can be used with solid supports having carboxamide or primary amine groups. In the latter case, the activated matrix is often coloured. Weston and Avrameas (1971) developed a method for the direct binding of affinants onto polyacrylamide gels using glutaraldehyde which, if present in excess, reacts *via* one of its two aldehyde groups with the free amide group present in the polyacrylamide gel. The remaining free active group then reacts with the amino group of the affinant added during the subsequent binding reaction. A firm bond is thus formed between the support and the affinant.

Bio-Gel P-300 is allowed to swell in water and is washed twice with a four-fold volume of 0.1 M phosphate buffer, pH 6.9. Then 19.4 ml of gel (1 g of dry beads per 45 ml) is mixed with glutaraldehyde solution (4.8 ml; 25%, v/v) and incubated at 37°C for 17 h. The gel is washed and centrifuged four times with a fourfold volume of 0.1 M phosphate buffer, pH 6.9, then three times with 0.1 M phosphate buffer, pH 7.7. The coupling of the protein is carried out after mixing of 3 ml of gel in 13.5 ml of a buffer, pH 7.7 with 0.3 ml of protein solution (20 mg/ml) at 4°C for 18 h on a shaker. After the reaction the gel is centrifuged and washed. Using this method, 70 mg of acid phosphatase could be coupled per gram of dry gel.

6-Aminohexyl-Sepharose 4B was activated with glutaraldehyde by Cambiaso *et al.* (1975) and used for the immobilization of immunoglobulins G and A, ferritin and albumin. The aminated gel was first washed with ten volumes of phosphate buffer (pH 8.5) on a sintered-glass filter. To 3 ml of packed gel, 7 ml of the same buffer containing one ml of 25% glutaraldehyde was added under stirring (final concentration: 2.5%). This represents a 100-fold molar excess of glutaraldehyde over the amino groups of the aminated gel (8 µmole NH_2/ml packed gel). A yellow-green colour soon developed after this addition. The reaction was allowed to proceed at room temperature ($\pm22°C$) for 10 min, after which the unreacted glutaraldehyde was eliminated by washing with five times 20 ml of buffer. Time was not found to play an important role at this stage. To 3 ml packed activated gel was added, under stirring, 7 ml of the protein solution in the same buffer as used for activation. The reaction was usually allowed to proceed at room temperature for fifteen minutes. After the incubation period, the gel was washed with five times 20 ml of buffer to allow the non-conjugated proteins to diffuse out of the gel beads. Further washing with 10 ml of 3 M ammonium thiocyanate was performed to remove non-covalently bound proteins. The protein content of both washings was estimated and subtracted from the amount of protein applied, in order to obtain the amount coupled per ml of packed gel.

When a moderate excess of protein (about 20%) was applied to the activated gel, it was not necessary to attempt to block unreacted aldehyde groups of the gel. However, when smaller amounts of protein were coupled, the gel was further incubated for 16 h at 4°C with 0.2 M glycine buffer pH 8.5 or with 0.2 M ethanolamine at pH 9.0. Such incubations were found to block unreacted aldehyde groups.

A number of other bifunctional derivatives are described by Turková (1993). However, when using bifunctional derivatives it should be born in mind that side reactions, such as cross-linking of the support may occur, and its permeability may decrease drastically (Mohr and Pommerening, 1985).

Cyanogen bromide activation

One of the first methods introduced to activate agarose, dextran, and less commonly of cellulose and hydroxyalkyl methacrylate gel, was the cyanogen bromide activation (Axén *et al.*, 1967). The mechanism of activation by CNBr and the subsequent coupling of the affinant was elucidated by Kohn and Wilcheck (1981) and is shown in Fig. 6.22.

The same investigators developed analytical methods for the determination of cyanate esters and imidocarbonates. Cyanate esters are most stable in acid, decreasing in stability as the pH is raised. Imidocarbonates behave in an opposite fashion: they are most stable in 0.1 M NaOH. During brief acid hydrolysis of an activated matrix, all imidocarbonates will be removed quantitatively, while over 95% of the cyanate esters will remain intact. On the other hand, brief hydrolysis in 0.1 M NaOH leads to a rapid hydrolysis of all cyanate esters, leaving a substantial amount of imidocarbonates. Based on the assumption that the coupling of an affinant to cyanate esters and to imidocarbonates occurs simultaneously and independently, the total coupling capacity of an activated support can be predicted according to the equation:

Total coupling capacity = 0.80 (cyanate esters) + 0.15 (imidocarbonates)

The initially formed cyanate esters are stable on Sepharose, but rearrange to cyclic imidocarbonates on Sephadex. The coupling of an affinant occurs predominantly *via* the free amines in the unprotonated state. The following pH values are appropriate for coupling: aliphatic amines, pH $\sim$ 10; amino acids, pH $\sim$ 9; aromatic amines,

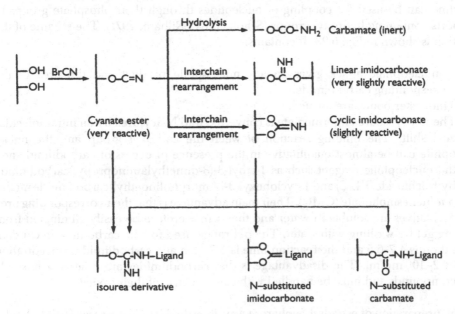

Figure 6.22 Mechanism of activation by CNBr and the subsequent coupling of the affinant.

pH 7–8. Ribonucleotides are coupled through their phosphate groups at pH 6 (Kempf et al., 1978).

The attachment of amines to cyanogen bromide-activated Sepharose produces an N-substituted isourea which is capable of protonation at neutral and alkaline pH values. This linkage is unstable in the presence of primary amines and ammonia (Wilchek et al., 1975), which is the primary flaw of this method. A review of cyano-based activation procedures for polysaccharides was published by Kohn and Wilchek (1984). Discussions of the mechanism for CNBr-activation and the difference between a freshly activated and commercially available CNBr-activated Sepharose (which is treated with acid in order to achieve better stabilization of activated resin) have been published by Wilchek and Miron (1986). CNBr-activated Sepharose was treated with 1 N hydrochloric acid for 1 h in order to form carbonate. This new type of activated Sepharose can be used to couple amino-containing ligands to the resin, yielding columns that consist of stable and uncharged carbonates. These activated resins will be useful for coupling of low-molecular-weight ligands such as diamino-hexane or aminocaproic acid, as the coupling to the resin has to be performed at high pH (ca. 9.5), because of the low reactivity of the carbonate formed. However, carbonate Sepharose also can be used to couple proteins under mild conditions and in high yields.

Coupling with condensation agents

One of the most frequent combinations of gel and spacer, used for the binding of low-molecular-weight affinity ligands, is Sepharose with attached hexamethylenediamine (trade name AH-Sepharose) or ε-aminocaproic acid (trade name CH-Sepharose). In order to couple affinants carrying primary aliphatic or aromatic amine or carboxyl groups to them, condensation via carbodiimide is used. Dicyclohexylcarbodiimide in pyridine can be used for coupling of nucleotides through their phosphate groups to supports containing hydroxyl groups (Schott, 1984; Gilham, 1971). The scheme of the reaction is shown in Fig. 6.23. It contains:

(a) A nucleophilic attack gives an acyl-nucleophile product and the urea of the corresponding carbodiimide.
(b) Thiol ester bonds are formed.
(c) The O-acylisourea intermediate is converted into N-acylurea by an intramolecular acyl shift. The binding reaction between the carboxyl group and the nucleophile can be almost quantitative in the presence of excess of carbodiimide and the nucleophilic reagent such as 1-ethyl-3-(3-dimethylaminopropyl)carbodiimide hydrochloride (EDC) and 1-cyclohexyl-3-(2-morpholinoethyl)carbodiimide metho-p-toluenesulphonate (CMC). Their main advantage is that their corresponding urea derivatives are soluble in water and they can therefore be easily eliminated from the gel by washing with water. The pH range used for the carbodiimide condensation is 4.7–6.5 and the reaction time is 1.5–72 h at a carbodiimide concentration of 2–100 mg/ml. The disadvantage is that carbodiimides are relatively unstable compounds and must be handled with care because of their toxicity.

The preparation of estradiol-Sepharose was described by Cuatrecasas (1970). A solution of 300 mg of 3-O-succinyl-[^{3}H]estradiol dissolved in 400 ml of dimethylformamide

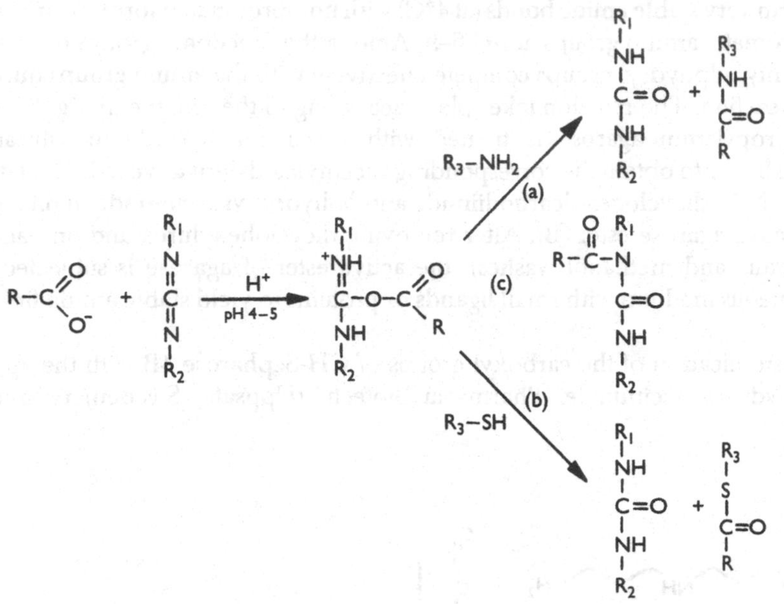

Figure 6.23 Scheme of the condensation reaction with a carbodiimide-promoted method.

is added to 40 ml of packed aminoethyl-Sepharose 4B. Dimethylformamide is needed in order to solubilize the estradiol. It is not required for affinants that are soluble in water. The suspension is maintained at pH 4.7 with 1 M hydrochloric acid. Then 500 mg (2.6 mmole) of 1-ethyl-3-(dimethylaminopropyl)carbodiimide, dissolved in 3 ml of water, is added to the suspension over 5 min and the reaction is allowed to proceed at room temperature for 20 h. Substituted Sepharose, after being transferred into the column, is washed with 50% aqueous dimethylformamide until the eluate is no longer radioactive. It is recommended that the derivative should be washed with about 10 l of the washing liquid over 3–5 days. Using this procedure, about 0.5 μmole of estradiol can be bound per millilitre of packed Sepharose.

Boschetti *et al.* (1978) published a comparative study of soluble carbodiimide (CMC) with a condensation agent: N-ethoxycarbonyl-2-ethoxy-1,2-dihydroquinoline (EEDQ). The latter catalyzes the reaction between spacer arm and ligand by forming a mixed anhydride on the carboxyl group of the spacer arm. The mixed anhydride then reacts with the complementary amine to form a stable amide bond. The mixed anhydride can also react with other nucleophilic groups such as sulphydryl and hydroxyl groups. EEDQ must be used in a water–ethanol mixture, which is an advantage when working with ligands that are only slightly soluble in water. EEDQ is a suitable condensation agent, being stable, non-toxic and cheap.

Active esters

Cuatrecasas and Parikh (1972) described the preparation of N-hydroxysuccinimide (NHS) esters of succinylated aminoalkyl agarose derivatives. These active ester derivatives of agarose, when stored in dioxane, are stable for several months. These derivatives form very stable amide bonds (at 4°C) with non-protonated forms of primary aliphatic or aromatic amino groups at pH 6–9. Among the functional groups of amino acids tested, only sulphydryl groups compete effectively with the amino groups during the coupling reaction. The reaction takes place according to the scheme in Fig. 6.24.

Diaminodipropylaminoagarose is treated with succinic anhydride in saturated sodium borate buffer to obtain the corresponding succinylated derivative (A). The latter is reacted with N,N'-dicyclohexylcarbodiimide and N-hydroxysuccinimide in dioxane to yield the active agarose ester (B). After removing dicyclohexylurea and unreacted reagents (dioxane and methanol washes), the active ester of agarose is subjected to reaction in aqueous medium with small ligands or proteins to yield stable amide-linked derivatives (C).

Using the esterification of the carboxyl groups of CH-Sepharose 4B with the application of N-hydroxysuccinimide, Pharmacia Biotech. (Uppsala, Sweden) produces

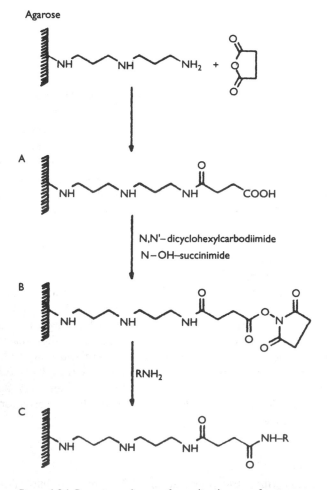

Figure 6.24 Reaction scheme of coupling by use of active esters.

activated CH-Sepharose 4B. The pH range suitable for binding to this derivative is indicated by Pharmacia to be 5–10, with an optimum of pH 8. The advantage of lower pH values is in the decreased esters hydrolysis but with a slower reaction rate. Buffers that contain amino acids cannot be used (Tris or glycine buffers) in the coupling reaction. Agarose derivatives containing N-hydroxysuccinimide ester have been introduced by Bio-Rad Labs. (Richmond, Calif., U.S.A.) under the name Affi-Gel 10 and Affi-Gel 15. As shown in Fig 6.25, Affi-Gel 10 couples proteins best at a pH near or below their isoelectric points, and Affi-Gel 15 couples proteins best near or above their isoelectric points. Therefore, when coupling at neutral pH (6.5–7.5), Affi-Gel 10 is recommended for proteins with isoelectric points of 6.5–11 (neutral or basic proteins) and Affi-Gel 15 is recommended for proteins with isoelectric points below 6.5 (acidic proteins). The difference in coupling efficiency of Affi-Gel 10 and Affi-Gel 15 for acidic and basic proteins can be attributed to interactions between the charge on the protein and charge on the gel. Hydrolysis of some of the active esters during aqueous coupling will impart a slight negative charge to Affi-Gel 10. This negative charge will attract positively charged proteins (proteins buffered at a pH below their isoelectric points) and enhance their coupling efficiency. Conversely, the negative charge will repel negatively charged proteins (proteins buffered at a pH above their isoelectric points) and lower their coupling efficiency. Affi-Gel 15, due to the tertiary amine incorporated into its arm, has a slight overall positive charge, and the effects are reversed. Coupling under anhydrous conditions is the preferred method whenever this is suitable for the ligand. Since there is no hydrolysis of active esters in the absence of water, the only reaction will be that of the ligand with the gel.

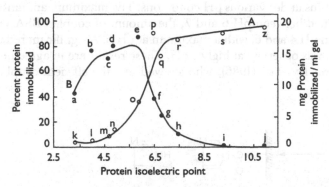

Figure 6.25 Immobilization of proteins to Affi-Gel 10 and Affi-Gel 15. Protein solutions were gently mixed at 0–4°C with 2 ml Affi-Gel 10 or Affi-Gel 15 for 2 h. The reaction was terminated by addition of ethanolamine, pH 8.0 to a concentration of 0.10 M, and after 30 min, transferred to 1 × 10 cm chromatography column. Unreacted protein was eluted with 7 M urea containing 1 M NaCl. Published values for the isoelectric points used to construct this figure were: fetuin (a,k), pH 3.3; human (α-antitrypsin (b,l), pH 4.0; human (γ-globulin (f,p), pH 5.8–7.3; human transferrin (e,o), pH 5.9; ovalbumin (c,m), pH 4.7; bovine serum albumin (d,n), pH 4.9; bovine hemoglobin (g,q), pH 6.8; equine myoglobin (h,r), pH 6.8–7.8; cytochrome c (i,s), pH 9.0–9.4; and lysozyme (j,z), pH 11.0. (o) Affi-Gel 10; (•) Affi-Gel 15. Reproduced with permission from R. G. Frost *et al.* (1981) *Biochim. Biophys. Acta*, **670**, 163–169.

Activation with carbonylating reagents

The reaction scheme for the covalent coupling of ligands to OH containg solid supports by use of 1,1'-carbonyldiimidazole (CDI) is depicted in Fig 6.26. The activated imidazolyl-carbamate supports react with primary amino groups at pH 8.5–10.0 and are more stable to hydrolysis compared to with N-hydroxysuccinimide ester-activated supports (Mohr and Pommering, 1985). CDI-activated agarose has a half-life of more than fourteen weeks when stored in dioxane. A further advantage of using CDI activated agarose is that the resulting N-alkylcarbamates are uncharged at normal pH ranges.

Activation of crosslinked agarose with CDI has been described by Bethell *et al.* (1981). CDI-activation has been performed for 15–30 min in dioxane, acetone, or dimethylformamide at room temperature. Optimization of protein immobilization on CDI-activated diol-bonded silica has been described by Crowley *et al.* (1986). Acetonitrile was used as the solvent in CDI-activation, since better coupling yields were obtained. It was found that extensive sonication and vacuum-degassing during the activation step significantly increased the amount of ligand coupled. In the coupling step, it was found that a subpopulation of active groups was resistant to hydrolysis and resulted in increased coupling yields of ligand over a six-day reaction time. The coupling and hydrolysis reactions were more rapid in carbonate buffer than in phosphate buffer, but the overall yields were the same. Coupling yields of several proteins (bovine serum albumin, immunoglobulin G, soybean trypsin inhibitor, Protein A, acetylcholine-esterase and horse liver alcohol dehydrogenase) were found to be relatively insensitive to pH over the range 4–8.

In order to determine the optimum coupling conditions, Ernst-Cabrera and Wilchek (1987) coupled trypsin and bovine serum albumin (BSA) to p-nitrophenyl chloroformate-activated resins under various pH conditions. The maximum amount of coupled trypsin was obtained between pH 6 and 7; the amount of coupled BSA was relatively constant between pH 4 and 6, with a maximum at pH 6. A significant reduction in coupling capacities was observed at higher pH. These results are in agreement with those reported by Crowley *et al.* (1986), who showed that the efficient coupling

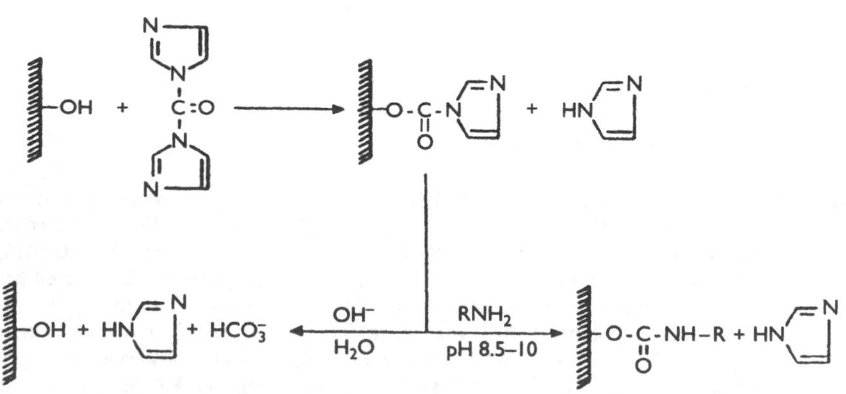

Figure 6.26 Reaction scheme for the covalent coupling of ligands by use of activation with carbonylating reagents.

of many proteins on carbonyldiimidazole-activated resins takes place at pH 4–5. Both results clearly indicate that it is preferable not to use basic conditions for coupling ligands to activated carbonates. CDI-activated glass matrices are commercially available for example from Pierce Chemical Co. (Rockford, Il., U.S.A.).

Triazine method

The covalent linkage of ligands to hydroxyl-containing supports activated with cyanuric chloride (2,4,6-trichloro-s-triazine = TCT) was developed by Kay and Crook (1967). An easily controllable variant for use with macroporous cellulose bead with TCT was developed by Beneš *et al.* (1991). Activation: 10 g of suction-filtered cellulose (water content 85%) was stirred with 20 ml of acetone for 30 min, 10 ml of aqueous acetone was removed after the stirring had been interrupted, 10 ml of acetone was added, stirring was continued for another 30 min, after which another 10 ml of aqueous acetone was withdrawn. Base was then added (10% NaOH or 20% K_2CO_3) and the stirring continued for one hour, after which the solution was cooled to 0°C and solution of TCT (1 mole per one equivalent of alkali) in acetone (5.5 ml/g) was added and left to react for 45 min. The product was washed in a column with 40 ml of acetone at 0°C and followed by 40 ml of ice-cold water. Preparation of the hydrazide derivative: to a solution of 233 mg of adipic acid dihydrazide in 17.5 ml 0.05 M borate buffer, pH 9, 20 g of cellulose activated with TCT was added. The mixture was stirred at room temperature for 4 h. The product was washed in a column with five volumes of distilled water. The final content of dihydrazide was 13.3 µmol/ml. Bílková *et al.* (1997) used this method of coupling for the immobilization of natural chymotrypsin inhibitor, antilysin. The amount of coupled antilysin was 6 µmol/g dry cellulose. The disadvantage of this method is that the activating reagents are highly toxic.

Kay and Lilly (1970) used the triazine method of protein coupling with a triazine derivative, in which a chlorine was replaced by a solubilizing NH_2 group. Fig. 6.27 shows the coupling 2-amino-4,6-dichloro-s-triazine to the hydroxyl group of cellulose and its reaction with the protein amine.

Reversible covalent immobilization of proteins by thiol-disulphide interaction

Carlsson *et al.* (1975) employed epoxide-activated agarose as the basis for the preparation of the mercaptohydroxypropyl ether of agarose gel, which they used for covalent immobilization of α-amylase and chymotrypsin by thiol-disulphide exchange. This technique consists of two steps: (a) thiolation of enzymes with methyl 3-mercaptopropioimidate; (b) binding of thiolated enzymes to a mixed disulphide derivative of agarose obtained by reaction of the mercaptohydroxypropyl ether of

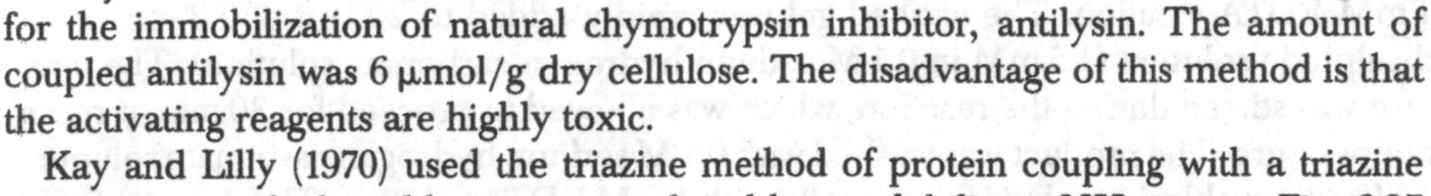

Figure 6.27 Reaction scheme of triazine method of coupling.

agarose with 2,2-dipyridyl disulphide. Immobilized α-amylase prepared in this fashion has been used for continuous hydrolysis of starch. When the preparation had lost its enzymatic activity, the inactive protein gel complex was reduced and the regenerated gel used for the coupling of a new active thiolated α-amylase.

Thiolation of the enzyme was carried out in the following manner: 30 mg of enzyme was dissolved in 5 ml of 0.1 M sodium hydrogen carbonate solution, pH 8.2. The solution was deaerated under nitrogen atmosphere for 15 min and 0.1–2 mg of methyl β-mercaptopropioimidate was added. The thiolation was carried out at room temperature under nitrogen for 60 min. Excess of imidate was eliminated by gel filtration on Sephadex G-25, using 0.1 M sodium hydrogen carbonate as the eluent. To prevent autooxidation of the thiolated enzymes, dithiothreitol (1 mM final concentration) was added to the solution before the gel filtration.

Activated thiol-Sepharose was prepared according to Brocklehurst *et al.* (1973). Epoxide-activated agarose (50 g) was washed on a glass filter with 0.5 M phosphate buffer (pH 6.3). Interstitial buffer was removed from the gel by suction, and the gel was resuspended in the same buffer to a final volume of 100 ml. A 2 M solution of sodium thiosulphate (50 ml) was added and the reaction mixture was shaken for 6 h at room temperature. The gel was washed free of sodium thiosulphate with distilled water. The resulting thiosulphate ester gel was suspended in 0.1 M sodium hydrogen carbonate solution (1 mM EDTA) to a total volume of 100 ml. Dithiothreitol (60 mg) in 4 ml of 1 mM EDTA solution was added to the suspension which was then incubated for 30 min at room temperature. The gel was washed on a glass filter with 0.1 M sodium hydrogen carbonate solution (1 M in sodium chloride and 1 mM in EDTA) and finally with 1 mM EDTA solution. The washed gel was rapidly added to 200 ml of 2,2'-dipyridyl disulphide solution (1.5 mM in 0.1 M sodium hydrogen carbonate solution). The mixture was stirred during the reaction, which was allowed to proceed for 30 min at room temperature. The product was washed with 0.1 M sodium hydrogen carbonate solution, 1 M sodium chloride solution and finally with 1 mM EDTA solution. The degree of substitution was determined by Kjeldahl nitrogen determination. The product, activated thiol-agarose, can be stored for a few days in 0.01 M deaereated sodium acetate buffer of pH 4 (1 mM in EDTA).

Coupling the thiolated enzyme was performed as follows: 1–20 mg of thiolated enzyme in 10 ml of 0.1 M sodium hydrogen carbonate solution was mixed with 3.0 ml of sedimented activated thiol-agarose (pre-washed with 0.1 M sodium hydrogen carbonate solution) and allowed to react at 23°C for 24 h, under constant stirring. The conjugate was washed on a sintered-glass funnel with 100 ml of 0.1 M sodium hydrogen carbonate solution, transferred into a column and washed at 10 ml/h with 240 ml of each of the following solutions: (1) 0.1 M sodium hydrogen carbonate containing 0.2 M sodium chloride; (2) 0.1 M sodium acetate, pH 5.4, containing 0.2 M sodium chloride; (3) 0.2 M sodium chloride.

The inactivated enzyme was removed from the carrier (0.5 ml) by washing the column with 50 ml of 20 mM dithiothreitol in 0.1 M sodium hydrogen carbonate solution at 20 ml/h. The reduced carrier was washed with 150 ml of 1 M sodium chloride and activated by passing 100 ml of a 1.5 mM solution of 2,2'-dipyridyl disulphide in 0.1 M sodium hydrogen carbonate. The activated thiol gel was washed with 100 ml of 1 M sodium chloride and 100 ml of 0.1 M sodium hydrogen carbonate solution and re-used for the immobilization of a new thiol ligand (enzyme).

Benzoquinone activation

The mechanism of the activation of hydroxyl-containing solid supports by means of benzoquinone and coupling of NH_2-containing compounds (Fig 6.28) was described by Brandt *et al.* (1975). Benzoquinone is a very active reagent and, presumably due to a secondary reaction, the immobilized compounds are usually strongly coloured. Brandt *et al.* (1975) determined the amount of bovine serum albumin and chymotrypsin coupled to benzoquinone-activated Sepharose 4B at various coupling pH values (Fig 6.29). The same proteins were immobilized at various pH *via* benzoquinone to hydroxy-alkyl methacrylate copolymer by Stambolieva and Turková (1980). In solid matrix supports section, 1 it was already noted that the pH optima for coupling different proteins on the epoxy-methacrylate copolymer and epoxy-activated agarose are different (Fig 6.13A and B). In contrast, when serum albumin and chymotrypsin were coupled

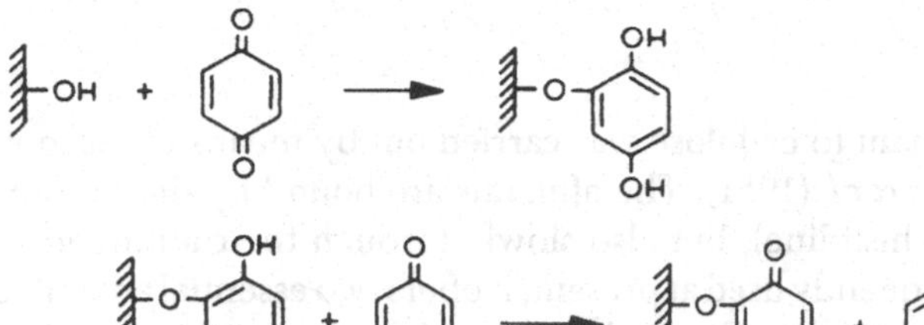

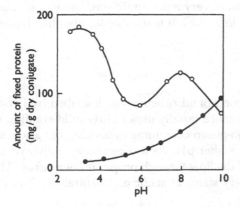

Figure 6.28 Reaction scheme of the activation of hydroxyl-containing solid supports by means of benzoquinone and coupling of NH_2-containing compounds.

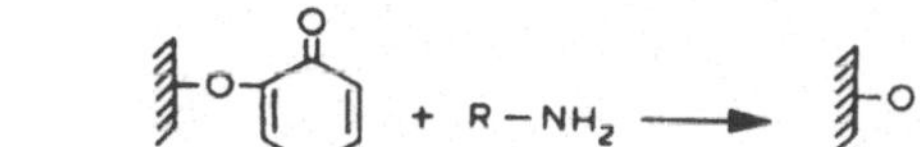

Figure 6.29 Amount of bovine serum albumin and chymotrypsin fixed to Sepharose 4B gel as a function of pH during the coupling reaction. (o), bovine serum albumin; (•), chymotrypsin. Reproduced with permission from J. Brandt et al. (1975) *Biochim. Biophys. Acta*, **386**, 196–202.

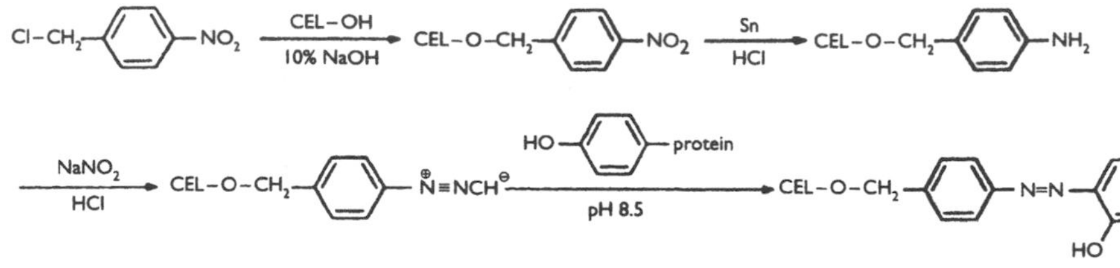

Figure 6.30 Reaction scheme for the attachment of aromatic residues of affinants by use of diazotization.

via benzoquinone, the pH optima were the same using methacrylate copolymer or Sepharose.

Diazotization

The first attachment of an affinant to cellulose was carried out by means of diazonium groups (Fig 6.30) by Campbell *et al.* (1951). The affinants are bound by their aromatic residues (mainly tyrosine and histidine), but also slowly through their amino groups. Although this method is not frequently used at present, it offers two essential advantages: (a) the bound ligand can easily be split off by reduction with sodium dithionite; (b) this reductive cleavage allows protein-inhibitor conjugates to be isolated intact under mild conditions (Mohr and Pommerening, 1985).

Sulphonyl chloride-containing supports

A simple method for the activation of supports carrying hydroxyl groups, such as agarose, cellulose, diol-silica, glycophase-glass or hydroxyalkyl methacrylate copolymer, with 2,2,2-trifluoroethanesulphonyl chloride (tresyl chloride), was introduced by Nilsson and Mosbach (1981).The advantage of tresyl chloride is that it is very reactive and it therefore allows efficient coupling under very mild conditions, and to a number of different matrices, including those used in HPLC. It is suitable for coupling ligands containing $-NH_2$ or $-SH$.

Other methods

The use of divinyl sulphone in the production of adsorbents was described by Porath and Sundberg (1972). The activation takes place rapidly under fairly mild conditions. The coupling can be performed with amino-group containing molecules, but also with carbohydrates, phenols and alcohols at a higher pH. As a consequence, divinyl sulphone crosslinking considerably improved the flow-through properties of agarose. The product coupled *via* divinyl sulphone is very stable at acidic and neutral pH, but it is labile under alkaline conditions.

   The activation of hydroxylic matrices by use of 2-fluoro-1-methylpyridinium toluene-4-sulfone (FMP) has been reported by Ngo (1988). FMP-activated gels can be used to couple ligands containing either amine or sulphydryl groups in slightly alkaline (pH 8–9) aqueous solutions or in organic solvents. The resulting linkages are stable and nonionic.

For more detailed information concerning matrix activation and ligand coupling to solid supports, the reader is refered to Hermannson *et al.* (1992) and Turková (1993).

Blocking of unreacted groups and washing out of noncovalently bou and ligands: recommendations

When the attachment of the affinity ligand onto the solid support is completed, it is necessary to eliminate any remaining reactive groups. The problem of excess of reactive groups is encountered in all coupling methods. This problem can be solved by one of two approaches:

1 By coupling a highly penetrable substance with no effect on the adsorption-desorption procedure.
2 By solvolysis. This method may be used when the affinants are stable to the conditions needed for the hydrolytic removal of the activated group. Excess epoxide groups may be hydrolysed to diols by treatment with 0.1 M perchloric acid or with 10 mM HCl.

In methods that use amino groups for the coupling of affinants, ethanolamine is most frequently used as an inactivating reagent. For example, Pharmacia recommends in the use of cyanogen-bromide activated Sepharose that remaining active groups can be deactivated by reaction with 1 M 2-aminoethanol at pH 9 and room temperature for 2 h, while, after binding to epoxide-activated Sepharose, 4 h are required. The buffer used is the same as the coupling buffer, for example 0.1 M sodium hydrogen carbonate containing 0.5 M sodium chloride. Turková *et al.* (1981) coupled 2-aminoethanol to hydroxyalkyl methacrylate copolymer containing 1.7 mmol of attached epichlorohydrin per gram of dry Separon to check the completeness of coupling and to quantify the number of epoxide groups. Figure 6.31 shows the coupling of 2-aminoethanol in relation to pH and coupling time. Blocking of epoxides proceeded slowly and required

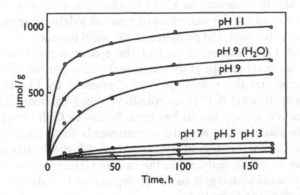

Figure 6.31 Coupling of 0.5 M 2-aminoethanol (in μmol/g dry conjugate) bound on Separon H 1000E$_{max}$ as a function of coupling time and pH. Britton-Robinson buffer were used for pH 3, 5, 7, 9, and 11, with the exception of pH 9, where an aqueous solution was also used. Coupling performed at room temperature. Data from J. Turková *et al.* (1981) *J. Chromatogr.*, **215**, 165–179.

a high pH. Practically complete removal of the epoxide groups could only be obtained by hydrolysis with 0.1 M perchloric acid.

Using Eupergit C oxirane acrylic beads, Fleminger *et al.* (1990b) obtained about 1.6 mmol of epoxide groups per gram of matrix by titration with thiosulphate. About half of these groups are readily available for reaction with amino or thiol groups, whereas the other half is much less reactive and requires hours to days to react. β-Mercaptoethanol was found to be an efficient blocker of residual oxirane groups. Blocking by ethanolamine and β-mercaptoethanol was investigated by Fleminger *et al.* (1990a). Eupergit C beads modified with adipic acid dihydrazide (ADH) and treated with 0.2 M ethanolamine, pH 9.5, tended to adsorb proteins at pH 5.5, apparently because of the positively charged secondary amine groups formed by the reaction. In contrast, when β-mercaptoethanol was used as a blocker, both protein adsorption at pH 5.5, as well as covalent protein binding to residual oxirane groups at pH 7.5, were markedly reduced. Consequently, ADH-modified beads were routinely treated with 0.2 M β-mercaptoethanol, pH 8.0, for 4 h at room temperature before protein binding. The blocking step eliminated most of the residual oxirane groups. The 10% of the original oxirane groups that still seem to remain active even after the blocking step most probably represent groups that are remote from the outer surface of the beads and are apparently not available for protein binding. Other low-molecular-weight molecules, for example, glucosamine, glycine, 2-amino-2-hydroxymethyl-propane-1,3-diol, etc. can also be used as blocking agents. The manufacturer of Sepharose states that, for the elimination of CNBr-activated groups from Sepharose, it is sufficient to suspend the gel in a Tris buffer of pH 8 for 2 h. The effect of the small number of charges introduced by the use of Tris or glycine can be overcome by using relatively high concentrations of salts during affinity chromatography. Almost complete elimination of these active groups can be achieved, however, even by merely incubating the gel overnight in a alkaline solution.

In gels that contain active ester groups (for example, Activated CH-Sepharose, Affi-Gel 10), the unreacted groups are eliminated by addition of 0.1 M Tris buffer, pH 8. After standing for 1 h virtually no groups capable of coupling proteins or peptides remain on the gel. In carriers that contain aldehyde groups as active binding groups, reduction with sodium borohydride may be used for the reduction of residual aldehyde groups and for the stabilization of the bond between the protein and the solid matrix.

If the affinity ligand is bound via a spacer, a part of the spacer arms – most commonly containing amino or carboxyl groups at their terminal – may remain unoccupied. Unreacted carboxyl groups on the spacer may be eliminated by blocking with 0.5 mM Tris and 1.6 mM N-cyclohexyl-N-[2-(4-morpholinyl) ethyl] carbodiimide metho-p-toluenesulphone. When the affinity ligand has been bound to CH- or AH-Sepharose by means of a carbodiimide, the supplier recommends that, after the coupling of the affinant, the reaction be continued by carrying out further carbodiimide reactions with glucosamine or 2-aminoethanol in the case of CH-Sepharose, or with acetic acid as blocking agent for the amino groups of AH-Sepharose. Unsubstituted amines can also be eliminated with acetic anhydride.

Another step in the preparation of specific sorbents for use in affinity chromatography consists in the thoroughly washing out all substances that are not covalently bound to the surface of the solid matrix. Most commonly the best results are obtained if the washing is carried out alternately with alkaline and acidic buffers of high ionic strength. To avoid the need for exhaustive and prolonged washing procedures, Santa-Colona *et al.* (1987) developed a cyclic system of bioaffinity chromatography for the purification of sex steroid binding protein. A charcoal column connected in series to the bioaffinity column allows the removal of any ligand that may be non-covalently bound to the matrix or released during its storage. This system could be particularly useful when difficulties arising from ligand leakage cannot be ignored.

General considerations in the choice of sorbents, coupling and blocking procedures

When choosing the carrier and the coupling procedure one should not only take account of the properties associated with the nature of affinity chromatography itself, but also its field of use. Kukongviriyapan *et al.* (1982) described the maximum binding of antibodies against *Naja naja siamensis* toxin 3 (T3) and operational half-life of T3 immobilized at various ligand densities (Table 6.9). The maximum binding capacity of antibody was obtained on immobilized T3 with the lowest half-life (19 days). The lowest antibody binding capacity was obtained on an adsorbent containing T3 coupled to albumin-Sepharose, where the half-life was 108 days. The investigation described was undertaken to study various parameters in the use of bioaffinity chromatography to purify antibodies against cobra postsynaptic toxin from horse refined globulin for therapeutic purposes.

The choice of coupling procedures and solid supports depends on the use to which the products will be put: analytical, semipreparation or preparation purposes. It is also necessary to take into consideration whether low-molecular-weight or high-molecular-weight affinity ligands are being used. It should also be born in mind that the toxicity of such reagents as hydrazine, cyanogen bromide, trichloro-s-triazine and divinylsulphone is high; that of epi-chlorohydrin, bisepoxiranes, glutaraldehyde, carbonyldiimidazole, benzoquinone, diazonium and tresyl chloride is moderate; only periodate is non-toxic.

For the binding of proteins, the most commonly used groups are the N-terminal α-amino group and ε-amino group of lysine, the C terminal carboxyl group and the carboxyl groups of glutamic and aspartic acids. Phenolic hydroxyl groups of tyrosine, imidazole anion of histidine or the −SH groups of cysteine residues, may also participate in the coupling. With carbohydrates and their derivatives, the groups that often take

Table 6.9 Ligand density, maximum antibody binding capacity and operational half-life of various adsorbents

Affinity sorbent[a]	Toxin immobilized (mg/ml packed gel[b])	Maximum binding capacity[c] (mg/mg immobilized toxin)	Half-life (days)
Seph-T3	2.60	4.75	43
Seph-Ae-Suc-T3	2.01	6.00	19
Seph-BSA-T3	1.50[d]	2.60	108
Biogel-Ae-Suc-T3	2.01	5.50	25

a Abbreviations: Seph, Sepharose 4B; Ae, aminoethyl; Suc, succinyl and T3 *N.n.siamensis* toxin 3.
b Volume of gel was measured in 0.15 N NaCl.
c Protein eluted at pH 2.05.
d Determined by using ^{125}I-labeled *N.n.siamensis* toxin 3.

Table 6.10 Summary of ligands bound and reaction

Active group	Ligands bound					
	−NH₂	−OH	−COOH	−SH	−CHO	phenolic-OH
Epoxide	+	+	+	+		+
Hydrazide			+		+	
Aldehyde (after periodate oxidation)	+					
Aldehyde (glutaraldehyde)	+					
CNBr	+					
Carbodiinide (EDC)	+		+			
N-ethoxycarbonyl-2-ethoxy-1,2-dihydroquinoline (EEDQ)	+		+			
N-hydroxysuccinimide (NHS)	+			+		
Carbodiimidazole (CDI)	+					
Triazine (Cyanuric Cl)	+	+				
Thiol				+		
Benzoquinone	+					
Diazotization						+
Tresyl chloride	+			+		
Divinyl sulfone (DVS)	+	+				
Fluoromethylperidinium (FMP)	+			+		

part in the coupling are the hydroxyl and the amino groups; in nucleic acids they are the phosphate groups, the sugar hydroxyl groups, and amino or enolate groups of the bases. If high-molecular-weight compounds, which possess several reactive functions, are coupled, they are attached at several places. As a consequence, the risk arising from the detachment of the coupled molecules decreases considerably, but, on the other hand, there is a certain risk that the multiple binding will induce a deformation of the native structure of the immobilized molecule and thus will also change its properties.

There is a dramatic increase in the recent production of commercially available activated solid supports and many biospecific adsorbents. Hermason *et al.* (1992) list 34 suppliers, their addresses and the products including affinity matrices, activated supports, activation reagents, immobilized ligands, prepacked columns, columns and accessoires and affinity purification kits. Turková (1993) lists addresses of 90 companies providing activated supports and biospecific adsorbents and examples of their products. A summary of the widely used coupling groups of ligands and their reaction with active groups of solid supports is given in Table 6.10.

Biospecific complex formation as a tool for oriented immobilization

Biotin and avidin or streptavidin

The binding of water-soluble vitamin biotin to the egg white protein, avidin, or to its bacterial counterpart, streptavidin, is accompanied by a large decrease in free energy compared to that observed for other noncovalent interactions. The change of enthalphy, ΔH, for biotin bound to avidin and streptavidin has been determined by Green (1966) as being −86 and −98.9 kJ/mol biotin, respectively. Each avidin or streptavidin molecule can bind four molecules of biotin. The change in entropy for this reaction is essentialy zero. The affinity constant for biotin-avidin determined by Green is approximately $10^{15}\,M^{-1}$.

In the past decade the interaction between biotin and avidin or streptavidin has provided the basis for establishing a new avidin-biotin technology. Methods for the biotinylation of membranes, nucleic acids, antibodies and other proteins have been developed in many laboratories. Figure 6.32 shows biotin and various derivatives, suitable for various types of bonds. However, a spacer arm should be used when proteins are modified by biotin. Detailed information on biotin-binding proteins, the preparation of biotin, avidin and streptavidin derivatives, assays for avidin and biotin, and applications are given in Volume 184 of "Methods in Enzymology" under the title "Avidin-Biotin Technology" edited by Wilchek and Bayer (1990).

The usefulness of an avidin–biotin complex in bioaffinity chromatography was demonstrated by the isolation of avidin from egg white on a biocytin-Sepharose column (Cuatrecasas and Wilchek, 1968). The conditions required for its dissociation were extremely drastic: requiring elution by 6 M guanidinium hydrochloride, pH 1.5. In order to decrease the strong affinity of avidin for biotin, Finn and Hofmann (1990) used immobilized succinylated avidin for the isolation of hormone receptor. Soluble receptor (R) is percolated through a bioafinity column to form the complex shown in the center of Fig. 6.33. The column is then exhaustively washed to remove contaminating materials. Alternatively, the biotinylated hormone ligand (B-H) can be added to a solution of solubilized receptor to form a soluble complex BHR. Applying a solution containing this complex to a column of immobilized succinylated avidin (SA) will result in the formation of the same complex (Fig. 6.33B). Both these schemes have been used

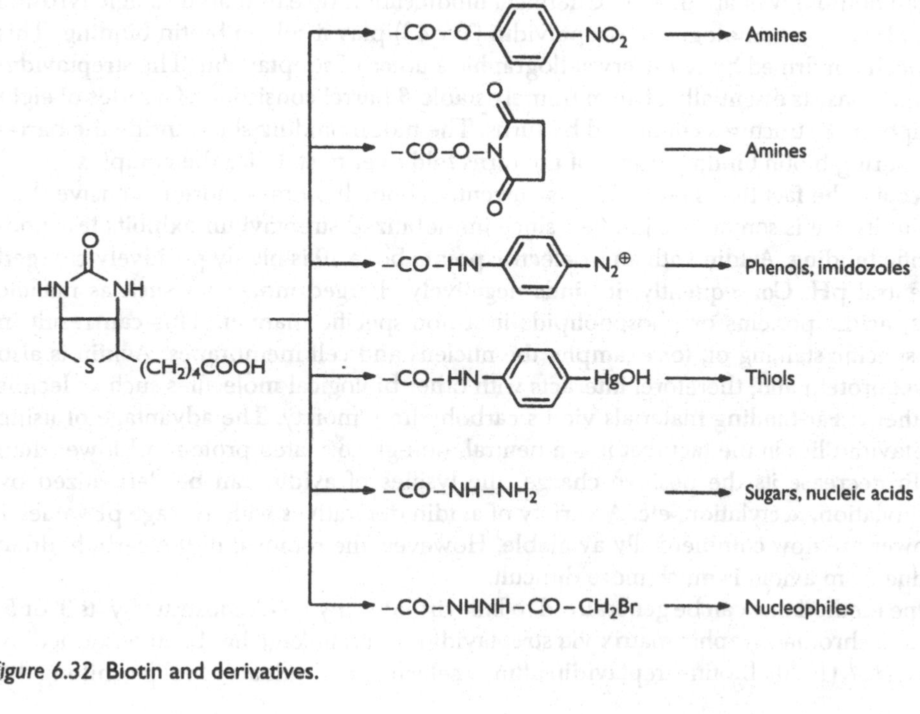

Figure 6.32 Biotin and derivatives.

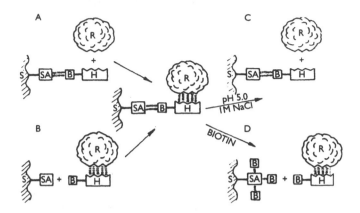

Figure 6.33 Application of the avidin-biotin system to the isolation of hormone receptors. Dashed lines represent noncovalent bonds. Reproduced with permission from F. M. Finn and K. Hofmann (1990) *Meth. Enzymol.*, **184**, 244–274.

for the isolation of insulin receptors from human placenta. Removal of active insulin receptor can be achieved by eluting the column with acetate buffer, pH 5 containing either 1 M NaCl or biotin.

Structural studies of avidin and streptavidin have been performed by Bayer and Wilchek (1990). Both proteins are tetramers with molecular weight 67 000. The genes for both proteins have been cloned and expressed in *Escherichia coli*. The primary sequences of both proteins are known. Avidin and the truncated form of streptavidin show an overall homology of about 40%. Chemical modification reveals that the single tyrosine (Tyr-33) and its homologue in streptavidin (Tyr-43) play a role in biotin binding. This has been confirmed by X-ray crystallographic studies of streptavidin. The streptavidin subunit consists essentially of an extremely stable β-barrel consisting of a series of eight juxtaposed β-structures connected by turns. The biotin binding site is inside the barrel and, during biotin binding, some of the turns fold over to stabilize the complex.

Despite the fact that streptavidin is currently about 100 times more expensive than avidin, its use is sometimes justified since immobilized streptavidin exhibits less non-specific binding. Avidin with an isoelectric point above 10 is highly positively charged at neutral pH. Consequently, it binds negatively charged molecules such as nucleic acids, acidic proteins or phospholipids in a non-specific manner. This can result in non-specific staining of, for example, the nucleus and cell membranes. Avidin is also a glycoprotein and, therefore, interacts with other biological molecules such as lectins or other sugar-binding materials via its carbohydrate moiety. The advantage of using streptavidin lies in the fact that it is a neutral, non-glycosylated protein (pI lower than 7). To decrease its the positive charge, the lysines of avidin can be derivatized by succinylation, acetylation, etc. A variety of avidin derivatives with average pI values 7 or lower are now commercially available. However, the removal of the carbohydrate residue from avidin is much more difficult.

One method that can be generalized to link virtually any DNA substrate by its 3′ or 5′ end to a chromatographic matrix via streptavidin-biotin linkage has been described by Fishel *et al.* (1990). Biotin-streptavidin affinity selection as a valuable tool permitting the analysis of the RNA components of splicing complexes assembled on a wide variety of pre-mRNA substrates has been reviewed by Grabowski (1990). A review of the isolation of cell surface glycoproteins by the use of biotinylated lectin was published by Cook and Buckie (1990). They demonstrated the use of immobilized streptavidin to achieve dissociation of complexes formed between biotinylated concanavalin A and membrane glycoproteins.

Isolation of detergent-solubilized membrane antigens (Updyke and Nicolson, 1984) is based on immunoaffinity adsorption, which employs the binding of biotinylated monoclonal antibodies with antigens in solution, followed by the adsorption of the antibody-antigen complexes to immobilized streptavidin. Antibodies were biotinylated using D-biotin-N-hydroxysuccinimide ester. The advantage of the biotinylation of antibody carbohydrate moieties using biotin hydrazine for use in immunoaffinity chromatography has been described by Phillips (1989). High performance immunoaffinity chromatography (HPIAC or HPIC) of specific phosphoryl-choline receptors can be employed using biotinylated mouse monoclonal antiidiotypic antibody adsorbed to streptavidin-coated glass beads (Fig 6.34). Using this technique HPIAC analysis was performed on isolated membranes from primed T cells obtained from mice immunized with phosphorylcholine (PC). These membranes were prepared by hypotonic lysis of the cells, followed by ultracentrifugation and detergent NP40 solubilization of the membrane-rich fraction. The preparation was passed through a Sephadex G25 column to remove excess detergent prior to injection into the HPIAC column. Using monoclonal anti-idiotype antibody as the immobilized ligand, a single peak was eluted by sodium thiocyanate gradient at 24 min. (Fig 6.34, peak B). This peak was shown to bind the antigen actively, although it demonstrated some cross-reactivity to other related antigens.

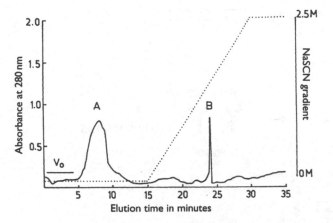

Figure 6.34 Isolation of specific T-cell PC receptors using a streptavidin-immobilized mouse monoclonal anti-idiotypic antibody HPIAC column. The column was 150 × 4.6 mm, run at 1 ml/min at 4°C. The receptors were recovered at 24 min using a sodium thiocyanate concentration gradient. V_o represents the void volume of the column. Detection was at 280 nm. The initial runninig buffer was 0.01 M phosphate, pH 7.0. Reproduced with permission from T. M. Phillips, in A. R. Kerlavage (ed.), The Use of HPLC in Receptor Biochemisry, Alan R. Liss, New York 1989, p. 148.

Oriented immobilization of immunoglobulin G by use of Protein A

Protein A covalently attached to Sepharose was the first reagent employed for oriented immobilization of immunoglobulin. Werner and Machleidt (1978) used N-ethyl-N'-(3-dimethylaminopropyl)-carbodiimide hydrochloride to couple IgG to immobilized Protein A, while Gersten and Marchalonis (1978) employed dimethylsuberamide as a crosslinking agent for covalent coupling of the same proteins. The binding of the IgG molecules through their Fc moiety was thus effected. This mode of binding makes the binding site of antibody well accesible for interaction with the antigen. The affinity constant of the complex created was high but the multiple use of immunoadsorbents under the conditions necessary for the elution of most antigens requires the cross-linkage of IgG with Protein A through a covalent bond.

Protein A-coated glass beads were developed as a universal support medium for HPIAC by Phillips *et al.* (1985). The preparation of IgG antibody binding is demonstrated in Fig 6.35. Protein A has the ability to bind to the Fc portion of IgG. Protein A is composed of five subunits, each with its own Fc receptor, althought three of these receptors become inactive when the molecule is bound. If Protein A is applied as a coating to either solid or controlled pore glass beads, its Fc receptors become points

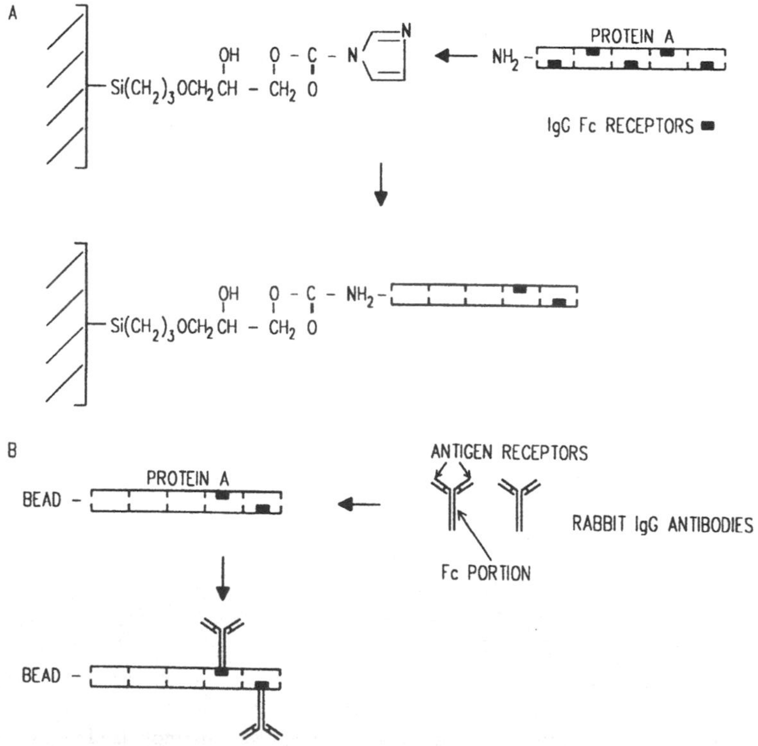

Figure 6.35 Diagrammatic representation of the process for binding rabbit antibodies to Protein A-coated glass beads. (A) Illustration of the chemistry used to couple Protein A to the carbonyl diimidazole-derivatized glass beads. (B) Mechanism of IgG antibody binding to the Fc receptors on the Protein A-coated glass beads. Reproduced with permission from T. M. Phillips *et al.* (1985) *J. Chromatogr.*, **327**, 213–219.

of attachment on which the antibody can be bound. The bound antibodies are then covalently immobilized on the Protein A covered surface by treatment with carbodiimide. This attachment in turn helps to orient the antigen receptors of the antibody toward the mobile phase of the column. In addition, the Protein A molecule becomes a spacer arm for the immobilized antibodies, thus preventing repulsion by the bead surface from inhibiting the formation of the antibody/antigen complex. However, only certain classes of immunoglobulin are able to bind to Protein A. Therefore Proten G, a bacterial cell wall protein isolated from a human group G streptococcal strain, was developed by Björck and Kronvall (1984) as a better reagent for IgG than Protein A.

In order to increase the specific IgG-binding activity of immobilized Protein A, Solomon *et al.* (1992) used tryptic digestion of Protein A for the preparation of its active fragments (FB). These FB fragments originate from almost identical five-repeated monoclonal Fc-binding units of 58 residues each. FB domain immobilized *via* glutaraldehyde to adipic dihydrazide-modified Eupergit CB6200 beads showed a higher antibody-binding capacity than intact Protein A, measured under the same experimental conditions.

Biospecific complex formations of enzymes

The occurence of several diverse binding sites on the surface of an enzyme molecule permits the formation of a relatively large number of biospecific complexes. These complexes can be utilized for efficient isolation of enzymes as well as for their oriented immobilization.

Figure 6.36 depicts the surface of an idealized enzyme molecule covered with several potential binding sites. Such an enzyme could be, for instance, carboxypeptidase Y containing the complementary binding site for glycyl-glycyl-p-aminobenzylsuccinic acid, a specific inhibitor. The active site of this enzyme contains a free SH$^-$ group. Carboxypeptidase Y is a glycoprotein whose carbohydrate moiety specifically interacts

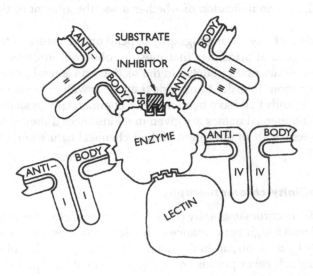

Figure 6.36 Possible ways in which an enzyme may form biospecific complexes.

with concanavalin A, a lectin. The antigenic sites of the enzyme can form the biospecific complexes with its antibodies. Enzymes also form complexes with substrates and their analogues, cofactor, allosteric effectors, metal ions, etc.

Turková *et al.* (1986) described affinity chromatography of carboxypeptidase Y by use of 3 biospecific adsorbents: Gly-Gly-p-aminobenzylsuccinic acid-Spheron, Mercury-Spheron and Spheron with attached concanavalin A. Carboxypeptidase Y after adsorption onto Con A-Spheron, was crosslinked with glutaraldehyde. The bound enzyme retained 96% of the native catalytic activity and showed very good operational stability. The advantages of the oriented immobilization of enzymes through their antibodies will be discussed in the section on Immobilization of enzymes on their immunosorbents.

Application of affinity chromatography

Affinity chromatography has increasingly become the method of choice for the isolation, determination, removal or oriented immobilization of biologically active substances. The use of biospecific adsorbents is described in an ever greater number of publications. Turková (1993) presents a bibliographic review of the use of affinity chromatography which covered more than 5 000 papers. Examples of classical, high-performance or large-scale affinity chromatography are shown in the following sections. The expansion of affinity chromatography has been largely due to developments in biotechnology.

Classical affinity chromatography

The preparation of bioadsorbents utilizing the exceptional properties of biologically active substances to form specific and reversible complexes has enormously facilitated the isolation of a number of natural substances. Some examples are presented in Table 6.11. In addition to these materials the table also lists affinity ligands, solid supports and the spacers used, with an indication of whether it was the affinant or the solid matrix that was modified.

The various conditions used in affinity chromatography depend on the nature of the substances to be isolated. The general principles that must be observed in order to achieve a successful isolation were discussed in detail in the section on General principles of affinant–substrate recognition. In order to provide the reader with information concerning individual affinity ligands that have been used, or commercially available immobilized affinity ligands, commercial names are given in all instances if they have been published. A review of these, with an indication of their chemical nature and the producer, is given in Table 6.13.

High-performance liquid affinity chromatography

In high performance liquid affinity chromatography (HPLAC) the specificity of affinity chromatography is combined with a high performance technology based on the use of rigid particles of uniform, small size (1–50 μm in diameter). The difference of affinity chromatography methods using soft gel or porous and nonporous small hard particles has been shown in Fig. 6.2.

The essential characteristic of HPLAC has been summarized by Ohlson *et al.* (1989). The separation times in HPLAC are short (minutes) compared with hours for traditional, soft-gel affinity chromatography. Time is saved not only in the application and elution phases but also during washing steps, and this can be of great importance when dealing with crude samples. In preparative applications, speed can also mean improvement in the quality of the isolated product, especially for labile biomolecules that may denature during prolonged chromatography. The peaks of purifed components are much sharper than those found with soft gel chromatography because of the reduced diffusion distances in the smaller HPLAC beads. Resolution is preserved by running the chromatography under HPLC conditions to minimize dead volumes and other extracolumn effects. The affinity aspect of HPLAC often makes it much more selective than standard separation modes, such as ion-exchange and hydrophobic interaction chromatography. The resulting sharper peaks simplify detection and the signal-to-noise ratio can be increased several fold. Furthermore, peak height (rather than area) can often be used to give quantitative estimates of sample components. HPLAC users have at their disposal a wide selection of HPLC equipment, including high-speed pumps, sophisticated injection units, detectors of various kinds, auto-sampling devices and data handling capabilities. This enables them to fine-tune the separation process and obtain increased productivity. HPLAC has been applied in almost all areas of traditional affinity chromatography. Some examples of HPLAC are presented in Table 6.12.

Trends in the application of HPLAC (Ohlson *et al.*, 1989) are directed toward improvement in analytical and preparative biotechnology. Processes such as the production of monoclonal antibodies or of recombinant DNA specified proteins and peptides have created a need for the rapid determination of specific biomolecules in complex mixtures during production. HPLAC can be used for monitoring biomolecules in complex mixtures, possibly providing on-line analysis in bioreactors and down-stream processing. Figure 6.37 shows the monitoring of Protein A in fermentation broth of *Staphylococus aureus.* The authors used HPLAC routinely to optimize the culture time and consumption of media in the fermentation. HPLAC has an important role in the quantitative and qualitative analysis of biologically active molecules, which leads to an assessment of their purity, potency and safety.

One form of high-performance membrane chromatography of serum and plasma membrane proteins (Josić *et al.*, 1992) used porous discs made of poly(glycidyl methacrylate). Rapid isolation of pepsin from human gastric juice or blood serum was achieved by Kučerová and Turková (1997) by batchwise use of Tyr(I$_2$) modified commercial membrane Immobilon™ AV. Rucklidge *et al.* (1996) used antibody against denatured collagen after adsorption to membrane with attached collagen for biotinylation. Biotinylation *in situ* may protect the variable region of the IgG compared to antibodies biotinylated in solution, thus increasing their antigen recognition.

Large-scale application of affinity chromatography

Large-scale affinity chromatography is usually performed in industrial laboratories and most information is thus proprietary. Large-scale protein purification was reviewed by Narayanan (1994). According to her the requirements of a large-scale purification protocol are largely determined by the nature and quality of the desired final product and its intended use. For example, proteins for therapeutic use need to be extremely

Table 6.11 Low-pressure affinity chromatography

Substances isolated	Affinity ligands	Solid supports or immobilized affinity ligands	References
Antibodies			
Antibodies against plant hormone abscisic acid (ABA) prepared from rabbits injected with conjugate ABA-bovine serum albumin	Conjugate of ABA with ovalbumin	Sepharose 4B	Wan and Hasenstein (1996)
–human immunoglobulin G	Human immunoglobulin G	Sepharose 4B	Guesdon and Avrameas (1976)
		Affi-Gel 10	Bober and Ownby (1988)
–myotoxin from rabbit	Myotoxin a from *Crotalus viridis* venom		
Anti-idiotypic antibody prepared from rabbits by use of complex anti-abscitic acid (ABA) IgG and cells *Staphylococcus aureus*	Anti-ABA IgG	Sepharose 4B	Wan and Hasenstein (1996)
Biologically active monomeric immunoglobulin A from human plasma fraction	Heparin and Protein G	Heparin-Sepharose CL-4B and Protein G Sepharose Fast Flow	Leibl et al. (1996)
F(ab′)₂ fragments from digestion of murine IgG1 monoclonal antibodies	Protein A	Sepharose-bound protein A	Khawli et al. (1996)
Monoclonal immunoglobulin G1 against Protein A	Protein A	Protein A Avi Gel F	Bloom et al. (1989)
Cells			
Cloned murine T helper (type II) cells	Anti-T cell receptor monoclonal antibodies	Polystyrene latex beads (3-μm average diameter)	De Bell et al. (1990)
Tumor cells from bone marrow	Polyclonal antibody	Dynabeads M-450	Ugelstad et al. (1988)
Enzymes			
Carboxypeptidase Y from *Saccharomyces cerevisiae*	Gly-Gly-p-aminobenzylsuccinic acid	Separon with epichlorohydrin	Turková et al. (1986)
α-Chymotrypsin	ε-Aminocaproyl-D-tryptophan methyl ester	Sepharose 4B	Cuatrecasas et al. (1968)
Galactose oxidase from *Dactylium dendroides*	Melibiose	Melibiose-polyacrylamide	Kelleher et al. (1988)
α-Glucosidase from yeast *Schizosaccharomyces pombe*	Antibodies against α-glucosidase	Perloza MT-200 activated wih 2,4,6-trichloro-1,3,5-triazine	Bílková et al. (1996)
Hexokinase from yeast	ATP complexed to immobilized boronic acid	Sepharose 6B with 6-aminocaproyl-3--aminophenylboronic acid	Bouriotis et al. (1981)
Human postheparin plasma lipases	m-Aminoboronate (m-APB)	m-APB immobilized on beaded agarose via nine-atom spacer	Uusi-Oukari et al. (1996)

Neuraminidase from influenza virus	p-Aminophenyloxamic acid	Copolymers of N-vinylpyrrolidone and acryloylchloride onto surface of γ-aminopro-pylsilylated porous glass	Ivanov et al. (1985)
Papain from dried papaya latex	Glutathione-2-pyridyl disulphide	Sepharose 2B	Brocklehurst et al. (1973)
Pepsin	ε-Aminocaproyl-L-Phe-D-Phe-Ome	Separon with epichlorohydrin	Turková et al. (1982)
Glycoproteins			
Cell surface glycoproteins from acute lymphoblastic leukemic cells	Biotinylated concanavalin A	CNBr-activated Sepharose 4B with streptavidin	Cook and Buckie (1990)
Decorin core protein (leucine-rich proteoglycan) from *Escherichia coli*	Amylose (eluted with maltose)	Amylose resin	Hering et al. (1996)
32Kd glycoprotein from rat sperm plasma membrane	Zona pellucida glycoprotein	CNBr-activated Sepharose 6MB	Hall et al. (1997)
Membrane glycoproteins (review)	Lectins	Mostly CNBr- or divinylsulfone activated hydroxylic supports	Caron et al. (1997)
Lectins			
Concanavalin A from jack bean seeds	Dextran	Sephacryl S-300	Nanderkar et al. (1987)
Concanavalin A	Mannan after periodate oxidation	Poly(acrylamide-allylamide)copolymer gel	Novotná et al. (1996)
Nucleic acids and nucleotides			
Biotinylated double-stranded DNA	Streptavidin	Streptavidin dynabead-coated paramagnetic beads	Cammas and Clark (1996)
Poly(A) mRNA from oviduct extract	Oligo(dT)	Ultrogel, Trisacryl or cellulose	Sene et al. (1982)
RNA components of splicing complexes	Biotinylated pre-m RNA	Streptavidin agarose beads	Grabowski (1990)
Proteins: transfer receptors and binding proteins			
Sex steroid binding protein	Androstanediol hemisuccinate	3,3'-Diaminopropylamine Sepharose	Santa-Coloma et al. (1987)
Streptavidin from *Streptomyces avidinii*	Iminobiotin hydrosuccinimide hydrobromide	CL-4B CL-Sepharose	Bayer et al. (1986)
Z-DNA-binding proteins from human lymphoblastic cell line	Biotinylated Z-DNA (left-handed conformation of the DNA double helix)	Biotin agarose and streptavidin	Fishel et al. (1990)
Viruses			
Soybean mosaic virus (SMV)	Monoclonal antibodies specific for SMV	Affi-Gel 10	Diaco et al. (1986)

Table 6.12 High-performance liquid affinity chromatography (HPLAC)

Substances isolated	Affinity ligands	Solid supports or immobilized affinity ligands	References
Antibodies			
Antibody against denaturated collagen (biotynylated after adsorption)	Denaturated collagen type II	Immobilon P	Rucklidge et al. (1996)
Human IgG	Protein A from *Staphylococcus aureus*	Non-porous silica from tetraamyl orthosilicate after modification with aminopropyltriethoxysilane activated with glutaraldehyde	Lee and Chuang (1996)
Immunoglobulin E (IgE) from serum of both adult and pediatric patients	Monoclonal antibodies against human IgE	Controlled-pore glass beads with carbonyl diimidazole-reactive side chains derived on their glycophase surface with attached Protein A	Phillips et al. (1985)
Polyclonal or monoclonal antibodies against carboxypeptidase A	Carboxypeptidase A	Eupergit C C30N	Fleminger et al. (1990b)
Cells			
Radiolabeled pathogenic *Escherichia coli*	Glycosphingolipids	PVDF membrane	Isobe et al. (1996)
Enzymes			
Alcohol dehydrogenase	Triazine dye	Blue Sepharose CL6B	Anspach et al. (1990)
Horse-radish peroxidase	Concanavalin A	Porous or nonporous silicas activated by use of 3-isothio-cyanatopropyltriethoxysilane (NCS-activated silicas)	Anspach et al. (1989)
Pig pancreatic elastase	tri-L-Alanine	NCS-activated nonporous silica	Anspach et al. (1989)
Plasminogen and plasmin from plasminogen activated by urokinase	p-Aminobenzamidine	Toyopearl HW 65S with chloroacetylglcylglycine	Shimura et al. (1984)
Pepsin from human blood serum or from gastric mucosa extract	3,5-Diiodo-L-tyrosine	IMMOBILON TM	Kučerová and Turková (1997)
Serine proteinase Thrombin from human Cohn fraction III	p-Aminobenzamidine	NCS-activated nonporous silica	Anspach et al. (1989)
Trypsin-family proteinases	m-Aminobenzamidine	Toyopearl HW-65	Kanamori et al. (1986)

Glycoproteins			
Glycated proteins in human serum	m-Aminophenyl boronic acid hemisulfate salt	Porous polymer gels composed of 2,3-dihydroxypropylmethacrylate monomer, poly(oxyethylenedimethacrylate) and dipentaerylthritolhexaacrylate as cross-linkers	Koyama and Teruchi (1996)
[125I]-labeled human chorionic gonadotropin	m-Aminophenylboronic acid	NCS-Activated nonporous silica	Anspach et al. (1989)
Lectins			
Galactose-binding lectins from human serum	3-Aminopropylglycosides of disaccharides galactosyl-N-acetylgalactosamine or fucosyl-galactose	Wide porous glass coated with poly(p-nitrophenylacrylate)	Rapoport et al. (1997)
Lectins: Ricinus communis agglutinin, concanavalin A, wheat germ agglutinin	Carbohydrates: lactose, galactose, mannose, glucose or N-acetylglucosamine	Polystyrene microtiter plates	Hatakeyama et al. (1996)
Nucleic acids and nucleotides			
Biotinylated DNA ranging in size from 100 to 5000 base pairs	Streptavidin	PS latex particles	Huang et al. (1996)
Nucleosides and nucleotides	m-Aminophenylboronic acid	NCS-activated nonporous silica	Anspach et al. (1989)
Proteins: transfer receptors and binding proteins			
Complement receptor s C3b from NP40-solubilized B-lymphocyte membranes	Anti-human C3 monoclonal antibody	Immobilized Protein A	Phillips (1989)
Transcription factor NF-kB from phorbol stimulated HeLa and Jurkat cells	Double stranded DNA	Crosslinked hydroxymethacrylate HEMA	Wheatley et al. (1996)
Other biologically active compounds			
Human serum amyloid P (hSAP) component from rat blood	Polyclonal anti-hSAP immunoglobulin	Cellulose membrane	Adachi et al. (1996)
Hydrophobic proteins from plasma membranes of Morris hepatoma	Heparin	Epoxy-activated poly(glycidyl methacrylate) disc	Josić et al. (1992)
Indolocarbazole derivatives	Human serum albumin	Immobilised HSA column	Ashon et al. (1996)
Phenylurea herbicides in plant material	Polyclonal antibodies	Glutaraldehyde-activated silica	Lawrence et al. (1996)
Phenylurea and triazine pesticides from environmental water	Polyclonal antisoproturon antibodies	Aldehyde-activated silica	Pichon et al. (1996)

Table 6.13 (a) Commercial names of solid supports

Trade name	Nature	Producer
Affi-Gel 10	Cross-linked agarose	Bio-Rad Laboratories, Richmond, CA, U.S.A.
Cellulose membrane		Sartorius, Gottingen, Germany
Dynabeads	Superparamagnetic polystyrene particles	Dynal A.S., Oslo, Norway
Eupergit	Glycidyl-methacrylate copolymer	Röhm Pharma GMBH, Damstadt, Germany
Eupergit C C30N	Nonporous Eupergit	Röhm Pharma GMBH, Damstadt, Germany
Glutardialdehyde activated silica		Boehringer, Mannheim, Germany
Immobilon P	Polyvinylidene difluoride (PVDF) membrane	Milipore Corp., Bedford, MA, U.S.A.
Immobilon TM	Membrane	Milipore Corp., Bedford, MA, U.S.A.
Perloza MT	Macroporous bead cellulose	Lovochemie a.s., Lovosice, Czech Republic
Polystyrene microtiter plates	(amino type)	Sumitomo Bakelite, Tokyo, Japan
PS latex particles	PS = polystyrene (diameters from 0.944 to 0.090 μm)	Seradyn or Bangs Laboratories
PVDF membrane	Polyvinylidene difluoride membrane	ATTO Co. Ltd., Tokyo, Japan
Separon	Hydroxyethyl methacrylate copolymer	TESSEK Ltd., Prague, Czech Republic
Sephacryl	Allyl-dextran after cross-linking with N,N'-methylene-bis-acrylamide	Pharmacia Biotech., Uppsala, Sweden
Sephadex	Dextran gels	Pharmacia Biotech., Uppsala, Sweden
Sepharose	Agarose	Pharmacia Biotech., Uppsala, Sweden
Sepharose CL	Agarose after cross-linking with 2,3-dibromopropanol and desulphurization	Pharmacia Biotech., Uppsala, Sweden
Toyopearl HW	Hydrophilic vinyl polymer	Toyo Soda Man. Co., Tokyo, Japan
Trisacryl	Hydrophilic acrylate polymer	Reactifs IBF, Villeneuve la Garenne, France
Ultrogel A	Agarose	Reactifs IBF, Villeneuve la Garenne, France
Ultrogel AcA	Polyacrylamide-agarose gel	Reactifs IBF, Villeneuve la Garenne, France

pure to minimize the risk of unwanted immunogenic responses. Four factors dictate at what stage affinity chromatography can best be exploited: (1) the concentration of the desired product in the starting material; (2) the composition of other components in the starting material, along with their physical and chemical properties; (3) the desired product purity; (4) the volume of the material to be processed. Each stage of an affinity chromatography process: adsorption, washing, elution and regeneration needs to be

Table 6.13 (b) Commercially available biosorbents

Trade name	Nature	Producer
m-Aminophenylboronate (m-APB)	m-APB immobilized on beaded agarose *via* nine-atom spacer	Sigma, St. Louis, MO, U.S.A.
Amylose	Amylose resin	New England Biolabs, Beverley, MA, U.S.A.
Biotin	Biotin -agarose	Sigma, St. Louis, MO, U.S.A.
Cibacron Blue F3G-A	Blue Sepharose CL-6B	Pharmacia Biotech., Uppsala, Sweden
Human serum albumin (HSA)	Immobilised HSA column	Shandon, Runcorn, UK
Melibiose	Melibiose-polyacrylamide	Pierce Chemical Co., Rockford, IL, U.S.A.
Protein A	Protein A AvidGel F	BioProbe International, Tustin, CA, U.S.A.
	Sepharose-bound protein A	Bio-Rad Laboratories, Richmond, CA, U.S.A.
Streptavidin	Streptavidin dynabead	Dynal A.S., Oslo, Norway

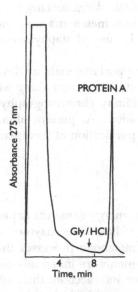

Figure 6.37 Monitoring of Protein A in a fermentation broth using an IgG-HPLAC column (10 μm, 10 × 0.5 cm). Conditions: mobile phase, initially 0.1 M NaH$_2$PO$_4$, pH 7.0, 0.15 M NaCl, changed to 0.1 M glycine/HCl, pH 2.2 (at arrow) to elute Protein A. Flow rate, 4 ml/min, sample, 0.96 fermentation broth, temperature, 22°C. Reproduced with permission from S. Ohlson *et al.* (1989) *Trends Biotechnol.*, **7**, 179–186.

optimized before the process is scaled up. Moreover, each step needs to be consistent and reproducible. Bioadsorbent stability is an important criterion since the ligands are often labile biological molecules. Affinity media can lose its effectiveness because of unstable ligands, microbial contamination, and column clogging due to the presence of insoluble matter in the sample and in the eluting buffers. Accumulation of denatured proteins, lipids, nucleic acids etc., that are not eluted during the regeneration process can also limit the lifetime of the column. A preparative column is exposed to more protein in three or four preparative cycles than an analytical column is exposed to in two or three hundred cycles. Under these conditions, maintenance of the affinity media becomes very important. Stringent cleaning-in-place procedures are recommended by the media manufactures to prolong their lifetime. The feasibility of such measures should be taken into consideration before a purification method is scaled up. Suitable affinity ligands for large-scale isolations are polyclonal or monoclonal antibodies, because they can be produced against any compound, even if the latter is only partially purified. Furthermore, monoclonal antibodies can be selected with any desired affinity, thereby making the use of biospecific columns, prepared by their immobilization, very attractive. Such antibodies, show absolute specifity for only one single epitope, the smallest immunologically sub-molecular group on an antigen. Monoclonal antibodies can be produced in large quantities by the hybridoma technology developed by Köhler and Milstein (1975). Tarnowski and Liptak (1983) used this antibody for the automated immunosorbent purification of interferon. Large-scale preparation of bovine and human fibronectins by affinity chromatography was described by Roulleau *et al.* (1982). Ohtsuru *et al.* (1982) used pepstatin-Sepharose for the purification of pepsin isozymes from large-scale culture of *Rhizopus chinensis.* Large-scale purification of monoclonal antibody, which recognized a human melanoma-associated 250 kDa proteoglycan, was isolated by Lee *et al.* (1986) by use of staphylococcal Protein A-Sepharose.

As improvements in the technology of chromatographic support materials are developed, the combination of the unique selectivity of an affinity interaction along with the improved performance of modern supports assures affinity chromatography a commanding position in the future of large-scale purification. At present affinity chromatography is already increasingly used in large-scale purification of therapeutic products.

Immobilization of enzymes on their immunosorbents

The high efficiency of most natural processes and their low energy demands depend on highly active and specific catalysts–enzymes. In nature, however, enzymes are produced by organisms for their own use: in regulated metabolic processes their low stability, narrow specificity and strictly defined requirements are inherently connected with their function. However, it is important to take into account that, after completion of their function in living cells, their denaturation and hydrolysis by proteinases occurs. For their stabilization, *in vivo*, as well as their function, hydrophobicity plays an important role. However, the contact of nonpolar amino acids with water is enthalpically disadvantageous and results in ice-like water structure. Such contact of water with hydrophobic surface clusters of proteins *in vitro* decreases protein stability. Hence, reduction of the nonpolar surface area should stabilize proteins. Shami *et al.* (1989) showed the dramatically increased activity of amylase complexed with their antibodies. Sheriff and coworkers (1987) used X-ray crystallography to determine the three-dimensional structure of antibody-antigen complex by use of anti-lysozyme Fab and lysozyme. They demostrated that more than 80 van der Waals bonds are formed during the antibody-lysozyme interaction. Formation of the complex resulted in exclusion of all molecules of water. The conclusion of cited data was, that oriented immobilization of enzymes by use of antigen-antibody interaction can result both in good steric accessibility of the enzyme's active site toward high-molecular-mass substrates and an increased stability. Moreover, biospecific adsorption of an enzyme to a suitable immunosorbent combines the isolation of molecules with their oriented immobilization.

To confirm this hypothesis, polyclonal antibodies suitable for the oriented immobilization of chymotrypsin were prepared by chromatography on a bioaffinity matrix which had the enzyme immobilized through its active site. This was prepared by the attachment of chymotrypsin to pancreatic trypsin inhibitor antilysin, covalently linked to bead cellulose (Fig. 6.38). The failure to detect any chymotryptic activity towards N-succinyl-L-phenylalanyl-p-nitroanilide showed that the enzyme was immobilized *via* its active site. After periodate oxidation of their carbohydrate moieties, the isolated antibodies were coupled to a hydrazide derivative of bead cellulose and used for the sorption of chymotrypsin (Bílková *et al.*, 1997). No decrease in proteolytic activity resulted from incubation of chymotrypsin with specific anti-chymotrypsin IgG in a 1 : 1 molar ratio. These isolated antibodies are thus suitable for the preparation of a biospecific affinity matrix bearing immobilized chymotrypsin orientated such that substrate proteins are accessible to its active site. The antigenic affinity of the anti-chymotrypsin antibodies was essentially unchanged by periodate oxidation of their carbohydrate moieties. Therefore this procedure was used to covalently attach isolated anti-chymotrypsin antibodies to a hydrazide derivative of beaded cellulose. The molar ratio of biospecifically adsorbed chymotrypsin molecules to immobilized antibody was 2 : 1, which is the value predicted for enzyme occupancy of each of the two Fab binding sites in IgG.

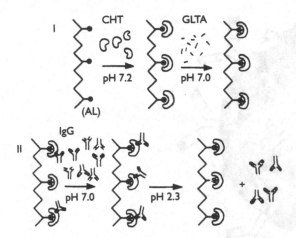

Figure 6.38 Schematic drawing (I) of oriented immobilization of chymotrypsin (CHT) by use of covalent crosslinking of its active site to immobilized natural polyvalent trypsin inhibitor antilysine (AL) with glutaraldehyde (GLTA) and (II) of use of this column for isolation of immunoglobulin G (IgG) against chymotrypsin (with antigenic sites outside the active site of CHT). Covalent bonds are shown as full lines. Reproduced from Z. Bílková *et al.* (1997) *J. Chromatogr. B*, **689**, 273–279.

The immobilized chymotrypsin retained practically 100% of the native catalytic activity determined by use of the high molecular substrate – denatured hemoglobin. Its proteolytic activity has not changed after more than one year.

In an analogy to non-enzymatic heterogeneous catalysis, in which an important role is played by the rate of diffusion of the reactants to the active surface of the catalyst, the rate of diffusion of the substrates to the binding site of the enzyme significantly affects the kinetic parameters of catalysis by an immobilized enzyme system. Very efficient columns packed with 1-μm non-porous spherical silica particles were described by Venema et al. (1996). In order to eliminate the kinetic limitation of chymotryptic hydrolysis of protein, porous bead cellulose was replaced by 1.2 μm non-porous hydroxyethyl methacrylate beads (Turková et al., 1997). Non-porous carrier was prepared by radical dispersion copolymerization of 2-hydroxyethyl methacrylate (HEMA) and ethylene dimethacrylate (EDMA) in the mixture of alcohol/toluene. The polymerization was initiated by dibenzoyl periodate and stabilized by cellulose butyrate. Isolated anti-chymotrypsin antibodies, attached to non-porous beads containing 1.9 μmol of dihydrazide groups per 1 g of dry product, was used for the coupling of anti-chymotrypsin antibodies. After the adsorption of chymotrypsin on the prepared immunosorbent 166.7 μg of chymotrypsin per 1 g of dry product was obtained (Fig 6.39). Immobilized chymotrypsin retained practically 100% of the native proteolytic activity. Monoclonal antibody (mAB) against horseradish peroxidase does not interfere with its enzyme activity. It also possesses a high affinity towards the enzyme and therefore was used for the preparation of a highly active immobilized enzyme by Solomon et al. (1991). They prepared the complex of peroxidase

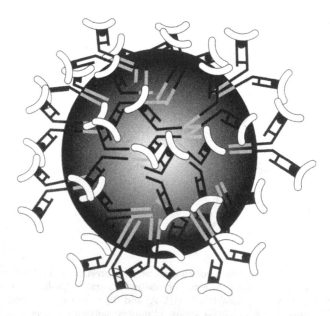

Figure 6.39 Schematic drawing of chymotrypsin prepared by use of adsorption on a suitable immunosorbent.

and mAB in solution and attached this immuno-complex to immobilized anti-Fc antibodies.

Conclusion

Affinity chromatography has increasingly become the method of choice for the purification or the determination of biologically active substances. It is used at both laboratory and industrial scale with a high degree of success. Many examples of classical, high-performance or large-scale applications were described in an ever greater number of publications. However, it is necessary to take into accout, that large-scale affinity chromatography is usually performed in industrial laboratories and most information is thus proprietary.

Because the basis of affinity chromatography is the biospecific complex formation of biologically active compounds, it is also useful for te study of their supramolecular structures in relation to their microenvironment. The use of biospecific adsorbents for oriented immobilization of proteins has been reviewed by Turková (1998). The advantages of this immobilization are good steric accessibilities of active binding sites and increased stability. This not only may help to increase the production of preparative procedures but is likely to promote current knowledge about how the living cells or tissues operate. Protein inactivation starts with unfolding of the protein molecule by the contact of water with hydrophobic clusters located on the surface of protein molecules or on the surface of solid support, which results in ice-like water structure. Reduction of nonpolar surface area by the formation of a suitable biospecific complex or by use of carbohydrate moieties thus may stabilize proteins. As an example can be mentioned antibody-antigen complexes which resulted in exclusion of all molecules of water. Biospecific adsorption of biologically active proteins to immunosorbents prepared by coupling through carbohydrate moieties of antibody can combine the isolation of molecules with their oriented immobilization.

References

Adachi, T., Mogi, M., Harada, M. and Kojima, K. (1996) Selective removal of human serum amyloid P component from rat blood by use of an immunoaffinity membrane in an extracorporeal circulation system. *J. Chromatogr.*, **682**, 47–54.

Amneus, H., Gabel, D. and Kasche, V. (1976) Resolution in affinity chromatography. The effect of the heterogeneity of immobilized soybean trypsin inhibitor on the separation of pancreatic proteases. *J. Chromatogr.*, **120**, 391–397.

Angal, S. and Dean, P. D. G. (1977) The effect of matrix on the binding of albumin to immobilized Cibacron Blue. *Biochem. J.*, **167**, 301–303.

Anspach, F. B., Johnston, A., Wirth, H. J., Unger, K. K. and Hearn, M. T. W. (1990) High-performance liquid chromatography of amino acids, peptides and proteins XCV. Thermodynamic and kinetic investigation on rigid and soft affinity gels with varying particle and pore sizes: comparison of thermodynamic parameters and the adsorption behaviour of proteins evaluated from batch and frontal analysis experiments. *J. Chromatogr.*, **499**, 103–124.

Anspach, F. B., Wirth, H. J., Unger, K. K., Stanton, P., Davis, J. R. and Hearn, M. T. W. (1989) High-performance liquid affinity chromatography with phenylboronic acid, benzamidine, tri-L-alanine and concanavalin A immobilized on 3-isothiocyanatopropylethoxysilane-activated nonporous monodisperse silicas. *Anal. Biochem.*, **179**, 171–181.

Arnott, S., Fulmer, A., Scott, W. E., Dea, I. C. M., Moorhouse, R. and Rees, D. A. (1974) The agarose double helix and its function in agarose gel structure. *J. Mol. Biol.*, **90**, 269–284.

Ashton, D. S., Beddell, C. R., Cockerill, G. S., Gohil, K., Gowrie, C., Robinson, J. E., Slater, M. J. and Valko, K. (1996) Binding measurements of indolcarbazole derivatives to immobilised human serum albumin by high-performance liquid chromatography. *J. Chromatogr. B*, **677**, 194–198.

Axén, R., Porath, J. and Ernback, S. (1967) Chemical coupling of peptides and proteins to polysaccharides by means of cyanogen halides. *Nature (London)*, **214**, 1302–1304.

Bayer, E. A., Ben-Hur, H., Gitlin, G. and Wilchek, M. (1986) An improved method for the single-step purification of streptavidin. *J. Biochem. Biophys. Methods*, **13**, 103–112.

Bayer, E. A. and Wilchek, M. (1990) Application of avidin–biotin technology to affinity-based separations. *J. Chromatogr.*, **510**, 3–11.

Belew, M., Porath, J., Fohlman, J. and Janson, J. C. (1978) Adsorption phenomena on Sephacryl S-200 Superfine. *J. Chromatogr.*, **147**, 205–212.

Beneš, M. J., Adámková, K. and Turková, J. (1991) Activation of beaded cellulose with 2,4,6-trichlortriazine. *Bioactiv. Compatible Polymers*, **6**, 406–413.

Bethell, G. S., Ayers, J. S., Hearn, M. T. W. and Hancock, W. S. (1981) Investigation of the activation of cross-linked agarose with carbonylating reagents and the preparation of matrices for affinity chromatography purifications. *J. Chromatogr.*, **219**, 353–359.

Bethell, G. S., Ayers, J. S., Hearn, M. T. W. and Hancock, W. S. (1981) Investigation of the activation of various insoluble polysaccharides with 1,1'-carbonyldiimidazole and of the properties of the activated matrices. *J. Chromatogr.*, **219**, 361–372.

Bílková, Z., Churáček, J., Kučerová, Z. and Turková, J. (1997) Purification of anti-chymotrypsin antibodies for the preparation of a bioaffinity matrix with oriented chymotrypsin as immobilized ligand. *J. Chromatogr. B*, **689**, 273–279.

Bílková, K., Králová, B. and Beneš, M. J. (1996) A new method for the purification of yeast α-glucosidase using immunoaffinity chromatography. *Intern. J. Bio-chromatogr.*, **2**, 101–108.

Björck, L. and Kronvall, G. (1984) Purification and some properties of streptococcal protein G, a novel IgG-binding reagent. *J. Immunol.*, **133**, 969–974.

Bloom, J. W., Wong, M. F. and Mitra, G. (1989) Detection and reduction of Protein A contamination in immobilized Protein A purified monoclonal antibody preparations. *J. Immunol. Methods*, **117**, 83–89.

Bober, M. A. and Ownby, C. L. (1988) Use of affinity-purified antibodies to measure the *in vivo* disapperance of antibodies to myotoxin *a*. *Toxicon*, **26**, 301–308.

Bonnafous, J. C., Dornand, J., Favero, J., Sizes, M., Boschetti, E. and Mani, J. C. (1983) Cell affinity chromatography with ligands immobilized through cleavable mercury-sulfur bonds. *J. Immunol. Methods*, **58**, 93–107.

Boschetti, E., Corgier, M. and Garelle, R. (1978) Immobilization of ligands for affinity chromatography. A comparative study of two condensation agents: 1-cyclohexyl-3-(2-morpholinoethyl)-carbodiimide-metho-*p*-toluene sulfonate (CMC) and N-ethoxycarbonyl-1,2-dihydroquinoline (EEDQ). *Biochimie*, **60**, 425–427.

Bouriotis, V., Galpin, I. J. and Dean, P. D. G. (1981) Applications of immobilised phenylboronic acids as supports for group-specific ligands in the affinity chromatography of enzymes. *J. Chromatogr.*, **210**, 267–278.

Brandt, J., Andersson, L. O. and Porath, J. (1975) Covalent attachment of proteins to polysaccharide carriers by means of benzoquinone. *Biochim. Biophys. Acta*, **386**, 196–202.

Brocklehurst, K., Carlsson, J., Kierstan, M. P. J. and Crook, E. M. (1973) Covalent chromatography. Preparation of fully active papain from dried papaya latex. *Biochem. J.*, **133**, 573–584.

Cambiaso, C. L., Goffinet, A., Vaerman, J. P. and Heremans, J. F. (1975) Glutaraldehyde-activated aminohexyl-derivative of Sepharose 4B as a new versatile immunosorbent. *Immunochem.*, 12, 273–278.

Cammas, F. M. and Clarc, A. J. L. (1996) S1 Nuclease protection assay using Streptavidin dynabeads-purified single-stranded DNA. *Anal. Biochem.*, 236, 182–184.

Campbell, D. H., Luescher, E. L. and Lerman, L. S. (1951) Immunologic adsorbents. I. Isolation of antibody by means of a cellulose-protein antigen. *Proc. Natl. Acad. Sci. U.S.A.*, 37, 575–578.

Carlsson, J., Axén, R. and Unge, T. (1975) Reversible, covalent immobilization of enzymes by thiol-disulphide interaction. *Eur. J. Biochem.*, 59, 567–572.

Caron, M., Chadli, A., Séve, A. P., Lutomski, D., Bladier, D. and Joubert-Caron, R. (1997) Glycobiology and bioaffinity chromatography. *Intern. J. Bio-chromatogr.*, 3, 111–122.

Charcosset, C. (1998) Purification of proteins by membrane chromatography (review). *J. Chem. Technol. Biotechnol.*, 71, 95–110.

Clemetson, K. J., Pfueller, S. L., Luscher, E. F. and Jenkins, C. S. P. (1977) Isolation of the membrane glycoproteins of human blood platelets by lectin affinity chromatography. *Biochim. Biophys. Acta*, 464, 493–508.

Cook, G. M. W. and Buckie, J. W. (1990) Lectin-mediated isolation of cell surface glycoproteins. *Meth. Enzymol.*, 184, 304–314.

Čoupek, J., Křiváková, M. and Pokorný, S. (1973) New hydrophilic materials for chromatography: glycol methacrylates. *J. Polymer. Sci. Symp.*, 42, 185–190.

Crowley, S. C., Chan, K. C. and Walters, R. R. (1986) Optimization of protein immobilization on 1,1'-carbonyldiimidazole-activated diol-bonded silica. *J. Chromatogr.*, 359, 359–368.

Cuatrecasas, P. (1970) Protein purification by affinity chromatography. Derivatizations of agarose and polyacrylamide beads. *J. Biol. Chem.*, 245, 3059–3065.

Cuatrecasas, P. and Parikh, I. (1972) Adsorbents for affinity chromatography. Use of *N*-Hydroxysuccinimide ester of agarose. *Biochemistry*, 11, 2291–2299.

Cuatrecasas, P. and Wilchek, M. (1968) Single-step purification of avidin from egg white by affinity chromatography on biocytin-Sepharose columns. *Biochem. Biophys. Res. Commun.*, 33, 235–239.

Cuatrecasas, P., Wilchek, M. and Anfinsen, C. B. (1968) Selective enzyme purification by affinity chromatography. *Proc. Natl. Acad. Sci. U.S.A.*, 61, 636–643.

DeBell, K. E., Taplits, M. S., Hoffman, T. and Bonvini, E. (1990) T Lymphocyte aggregation with immobilized anti-TCR-antibodies is dependent upon energy and microfilament assembly. *Cell. Immunol.*, 127, 159–171.

Diaco, R., Hill, J. H. and Durand, D. P. (1986) Purification of soybean mosaic virus by affinity chromatography using monoclonal antibodies. *J. Gen. Virol.*, 67, 345–351.

Doley, S. G., Harvey, M. J. and Dean, P. D. G. (1976) The potential of Ultrogel, an agarose-polyacrylamide copolymer, as a matrix for affinity chromatography. *FEBS Lett.*, 65, 87–91.

DuVal, G., Swaisgood, H. E. and Horton, H. R. (1984) Preparation and characterization of thionyl chloride-activated succinamidopropyl-glass as a covalent immobilized matrix. *J. Appl. Biochem*, 6, 240–250.

Ernest-Cabrera, K. and Wilchek, M. (1987) Coupling of ligands to primary hydroxyl-containing silica for high-performance affinity chromatography. Optimization of conditions. *J. Chromatogr.*, 397, 187–196.

Finn, F. M. and Hofmann, K. (1990) Isolation and characterization of hormone receptors. *Meth. Enzymol.*, 184, 244–274.

Fishel, R., Anziano, P. and Rich, A. (1990) Z-DNA affinity chromatography. *Meth. Enzymol.*, **184**, 328–340.

Fleminger, G., Solomon, B., Wolf, T. and Hadas, E. (1990a) Single step oxidation binding of antibodies to hydrazide-modified Eupergit C. *Appl. Biochem. Biotech.*, **23**, 123–137.

Fleminger, G., Wolf, T., Hadas, E. and Solomon, B. (1990b) Eupergit C as a carrier for high-performance liquid chromatographic-based immunopurification of antigens and antibodies. *J. Chromatogr.*, **510**, 311–319.

Frost, R. G., Monthony, J. F., Engelhorn, S. C. and Siebert, C. J. (1981) Covalent immobilization of proteins to *N*-hydroxysuccinimide ester derivatives of agarose. Effect of protein charge on immobilization. *Biochim. Biophys. Acta*, **670**, 163–169.

Gersten, D. M. and Marchalonis, J. J. (1978) A rapid, novel method for the solid-phase derivatization of IgG antibodies for immune-affinity chromatography. *J. Immunol. Methods*, **24**, 305–309.

Gierasch, L. M., Lacy, J. E., Thompson, K. F., Rockwell, A. L. and Watnick, P. I. (1982) Conformaton of model peptides in membrane-mimetic environments. *Biophys. J.*, **37**, 275–284.

Gilham, P. T. (1971) The covalent binding of nucleotides, polynucleotides and nucleic acids to cellulose. *Meth. Enzymol.*, **21**, 191–197.

Grabowski, P. J. (1990) Isolation and analysis of splicing complexes. *Meth. Enzymol.*, **184**, 319–327.

Green, N. M. (1966) Thermodynamics of the binding of biotin and some analogues by avidin. *Biochem. J.*, **101**, 774–780.

Groman, E. V. and Wilchek, M. (1987) Recent developments in affinity chromatography supports. *Trends Biotechnol.*, **5**, 220–224.

Guesdon, J. L. and Avrameas, S. (1976) Polyacrylamide-agarose beads for the preparation of effective immunoabsorbents. *J. Immunol. Methods*, **11**, 129–133.

Guesdon, J. L. and Avrameas, S. (1977) Magnetic solid phase enzyme-immunoassay. *Immunochemistry*, **14**, 443–447.

Gustavsson, P. E. and Larsson, P. O. (1996) Superporous agarose, a new material for chromatography. *J. Chromatogr.*, **734**, 231–240.

Hall, J. C., Tubbs, C. E., Li, Y., Ashraf, S. and Lamarche, M. D. (1997) Affinity purification and characterization of a 32 Kd glycoprotein from rat sperm plasma membrane that is required for egg zona pellucida binding. *Int. J. Bio-chromatogr.*, **3**, 155–176.

Harvey, M. J., Lowe, C. R., Craven, D. B., and Dean, P. D. G. (1974) Affinity chromatography on immobilised adenosine 5′-monophosphate 2. Some parameters relating to the selection and concentration of the immobilised ligand. *Eur. J. Biochem.*, **41**, 335–340.

Hatakeya, T., Murakami, K., Miyamoto, Y. and Yamasaki, N. (1996) An assay for lectin activity using microtiter plate with chemically immobilized carbohydrates. *Anal. Biochem.*, **237**, 188–192.

Hering, T. M., Kollar, J., Huynh, T. D. and Varelas, J. B. (1996) Purification and characterization of decorin core protein expressed in *Escherichia coli* as a maltose-binding protein fusion. *Anal. Biochem.*, **240**, 98–108.

Hermanson, G. T., Mallia, A. K. and Smith, P. K. (1992) *Immobilized affinity ligand techniques*, Academic Press, INC, San Diego, New York, Boston, London, Sydney, Tokyo, Toronto.

Hou, K. C. and Mandaro, R. M. (1986) Bioseparation by ion exchange cartridge chromatography. *Biotechniques*, **4**, 358–367.

Huang, S. C., Stump, M. D., Weiss, R. and Caldwell, K. D. (1996) Binding of biotinylated DNA to streptavidin-coated polystyrene latex: effects of chain length and particle size. *Anal. Biochem.*, **237**, 115–122.

Huse, K., Himmel, M., Gärtner, G., Kopperschläger, G. and Hofmann, E. (1990) Use of an activated nylon membrane (Immunodyne) as an affinity adsorbent for the purification of phosphofructokinase and phosphoglycerate kinase from yeast. *J. Chromatogr.*, **502**, 171–177.

Inman, J. K. and Dintzis, H. M. (1969) The derivatization of cross-linked polyacrylamide beads. Controlled introduction of functional groups for the preparation of special-purpose, biochemical adsorbents. *Biochemistry*, **8**, 4074–4082.

Isobe, T., Naiki, M., Handa, S. and Taki, T. (1996) A simple assay method for bacterial binding to glycosphingolipids on a polyvinylidene difluoride membrane after thin-layer chromatography *in situ* mass spectrometric analysis of the ligands. *Anal. Biochem.*, **236**, 35–40.

Ivanov, A. E., Zhigis, L. S., Chekhovskykh, E. A., Reshetov, P. D. and Zubov, V. P. (1985) Carbonylchloride-containing compositional matrices for immobilization of biospecific ligands. *Bioorg. Khim.*, **11**, 1527–1532.

Jakoby, W. B. and Wilchek, M. (1974) Affinity Chromatography. *Meth. Enzymol.*, **34**, 1–810.

Josić, D., Reusch, J., Löster, K., Baum, O. and Reutter, W. (1992) High-performance membrane chromatography of serum and plasma membrane proteins. *J. Chromatogr.*, **590**, 59–76.

Kanamori, A., Seno, N. and Matsumoto, I. (1986) Preparation of high-capacity affinity adsorbents using formyl carriers and their use for low- and high-performance liquid affinity chromatography of trypsin-family proteases. *J. Chromatogr.*, **363**, 231–242.

Kay, G. and Crook, E. M. (1967) Coupling of enzymes to cellulose using chloro-*s*-triazines. *Nature (London)*, **216**, 514–515.

Kay, G. and Lilly, M. D. (1970) The chemical attachment of chymotrypsin to water-insoluble polymers using 2-amino-4,6-dichloro-*s*-triazine. *Biochim. Biophys. Acta*, **198**, 276–285.

Kelleher, F. M., Dubbs, S. B. and Bhavanandan, V. P. (1988) Purification of galactose oxidase from *Dactylium dendroides* by affinity chromatography on melibiose-polyacrylamide. *Arch. Biochem. Biophys.*, **263**, 349–354.

Kempf, J., Pfleger, N. and Egly, J. M. (1978) Coupling of nucleic acids to agarose: a biospecific support for the purification and/or study of the interactions of related compounds. *J. Chromatogr.*, **147**, 195–204.

Khawli, L. A., Milkie, M. N., Hornick, J. L., Glasky, M. S., Sharifi, J., Hu, P. and Epstein, A. L. (1996) Production of immunoreactive F(ab')₂ fragments in high yield from murine IgG₁ monoclonal antibodies. *Intern. J. Bio-chromatogr.*, **2**, 89–99.

Klein, E. (1991) *Affinity Membranes, Their Chemistry & Performance in Adsorption Separation Processes*, Wiley, New York.

Koelsch, R., Fusek, M., Hostomská, Z., Lasch, J. and Turková, J. (1986) Coupling of ligands to insoluble matrices *via* aldehyde groups. *Biotechnol. Lett.*, **8**, 283–286.

Köhler, G. and Milstein, C. (1975) Continuous cultures of fused cells secreting antibody of predefined specificity. *Nature*, **256**, 495–497.

Kohn, J. and Wilchek, M. (1981) Procedures for the analysis of cyanogen bromide-activated Sepharose or Sephadex by quantitative determination of cyanate esters and imidocarbonates. *Anal. Biochem.*, **115**, 375–382.

Kohn, J. and Wilchek, M. (1984) The use of cyanogen bromide and other novel cyanylating agents for the activation of polysaccharide resins. *Appl. Biochem. Biotech.*, **9**, 285–305.

Koyama, T. and Teruchi, K. (1996) Synthesis and application of boronic acid-immobilized porous polymer particles: a novel packing for high-performance liquid affinity chromatography. *J. Chromatogr. B*, **679**, 31–40.

Krämer, D. M., Lehmann, K., Pennewiss, H. and Plainer, H. (1978) *Enzyme Eng.*, **4**, 153–154.

Kučerová, Z. and Turková, J. (1997) Isolation of human pepsin by use of membrane based bioadsorbent. *Int. J. Bio-chromatogr.*, **2**, 145–151.

Kukongviriyapan, V., Poopyruchpong, N. and Ratanabanangkoon, K. (1982) Some parameters of affinity chromatography in the purification of antibody against *Naja naja siamensis* toxin 3. *J. Immunol. Methods*, **49**, 97–104.

Lamed, R., Levin, Y. and Wilchek, M. (1973) Covalent coupling of nucleotides to agarose for affinity chromatography. *Biochim. Biophys. Acta,* **304**, 231–235.

Lawrence, J. F., Ménard, C., Hennion, M. C., Pichon, V., Le Goffic, F. and Durand, N. (1996) Use of immunoaffinity chromatography as a simplified cleanup technique for the liquid chromatographic determination of phenylurea herbicides in plant material. *J. Chromatogr. A,* **732**, 277–281.

Lee, W.-C. and Chuang, C-Y. (1996) Performance of pH elution in high-performance affinity chromatography of proteins using non-porous silica. *J. Chromatogr. A,* **721**, 31–39.

Lee, S. M., Gustafson, M. E., Pickle, D. J., Flickinger, M. C., Muschik, G. M. and Morgan, A. C. (1986) Large-scale purification of a murine antimelanoma monoclonal antibody. *J. Biotechnol.,* **4**, 189–204.

Leibl, H., Tomasits, R., Wolf, H. M., Eibl, M. M. and Mannhalter, J. W. (1996) Method for the isolation of biologically active monomeric immunoglobulin A from a plasma fraction. *J. Chromatogr. B,* **678**, 173–180.

Liu, Y. C. and Stellwagen, E. (1987) Accessibility and multivalency of immobilized Cibacron Blue F3GA. *J. Biol. Chem.,* **262**, 583–588.

Lowe, C. R. and Dean, P. D. G. (1974) *Affinity Chromatography,* Wiley, New York, London.

Luna, E. J., Goodloe-Holland, C. M. and Ingalls, H. M. (1984) A membrane cytoskeleton from *Dictyostelium discoideum.* II. Integral proteins mediate the binding of plasma membranes to F-actin affinity beads. *J. Cell Biol.,* **99**, 58–70.

Matsumoto, I., Ito, Y. and Seno, N. (1982) Preparation of affinity adsorbents with Toyopearl gels. *J. Chromatogr.,* **239**, 747–754.

Miron, T. and Wilchek, M. (1981) Polyacrylhydrazido-agarose: preparation *via* periodate oxidation and use for enzyme immobilization and affinity chromatography. *J. Chromatogr.,* **215**, 55–63.

Mohr, P. and Pommerenig, K. (1985) *Affinity Chromatography: Practical and Theoretical Aspects.* Marcel Dekker, New York.

Morehead, H. W., Talmadge, K. W., O'Shannessy, D. J. and Siebert, C. J. (1991) Optimization of oxidation of glycoproteins: an assay for predicting coupling to hydrazide chromatographic supports. *J. Chromatogr.,* **587**, 171–176.

Nandedkar, U. N., Sawhney, S. Y., Bhile, S. V. and Kale, N. R. (1987) Sephacryl S-300 – an affinity matrix which distinguished concanavalin A from other D-mannose/D-glucose-specific lectins. *J. Chromatogr.,* **396**, 363–368.

Narayanan, S. R. (1994) Preparative affinity chromatography of proteins. *J.Chromatogr. A,* **658**, 237–258.

Narayanan, S. R., Knochs, S., Jr. and Crane, L. J. (1990) Preparative affinity chromatography of proteins. Influence of the physical properties of the base matrix. *J. Chromatogr.,* **503**, 93–102.

Ngo, T. T. (1986) Facile activation of Sepharose hydroxyl groups by 2-fluoro-1 methylpyridinium toluene-4-sulfonate: preparation of affinity and covalent chromatographic matrices. *Biotechnology,* **4**, 134–137.

Nilsson, K. and Mosbach, K. (1981) Immobilization of enzymes and affinity ligands to various hydroxyl group carrying supports using highly reactive sulfonyl chlorides. *Biochem. Biophys. Res. Commun.,* **102**, 449–457.

Noppen, C., Spagnoli, G. C. and Schaefer, C. (1996) Isolation of Multiple mRNAs from a few, eukaryotic cells: a fast method to obtain templates for RT-PCR. *Biotechniques,* **21**, 394–396.

Novotná, V., Mikeš, L., Horák, P., Jonáková, V. and Tichá, M. (1996) Preparation of water-soluble and water-insoluble poly(acrylamide-allylamine) derivatives of polysaccharides. *Intern. J. Bio-chromatogr.,* **2**, 37–47.

Ohlson, S., Hansson, L., Glad, M., Mosbach, K. and Larson, P.-O. (1989) High performance liquid affinity chromatography: a new tool in biotechnology. *Trends Biotechnol.*, 7, 179–186.

Ohtsuru, M., Tang, J. and Delaney, R. (1982) Purification and characterization of rhizopus-pepsin isozymes from a liquid culture of *Rhizopus chinensis*. *Int. J. Biochem.*, 14, 925–932.

O'Shannessy, D. J. (1990) Hydrazido-derivatized supports in affinity chromatography. *J. Chromatogr.*, 510, 13–21.

Petkov, L., Sajdok, J., Rae, K., Šuchová, M., Káš, J. and Turková, J. (1990) Activation of galactose-containing glycoprotein and solid supports by galactose oxidase in presence of catalase for immobilization purposes. *Biotechnol. Techniques*, 4, 25–30.

Phillips, T. M. (1989) Isolation and recovery of biologically active proteins by high performance immunoaffinity chromatography. In A. R. Kerlavage (ed.), *The Use of HPLC in Receptor Biochemistry*, Alan R. Liss, Inc., New York, pp. 129–154.

Phillips, T. M., Queen, W. D., More, N. S. and Thompson, A. M. (1985) Protein A-coated glass beads. Universal support medium for high-performance immunoaffinity chromatography. *J. Chromatogr.*, 327, 213–219.

Pichon, V., Chen, L., Durand, N., Le Goffic, F. and Hennion, M. C. (1996) Selective trace enrichment on immunosorbents for the multiresidue analysis of phenylurea and triazine pesticides. *J. Chromatogr. A*, 725, 107–119.

Porath, J. (1974) General methods and coupling procedures. *Meth. Enzymol.*, 34, 13–30.

Porath, J., Aspberg, K., Drevin, H. and Axén, R. (1973) Preparation of cyanogen bromide-activated agarose gels. *J. Chromatogr.*, 86, 57–64.

Porath, J., Carlsson, J., Olsson, I. and Belfrage, G. (1975) Metal chelate affinity chromatography, a new approach to protein fractionation. *Nature*, 258, 598–599.

Porath, J. and Sundberg, L. (1972) High capacity chemisorbents for protein immobilization. *Nature New Biol.*, 238, 261–262.

Rapoport, E. M., Zhigis, L. S., Ivanov, A. E., Korchagina, E. J., Ovchinikova, T. V., Zubov, V. P. *et al.* (1997) Isolation and characterization of galactose-binding lectins from human serum. *Intern. J. Bio-chromatogr.*, 3, 57–67.

Roulleau, M. F., Boschetti, E., Burnouf, T., Kirzin, J. M. and Saint-Blancard, J. (1982). In T. C. J. Gribnau, J. Visser and J. F. Nivard, (eds), *Affinity Chromatography and Related Techniques*, Elsevier, Amsterdam, pp. 323–331.

Rucklidge, G. J., Milne, G., Chaudhry, M. and Robins, S. P. (1996) Preparation of biotinylated, affinity-purified antibodies for enzyme-linked immunoassays using blotting membrane as an antigen support. *Anal. Biochem.*, 243, 158–164.

Ruhn, P., Garver, S. and Hage, D. S. (1994) Development of dihydrazide-activated silica supports for high-performance affinity chromatography. *J. Chromatogr.*, 669, 9–19.

Saito, T. and Nagai, F. (1983) Immobilization of antibody to a plastic surface by toluene 2,4-diisocyanate and its application to radioimmunoassay. *Clin. Chim. Acta*, 133, 301–310.

Sanderson, C. J. and Wilson, D. V. (1971) A simple method for coupling proteins to insoluble polysaccharides. *Immunology*, 20, 1061–1065.

Santa-Coloma, T. A., Garraffo, H. M., Gross, E. G. and Charreau, E. H. (1987) A cyclic affinity chromatography method for the purification of the sex steroid binding protein. *J. Chromatogr.*, 415, 297–304.

Schott, H. (1984) *Affinity Chromatography – Template Chromatography of Nucleic Acids and Proteins*, Marcel Dekker, New York.

Scouten, W. H. (1981) *Affinity Chromatography: Bioselective Adsorption on Inert Matrices*, Wiley, New York.

Sene, C., Girot, P., Boschetti, E., Plassat, J. L., Bloch, J. and Egly, J. M. (1982) Purification of polyadenylated mRNA on three oligo(dT)-substituted gels: a comparative study. *J. Chromatogr.*, 248, 441–445.

Shami, E. Y., Rothstein, A. and Ramjeesingh, M. (1989) Stabilization of biologically active proteins. *Trends Biotechnol.*, 7, 186–190.

Sheriff, S., Silverton, E. A., Padlan, E. A., Cohen, G. H., Smith-Gill, S. J., Finzel, B. C. and Davis, D. R. (1987) Three-dimensional structure of an antibody-antigen complex. *Proc. Natl. Acad. Sci. U.S.A.*, 84, 8075–8079.

Shimura, K., Kazama, M. and Kasai, K. I. (1984) High-performance affinity chromatography of plasmin and plasminogen on a hydrophilic vinyl-polymer gel coupled with p-aminobenzamidine. *J. Chromatogr.*, 292, 369–382.

Smalla, K., Turková, J., Čoupek, J. and Hermann, P. (1988) Influence of salts on the covalent immobilization of proteins to modified copolymers of 2-hydroxyethyl methacrylate with ethylene dimethacrylate. *Biotechnol. Appl. Biochem.* 10, 21–31.

Solomon, B., Hadas, E., Koppel, R., Schwartz, F. and Fleminger, G. (1991) Highly active enzyme preparations immobilized *via* matrix-conjugated anti-Fc antibodies. *J. Chromatogr.*, 539, 335–341.

Solomon, B., Koppel, R., Schwartz, F. and Fleminger, G. (1990) Enzymatic oxidation of monoclonal antibodies by soluble and immobilized bifunctional enzyme complexes. *J. Chromatogr.*, 510, 321–329.

Solomon, B., Raviv, O., Leibman, E. and Fleminger, G. (1992) Affinity purification of antibodies using FB domain of protein A. *J. Chromatogr.*, 597, 257–262.

Stambolieva, N. and Turková, J. (1980) Covalent attachment of proteins to Spheron by means of benzoquinone. *Collect. Czech. Chem. Commun.* 45, 1137–1143.

Staudenbauer, W. L. and Orr, E. (1981) DNA gyrase: affinity chromatography on novobiocin-Sepharose and catalytic properties. *Nucleic Acid. Res.*, 9, 3589–3603.

Tarnowski, S. J. and Liptak, R. A. (1983) Automated immunosorbent purification of interferon. In A. Mizrahi and A. L. van Wezel, (eds.), *Advances in Biotechnical Processes*, Alan R. Liss, Inc., New York, pp. 271–287.

Turková, J. (1978) *Affinity Chromatography*, Elsevier, Amsterdam.

Turková, J. (1993) *Bioaffinity Chromatography*, Elsevier, Amsterdam.

Turková, J. (1999) Oriented immobilization of biologically active proteins as a tool for revealing protein interaction and function. *J. Chromatogr. B*, 722(1–2), 11–31.

Turková, J., Bílková, Z., Mazurová, J. and Horák, D. (1997) Oriented immobilization of chymotrypsin by use of suitable antibodies coupled to porous or non-porous solid support. *12th International Symposium on Affinity Interaction: Fundamentals and Applications of Biomolecular Recognition*, Kalmar, June 1997, PA34.

Turková, J., Bláha, K. and Adamová, K. (1982) Effect of concentration of immobilized inhibitor on the biospecific chromatography of pepsins. *J. Chromatogr.* 236, 375–383.

Turková, J., Bláha, K., Horáček, J., Vajčner, J., Frydrychová, A. and Čoupek, J. (1981) Hydroxyalkyl methacrylate gels derivatized with epichlorohydrin as supports for large-scale and high-performance affinity chromatography. *J. Chromatogr.* 215, 165–179.

Turková, J., Bláha, K., Malaníková, M., Vančurová, D., Švec, F. and Kálal, J. (1978) Methacrylate gels with epoxide groups as supports for immobilization of enzymes in pH range 3–12. *Biochim. Biophys. Acta.*, 524, 162–169.

Turková, J., Bláha, K., Valentová, O., Čoupek, J. and Seifertová, A. (1976) Affinity chromatography on hydroxyalkyl methacrylate gels III. Adsorption of chymotrypsin to poly(hydroxyalkyl methacrylates) with covalently bound benzyloxycarbonyl-glycyl-D-phenylalanine and -D-leucine as function of pH and ionic strength. *Biochim.Biophys.Acta.*, 427, 586–593.

Turková, J., Fusek, M., Maksimov,J. J. and Alakhov, Y. B. (1986) Reversible and irreversible immobilization of carboxypeptidase Y using biospecific adsorption. *J.Chromatogr.*, **376**, 315–321.

Turková, J., Hubálková, O., Křiváková, M. and Čoupek, J. (1973) Affinity chromatography on hydroxyalkyl methacrylate gels. I. Peparation of immobilized chymotrypsin and its use in the isolation of proteolytic inhibitors. *Biochim. Biophys. Acta.*, **322**, 1–9.

Turková, J., Kučerová, Z., Vaňková, H. and Beneš, M. J. (1997) Stabilization and oriented immobilization of glycoproteins. *Int. J. Bio-chromatogr.*, **3** , 45–55.

Ugelstad, J., Berge, A., Ellingsten, T., Aune, O., Kilaas, L., Nilsen, T. N., Schmid, R., Stenstad, P., Funderud, S., Kvalheim, G., Nustad, K., Lea, T., Vartal, F. and Danielsen, H. (1988) Monosized magnetic particles and their use in selective cell separation. *Makromol. Chem., Macromol. Symp.*, **17**, 177–211.

Unger, K. K., Jilge, G., Kinkel, J. N. and Hearn, M. T. W. (1986) Evaluation of advanced silica packings for the separation of biopolymers by high-performance liquid chromatography II. Performance of non-porous monodisperse 1.5-µm silica beads in the separation of proteins by reversed-phase gradient elution high-performance liquid chromatography. *J. Chromatogr.*, **359**, 61–72.

Updyke, T. V. and Nicolson, G. L. (1984) Immunoaffinity isolation of membrane antigens with biotinylated monoclonal antibodies and immobilized streptavidin matrices. *J. Immunol. Methods*, **73**, 83–95.

Uusi-Oukari, M., Ehnholm, C. and Jauhiainen, M. (1996) Inhibition of hepatic lipase by *m*-aminophenylboronate. Application of phenylboronate affinity chromatography for purification of human postheparin plasma lipases. *J. Chromatogr. B*, **682**, 233–242.

Van Sommeren, A. P. G., Machilsen, P. A. G. M. and Gribnau, T. C. J. (1993) Comparison of three activated agaroses for use in affinity chromatography: effects on coupling performance and ligand leakage. *J. Chromatogr.*, **639**, 23–31.

Venama, E., Kraak, J. C., Poppe, H. and Tijssen, R. (1996) Packed-column hydrodynamic using 1-µm non-porous silica particles. *J. Chromatogr.*, **740**, 159–167.

Vijayalakshmi, M. A. and Bertrand, O., (eds), (1989) *Protein-Dye Interations: Developments and Applications*, Elsevier Applied Science, London and New York.

Vijayalakshmi, M. A. (1989) Pseudobiospecific Ligand Affinity Chromatography, *Trends Biotechnol.*, **7**(3), 71–76.

Wan, Y. and Hasenstein, H. (1996) Preparation and characterization of anti-idiotypic antibody to probe putative abscisic acid receptors. *Intern. J. Bio-chromatogr.*, **2**, 77–88.

Weetall, H. H. and Filbert, A. M. (1974) Porous glass for affinity chromatography application. *Meth. Enzymol.*, **34**, 59–72.

Weetall, H. H. and Lee, M. J. (1989) Antibodies immobilized on inorganic supports. *Appl. Biochem. Biotech.*, **22**, 311–330.

Werner, S. and Machleidt, W. (1978) Isolation of precursors of cytochrome oxidase from *Neurospora crassa*: application of subunit-specific antibodies and Protein A from *Staphylococcus aureus*. *Eur. J. Biochem.*, **90**, 99–105.

Weston, P. D. and Avrameas, S. (1971) Proteins coupled to polyacrylamide beads using glutaraldehyde. *Biochem. Biophys. Res. Commun.*, **45**, 1574–1580.

Wheatley, J. B., Lyttle, M. H., Hocker, M. D. and Schmidt, Jr. D. E. (1996) Salt-induced immobilization of DNA oligonucleotides on an epoxide-activated high-performance liquid chromatographic affinity support. *J. Chromatogr. A*, **726**, 77–90.

Wilchek, M. and Bayer, E. A. (1990) Avidin–Biotin Technology. *Meth. Enzymol.*, **184**, 1–746.

Wilchek, M. and Miron, T. (1986) Origin of the carbamate functional groups in cyanogen bromide-activated, alkylamine-substituted Sepharose. *J. Chromatogr.*, **357**, 315–317.

Wilchek. M., Oka, T. and Topper, Y. (1975) Structure of a soluble super-active insulin is revealed by the nature of the complex between cyanogenbromide-activated Sepharose and amines. *Proc. Natl. Acad. Sci. U.S.A.*, **72**, 1055–1058.

Zemanová, I., Turková, J., Čapka, M., Nakhapetyan, L. A., Švec, F. and Kálal, J. (1981) Effect of the nature of proteins on their coupling to different epoxide-containing supports. *Enzyme Microb. Technol.*, **3**, 229–232.

Chapter 7

Dye ligand affinity chromatography

Robert K. Scopes

Discovery of dye adsorption

One of the most successful, yet perhaps the least understood method of biochromatography is variously known as dye ligand chromatography, pseudo-affinity chromatography or biomimetic affinity chromatography. The ligand is a dye molecule such as those developed for the colouring of clothing. Most important discoveries in science occur accidentally, and dye ligand chromatography is one of these. In the late 1960s, scientists purifying kinase enzymes were initially puzzled when, on gel filtration, their enzyme seemed to elute with the void volume marker molecule, Blue Dextran. But in the absence of marker, the elution position was later, at the expected volume (Haeckel *et al.*, 1968; Kopperschläger *et al.*, 1968). This was found to be due to an interaction between the enzymes and the dye itself, which was identified as the reactive dye known as Cibacron Blue F3G-A, from Ciba-Geigy (Fig. 7.1). By immobilising the dye on a suitable matrix, various Blue adsorbents were produced and marketed. These have been particularly suitable for adenine nucleotide-binding proteins, with NAD-utilising dehydrogenases suggested as the most likely to adsorb. However, it was soon found that many other proteins, including non-enzyme proteins were selectively bound to these Blue adsorbents, in particular human serum albumin (Gianazza and Arnaud, 1982) and some interferons (Jankowski *et al.*, 1976). Since then, many hundreds of protein purification procedures have included a Cibacron Blue adsorption step.

Alternative dyes

It is particularly fortunate that Pharmacia chose Cibacron Blue F3G-A as the dye to stain their void volume marker, because of all the hundreds of different dyes, this one does seem to be particularly effective at binding certain proteins rather specifically. But is was not long before workers began to investigate other dyes for protein-binding properties. Since the Reactive dyes, to which class the Cibacron series belongs, have a built-in reactivity which enables simple covalent attachment to a hydroxylated matrix such as beaded agarose, these have been the most investigated. Dyes manufactured by ICI Ltd. (Manchester, U.K.), the Procion series, were most studied initially by a group in Liverpool University, and later by many others. Additionally, the Ciba-Geigy Cibacron, Hoechst Remazol, Sandoz Drimarene and Bayer Levafix series have been investigated (Stead, 1991). Some of these propriety dyes differ only by the reactive mode of attachment, the chromaphore being identical (Fig. 7.2). This may not greatly

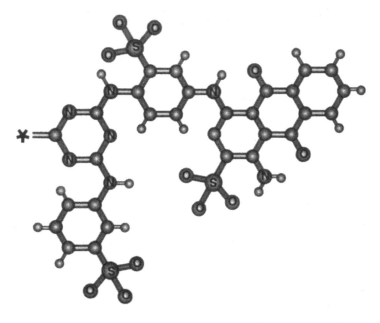

Figure 7.1 Two-dimensional structural diagram of Cibacron Blue F3G-A. The attachment to the matrix occurs at the starred linkage, by replacement of a chlorine at this position in the dye with the oxygen of a primary hydroxyl group in the matrix, or a nitrogen if coupling through an amine on the matrix.

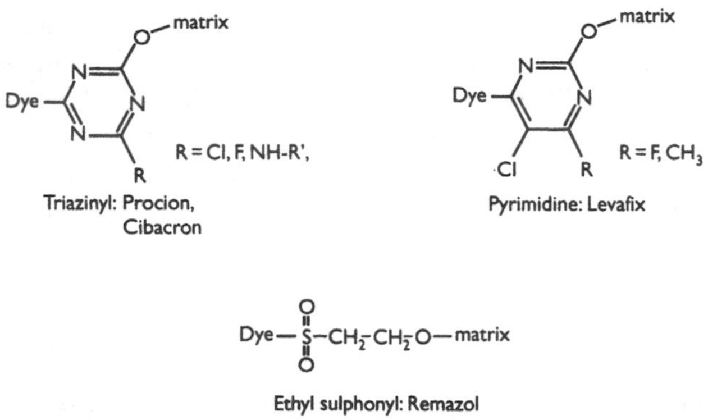

matrix
Dye
R = Cl, F, NH-R',
R
Triazinyl: Procion, Cibacron
matrix
Dye
R = F, CH3
Cl
R
Pyrimidine: Levafix
Dye — S–CH2–CH2–O— matrix
Ethyl sulphonyl: Remazol

Figure 7.2 Three examples of reactive groups on dyes used in dye–ligand chromatography. Illustrated after reaction has occurred with a hydroxyl matrix.

affect their specificity towards proteins; however, the structural details of many of the dyes have not been generally released. It was found that many of the dye adsorbents bound proteins (not always the same proteins as Cibacron Blue), and showed surprising selectivity in some cases. The general rule that Cibacron Blue was most suited to NAD-dehydrogenases was extended to include a claimed NADP-specific dye, Procion Red HE-3B (Watson *et al.*, 1978). It must be stated that although this red dye has been successfully used for many NADP enzymes, this is more because workers have used it as first choice, rather than after a screening of other potential dyes for selectivity. In our experience, Procion Red HE-3B is equally successful with NAD-enzymes, and other dyes can be superior for particular NADP-enzymes.

Some personal observations and developments

The key to dye ligand chromatography, as with any affinity technique, is selectivity. Resolution of adsorbed components by gradients is never sharp, certainly nothing like that achievable with ion exchangers. So much of the purification should occur at the adsorption step, with the bulk of the unwanted proteins not adsorbing to the dye. In our laboratory we carried out several screenings of 50 dye adsorbents to find out not only which proteins (enzymes) bound to which dyes, but also how much protein altogether bound, since this is important to the purification achieved during adsorption. The first screening included 5 mM manganous ions: the reason was that the particular enzyme we were trying to purify, 6-phosphogluconate dehydratase, was known to be stabilised by manganous ions (Kovachevich and Wood, 1955). The proportion of protein bound, from bacterial, yeast and rabbit muscle extracts, ranged from 10% to 90% (Fig. 7.3). However, when we repeated the screenings in 20 mM K-phosphate buffer without manganous ions, the dyes behaved in much the same way relative to each other, but the amount of protein ranged from only 3% to 40%. Thus the nature of the buffer was greatly affecting the quantity of protein binding. It had already been reported that divalent metal ions, particularly transition metals, strengthen the interactions, probably by forming metal bridges between the sulfonate groups (which are present on all of these dyes), and carboxyls in the proteins (Hughes and Sherwood, 1987).

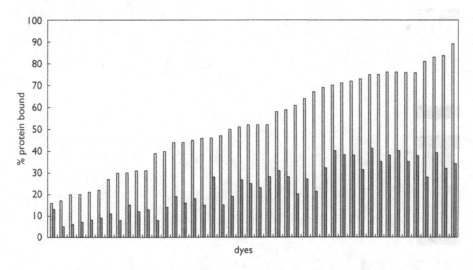

Figure 7.3 The binding of proteins from a crude bacterial extract to a range of 44 dyes. In light shading, the buffer used consisted of 20 mM K-Mes + 50 mM NaCl + 2 mM $MgCl_2$ + 5 mM $MnCl_2$, pH 6.5 ($I = 0.08$). In dark shading, the buffer consisted of 20 mM K-phosphate, pH 6.6 ($I = 0.03$). Despite the lower ionic strength, the amount of protein binding in phosphate buffer was less than half that binding in the buffer containing metal ions. Dyes are arranged in order of binding to the metal ion buffer.

The conclusions reached were that in some conditions, many of these dyes were not at all selective, binding a large proportion of the proteins present. If elution was not very resolving, then the degree of purification was going to be modest from these dyes. We grouped the dyes according to the range of binding that they came in, group 1 binding little, and group 5 the most (Scopes, 1993). However subsequent work has shown that these groupings are dependent not only on the nature of the dye, but also on the degree of substitution of the matrix, which varies very widely when using simple coupling reaction conditions.

Three procedures have enabled high degrees of purification even when using group 5 dye adsorbents. The first is affinity elution, in which introduction of the natural ligand to the buffer causes displacement of the enzyme/protein that interacts with that ligand (Scopes, 1977). Typically, dehydrogenases can be eluted with buffers containing NAD, NADH or NADP at quite low concentrations if the buffer conditions have been optimised. The second procedure is to optimise the degree of purification at the adsorption stage. This is done first by screening a substantial number of dyes so that the best can be selected, and second by using a tandem column procedure in which the first column adsorbs unwanted proteins (which otherwise would have adsorbed to the chosen dye) (Fig. 7.4) (Scopes, 1984). In this way, the dye adsorbent which binds the desired protein might bind 50% of the proteins in the sample, but may only bind 10% if 40% are removed on the first column – giving a 10-fold purification, rather than 2-fold, at the adsorption step. The tandem column (differential adsorption) procedure can of course be used with any combination of adsorbents, but with dyes it is particularly useful

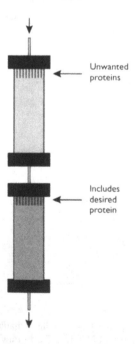

Figure 7.4 Principle of tandem column operation. The sample is passed through both columns and washed through with buffer. The desired protein is bound only on the second (positive) column, while most unwanted proteins are removed on the first (negative) column.

because of the similarity of the binding principles and the use of a common buffer for the whole process. The third procedure relies on displacement of weakly-bound proteins by more strongly-binding proteins, and the desired protein must be among the latter (O'Shannessy *et al.*, 1996). This technique is more suited to batch processing, as the displacement process can be relatively slow.

The nature of the dye–protein interaction

The dyes that have been most used for protein purification are complex molecules. As dyes, they have chromophores which include aromatic rings and conjugated double bonds responsible for their absorption of visible light. In order for them to be soluble in aqueous solvents, most have sulfonate groups attached, which are negatively charged at all pH. Additionally, many have nitrogen atoms capable of acting as electron donors and forming hydrogen bonds, as well as a variety of other substituents including hydroxyl, chloride and metal-ion complexing groups. Consequently there is a wide variety of possible interactions that can assist with protein binding. Chief amongst these are expected to be: (1) Electron donor–acceptor interactions between the conjugated electrons in the chromophore, and peptide bonds, carboxylate and amide side chains in the protein molecule. (2) The ion exchange character of the negatively-charged ligands cannot be ignored, and although the adsorbing proteins do not necessarily have a high isoelectric point, it helps. However, whereas with simple ion exchangers the binding reduces rapidly with increasing ionic strength, with dyes there is relatively little effect of ionic strength up to about 0.1 M. (3) Hydrogen bond formation: here are many opportunities for hydrogen bonds between atoms in the dyes and on the proteins. (4) Hydrophobic interactions. Some dyes have a greater hydrophobic character which can selectively attract the more hydrophobic proteins. This can result in difficulties in elution, especially if salt elution is attempted.

Elution of proteins from dyes is commonly carried out with salt, and/or an increase in pH, which suggests cation-exchange behaviour. But a typical dye–protein interaction will consist of several separate weak interactions which together add up to a binding energy sufficient to retain the protein on a column (>25 kJ/mol). Reduction of one or more of these by, for instance, addition of salt, may reduce the total binding energy to a value insufficient to keep the protein bound.

In many instances the main dye–protein interaction is located at the active site of an enzyme. This is commonly described as a biomimetic or pseudo-bioaffinity interaction, in which it is assumed that the dye mimics the structure of the substrate(s). However, it can equally be argued that the active site is a location on the protein which is particularly susceptible to binding complex molecules, which do not necessarily resemble the natural ligand structurally. Whichever is true, it means that the dye is occupying the substrate site as a competitive inhibitor, and the presence of substrate has the potential of displacing the dye. This is the basis of affinity elution, which enables selective displacement of the desired protein without eluting other unwanted material. It is this feature, more than any other, that has established dye ligand chromatography as a valuable selective affinity method, without having the high cost of conventional affinity adsorbents.

Purity, reproducibility and availability of dye adsorbents

The full use of dye–ligand chromatography has only been practised in a few laboratories that are engaged in many different protein purification projects. This is partly because of the difficulty of obtaining a suitable range of adsorbents of guaranteed consistency and reliability. In 1980 Amicon Corp. produced a small range of five dyes, which continue to be used in many laboratories. In 1990 Affinity Chromatography Ltd. produced a 10-dye kit (MIMETIC™) of superior quality, having negligible dye leakage, and consistent ligand density. Other "non-commercial" distributions of dye kits containing up to 40 different dyes have been made from time to time.

The problems with reproducibility arise mainly from several features of the raw material, the dyes themselves. These are manufactured on a very large scale; their availability and quality control is based on colour fashion and their suitability for dyeing cloth, not for purifying proteins. As a result the crude dyes may contain more than one reactive component, as well as impurities that do not end up on the adsorbent. If the reactive components have the same colour, then the relative proportions of these may vary from batch to batch. The original Cibacron Blue F-3GA contained two isomers of identical colour, and in some cases it may be that only one of these is active in binding a particular protein (Hanggi and Carr, 1985). And some dye colours go out of fashion and become unobtainable. Storage of dyes, especially the more reactive dichlorotriazinyl (Procion MX-) and Remazol series, can lead to loss of reactivity, resulting in reduced ligand density of the adsorbent. This final property, the ligand density, can be very variable depending on the method used for reaction with the matrix, and is not easily controllable. Consequently purification procedures described using dye ligand chromatography are not always immediately reproducible. In most cases it is a quantitative variation rather than qualitative: specificity remains, but loading and buffer conditions may need modification.

These problems can be addressed by specific manufacture of the dyes to guarantee purity, and by changing the method for coupling the dyes to the matrix. The MIMETIC™ adsorbents have been manufactured with these features in mind. We have recently switched to using dyes that are attached through an amino group introduced to the matrix under controlled conditions (Scoble and Scopes, 1996). Particular attention has been given to the nature of the covalent coupling to minimise leakage of dyes during the purification procedure. Partly because it is so obvious, leakage of dye has been a concern when using dye adsorbents, and is especially so when producing therapeutic proteins (Santambien et al., 1992).

Protocols for developing a dye ligand step in a protein purification procedure

Although the main thrust of protein purification is currently to use recombinant products, especially with built-in tags such as hexahistidine for affinity adsorption, there are still many processes in which a dye adsorption can be used as the major step in a purification, or as one of several in a more complex process. Because of their robustness, high capacity and relative cheapness, dye adsorbents can be used at the first step with a relatively crude tissue extract. One advantage of this is that there is usually no need to have any buffer change before starting; the clarified extract can be applied directly to the dye, or sometimes more conveniently, the dye adsorbent added to the extract in a batch-wise fashion. However, it is important to have high selectivity at this stage, to minimise the amount of adsorbent needed. In a few cases, a dye can be found that is highly selective for the desired protein, and the adsorption can be done in a displacement mode, preferably by batch adsorption (O'Shannessy *et al.*, 1996). In this mode, although many other proteins in the extract may bind to the dye, they are subsequently displaced by the more tightly-binding desired protein, until nearly all of the available binding sites are so occupied. This enables a relatively small amount of adsorbent to be used despite the large quantity of protein. To find the optimum adsorbent for such a process, it may be necessary to screen many dyes (and other materials), but there is no certainty that sufficient high selectivity will be found. The alternative is to use the "negative–positive" tandem system outlined above.

The first thing to be determined is whether the protein you are interested in has an affinity for dyes at all. A screening process using columns (Fig. 7.5) or batch-wise on a small scale with microfuge tubes (Fig. 7.6) will find the dye that the protein binds to most avidly. But if it does not bind at all, then the only useful dye step will be a negative one: passage of your sample through a dye column will remove some unwanted proteins. To maximise the chance of adsorbing, the pH should be reasonably low, e.g. 5.5–6.0, a few mM divalent metals ions should be present, preferably a transition metal such as Co, Ni, Zn or Mn, and the ionic strength should be no more than about 0.05. If your protein does bind to a lot of dyes in these conditions, then a decision needs to be made as to whether the buffer conditions should be relaxed, or whether to continue with the

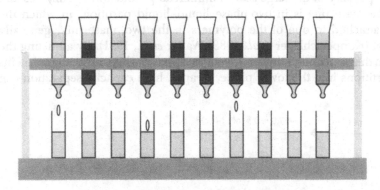

Figure 7.5 Screening of columns to find the optimum one for binding. Generally the minimum practical column size is 1 ml, to which 5–30 mg of protein should be applied.

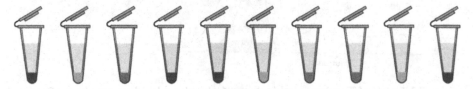

Figure 7.6 Screening of dye adsorbents batch-wise in microfuge tubes. About 20–30 mg of adsorbent is placed in the tubes, and a sample containing between 0.5 and 2 mg protein added.

conditions but look into tandem adsorbents or even displacement batch processes. The questions of loading and capacity may also influence your decision.

Having found satisfactory binding conditions, the protein now needs to be eluted. Elution should be as specific as possible, and preferably sharp and quick with high recovery. Change of buffer conditions may be sufficient, and this may be by removing metal ions, increasing salt (NaCl), increasing pH, introduction of phosphate ions, or a combination of all four. Gradients are sometimes useful, but stepwise elution generally achieves much the same degree of purification in a smaller elution volume. Affinity elution is much preferred, provided that the ligand to be used is not too expensive. However, for affinity elution to succeed, it is necessary to ensure that the protein is not too strongly bound, otherwise the introduction of ligand may not make sufficient difference to the binding strength. First, adjust the buffer to conditions where the protein is only just staying bound, then add the ligand. Many workers have used quite high concentrations of ligand (at great expense) because they have not attended to this point. A small ligand like ATP or NAD needs only to be used at a concentration of about 10 times its dissociation constant, and so values of less than 1 mM can be successful if the buffer conditions are right (Fig. 7.7).

Other affinity methods using dyes

Dyes have principally been used in column chromatographic processes. There are several other applications relying on the interactions between dyes and proteins that have found uses, especially in the large-scale commercial production of enzymes and other proteins. The main one is in two-phase liquid–liquid partition, in which the dye is covalently attached to one of the polymers in the two-phase mix, generally polyethylene glycol (Kopperschläger *et al.*, 1983; Walter *et al.*, 1991). By attracting the desired protein into the upper polyethylene glycol-rich phase, while most other proteins and cell debris partitions into the lower phase, a rapid, high capacity separation can

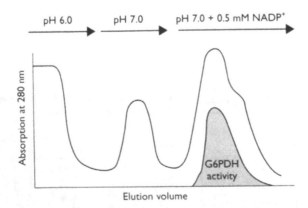

Figure 7.7 Elution of *Zymomonas mobilis* glucose 6-phosphate dehydrogenase from a Procion Yellow HE-3G column using $NADP^+$. Efficient elution at pH 7 (0.1 M phosphate) can be achieved with as little as 0.5 mM nucleotide, which is approximately 10 times its K_m value.

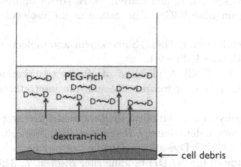

Figure 7.8 Principle of affinity phase partition. The dye molecules (D) are covalently attached to polyethylene glycol (PEG) molecules, which partition in the upper layer.

be achieved (Fig. 7.8). Although applicable to any affinity ligands, dyes have found the most use in affinity partition, their cheapness being a major attraction.

The other main application is closely related to the chromatographic process: the use of membranes for affinity adsorption. Membranes which are permeable to proteins are used, and the affinity ligands are covalently attached to the membrane material. These have an advantage over column systems in speed of processing, because of the minimal diffusion distances required of the proteins. Dyes are easy to attach to membrane material, and have been widely investigated (Gerstner *et al.*, 1992; Champluvier and Kula, 1992). Stacked membranes used in this way resemble squat columns, and have similar volumetric capacities. Alternatively, membranes have been used in a combination of filtration and adsorption, with unwanted proteins passing through, cellular debris excluded and washed away, and the desired protein remaining on the membrane. This technology has not yet developed far, because of the limited capacity of a single filter-membrane, and quick fouling of the membrane by cellular debris. Dyes have also been employed in affinity precipitation procedures (Pearson *et al.*, 1986), and as reactive affinity labels (Labrou *et al.*, 1996).

References

Champluvier, B. and Kula, M.-R. (1992) Sequential membrane-based purification of proteins applying the concept of multidimensional liquid chromatography (MDLC). *Bioseparation*, 2, 343–351.

Gerstner, J. A., Hamilton, R. and Cramer, S. M. (1992) Membrane chromatographic systems for high throughput protein separations. *J. Chromatogr.*, 596, 173–180.

Gianazza, E. and Arnaud, P. (1982) A general method for fractionation of plasma proteins. Dye-ligand affinity chromatography on immobilized Cibacron Blue F3-GA. *Biochem. J.*, 201, 129–136.

Haeckel, R., Hess, B., Lauterborn, W. and Wurster, K.-H. (1968) Purification and allosteric properties of yeast pyruvate kinase. *Hoppe-Seyler's Z. Physiol. Chem.*, 349, 699–714.

Hanggi, D. and Carr, P. (1985) Analytical evaluation of the purity of commercial preparations of Cibacron Blue F3G-A and related dyes. *Anal. Biochem.*, 149, 91–105.

Hughes, P. and Sherwood, R. F. (1987) Metal ion-promoted dye-ligand chromatography. In Y. D. Clonis, A. Atkinson, C. J. Bruton and C. R. Lowe (eds), *Reactive Dyes in Protein and Enzyme Technology*, Macmillan, London pp. 125–160.

Jankowski, W. J., von Muenchenhausen, W., Sulkowski, E. and Carter, W. A. (1976) Binding of human interferons to immobilized Cibacron Blue F3GA: The nature of the molecular interaction. *Biochemistry*, **15**, 5182–5187.

Kopperschläger, G., Freyer, R., Diezel, W. and Hofmann, E. (1968) Some kinetic and molecular properties of yeast phosphofructokinase. *FEBS Lett.*, **1**, 137–141.

Kopperschläger, G., Lorenz, G. and Usbeck, E. (1983) Application of affinity partitioning in an aqueous two-phase system to the investigation of triazine dye–enzyme interactions. *J. Chromatogr.*, **259**, 97–105.

Kovachevich, R. and Wood, W. A. (1955) Carbohydrate metabolism *by Pseudomonas fluorescens.* Purification and properties of a 6-phosphogluconate dehydrase. *J. Biol. Chem.*, **213**, 745–756.

Labrou, N. E., Eliopoulos, E. and Clonis, Y. D. (1996) Dye-affinity labelling of bovine heart mitochondrial malate dehydrogenase and study of the NADH-binding site. *Biochem. J.*, **315**, 687–693.

O'Shannessy, K., Scoble, J. and Scopes, R. K. (1996) A simple and economical procedure for purification of muscle lactate dehydrogenase by batch dye-ligand adsorption. *Bioseparation*, **6**, 77–80.

Pearson, J. C., Burton, S. J. and Lowe, C. R. (1986) Affinity precipitation of lactate dehydrogenase with a triazine dye derivative: selective precipitation of rabbit muscle lactate dehydrogenase with a Procion Blue H-B analog. *Anal. Biochem.*, **158**, 382–389.

Santambien, P. Hulak, I., Girot, P. and Boschetti, E., (1992) Elisa-based quantification of Cibacron Blue F3G-A used as ligand in affinity chromatography. *Bioseparation*, **2**, 327–334.

Scoble, J. and Scopes, R. K. (1996) Well defined adsorbents for protein purification. *J. Mol. Rec.*, (in press).

Scopes, R. K. (1977) Purification of glycolytic enzymes by affinity elution chromatography. *Biochem. J.*, **161**, 253–263.

Scopes, R. K. (1984) Use of differential dye-ligand chromatography with affinity elution for enzyme purification: 2-keto 3-deoxy 6-phosphogluconate aldolase from *Zymomonas mobilis*. *Anal. Biochem.*, **136**, 525–529.

Scopes, R. K. (1993) *Protein Purification, Principles and Practice*. 3rd edn. Springer, New York. p. 221.

Stead, C. V. (1987) The chemistry of reactive dyes. In: Y. D. Clonis, A. Atkinson, C. J. Bruton, and C. R. Lowe (eds), *Reactive dyes in protein and enzyme technology*, Macmillan, London, pp. 13–32.

Walter, H., Johansson, G. and Brooks, D. E. (1991) Partitioning in aqueous two-phase systems; recent results. *Anal. Biochem.*, **197**, 1–18.

Watson, D. H., Harvey, M. J. and Dean, P. D. G. (1978) The selective retardation of NADP + − dependent dehydrogenases by immobilized Procion Red HE-3B. *Biochem. J.*, **173**, 591–596.

Chapter 8

Immobilized synthetic dyes in affinity chromatography

Nikos E. Labrou and Yannis D. Clonis

Introduction

Affinity chromatography (Clonis, 1990, 2000; Labrou and Clonis, 1994; Garg *et al.*, 1996; Finette *et al.*, 1997; Keller *et al.*, 2001; Lowe, 2001) is the most powerful technique used in protein purification, especially in cases where the quality criteria imposed on the final product are stringent. In principle, affinity chromatography exploits natural bio-recognition phenomena for the formation of specific reversible complexes between a ligand, immobilized on an insoluble porous support packed in a column, and the complementary ligand-binding sites on the biomolecule to be isolated.

Some of the most widely used ligands in affinity chromatography have been several reactive chlorotriazine dyes (Clonis, 1990, 1991, 2000; Labrou and Clonis, 1994; Garg *et al.*, 1996, Clonis *et al.*, 2000). In particular, immobilized Cibacron Blue 3GA (CB3GA) or F-3GA is widely used in affinity chromatography (Labrou and Clonis, 1994; Garg *et al.* 1996; Clonis *et al.*, 2000), because of its broad spectrum of interaction with many proteins.

Structure and chemistry of triazine dyes

Triazine dyes can be considered to consist of two structurally distinct units joined together via an amino-bridge (Fig. 8.1A). One unit, the chromophore, contributes the colour and the other, the reactive unit, provides the site for covalent attachment to the insoluble support. The first and most successful reactive unit that was explored in dye chemistry was cyanuric chloride (1,3,5-*sym*-trichlorotriazine). The high reactivity of cyanuric chloride stems from the deficiency of electrons on the ring carbon atoms, and from the contribution of the polarization of the carbon–chlorine bond which arises from the greater electronegativity of the halogen atom (Fig. 8.1) (Stead, 1987). In general, dichlorotriazinyl dyes are prepared by condensation of amino-containing chromophores with an excess of cyanuric chloride in acetone for 0.5–1 h at pH 5–6 and 0–5°C (Fig. 8.1A). Monochlorotriazinyl-dyes are conveniently prepared by nucleophile substitution of the second chlorine of the triazinyl ring of dichlorotriazinyl dyes by an alkoxy, aryloxy, amino, or arylamino group at pH 6–8 and 25–40°C.

The chromophore must contain an amino group to which a reactive unit can be attached, and a number of sulphonic acid groups to provide aqueous solubility (Stead, 1987). The commercial dyes contain anthraquinone, azo, and/or phthalocyanine chromophores. Anthraquinone dyes give rise to bright blue and the phthalocyanines to bright turquoise shades. The mixed chromophores of the anthraquinone-stilbene, anthraquinone-azo or pthalocyanine-azo classes generate green shades. Ruby, violet, brown and black dyes are generally metal complexes of o,o'-dihydroxyazo or o-carboxy-o'-hydroxyazo dyes. The λ_{max} of these dyes covering the entire visible spectral range (350–750 nm) and their molar extinction coefficients, typically fall in the range of $4\,000$–$60\,000 \text{ mol}^{-1}\text{l cm}^{-1}$. The structures of six typical dyes are given in Fig. 8.2. Anthraquinone triazine dyes are probably the most widely used dye–ligands in enzyme and protein purification, and especially the triazine dye CB3GA has received by far

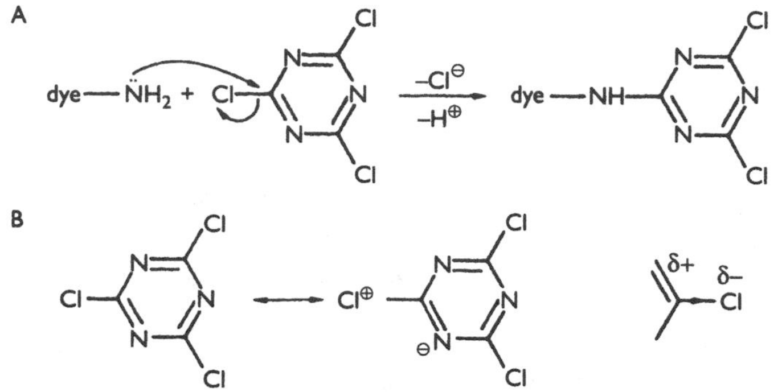

Figure 8.1 (A) Synthetic route to chlorotriazine dyes. (B) Electron phenomena of trichlorotriazine group (Stead, 1987).

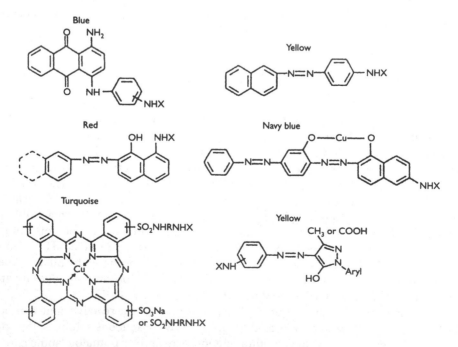

Figure 8.2 Partial structure of some triazine dyes (Stead, 1987).

most attention. Therefore, in the next pages of this review we will focus our attention primarily on this dye and its analogs.

Synthesis and purification of triazine dyes

The anthraquinone chromogen, the basic building block of most blue dyes, is synthesized from bromaminic acid (Burton *et al.*, 1988). In the presence of a copper catalyst, aromatic amines may substitute the halogen atom of bromaminic acid to produce the characteristic blue chromogen, Fig. 8.3. The blue colour of the chromogen is generated by the presence of 1,4-diamino groups on the anthraquinone ring which produces, a charge-transfer adsorption peak in the adsorption spectrum of the anthraquinone chromophore. The reaction with cyanuric chloride is straightforward at 0–5°C, as long as, acidic to neutral pH is maintained in order to protect the reactive chloride from solvolysis. The reaction of cyanuric chloride with the anthraquinone ring 1-amino group is sterically hindered by the adjacent carbonyl and sulphonyl groups, therefore the only feasible reaction is that with the 4-amino group of the anilino residue. The terminal ring of the dye is synthesized by nucleophilic substitution of the second chlorine atom of the dichlorotriazine by an aminobenzene sulphonic acid. The course of the reaction and the product yield may be followed by analytical TLC on silica gel or HPLC using the ion pair reagent N-cetyltrimethylammonium bromide (Burton *et al.*, 1988; Labrou and Clonis, 1995a).

Commercially available dyes are chromophoretically heterogeneous and usually contain a number of stabilizing agents (Burton *et al.*, 1988; Labrou and Clonis, 1995a). Application of these dye preparations in affinity chromatography, in most cases, is acceptable since most of the minor chromophoric impurities are not reactive, therefore, do not bind covalently to the support matrices. However, for analytic application,

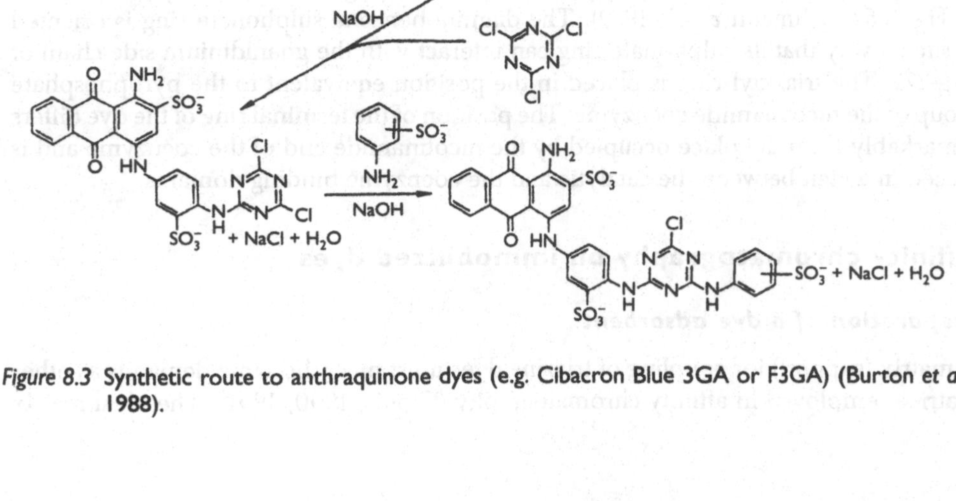

Figure 8.3 Synthetic route to anthraquinone dyes (e.g. Cibacron Blue 3GA or F3GA) (Burton *et al.*, 1988).

for example, when studying dye-protein interactions or for producing dyes of high specificity (i.e. biomimetic dyes), it is necessary that the dye be of the highest purity possible (Labrou and Clonis, 1995a; Bohacova *et al.*, 1998; Labrou *et al.*, 1999). Purification may be achieved by conventional column chromatography on silica gel, cellulose, alumina or Sephadex LH-20 which provides the high-quality dye preparation with high degree of purity (>98%) (Burton *et al.*, 1988; Labrou and Clonis, 1995a; Labrou *et al.*, 1999).

Interaction of triazine dyes with proteins

Why reactive dyes are able to interact, often specifically, with several enzymes and proteins? Considerable dedicated studies, employing, electrophoresis, enzyme inhibition, difference spectral titration, circular dichroism, NMR spectra, molecular modeling, and X-ray diffraction, have been conducted in order to elucidate the mode of interaction between a variety of dyes and of proteins. As a result of these studies it has been suggested that the presence of hydrophobic, hydrogen bonding and charge groups on the dye molecule, promote the interaction with the amino acid side chains of substrate, prosthetic group or coenzyme binding sites (Biellmann *et al.*, 1979; Small *et al.*, 1982; Labrou and Clonis, 1995a; Labrou *et al.*, 1996a,b; Bohacova *et al.*, 1998; Labrou *et al.*, 1999; Aaron *et al.*, 1999; Li *et al.*, 1995).

Enzyme inhibition and affinity labeling studies produced comprehensive evidence for the nature of dye-protein interaction. For example, the reactive dichlorotriazine analogue of CB3GA, Procion Blue MX-R, specifically inactivates horse liver alcohol dehydrogenase after covalent attachment to the thiol side-chain Cys-174 which lies at the bottom of the active site crevice in the nucleotide binding domain of the enzyme (Small *et al.*, 1982). Another example is the affinity labeling of bovine heart L-malate dehydrogenase with the reactive dichlorotriazine dye Vilmafix Blue A-R (Labrou *et al.*, 1996b). In this case, by combining chemical and molecular-modeling studies it became evident that the reactive dye reacts with the side chain of Lys-81 and or of Lys-217 which are located at the nucleotide binding site of the enzyme, Fig. 8.4.

X-ray diffraction studies have given more detailed and direct information on the dye-protein interaction. From studies on the crystal structure of the CB3GA-horse liver alcohol dehydrogenase complex (0.27 nm resolution), it was concluded that the anthraquinone ring binds in the apolar adenine binding site of the enzyme as shown in Fig. 8.5 (Biellmann *et al.*, 1979). The diaminobenzene sulphonate ring is oriented in such a way that its sulphonate ring can interact with the guanidinium side-chain of Arg-271. The triazinyl ring is placed in the position equivalent to the pyrophosphate group of the nicotinamide coenzyme. The position of the terminal ring of the dye differs remarkably from the place occupied by the nicotinamide end of the coenzyme and is placed in a cleft between the catalytic and the coenzyme binding domains.

Affinity chromatography on immobilized dyes

Preparation of a dye adsorbent

A matrix (support) for coupling of triazine dyes must meet the same demands as other matrices employed in affinity chromatography (Clonis, 1990, 1991). The ideal matrix

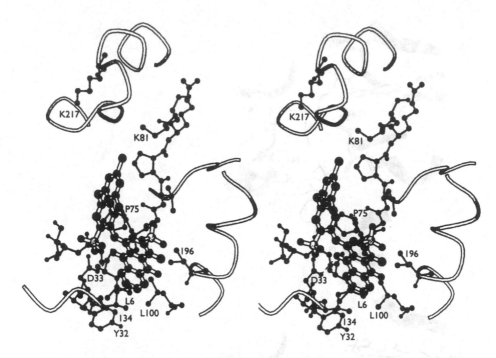

Figure 8.4 Stereodiagram of dichlorotriazinyl dye Vilmafix Blue A-R in the coenzyme-binding site of pig heart mitochondrial L-malate dehydrogenase (Labrou *et al.*, 1996b).

should be hydrophilic, chemically and biologically stable and have sufficient modifiable groups to permit an appropriate degree of substitution with dye (Boyer and Hsu, 1992). Various types of beaded supports have been used successfully in dye–ligand affinity chromatography, for example, natural polymers (e.g. agarose, dextran and cellulose), synthetic polymers (e.g. perfluorocarbons, polyacrylamide, polyacryloyl trihydroxymethylacrylamide), inorganics (e.g. silica, metal oxides, controlled pore glass) and microporous flat membrane. Of these, beaded cross-linked agarose is the best general-purpose matrix and its popularity is primarily due to its macroporocity, low non-specific interactions, and good chemical stability (Clonis, 1991).

Covalent attachment of a triazine dye onto a carbohydrate support is achieved under alkaline conditions with nucleophilic displacement of the dye's chlorine atom by the polymer hydroxyls (Labrou *et al.*, 1995a; Scoble and Scopes, 1996). A typical protocol is as follows: to washed agarose gel (1 g) a solution of purified dye in water (1 ml, 5–20 mg dye) is added and followed by NaCl solution (22% w/v, 0.2 ml). The suspension is tumbled for 30 min at room temperature prior to adding solid sodium carbonate (at a final concentration 1%). The reaction continues under shaking, at 60°C for monochlorotriazine dyes, and at room temperature for dichlorotriazine dyes. The time of immobilization reaction and the amount of dye in the reaction mixture depend on the reactivity of a particular dye molecule (Labrou *et al.*, 1995a). In general, 4–8 h incubation, yields substitution in the range of 2–4 μmol dye/g moist wet gel. The presence of electrolytes (e.g. NaCl) during the coupling procedure is used, in order to "salt out" the dye molecules onto the matrix (Clonis, 1990). When satisfactory adsorption of

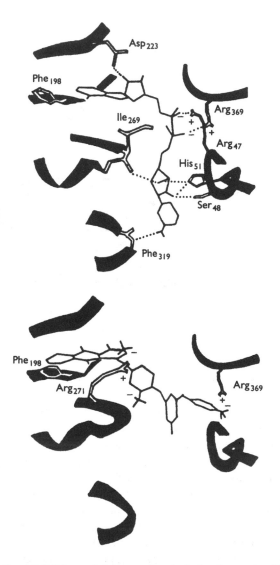

Figure 8.5 Schematic presentation depicting the mode of binding of coenzyme NAD⁺ (top) and Cibacron Blue 3GA (bottom) to the nucleotide binding site of horse liver alcohol dehydrogenase.

the dye has been achieved, the pH is raised to 10–11 by adding base (e.g. sodium carbonate) in order to activate the hydroxyl groups of the support to act as a nucleophile. Other alkali, such as NaOH (0.01–0.2 M) or LiOH (0.2% w/v), may be used instead of Na_2CO_3 in the above protocol. After immobilization of dichlorotriazine dyes the residual unreacted chlorines may be converted to hydroxyl groups by incubating the matrix at pH 8.5 for 2–3 days at room temperature, or to amino groups by incubating with 2 M NH_4Cl at pH 8.5 for 8 h at room temperature (Labrou *et al.*, 1995a). After immobilization of the reactive dye, the gel is washed with distilled water, 1 M KCl, 20%

DMSO, until the washings are colorless. Gels are stored as a suspension in 20% ethanol at 4°C.

Immobilized dye concentrations have been determined by spectrophotometric measurements of, (a) the gel, (b) the dye released after acid hydrolysis (HCl or acetic acid) of the gel, and (c) by the difference between added and unbound dye at the time the gel is made. The immobilized dye concentration is best determined by the acid hydrolysis method (Labrou et al., 1995a) as follows: the dye-substituted gel (30 mg) is suspended in HCl (5 M, 0.6 ml) and hydrolyzed at 70°C. The hydrolysate is neutralized by the addition of NaOH (10 M, 0.3 ml) and potassium phosphate buffer (1 M, pH 7.6, 2.1 ml), before its absorbance is read (at 620 nm) against an equal amount of hydrolyzed unsubstituted gel. The concentration of immobilized dye is calculated as micromoles of dye per gram moist gel.

Alternatively to the direct coupling of dyes to polyhydroxyl matrices is coupling of the dye to a support via a spacer molecule. This give the advantage to extend the immobilized dye away from the matrix microenvironment so that the interaction with a macromolecule will not be sterically hindered by the matrix. Chromatographic studies have shown that coupled dyes via alkyl spacers lead to increased selectivity over directly coupled dyes (Naumann et al., 1989). On a purely empirical basis a hexamethylene spacer arm would normally be inserted between the ligand and matrix backbone to reduce steric hindrance (Naumann et al., 1989). A hexyl spacer may be inserted by substitution of 1,6-diaminohexane at one of the chlorine atoms, of the triazinyl group, whence the dye-spacer conjugate may be immobilized to CNBr or 1,1-carbonyldiimidazole-activated agarose (Burton et al., 1988) (Fig. 8.6). Alternatively, anthraquinone dyes may be covalently attached through the anthraquinone 1-amino group by reacting with chloroacetyl chloride and ethylenediamine (Burton et al., 1990) (Fig. 8.6). Chromatographic studies have shown that, adsorbents having dyes immobilized via the anthraquinone rings were more effective in the isolation of horse liver alcohol dehydrogenase and other adenine nucleotide-requiring enzymes, compared to the adsorbents comprising triazine ring-immobilized dyes (Burton et al., 1990). Nevertheless, direct coupling of the reactive dyes onto polyhydroxylic matrices still remains the most favored methodology due to its simplicity and economy.

Dye screening: selection of dyes as ligands for affinity chromatography

The selection of a dye adsorbent for the isolation of a particular target macromolecule still remains an empirical undertaking (Scoble and Scopes, 1996). The suitability of a range of dye-adsorbents may be assessed by using small columns, each containing adsorbent to give a bed volume of 0.5–1 ml. The protein sample applied to a column must be of an equivalent ionic strength and pH to the column equilibration buffer. Total protein concentration of the applied sample may vary widely. Ideally 20–30 mg total protein/ml of adsorbent in a volume of 1–5 ml should be applied to each column. Nonadsorbed protein is washed with 5–10 ml of the equilibration buffer. Elution of bound protein may be achieved non-specifically with KCl (1 M), or specifically with substrate/cofactor or inhibitor (1–5 mM). Salt elution leads to practically total protein desorption. Specific elution of an enzyme leaves most unwanted proteins still bound. Eluted protein is collected as a single fraction. Both the void and the eluate fractions are

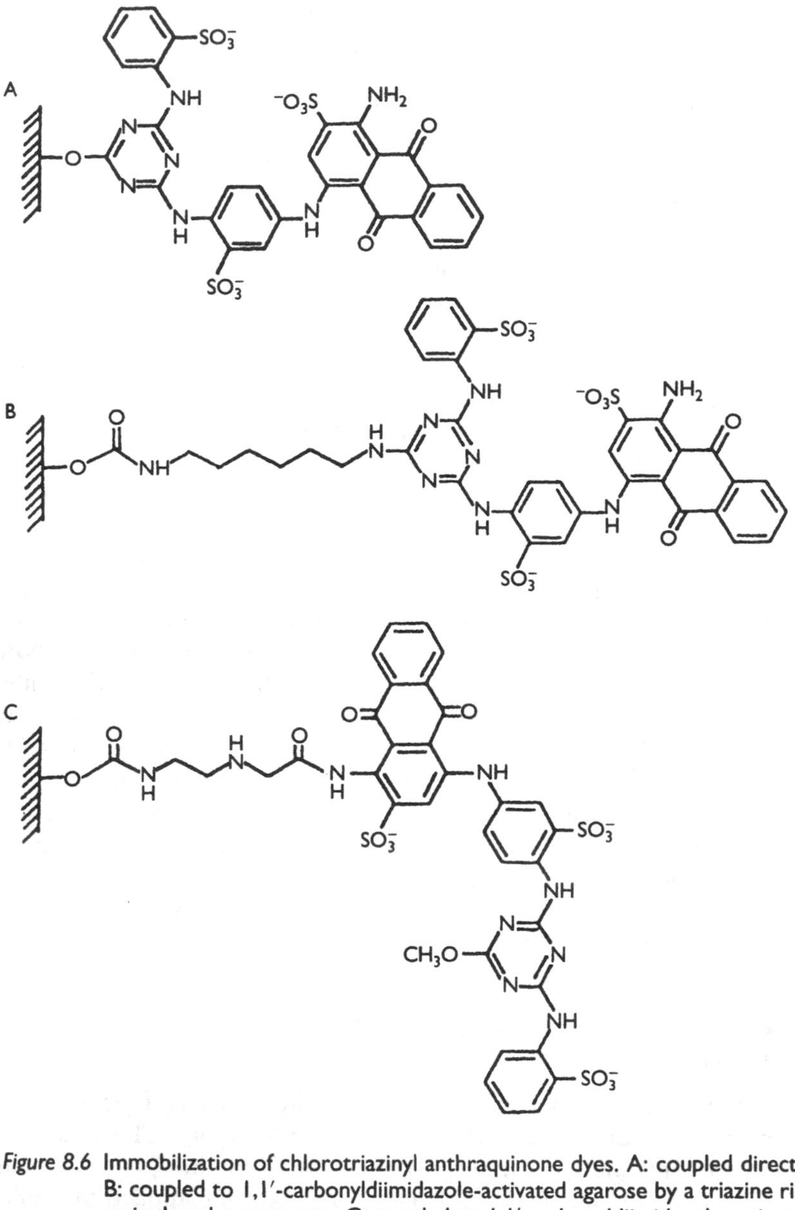

Figure 8.6 Immobilization of chlorotriazinyl anthraquinone dyes. A: coupled directly to agarose; B: coupled to 1,1'-carbonyldiimidazole-activated agarose by a triazine ring-coupled 6-aminohexyl spacer arm; C: coupled to 1,1'-carbonyldiimidazole-activated agarose by an anthraquinone 1-amino group.

assayed for protein and enzyme activity in order to determine the purification (fold), the binding capacity (mg protein/μmol immobilized dye), and the yield (%). The results from such screening generally reveal several dye-adsorbent as being worth of further study and chromatographic optimization (Scoble and Scopes, 1996; Labrou, 2000).

Alternatively, dye adsorbent screening may be accomplished by frontal analysis. In this method the column is continuously loaded with sample until the protein concentration of the eluate is equivalent to the applied onto the column. Using frontal analysis approach for screening, usually reveals information with regards to the relative affinities of different proteins in the mixture for the adsorbent (Labrou et al., 1995b). This approach for screening is successfully applied in the cases where the target protein is present at low concentration in a crude protein mixture.

Another procedure for screening dyes, called dye–ligand centrifugal affinity chromatography (Berg and Scouten, 1990), uses centrifugal force rather than gravity to pass solutions through a column. Using this technique a large number of dye-columns can be screened simultaneously and was shown to be both satisfactory and much faster compared with conventional gravity flow dye–ligand chromatography.

Characterization of dye–protein interactions in terms of kinetic inhibition constants or dissociation constants for immobilized or free dyes, sometimes is used as an alternative method for dye screening (Labrou et al., 1995; Bohacova et al., 1998). These methods, in addition, allow the evaluation of kinetic constants and isotherms of adsorption and the elucidation of the mode of dye–protein interaction.

The development and optimization of a protein purification, based on dye–ligand adsorbents

The development and optimization of a dye–ligand purification step can be accomplished by performing small scale trial purification experiments (using 0.5–1 ml adsorbent) prior to scaling of the procedure. Attention should be paid to the variables such as: the ligand concentration, pH, ionic strength, temperature, buffer composition, and sample size (Labrou and Clonis, 1996; Labrou et al., 1999). The pH, ionic strength, and temperature of equilibration buffer are important factors which influence the chromatographic behavior (e.g. adsorption and elution) of bound proteins, reflecting the mixed electrostatic-hydrophobic character of the dyes. Generally, low pH and low ionic strength, absence of phosphate ions, and the presence of divalent metal ions increase the binding (Scoble and Scopes, 1996). The influence of the first two factors stem from the degree of cation-exchange character of the dye, due to the presence of negative charged sulphonic groups (Sebastian et al., 2001). However, hydrophobic interactions with the dyes usually are increased at lower pH, but decreased at lower ionic strength. Molarities in the range of 5–50 mM and pH values of 5.5–8.5 of the equilibration buffer should be used in most cases. For stronger binding proteins, higher pH values and higher ionic strengths may be worth exploring in order to improve the selectivity of the dye (Scoble and Scopes, 1996).

In general, most of the buffers may be used in dye–ligand chromatography, but low conductivity buffers (e.g. MOPS, MES, HEPES) are often used, especially in those cases, where an increase in protein binding is advisable (Worall, 1996). Phosphate salts usually reduce the binding and in particular favor reduction of non-specific protein dye interactions. Metal ions (e.g. Mg^{+2}, Ca^{+2}, Zn^{+2}, Mn^{+2}, Cu^{+2}, Co^{+2}, Fe^{+3} and Al^{+3}) may be added at concentrations in the range of 0.1–10 mM to promote protein binding. It has been suggested that metal ions act as bridges and help the formation of a specific ternary complex that would not otherwise occur (Hughes et al., 1982).

The buffer system must be properly selected when multivalent metal ions are added, otherwise precipitation problems may arise (e.g. calcium phosphate formation).

The binding strength for a protein of a dye adsorbent is usually enhanced by increasing immobilized dye concentration. However, it is worth mentioning that at high dye concentration the adsorbent looses its selectivity and binding capacity, owing to steric effects caused by the dye molecules or may act as a nonspecific strong ion-exchanger (Finette *et al.*, 1997). Therefore, the dye concentration must be carefully controlled. In general, immobilized dye concentration of about 2–5 μmol/g moist gel is commonly employed.

Temperature is yet another factor that frequently influences the behavior of proteins in dye–ligand chromatography. The effect of temperature is variable: it may enhance or weaken protein binding depending on the contribution of hydrophobic or electrostatic forces on protein–dye complex. Temperatures within the range of 0–50°C have been exploited (Worall, 1996).

Special consideration should be given to the sample size since it frequently influences the purification potential and the capacity of the adsorbent. Increasing the amount of a sample of complex protein mixture applied to the column, usually is expected to weaken the binding, due to the competing phenomena arising between different macromolecules. Therefore, it may diminish the extent of purification of a target protein. However, if the dye–target protein interaction is strong and specific, then one may increase the amount of applied sample without affecting the extent of purification and the binding capacity of the adsorbent. Sample size can be readily determined by frontal analysis, where the sample solution is pumped continuously onto the column until the desired protein is detectable in the eluate (Clonis *et al.*, 1987).

The elution conditions of the bound macromolecule, should be both, well tolerated by the dye–ligand affinity adsorbent and effective in desorbing the biomolecule in good yield and in the native state. Elution of bound proteins is performed in a non-specific and biospecific manner. Non-specific elution usually involves: (1) changing the ionic strength (usually by increasing the buffer's molarity or including salt, e.g. KCl or NaCl) and the pH (adsorption generally weakens with increasing pH) altering the polarity of the irrigating buffer by employing, for example, ethylene glycol or other organic solvents, if the hydrophobic contribution in protein–dye complex is large. Non-specific elution methods, although economical, generally give lower degrees of purification due to the coelution of non-specifically bound proteins. For group-specific affinity adsorbents, as for dye–ligand adsorbents, biospecific elution methods are recommended (Clonis, 1988, 1990, 1991; Labrou and Clonis, 1994; Garg *et al.*, 1996; Labrou, 2000). Biospecific elution is achieved by inclusion in the equilibration buffer of a suitable ligand which competes with the immobilized ligand for the same binding-site on the enzyme/protein. Any competing ligand may be used. For example, substrates, products, cofactors, inhibitors or allosteric effector are all potential candidates as long as they have higher affinity for the macromolecule than the dye. Furthermore, in more than a few cases it has been observed that a suitable combination of substrates and coenzymes is better than an individual component. Desorption of proteins whose binding is enhanced by metal ions is often facilitated by the addition of chelating agents (e.g. EDTA) (Hughes *et al.*, 1982).

The high stability of dye–ligand gels allows their multiple use several times without affecting their purification potential. However, repeated use of the columns, especially with crude protein extracts can result in the accumulation of various contaminants (denatured proteins, lipids, lipoproteins). This may diminish the column's performance, i.e. the flow rate, purification, binding capacity. Regeneration of dye–ligand adsorbents is accomplished conveniently with NaOH (1 M), and chaotropes: urea (6 M), guanidine hydrochloride (6–8 M) or sodium thiocyanate (1–3 M) (Labrou, 2000).

Large-scale dye–ligand affinity chromatography

Triazine dyes are the most promising pseudoaffinity ligands for large-scale applications, due to the numerous advantages they offer (Clonis, 1991). For example, they are comparatively inexpensive and available in large quantities, easily immobilized directly to chromatographic support via a stable bond, and completely resistant to chemical and biological degradation. Their ability to withstand caustic alkali is very important, especially in industrial applications since sodium hydroxide provides an economic means for cleaning, sterilizing and removing pyrogens from chromatography columns. Furthermore, dye–ligand adsorbents have high binding capacities for many proteins that can be eluted under mild conditions with good yields. The advantages offered by dye–ligands stimulated workers to employ affinity chromatography with dyes on a large scale. As an example of successful large-scale application one can mention the purification of human serum albumin on Blue-Trisacryl column, an affinity derivative obtained by coupling Reactive blue 2 to macroporous Trisacryl GF 2000. A 50 l column was used for over 500 cycles, maintaining a productivity of more than 2400 g albumin per liter (Allary et al., 1991). A detailed description of large-scale applications of dye–ligands in downstream processing has been presented elsewhere (Clonis, 1990, 1991).

Purpose-designed dye–ligands: the generation of biomimetic dye–ligands

As mentioned earlier, triazine-dyes offer clear advantages over biological ligands. However, the main drawback of these compounds appears to be their lack of selectivity. Fortunately, considerable experimental work has improved our understanding on dye–protein interactions and enabled the design and synthesis of novel synthetic dye–ligands with improved selectivity, the so-called biomimetic dye–ligands. According to the biomimetic dye concept, the presence of a purpose-designed structural alteration on the parent dye can lead to a new dye which closely resembles the structure and function of biological ligands, or mimic their interaction with the binding sites of proteins. Such biomimetic dyes display increased specificity for target enzymes and herald a new trend in this area of biotechnology. In fact, biomimetic dyes have signaled the beginning of a new era in affinity separation (Clonis et al., 1987; Lindner et al., 1989; Labrou and Clonis, 1994, 1995a; Labrou et al., 1995, 1996a, 1999; Clonis et al., 2000).

As can be seen in Fig. 8.7 the structure of CB3GA may be divided into four structural components: the sulfonated anthraquinone group I, the bridging sulfonated benzene ring II, the triazine ring III, and the terminal sulfonated benzene ring IV. Kinetic and affinity chromatography experiments with various NAD(H) and ATP-dependent enzymes established that only the I and II ring portions of the CB3GA molecule are required for inhibition of, and binding to, enzymes (Bohacova et al., 1998). Ring I alone was a relatively poor inhibitor, whilst an analogue comprising rings I and II

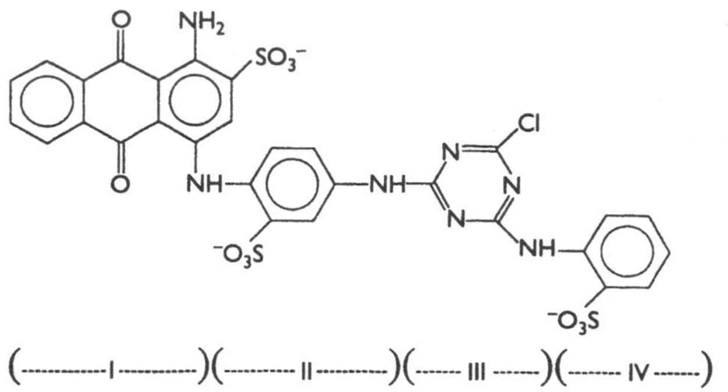

Figure 8.7 The principal structural elements of the anthraquinone dye Cibacron Blue 3GA. (I): Sulphonated anthraquinone moiety, (II): bridging diaminobenzene sulphonate ring, (III): reactive chlorotriazine group, (IV): terminal o-aminobenzene soulphonate ring.

was only marginally less inhibitory than the complete parent dye itself. Furthermore, the binding of CB3GA to horse liver alcohol dehydrogenase (as investigated by X-ray crystallography) resembles ADP binding but differs at the nicotinamide end of the coenzyme, with the aminobenzenesulphonic ring IV of the bound dye to be away by about 10 Å to that normally occupied by NAD^+ (Biellmann *et al.*, 1979), Fig. 8.5. Thus, based on the kinetic, affinity chromatography and X-ray crystallography studies, it was evident that structural modifications of the terminal ring IV of CB3GA would generate remarkable variations in the affinity toward proteins.

The first example of a design, synthesis and application of a biomimetic dye was the terminal ring modification of the parent dye CB3GA, and the study of interaction of these analogues with horse liver alcohol dehydrogenase (Lowe *et al.*, 1986). Studies by difference spectroscopy showed that analogues with terminal carboxylated structures (e.g. *m*-aminobenzoic acid) displayed higher affinities for horse liver enzyme than dyes with more bulky sulfonate substituents. Dyes with para-orientated anionic groups displayed reduced affinity compared to dyes with ortho- or meta-orientated equivalent anionic groups. Furthermore, dye analogue with cationic substituents on the terminal ring were bound with a reduced affinity. Unfortunately, the difference in the affinity between the analogues toward liver alcohol dehydrogenase in solution was not translated in corresponding chromatographic behavior of the enzyme when the dyes were immobilised to beaded agarose. Molecular modeling studies have shown that the parent dye CB3GA is too short and rigid to adopt the same conformation as the natural coenzyme. To cope with this problem a new analogue with a central ethyl-spacer between the bridging diaminobenzene sulphonate ring and the reactive triazine ring (Fig. 8.8b) was synthesized in order to increase the length and flexibility of the dye. This analogue, although it does not structurally mimic the native substrate of ADH, was effective in resolving the commercial sample of horse liver alcohol dehydrogenase into two active components, whereas CB3GA under identical conditions was unable to do so (Lowe *et al.*, 1986).

In the case of the biomimetic dye for alkaline phosphatase (Lindner *et al.*, 1989), this new dye is designed by substituting the terminal ring of CB3GA with 4-aminobenzene phosphonate ring, a known inhibitor of alkaline phosphatase (Fig. 8.8c). When this

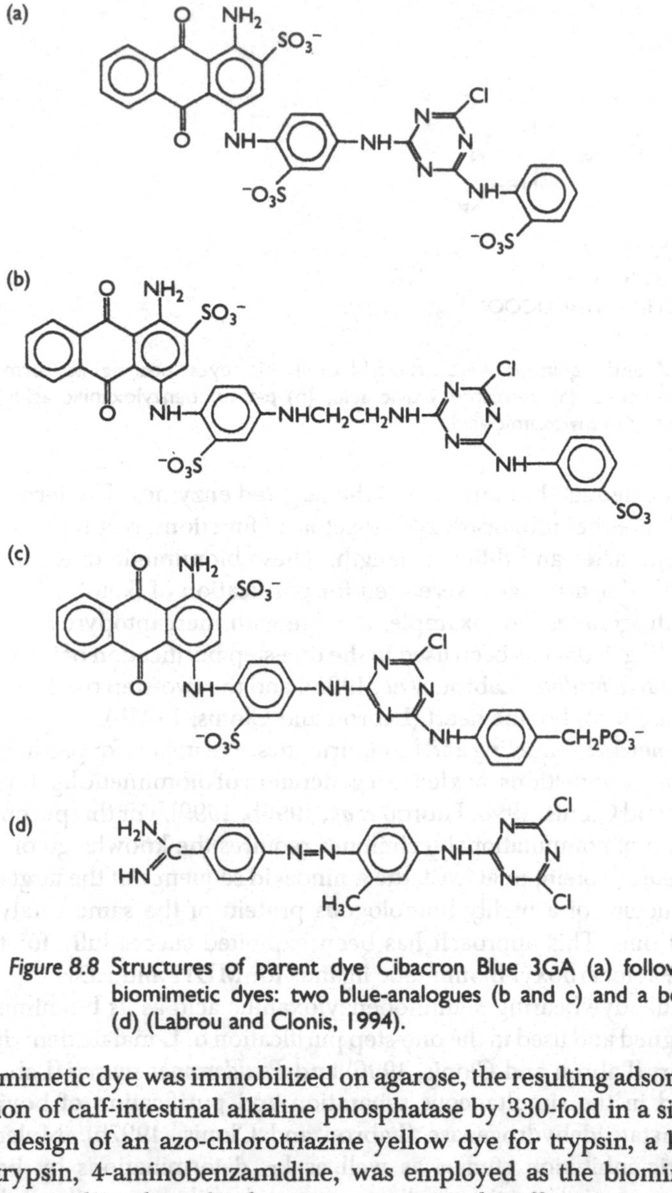

Figure 8.8 Structures of parent dye Cibacron Blue 3GA (a) followed in sequence by three biomimetic dyes: two blue-analogues (b and c) and a benzamidino-cationic yellow (d) (Labrou and Clonis, 1994).

biomimetic dye was immobilized on agarose, the resulting adsorbent enabled the purification of calf-intestinal alkaline phosphatase by 330-fold in a single step. Likewise, for the design of an azo-chlorotriazine yellow dye for trypsin, a known potent inhibitor of trypsin, 4-aminobenzamidine, was employed as the biomimetic component. The corresponding dye adsorbent was proven to be effective in separation of trypsin and chymotrypsin, and purifying of trypsin in a single step (Clonis et al., 1987).

More recently a new family of biomimetic dyes, the anthraquinone ketocarboxyl-biomimetic dyes, has been introduced (Labrou and Clonis, 1995a; Labrou et al., 1995, 1996a, 1999; Labrou 2000). In this case, purpose-modifications of the terminal ring of CB3GA yielded new members of the family of "blue" dyes. These dyes are composed of two enzyme-recognition moieties, joined together via the chlorotriazine group: the variable terminal moiety bearing a (keto)carboxylated structure (Fig. 8.9a), that mimicks natural organic acid substrates, and the chromogen anthraquinone moiety that is used as

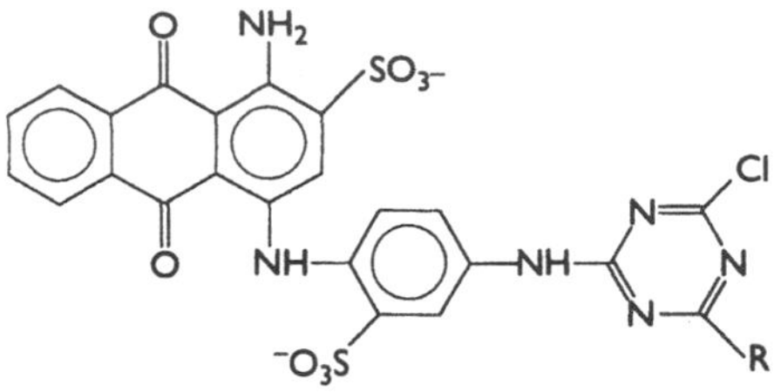

Where R: (a) –SCH$_2$COCOO$^-$
           (b) –NHC$_6$H$_4$COCOO$^-$
           (c) –NHC$_6$H$_4$CH$_2$CH$_2$NHCOCOO$^-$

Figure 8.9 Structures of anthraquinone ketocarboxyl-biomimetic dyes bearing as terminal biomimetic moieties: (a) mercaptopyruvic acid; (b) *p*-aminobenzyloxanilic acid; (c) 2-(4-aminophenyl)-ethyloxamic acid.

pseudoanalogue for the nucleotide-binding area of the targeted enzymes. The terminal biomimetic moiety exhibits either monocarboxyl or ketoacid functions, combined with aromatic and aliphatic character and different length. These biomimetic dyes, when immobilized on cross-linked agarose gel, were used for purification of (keto)carboxyl-group-recognizing dehydrogenases. For example, the dye with mercaptopyruvic acid as its biomimetic moiety (Fig. 8.9a) has been used in the one-step purification of formate dehydrogenase from *Candida boidinii* (Labrou *et al.*, 1995), and the two-step purification of L-lactate dehydrogenase from bovine heart (Labrou and Clonis, 1995b).

The introduction of molecular modeling and bioinformatics, as a means for predicting and studying protein-ligand interactions, has led to a generation of biomimetic ligands of superior affinity (Labrou and Clonis, 1996; Labrou *et al.*, 1996b, 1999). For this purpose, the successful exploitation of computational techniques requires the knowledge of the 3-D structure of the targeted protein, or at least, the aminoacid sequence of the targeted protein and the 3-D structure of a highly homologous protein of the same catalytic function as the targeted one. This approach has been exploited successfully for the design of anthraquinone ketocarboxyl-biomimetic ligands for MDH and LDH.

An anthraquinone 'blue' dye bearing *p*-aminobenzyloxanilic acid as its biomimetic moiety (Fig. 8.9b) is designed and used in the one-step purification of L-malate dehydrogenase from bovine heart (Labrou and Clonis, 1996) and *Pseudomonas stutzeri* (Labrou and Clonis, 1997a), and in the simultaneous separation and purification of bovine heart L-malate and L-lactate dehydrogenase (Labrou and Clonis, 1997b). Molecular modeling and kinetic inhibition studies as well as k_D determinations by both difference-spectra and enzyme-inactivation studies, were employed to assess the ability of the (keto)carboxyl-biomimetic dyes to act as affinity ligands for L-malate dehydrogenase. In general, biomimetic dyes interacted specifically with MDH, exhibiting higher affinity (10-fold) over non-biomimetic dyes (e.g. CB3GA) (Labrou *et al.*, 1996a). Furthermore, molecular modeling studies (Fig. 8.10) were employed to reveal the possible nature of interaction between L-malate dehydrogenase and the dye bearing *p*-aminobenzyloxanilic acid as its biomimetic moiety (Fig. 8.9b) (Labrou *et al.*, 1996a). These computational studies have shown that the anthraquinone moiety was placed in the position of the pyrimidine of NAD$^+$ in a hydrophobic crevice formed by the

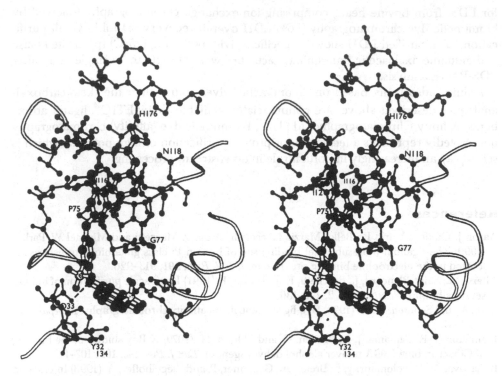

Figure 8.10 Stereodiagram of p-aminobenzyloxanyl-biomimetic blue dye in the coenzyme-binding site of pig heart mitochondrial L-malic dehydrogenase (Labrou et al., 1996a).

enzyme's 6–10, 33–36, 76–79, and 94–104 chain regions. The triazine ring binds in the region where the coenzyme pyrophosphate binds. The benzene ring (of the biomimetic moiety) is placed in the space occupied by the second ribose ring (linked to the nicotinamide) in the hydrophobic cavity formed by Ile-12, Ile-116, Asn-118, Pro-75 and fragment of the main chain of the enzyme. The ketocarboxyl moiety superimposes readily on the amide group of the nicotinamide moiety, that interacts with His-176 of the active site.

The latest addition to the family of ketocarboxyl-biomimetic dyes is a new anthraquinone bifunctional dye which was designed by means of molecular modeling specifically for L-lacatate dehydrogenase (Labrou et al., 1999). This dye features 2-(4-aminophenyl)-ethyloxamic acid as its biomimetic moiety (Fig. 8.9c). The positioning of the dye in the enzyme binding site is primarily achieved by the recognition and positioning of the pseudomimetic anthraquinone moiety. The positioning of the biomimetic ketocarboxylic moiety is based on a match between the polar and hydrophobic regions of the enzyme binding site with those of the biomimetic moiety of the ligand. The length of the biomimetic moiety is predetermined for the ketoacid to approach the enzyme catalytic site and form charge–charge interactions. When this new ligand was immobilised on agarose, the derived affinity adsorbent shown an approximately 200% higher purifying ability for LDH from bovine heart, bovine pancreas, porcine muscle, chicken liver, chicken muscle, and pea seeds, compared to the "control" CB3GA adsorbent. Based on the new biomimetic adsorbent, a facile purification procedure was designed for LDH from bovine heart, comprising ion-exchange chromatography followed by biomimetic dye chromatography (56% LDH overall recovery, 44-fold overall purification). The purified LDH shows a specific activity 600 u/mg (25°C) (pyruvate kinase and glutamic-oxaloacetic transaminase activities were absent) and a single band after SDS-PAGE analysis.

Affinity adsorbents based on "biomimetic" dyes, other than the (keto)carboxyl-analogues described above, are commercially available (MIMETIC® ligand adsorbents, Affinity Chromatography Ltd., UK). Biomimetic dye (affinity) chromatography undoubtedly represents a technique for protein purification of high potential which is set to play an increasingly important role in downstream processing.

References

Aaron J. Oakley, Mario Lo Bello, Marzia Nuccetelli, Anna P. Mazzetti and Michael W. Parker (1999) The ligandin (non-substrate) binding site of human Pi class glutathione transferase is located in the electrophile binding site (H-site). *J. Mol. Biol.*, **291**, 913–926.

Allary, M., Saint-Blancard, J., Boschetti, E. and Girot, P. (1991) Large scale purification of human serum albumin. *Bioseparation*, **2**, 121–130.

Berg, A. and Scouten, W. H. (1990) Dye-ligand centrifugal affinity chromatography. *Bioseparation*, **1**, 23–31.

Biellmann, J.-F., Samama, J.-P., Braden, C. and Eklund, H. (1979) X-Ray studies of the binding of Cibacron blue F3GA to liver alcohol dehydrogenase. *Eur. J. Biochem.*, **102**, 107–110.

Bohacova, A., Docolomansky, P., Breier, A., Gemeiner, P. and Ziegelhoffer, A. (1998) Interaction of lactate dehydrogenase with anthraquinone dyes: characterization of ligands for dye-ligand chromatography. *J. Chromatogr. B. Biomed. Sci. Appl.*, **715**, 273–281.

Burton, S. J., Stead, C. V. and Lowe C. R. (1988) Design and application of biomimetic dyes II: The interaction of C.I. Reactive Blue 2 analogues bearing terminal ring modifications with horse liver alcohol dehydrogenase. *J. Chromatogr.*, **455**, 201–206.

Boyer, P. M. and Hsu, J. T. (1992) Effects of ligand concentration on protein adsorption in dye-ligand adsorbents. *Chem. Eng. Sci.*, **47**, 241–251.

Clonis, Y. D. (1990) Process-scale affinity chromatography. In: J. Asenjo (ed.), *Separation Processes in Biotechnology*, Mercel-Dekker, New York, pp. 401–445.

Clonis, Y. D. (1991) Preparative dye-ligand chromatography. In: M. Hearn (ed.), *HPLC of Proteins, Peptides, and Polynucleotides*, VCH, New York, pp. 453–468.

Clonis, Y. D. (2000) Affinity separation: dye-ligands. In: I. Wilson (ed.), *Encyclopaedia of Separation Science*, Academic Press Ltd., London, pp. 259–265.

Clonis, Y. D., Stead, C. V. and Lowe, C. R. (1987) Novel cationic triazine dyes for protein purification. *Biotechnol. Bioeng.*, **30**, 621–627.

Finette G. M., Mao, Q. M. and Hearn, M. T. (1997) Comparative studies on the isothermal characteristics of proteins adsorbed under batch equilibrium conditions to ion-exchange, immobilised metal ion affinity and dye affinity matrices with different ionic strength and temperature conditions. *J. Chromatogr.*, **763**, 71–90.

Garg, N., Galaev, I. and Mattiasson, B. (1996) Dye-affinity techniques for bioprocessing: recent developments. *J. Mol. Recognit.*, **9**, 259–274.

Hughes, P., Sherwood, R. and Lowe, C. R. (1982) Metal ion-promoted binding of proteins to immobilized triazine dye affinity adsorbents. *Biochim. Biophys. Acta.*, **700**, 90–100.

Keller, K., Friedman, T. and Boxman, A. (2001) The bioseparation needs for tomorrow. *Trends Biotechnol.*, **19**, 438–441.

Labrou, N. E. (2000) Dye-ligand affinity chromatography for protein separation and purification. *Methods Mol. Biol.*, **147**, 129–139.

Labrou, N. E. and Clonis, Y. D. (1994) The affinity technology in downstream processing. *J. Biotechnol.*, **36**, 95–119.

Labrou, N. E. and Clonis, Y. D. (1995a) The interaction of *Candida boidinii* formate dehydrogenase with a new family of chimeric biomimetic dye-ligands. *Arch. Biochem. Biophys.*, **316**, 169–178.

Labrou, N. E. and Clonis, Y. D. (1995b) Biomimetic-dye affinity chromatography for the purification of bovine heart lactate dehydrogenase. *J. Chromatogr.*, **718**, 35–44.

Labrou, N. E. and Clonis, Y. D. (1996) Biomimetic-dye affinity chromatography for the purification of L-malate dehydrogenase from bovine heart. *J. Biotechnol.*, **45**, 185–194.

Labrou, N. E. and Clonis, Y. D. (1997a) L-malate dehydrogenase from *Pseudomonas stutzeri*: Purification and characterization. *Arch. Biochem. Biophys.*, **337**, 103–114.

Labrou, N. E. and Clonis, Y. D. (1997b) Simultaneous purification of L-malate dehydrogenase and L-lactate dehydogenase from bovine heart by biomimetic-dye affinity chromatography. *Bioprocess Eng.*, **593**, 157–161.

Labrou, N. E., Eliopoulos, E. and Clonis, Y. D. (1996a) Molecular modelling for the design of chimaeric biomimetic dye-ligands and their interaction with bovine heart mitochondrial malate dehydrogenase. *Biochem. J.*, **315**, 695–703.

Labrou, N. E., Eliopoulos, E. and Clonis, Y. D. (1996b) Dye-affinity labelling of bovine heart malate dehydrogenase and study of the NADH-binding site. *Biochem. J.*, **315**, 687–693.

Labrou, N. E., Eliopoulos, E. and Clonis, Y. D. (1999) Molecular modeling for the design of a biomimetic chimeric ligand. Application to the purification of bovine heart L-lactate dehydrogenase. *Biotechnol. Bioeng.*, **63**, 322–332.

Labrou, N. E., Karagouni, A. and Clonis, Y. D. (1995) Biomimetic-dye affinity adsorbents for enzyme purification: Application to the one-step purification of *Candida boidinii* formate dehydrogenase. *Biotechnol. Bioeng.*, **48**, 278–288.

Li, R., Bianchet, M. A., Talalay, P., Amzel, L. M. (1995) The three-dimensional structure of NAD(P)H: quinone reductase, a flavoprotein involved in cancer chemoprotection and chemotherapy: mechanism of the two-electron reduction. *Proc. Natl. Acad. Sci. USA*, **92**, 8846–8851.

Lindner, N. M., Jeffcoat, R. and Lowe, C. R. (1989) Design and application of biomimetic dyes: Purification of calf intestinal alkaline phosphatase with immobilized terminal ring analogues of C.I. Reactive Blue 2. *J. Chromatogr.*, **473**, 227–240.

Lowe, C. R. (2001) Combinatorial approaches to affinity chromatography. *Curr. Opin. Chem. Biol.*, **5**, 248–256.

Lowe, C. R., Burton, S. J., Pearson, J., Clonis, Y. D. and Stead, C. V. (1986) Design and application of biomimetic dyes in biotechnology. *J. Chromatogr.*, **376**, 121–130.

Naumann, M., Reuter, R., Metz, P. and Kopperschlager, G. (1989) Affinity chromatography of bovine heart lactate dehydrogenase using dye ligands linked directly or spacer-mediated to bead cellulose. *J. Chromatogr.*, **466**, 319–329.

Raya-Tonetti, G. and Perotti, N. (1999) Rapid screening of textile dyes employed as affinity ligands to purify enzymes from yeast. *Biotechnol. Appl. Biochem.*, **29**, 151–156.

Scoble, J. and Scopes, R. (1996) Well defined dye adsorbents for protein purification. *J. Mol. Recognit.*, **9**, 728–732.

Sebastian, D. Friess and Renato Zenobi (2001) Protein structure information from mass spectrometry? Selective titration of arginine residues by sulfonates. *J. Amer. Soc. Mass Spectr.*, **12**, 810–818.

Small, D. A., Lowe, C. R., Atkinson, T. and Bruton, C. J. (1982) Affinity labelling of enzymes with triazine dyes. Isolation of a peptide in the catalytic domain of horse liver alcohol dehydrogenase using Procion Blue MX-R as a structural probe. *Eur. J. Biochem.*, **128**, 119–123.

Stead, V. (1987) The chemistry of reactive dyes. In: Clonis, Y. D., Atkinson, T., Bruton, C. and Lowe, C. R. (eds), *Reactive dyes in protein and enzyme technology*, Macmillan Press, Basingstoke, U.K., pp. 13–32.

Worrall, D. M., (1996) Dye-ligand affinity chromatography. *Methods Mol. Biol.*, **59**, 169–176.

Chapter 9

Immobilized histidine ligand affinity chromatography

Olivier Pitiot and Mookambeswaran A. Vijayalakshmi

Introduction

Affinity chromatography is based on adsorption mechanisms which exploit the recognition between an immobilized ligand and a molecule to be separated. The selective retention of molecules displaying specific recognition allows at the removal of all the others during the adsorption phase of chromatography. Moreover, fine tuning of the elution will result in separation of the differentially retained molecules.

The majority of affinity chromatography ligands is of biological origin. In fact, their use as immobilized ligands is based on the knowledge of molecular interactions in living systems (Hormones/Receptors, Antigens/Antibodies, Enzymes/Inhibitors, Lectins/Sugars . . .). However, many of these biological ligands are macromolecular and fragile. They are frequently difficult to immobilize on a support and often expensive. These factors should be considered in a large scale operation.

Biological molecules of interest display often affinities for simpler chemical ligands. The term "pseudobiospecific affinity ligands", introduced by Vijayalakshmi (1989), encompasses these simpler biological or non-biological ligands, such as amino acids, hydrocarbons, metal ions chelates and triazine dyes. They represent promising alternatives, because of their resistance to harsh chemicals and high temperatures (sterilization conditions) and their low cost.

Pseudobiospecific ligands interact with soluble molecules via the same forces as biological ligands (but may differ in their relative magnitude), based on complementarity of charges, hydrophobicity, shape . . ., and they are sometimes very fittingly called "biomimetic ligands".

Pseudobiospecific ligands display, in general, weaker affinity and broader specificity compared to biospecific ligands. However, these drawbacks can be readily overcome: the specificity could be increased by fine tuning of the adsorption and elution conditions to attain resolutions and degrees of purification comparable, or at times superior, to biological ligands such as antibodies. The weak affinity is often advantageous, as it allows gentler elution conditions and, therefore, ensures the structural integrity of the purified molecules, without any denaturation usually caused by low pH elution conditions (Buchner *et al.*, 1991).

The hitherto well established pseudobiospecific ligands – namely amino acids, metal chelates and dyes – recognize protein molecules through somewhat similar mechanisms. These immobilized ligands all act as electron acceptors of NH, SH or OH groups of protein amino acid residues (histidine, cysteine, tryptophan, and perhaps serine).

The feasibility of these interactions with the ligand will depend on the protein surface amino acids accessibility, pH, buffer, temperature, ionic strength and support matrix.

Histidine residues of proteins are involved in the interactions in Immobilized Metal Affinity systems, and sometimes in the dye–ligand system. But, histidine itself can also be immobilized and act as a pseudobiospecific ligand to adsorb biomolecules. In this chapter, we give a brief account of the potential of Histidine Ligand Affinity Chromatography (HLAC) both for the isolation and analysis of proteins.

Histidine as a pseudobiospecific ligand

Histidine is a less frequent amino acid in proteins, at about 2% of total amino acid composition (Klapper, 1977). This may indicate nature's selection of this amino acid to play very specific functions. Histidine is often involved in the catalysis of many enzymes and also in certain biorecognition events (Table 9.1).

Figure 9.1 presents the different protonation states of histidine. In addition to ionogenic COOH and NH_2 groups common to all amino acids, its side chain is the polar imidazole ring which conferes aromaticity to histidine at basic and acid pH.

Due to its imidazole group, histidine is the only amino acid to have a good buffering capacity at physiological pH. In proteins, as a result of the microenvironment, pK_a of histidine imidazole group can vary between 5.5 and 7.0 (Schellenberger, 1990). Moreover, histidine is an ideal amino acid for the formation of hydrogen bonds, because its imidazole ring is potentially a proton acceptor (N_3) and/or a proton donor (highly nucleophilic N_1), at neutral pH. Histidine residues also play a charge relay role in acid–base catalysis.

These properties mean that it can interact in many ways with proteins depending on conditions, such as pH, temperature, and ionic strength.

Table 9.1 Examples illustrating the role of histidine in biological phenomena

Biological system	Role of histidine	Reference
RNase A	His 12 proton donor	Nishikawa et al., 1987 (30)
RNase T	His 119 proton acceptor	Steyaert et al., 1990 (31)
Serine protease	Acylation by the triad His-Asp-Ser	Blow et al., 1969 (32)
Antigen, pH dependent epitope	pH dependence of immuno-adsorption equilibrium	Sada et al., 1988 (33)
Collagenase	Inhibition	Harper, 1979 (34)
Phosphoglycerate kinase	Contribution to the mechanism of phosphorylation of phosphoglycerate to diphosphoglycerate	Fairbrother et al., 1989 (35)
Human liver alcohol dehydrogenase	General catalysis	Tosten et al., 1991 (36)
Diphteria toxin	Binding of NAD+	Papini et al., 1989 (37)
Thymidylate synthase	Catalysis	Dev et al., 1989 (38)
Mitochondria F1F0-ATPase	Nucleophilic attack between His245 and Glu219	Cain et al., 1988 (39)

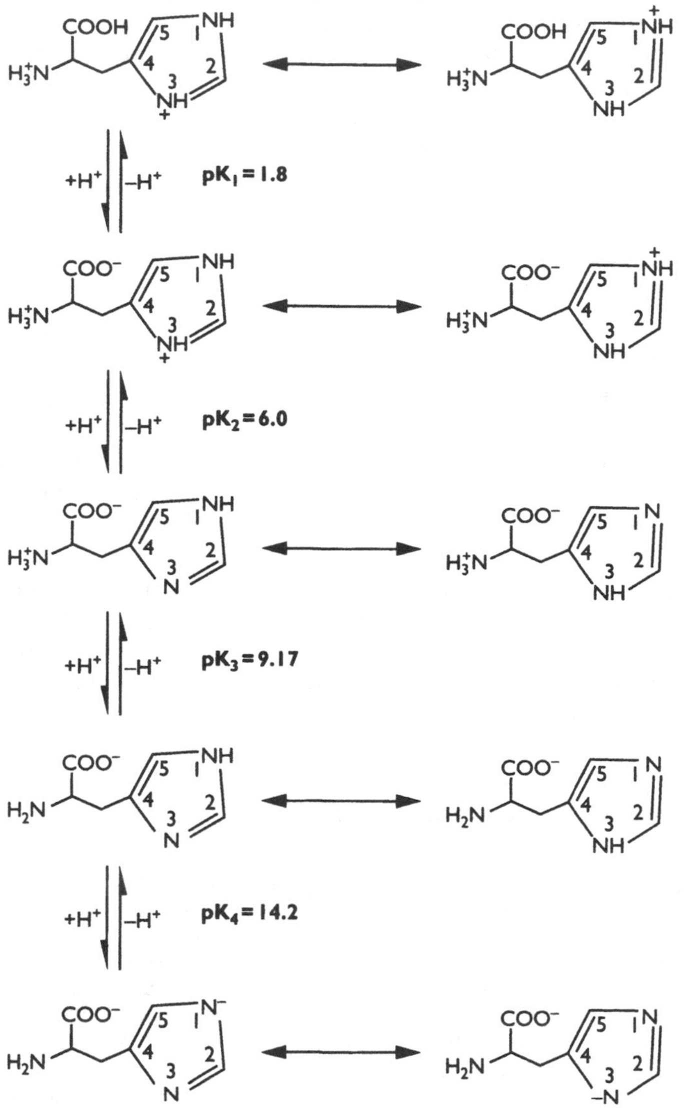

Figure 9.1 Protonation states and tautomeric forms of histidine. Modified from Schellenberger, 1990.

Since 20 years, histidine has been extensively studied as pseudobiospecific ligand in affinity chromatography. Several proteins and peptides have been purified using HLAC, both in analytical HPLC systems (Wu *et al.*, 1992) and on preparative scales (Table 9.2).

In all cases, the molecules were retained on HLAC at pH at or near their isoelectric points. The adsorption mechanism(s) seem(s) to involve different non covalent interactions resulting in a weak affinity with proteins. Due to the preponderant role played by dipole mediated interactions, the matrix–ligand interface should be considered rather

Table 9.2 Examples of proteins and peptides purified by HLAC

Proteins	Organism	Reference
IgG	Human	Kanoun et al., 1986
polyclonal	Mouse	Mdiba et al., 1989
monoclonal	Mouse (ascites fluid)	El kak and Vijayalakshmi, 1991
from plasma	Human	El kak and Vijayalakshmi, 1992
Chymosin	Kid	Amourache and Vijayalakshmi, 1984
Factor VIII	Human	Ezzedine et al., 1993
Endotoxin removal	Gram(−)ve bacterial contamination	Legallais et al., 1996
from IgG	in IgG	
Collagenase	Clostridium histolyticum	Emöd et al., 1977
Myxalin	Myxococcus xanthus	Akoum et al., 1987
Interferon	Human	Sulkowski et al., 1976

than the ligand (histidine) alone. Moreover, the chromatographic conditions could be adjusted as a function of molecules to be separated. These elements are discussed by Vijayalakshmi who named histidine an universal ligand (Vijayalakshmi, 1993).

Preparation of HLAC adsorbents

Selection of matrices for ligand immobilization

Many matrices containing OH group have been successfully used for coupling of histidine. Silica or agarose beads are usually used as support matrices. Recently, we have also developed flat or hollow fiber membranes of different chemical composition such as nylon, nylon metacrylate composite and poly(ethylenvinylalcohol): PEVA (Manjini and Vijayalakshmi, 1993; Bueno et al., 1995). These supports allow large-scale applications without limitation in terms of compressibility and pore diffusion as is the case with soft gels.

Influence of support matrix

The specific retention capacities of the histidyl-liganded adsorbents vary from one protein to another. Table 9.3 summarizes the capacities obtained for different proteins with a histidyl-Sepharose 4B adsorbent having 10 μmol histidine/mL gel. It is to be noted that this adsorbent, though very specific to certain groups of IgG_1 subclass from the human placental sera, shows rather a low capacity (Kanoun et al., 1986).

Moreover, for a given protein, large differences in capacity were described for different supports. As an example, histidyl-PEVA hollow fiber membranes (Haupt et al., 1995) showed, under the same chromatographic conditions, a much better adsorption of IgG (76 mg IgG/g support) than the one reported for the histidyl-Sepharose 4B (12 mg IgG/g support; El kak and Vijayalakshmi, 1992). In the case of Sepharose, the ligand distribution and orientation is a random event, that may result in interaction between ligand–ligand or ligand and hydroxyl groups of the polysaccharide material. Histidine may then form hydrogen bonds within the adsorbent, which will reduce its affinity for the IgGs.

Table 9.3 Capacity of the histidyl-Sepharose 4B for different proteins tested[a]

Protein	Capacity (mg protein/mL gel)
IgG1	0.5
Myxaline	0.5–1.0
Chymosin	1.0

[a] Capacity is calculated from the amount of pure product recovered in experiments where crude fractions containing other proteins/peptides and molecules were injected.

Table 9.4 Comparison of different membranes for their IgG purification characteristics

Membrane[a] support matrices	Capacity for IgG ($\mu g/cm^2$ support)	Dissociation constant, K_D (M)
Histidine liganded		
Silica FMC	145	9.67×10^{-5}
Nylon-methacrylate Composite	117	4.07×10^{-5}
PAL nylon	103	2.57×10^{-5}
PEVA (Hollow fiber membrane)	150	2.50×10^{-5}
Protein A liganded		
Nygene	173	5.69×10^{-5}

[a] PAL, FMC and Nygene are trade names supplied respectively by PAL Biproduct, N.J., USA; FMC bioproducts, M.E., USA; Nygene Corporation, N.Y., USA.

Another explanation could be that ligand molecules may not be accessible for IgG when coupled onto Sepharose because of diffusion limitation in the gel beads, as activation with oxirane group of spacer arm may result in the cross-linking of agarose.

By contrast, the high surface area and perhaps also the position of the available OH groups favorable for the accessibility of ligand (histidine) coupled to them may also explain the higher protein capacity of the membrane matrix supports, such as PEVA, as compared with gels. Moreover, the mild hydrophobic nature of PEVA hollow fiber membranes could also favor adsorption of IgG. IgG purification on different membrane types to which histidine has been chemically attached is presented in Table 9.4. PEVA based hollow fiber or silica based flat sheet membranes coupled with histidine showed the best capacities and were comparable to membranes coupled with Protein A. Hence, histidine is promising as an alternative ligand to Protein A, which is expensive and vulnerable to proteolysis.

Choice of coupling chemistry

Histidine can be immobilized onto OH-containing matrices through its α-NH$_2$ or through its COOH groups, with or without introduction of a spacer arm. However, the chemistry used is different in each case. With the conventional polysaccharide gel or polymer membrane based-OH containing matrices, the coupling through α-NH$_2$ group of histidine is best achieved by the oxiran chemistry using either epichlorhydrin or 1, 4 butanediol-diglycidyl-ether. For coupling of histidine through its −COOH group, the best adapted method is the use of water soluble carbodiimides, after introducing a primary amine group on the matrix prior to carbodiimide reaction (El kak and Vijayalakshmi, 1991). In the case of silica or nylon membranes, oxirane group is introduced by reacting with γ-glycidoxy trimethoxy silane according to Chang *et al.* (1976). The structures of the resultant activated matrices in all these cases are schematically represented in Fig. 9.2.

The amount of ligand coupled can be determined by the nitrogen estimation of an aliquot of the matrix using a micro Kjedahl method (Hajmarsson and Akesson, 1983)

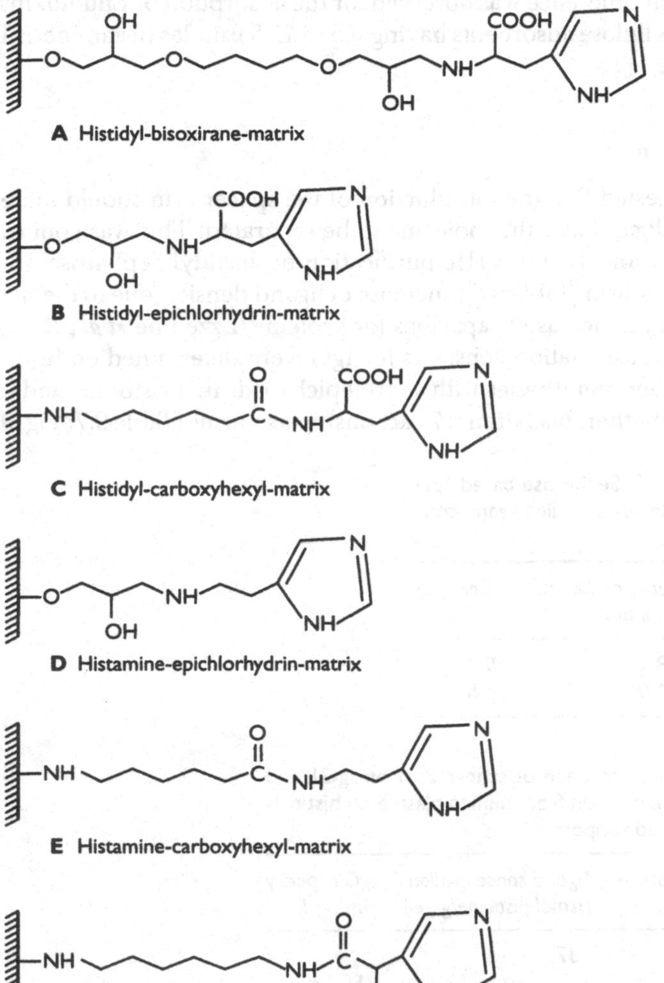

A Histidyl-bisoxirane-matrix

B Histidyl-epichlorhydrin-matrix

C Histidyl-carboxyhexyl-matrix

D Histamine-epichlorhydrin-matrix

E Histamine-carboxyhexyl-matrix

F Histidyl-aminohexyl-matrix

Figure 9.2 Proposed schematic structures of various histidine or histamine liganded matrix. Adapted from Haupt *et al.*, 1993.

or using the Pauly's reagent. Histidyl-Sepharose 4B adsorbent normally had a ligand concentration of 10 μmoles histidine/mL of gel.

Influence of ligand concentration

In an exploratory study, Sepharose based adsorbents with different histidine concentrations were compared for their capacity to retain IgG_1 from the placental serum (El kak and Vijayalakshmi, 1991). The results, presented in Table 9.5, showed that the lower ligand concentration gives a higher recovery and a higher purity compared to a gel with a higher ligand concentration. These results confirm our opinion that in Sepharose-based support, ligand accessibility is a limiting factor for large molecules such as IgG.

However, no significant difference was observed for the adsorption of Endotoxins on histamine-aminohexyl-cellulose adsorbents having 0.5 to 15.5 μmoles histamine/mL of gel (Minobe *et al.*, 1982).

Influence of spacer arm

Many authors have suggested that the introduction of the spacer arm should increase the interaction between ligand and the molecule to be separated. This was confirmed by the examples of IgG1 and Factor VIIIc purification on histidyl-Sepharose 4B gel with, or without, the spacer arm (Table 9.6). Increase of ligand density (due to the spacer arm) was correlated with an increased capacities for proteins (Ezzedine *et al.*, 1993).

In a more recent study, association constants for IgG were determined on histidine coupled PEVA hollow fiber membranes with short (epichloridrin: 3 carbons) and long (1,4 butanediol-diglycidyl-ether: bisoxirane: 7 carbons) spacer arms (Table 9.7; Fig. 9.2),

Table 9.5 Comparison of Sepharose-based gel capacity at different histidine ligand concentrations

Ligand concentration (μM/g dry gel)	Purity of the IgG I final product (%)	Yield (%)
10.5	98.9	9.2
24.3	92.0	4.5

Table 9.6 Influence of the presence of spacer arm on IgG I and Factor VIIIc purification from human plasma on histidyl-Sepharose based support

Sepharose 4B support matrice	Ligand concentration (μmol histidine/g gel)	IgG capacity (/mL gel)
Without spacer	37	
IgG I		150 μg
Factor VIII		30 IU
With spacer (bisoxirane)	150	
IgG I		350 μg
Factor VIII		60 IU

Table 9.7 Influence of the ligand concentration on dissociation constant (K_D) and maximum binding capacity (Q_x) of IgG on
histidyl-PEVA hollow fiber membranes

Support matrice	Ligand density (μmol/g support)	K_D (10^{-5})	Q_x (mg/g)
H-E-PEVA	60	2.5 +/− 0.2	79.8 +/− 2.9
H-B-PEVA	126	2.0 +/− 0.2	70.0 +/− 2.8

H-E-PEVA = histidyl-epichlorhyhdrin polyethylenvinyl alcohol
H-B-PEVA = histidyl-bisoxirane polyethylenvinyl alcohol

Table 9.8 Comparative efficiencies of the differents gels used for mouse
monoclonal antibodies (IgG1) purification

Support	Retained IgG1 (%)	IgG1 Capacity/ mL of gel (μg)
Histidyl-epichlorhydrin-Sepharose	37	50
Histamine-epichlorhydrin-Sepharose	87	117
Histidyl-aminohexyl-Sepharose	90	123

respectively. Increase in the ligand distance from the membrane seems to be of critical
importance, because histidine-bisoxirane-PEVA membranes presented a greater IgG
binding capacity than histidine-epichloridrin-PEVA, despite its lower ligand density.

Influence of ligand orientation

As we had previously noted, histidine could be coupled to matrices via its α-NH$_2$
or COOH groups. The resultant adsorbents will thus have either free NH$_3^+$ (positive
charge) or free COO$^-$ (negative charge) available. They may contribute significantly to
the protein recognition. Histamine was also coupled to the matrix via its α-NH$_2$ group
in order to obtain an adsorbent without either free NH$_2$ or COOH group (Fig. 9.2).

The adsorption of human IgG on these different adsorbents showed that, while the
specificity of adsorption and adsorption/desorption parameters was not significantly
altered, the capacity was influenced by the remaining free NH$_2$ or COOH groups on
the ligand (El kak and Vijayalakshmi, 1992). Results, presented in Table 9.8 indicate a
repulsion by the free COOH group of histidine in IgG adsorption on Sepharose-based
gels. Furthermore, these residual charge effects were different for different matrices and
different proteins.

In the case of Catechol-2,3-Dioxygenase (C-2,3-D) from *Pseudomonas putida*,
one-step purification showed a higher affinity of this enzyme for histamine-
carboxyhexyl-Sepharose and histidyl-carboxyhexyl-Sepharose, as compared to the
histidyl-aminohexyl-Sepharose (Haupt and Vijayalakshmi, 1993). These two adsorbents have either a free carboxylic group or no charge at all (Fig. 9.2). In any
case, there is no remaining positive charge in contrast to the histidyl-aminohexyl-
Sepharose (Table 9.9). These results suggested an electrostatic repulsion of C-2,3-D
by the positively charged NH$_2$ of aminohexyl spacer arm.

Table 9.9 Retention at different pH, of Catechol-2,3-Dioxygenase, on different supports

Support	Retained activity at pH6 (%)	Retained activity at pH7 (%)	Retained activity at pH8 (%)
Histidyl-E-Sepharose	20	0	0
Histidyl-AH-Sepharose	23	0	0
Histidyl-CH-Sepharose	100	5	0
Histamine-CH-Sepharose	100	100	100
CH-Sepharose	0	0	0

E = Epichlorhydrin; AH = Aminohexyl and CH = Carboxyhexyl.

Table 9.10 Adsorption of different IgG fragments (obtained after pepsin and papaïn digestion) on histidyl-bisoxirane-PEVA (H-B-PEVA) and histidyl-aminohexyl-Sepharose (H-AH-Sepharose)

Digestion by	Fragments	Retention on H-B-PEVA	Retention on H-AH-Sepharose
Pepsin	$(F_{ab'})^2$	Yes	ND
+ β-SH	$F_{ab'}$	Yes	ND
Papaïn	F_{ab}	Yes	No
	F_c	No	Yes

ND = not determined.

Moreover, recent experiments on PEVA hollow fibers or silica membrane showed the possibility to purify IgG from human serum on larger scale compared to Sepharose-based gels (as discussed above) despite the presence of the free COOH group of histidine (Manjini *et al.*, 1993; Bueno *et al.*, 1995; Fig. 9.3).

El kak *et al.* (1992) and Haupt *et al.* (1995), respectively, explain this difference between Sepharose and PEVA hollow fiber based adsorbent, in terms of the binding sites (Fc and Fab, respectively) of IgG involved in the interaction with the immobilized histidine on these adsorbents (Table 9.10).

These results seem to indicate that the nature of support matrix, presence of spacer arm and/or free charged group could influence independently of the recognition specificity of the protein, the capacity and the interaction sites of the adsorbed protein. The charge–charge interaction by the induced dipole both at the adsorbent–solvent interface and on the protein due to the pH effect, perhaps brings the solute molecule close enough to the immobilized ligand (histidine). This results in the selective adsorption of the solutes due to the specific interaction mediated by imidazole.

Adsorption conditions: a critical step in HLAC

As we had previously observed, HLAC involves in general a weak affinity and broader specificity compared to biospecific ligands (Vijayalakshmi, 1989).Thus, different ligates may compete for the immobilized histidine which, in turn, will decrease the binding capacity for the molecule of interest. As a consequence, adsorption conditions, such as sample preparation and composition, buffer and pH, temperature, additives such as salts, could be modulate to accomodate molecule to be separated. We will discuss

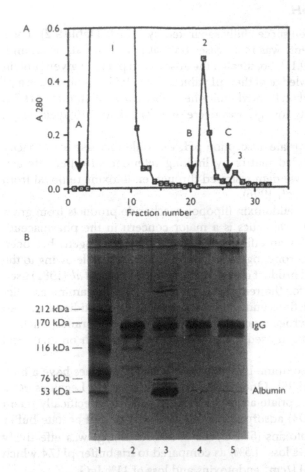

Figure 9.3 Separation of IgG from Plasma on hystidyl-bisoxirane-PEVA hollow fiber membranes. (A) Conditions (a) 25 mM Tris-HCl buffer (b) 25 mM Tris-HCl buffer + 100 mM NaCl (c) 25 mM Tris-HCl buffer + 1 M NaCl. (B) SDS-PAGE under non reducing conditions of the fraction of the chromatography. (1) Standard markers (2) prepurified IgG (3) peak 1 (4) peak 2 (5) peak 3. From Bueno *et al.*, 1995 with permission of the editor.

through the following examples, the role of these various parameters in achieving an optimum capacity/specifity toward the target molecule.

Importance of the upstream extraction methods

The method used to prepare the crude extract of the protein to be isolated may play an important role in its retention behavior. The complexity of the extract used for the chromatographic step is also an important factor, as illustrated during the purification of Factor VIIIc on histidyl-Sepharose 4B columns (Ezzedine *et al.*, 1991). While a starting material – cryoprecipitate – with a specific activity of 1.59 U/mg can yield a final product with a specific activity of only 29.5 U/mg, another partially purified material, with a specific activity of 159 U/mg, can yield a final product with a specific activity of 875 U/mg.

Influence of the adsorption pH

Many peptides/proteins have been successfully separated by HLAC (Table 9.2). Their specific retention on the adsorbents was in all cases only at pH values at, or around, their isoelectric points: pI (Table 9.11). So, ideally, the adsorption pH for a given protein can be chosen, based on the knowledge of their pI values. Thus, IgG_1s, which have a pI around 7.8 are selectively retained on histidyl-aminohexyl-Sepharose column at pH 7.4. Below and above pH 7.4, capacity for IgG was decreased (El kak and Vijayalakshmi, 1992).

As a consequence, at an appropriate adsorption pH, we could increase the capacity and specificity on histidine-liganded matrix by limiting retention of other interacting proteins with different pI, as we demonstrated through endotoxins removal from different IgG samples (Legallais et al., 1996).

The pyrogen contamination by endotoxin (lipopolysaccharide products from gram negative bacteria) of injectable therapeutics is a major concern in the pharmaceutical industry. Many approaches for an efficient removal of these pyrogens has been developed and it is obvious that chromatographic methods are preferable owing to the minimum denaturation of the end product during the process. Minobe et al. (1982) used histamine coupled to Sepharose for the removal of pyrogens. But, histamine as a ligand suffers from regulatory restrictions and we therefore developed histidine-liganded matrices as an alternative for pyrogen removal. Hollow fiber membranes, such as histidyl-bisoxirane-PEVA, have been used for endotoxin removal both on analytical level and on preparative scales.

As we have shown, histidyl-bisoxirane-PEVA hollow fiber membranes have a high affinity for IgGs (Bueno et al., 1995). One of the strategies, used by Legallais et al. (1996), was to test the more appropriate adsorption pH in order to specifically retain endotoxins without IgG (MacCD4) adsorption (Table 9.12). In 25 mM acetate buffer at pH5, higher removal of endotoxins ($63\,EU/cm^2 = 33000\,EU/g$) was effectively observed with a minimum of IgGs loss (1.5%) as compared toTris buffer pH7.4 which resulted in the retention of $47.5\,EU/cm^2$ endotoxins and loss of 11% IgG.

Influence of buffer composition

The study of IgG adsorption onto histidyl-bisoxirane-PEVA hollow fiber membranes showed that adsorption over a broad pH range was possible depending on the nature of the buffer ions. Zwitterionic buffers like MOPS and HEPES yielded much higher

Table 9.11 Isoelectric points and optimal pH adsorption of some proteins and peptides purified by HLAC

Substance purified	pI	Adsorption pH
Goat Chymosin	6.0	5.5
Acid protease A. niger	3.6	3.0–4.0
Yeast carboxypeptidase	3.6	3.0–4.0
Human placental IgGI	6.8–7.2	7.4
Myxaline (bacterial human blood anticoagulant)	4.0	5.5
Phycocyanin chromopeptides	5.8	5.0–6.0

adsorption capacities toward IgG than other buffers e.g. Tris-HCl. Phosphate buffers showed the least adsorption capacities. These zwitterionic buffers could be used at much higher concentration without jeopardising the IgG adsorption. An inhibition analysis revealed that non-zwitterionic buffers competitively inhibit IgG binding (by masking the binding site for histidine), whereas MOPS and HEPES in their zwitterionic form do not (Haupt *et al.*, 1995).

So, in the case of non-zwitterionic buffers used for adsorption, an *in situ* gradient of ligand accessibility could be generated and this in turn can result in selective adsorption of closely related molecules, such IgG subclasses (Table 9.13). As an example, histidyl-bisoxirane-PEVA membrane with a Tris buffer (pH7.4) could be used for the selective retention of IgG_3 subclass while the MOPS buffer facilitated the adsorption of total IgGs without any restriction. One should note that IgG_3 is not retained on Protein A (Van loghem *et al.*, 1982). Thus this use of appropriate buffers is an added advantage of this histidine coupled membrane.

Table 9.12 Endotoxin adsorption on histidyl-bisoxirane-PEVA hollow fiber membrane mini-cartridge (41 cm²) in IgG solution (1 mg/mL)

Buffer	pH	C_i (EU/mL)	Quantity adsorbed (EU/cm²)	Endotoxins remaining in solution		IgG removal (%)
				C_{eq} (EU/mL)	% of C_i	
Tris 25 mM	7.4	255	47.5	115	45	11
Phosphate 25 mM	6.0	39	7	17	43	3
MES 10 mM	5.5	75.6	11.2	42.7	56	4.5
Acetate 25 mM	5.0	228	63	44	19	1.5
Acetate 25 mM	5.0	25	8.5	0*	0	1

C_i: Initial concentration in the tank.
C_{eq}: Tank concentration at the end of the experiment (after 1 h).
* Below the detectable limit.

Table 9.13 Isoelectric points of IgG subclasses in the non-retained and the adsorbed fractions on Sepharose and PEVA matrices coupled with L-Histidine

Support matrice	Buffer (25 mM)	Fractions	pI	IgG subclass		
				IgG1	IgG2	IgG3
H-AH-Sepharose (free NH2)	Tris-HCl, pH7.4	Non-retained	4.8–6.7; 7.1–8; 8.3–10.2	+	+	+
		Eluted at				
		0.2 M NaCl	7.9–8.2	+	+	−
		1 M Nacl	6.8–7.2	−	+	−
H-B-PEVA (free COOH)	Tris-HCl, pH7.4	Non-retained	6–8	+	+	−
		Eluted at				
		0.2 M NaCl	8–9.5	+	−	+
H-B-PEVA (free COOH)	MOPS pH6.5	Non-retained	BT	−	−	−
		Eluted at				
		0.2 M NaCl	6.6–9.3	+	+	+

With BT: Below threshold; H: Histidine; AH: Aminohexyl and B: Bisoxirane.

Role of adsorption temperature

The theoritical consideration and understanding of the mechanism(s) of interaction between the proteins/peptides and the matrix coupled histidine ligands have shown the mechanism to be water-mediated, involving the changes in the dielectric constants at the adsorption interface owing to the combined electrostatic, hydrophobic, hydrogen bond and to some extent, charge transfer interactions between histidine and the specific amino acid residues available on the protein surface (e.g. Tyr, His and so on).

These low energy interactions are well known to be temperature dependant. While the hydrophobic interaction is favored by increased temperatures, the others are favored by lower temperatures. Thus an additional parameter of discriminating between different molecules, is the possibility of adjustment of adsorption temperature, both as a function of support matrix and of the biomolecule on a case by case basis. A few examples discussed below will elucidate this.

A detailed study was carried out in the case of the milk-clotting enzyme: Chymosin. It showed that its selective adsorption in the presence of other proteases, such as Pepsin, was favored at +4°C, whereas at a higher temperature of +20°C, both Pepsin and Chymosin are equally retained on a histidyl-epichlorhydrin-Sepharose gel (Amourache and Vijayalakshmi, 1984). On the contrary, in the case of IgG specific adsorption onto a histidyl-silica was favored at +20°C rather than at +4°C.

With histidyl-bisoxirane-PEVA hollow fiber membranes, determination of dissociation constants at different temperatures allowed calculation of thermodynamic adsorption parameters (Haupt et al., 1995). Decrease in K_D with increasing temperature and a positive entropy value between 20°C and 35°C (in Mops buffer, 25 mM) indicated that adsorption is partially governed by hydrophobic forces in that temperature range, whereas at lower temperatures, electrostatic forces (and perhaps hydrogen bonding) are more important for adsorption.

In the case of purification of C-2,3-D from *Pseudomonas pubida*, this temperature dependent adsorption was different for histamine-carboxyhexyl-Sepharose and histidine-carboxyhexyl-Sepharose, the later presenting a free COOH group (Table 9.14). While the histamine-carboxyhexyl-Sepharose showed a significant increase in affinity for C-2,3-D with increasing temperature, the histidine-carboxyhexyl-Sepharose showed much smaller increase in affinity with decreasing temperature. This

Table 9.14 Dissociation constants (K_D) and maximum binding capacities (L_t) for Catechol-2,3-Dioxygenase determined at different temperatures for histamine or histidyl-carboxyhexyl-Sepharose

Parameter	Histamine-CH-Sepharose				Histidyl-CH-Sepharose		
	4°C	15°C	26°C	37°C	4°C	20°C	37°C
$K_D(10^{-7})$	2.8	2.3	1.6	0.95	2.6	3.2	4.0
L_t (mg/ml)	4.5	4.3	6.0	5.6	1.9	2.0	2.2
$\Delta H°$ (kcal/mol)		5.6				−2.2	
$\Delta S°$ (cal/mol.K)		49.8				22.2	
$\Delta G°$ (kcal/mol)	−8.2	−8.7	−9.3	−9.8	−8.3	−8.7	−9.2

$\Delta H°$ is the standard enthalphy change, $\Delta S°$ the standard entropy change $\Delta G°$ the standard free energy change calculated from the dissociation constants. CH: Carboxyhexyl.

perhaps, indicates the additional charge (electrostatic and hydrogen bond) contribution from the free COOH group involved in the protein–ligand recognition.

Influence of additives: salt and chaotropic agents

As a general rule, low ionic strength of the chosen buffer (in the range of 20–50 mM) is favorable for the protein retention on the histidine-coupled matrices. Moreover, desorption of a molecule adsorbed on immobilised histidine is invariably achieved by the addition of sodium chloride (0.2–1 M NaCl) to the irrigation buffer.

This parameter is very important. The conductivity of the injected sample should be kept at a minimum in order to achieve maximum adsorption. This was illustrated in the case study of FVIIIC purification from human serum. A resistance of 1100 Ohms (8 mM NaCl) ensured good adsorption onto histidyl-aminohexyl-Sepharose but even as low as 20 mM added NaCl concentration decreased the adsorption capacity for FVIIIC (Ezzedine et al., 1993).

Similar observations were reported for both endotoxin (Minobe et al., 1983) and IgG (El kak et al., 1992) adsorption. Minobe et al. have made a systematic investigation of added NaCl effects on the adsorption of endotoxin onto histamine-Sepharose. The data shown in Table 9.15, confirm that adsorption of endotoxin onto histamine supports was maximal in low ionic strength conditions but when the salt concentration was higher than 1.5 M, the affinity once again, increased slightly.

In the case of IgG adsorption, El kak et al. (1992), observed a maximum adsorption at <0.1 mM NaCl and no adsorption at all between 0.2 and 1.0 M NaCl. At concentrations of 3.0 and 5.0 M NaCl, adsorption occured once again, though to a lesser extent as compared to the capacities observed at <0.1 M NaCl. Further, the addition of

Table 9.15 Effect of salt concentration on the adsorption of pyrogen on immobilized histamine-Sepharose based support

NaCl concentration (M)	Non-retained pyrogen concentration (ng/mL)
0	0.005
0.05	0.20
0.075	0.85
0.1	9.2
0.15	43
0.2	360
0.3	390
0.5	400
1.0	380
1.5	290
2.0	160
3.0	150
4.0	120
5.0	82

Pyrogen (E. coli, LPS) was at 1000 ng/mL in the starting material. Modified from Minobe et al., 1983.

chaotropic agents such as urea and ethylene glycol prevented the retention of IgG on the adsorbent.

This, in addition to the observation of highly aromatic molecules, such as bioamines, being retained at high salt concentrations (Vijayalakshmi, unpublished data) and that of C-2,3-D show an enhanced adsorption in the presence of a cosmotropic salt $(NH_4)_2SO_4$ onto the histidyl/histamine liganded matrices strongly suggest a water mediated adsorption mechanism (Haupt and Vijayalakshmi, 1993).

Elution conditions: fine tuning

If the adsorption conditions are critical for the selectivity of retention, the elution conditions can significantly contribute to good separation in HLAC. Furthermore, within the possibilities of using mild elution conditions, further fine tuning is possible to separate closely related molecules. The major parameters studied for efficient separation by fine tuning elution conditions are discussed below.

Salt desorption

Desorption of proteins in HLAC is generally achieved by the addition of sodium chloride to the mobile phase. The optimal concentration of sodium chloride varies from 0.2 to 1 M for different proteins. As an example, IgG_1s were successfully eluted by adding 0.2 M sodium chloride to the buffer whereas IgG_2 eluted at higher salt concentration (1 M) (El kak and Vijayalakshmi, 1992).

"Myxaline" is a microbial glycopeptide showing blood anticoagulant activity. It was isolated from the culture medium of *Myxococcus xanthus*. Myxaline was eluted with 0.5 M and with 1.0 M sodium chloride, using a stepwise gradient from 0 to 1 M sodium chloride while the contaminants were eluted at a lower sodium chloride concentration (Akoum *et al.*, 1989).

pH desorption

In the case of human IgG purification on histidyl-PEVA hollow fiber membranes, the desorption by either increasing NaCl concentration added to the starting buffer or by decreasing pH could be achieved. The decreasing pH, using discontinuous step gradient, allowed to separate the IgG subclasses into IgG2, part of IgG, subsets IgG, subsets IgG3 and others (Bueno *et al.*, 1995).

Amino acid elution

Amino acid elution studies were performed on histidyl-aminohexyl-Sepharose (data not published). Results, presented in Table 9.16, show that only amino acids with a net charge (negative: Glu, Asp or positive: Lys, Arg) were able to efficiently desorb IgGs. This phenomenon could be related to the competition of non-zwitterionic buffer used during adsorption of IgG.

Moreover, elution with a zwitterionic salt, such as glycine-betaine, was not possible, even at high concentration (1 M). Other amino acids, tested, Met and His, allowed only a partial desorption (15% and 14% of total adsorbed IgG, respectively).

Table 9.16 Elution by different amino acids of the IgG absorbed onto histidyl-aminohexyl Sepharose

Amino acid	Eluted IgG with amino acid (%)	Eluted IgG with 1 M NaCl (%)
Met	14	86
Lys	74	26
Ser	0	100
Glu	84	16
Arg	94	6
Leu	0	100
Asp	80	20
His	15	85
Gly	0	100

Amino acid was at 50 mM each and IgG solution of starting material was at 4 mg/mL. Adsorption was performed in Tris solution 25 mM, pH 7.4 with 4 mL of gel.

Example of a combination of these elution parameters

When endotoxin spiked samples of Factor VIIIc were tested (Ezzedine *et al.*, 1993), the retention of endotoxins is optimum at pH 6.0–6.1 which is at the same pH optimum for the retention of Factor VIIIc. However, the desorption optima were different for Factor VIIIc and for endotoxins. Selective desorption of these two products was achieved by both increasing the ionic strength with $0.3\,M$ $CaCl_2$ + $0.1\,M$ Gly + $0.3\,M$ Lys and the pH from 6.0 to 7.0. Under these conditions the retained endotoxins were not coeluted with the Factor VIIIc. This eluting buffer composition, in addition, helps to avoid any activation of Factor VIIIc and hence its denaturation (Ruttyn *et al.*, 1989).

What is the basis for the selective retention of proteins on immobilized histidine?

From the above discussed chromatographic conditions of different proteins, and especially those studied for IgG adsorption, we will attempt to explain the underlying mechanisms involved in protein recognition by the immobilized histidine.

At the first glance, the absolute necessity for low ionic strengh for adsorption and the elution by simple increase in the ionic strength, may suggest a simple ion exchange phenomenon.

However, the optimal pH for adsorption of different proteins was close to their pI values indicating that the electrostatic interaction between the immobilized ligand and the protein is not based on the net charge of the protein. Furthermore, the efficient desorption with charged amino acids both basic (Arg, Lys) and acidic (Glu, Asp) indicates the involvement of localized charges on the protein surface, in the interaction with the adsorbent (Table 9.16).

Water mediated adsorption is indicated from the data described by El kak *et al.*, 1992, where the influence of urea and ethylene glycol on the IgG adsorption were studied. 1 M Urea abolished ~60% of the adsorption. The adsorption decreased up to 30% of ethylene glycol and increased above this concentration to reach the maximum adsorption at 50% ethylene glycol.

Similary, the studies with C.2.3.D. (Haupt and Vijayalakshmi, 1993) and IgG adsorption (Haupt *et al.*, 1995) indicated the hydrophobic interactions of these protein molecules with the histidine coupled adsorbents in the presence of ammonium sulfate and sodium chloride, respectively.

The temperature parameters for the optimal adsorption of two proteins (IgG and C.2.3.D.) on different matrices coupled with histidine were studied. The adsorption decreased with increasing temperatures in the case of histidyl-Sepharose adsorbents.

All in all, we can conclude that the recognition of different proteins studied by the matrix immobilized histidine is due to a concerted action of different interactions such as electrostatic, hydrophobic, hydrogen bonding and Van der Waals forces.

Specificity of the recognition sites in proteins?

To exert this concerted action, are specific structural features on the protein surface necessary? Some efforts to pin point the involvement of specific amino acid residues or peptide segment structures on the protein surfaces for the specific adsorption of these proteins onto immobilized histidines using homologous peptide sequence consisting of Asp, Tyr and Ser did not lead to any unequivocal conclusions.

In an attempt to address the question of whether or not there is a structural specificity of protein recognition by immobilized histidine we will now consider a typical example of a protein showing strong bioaffinity to histidine.

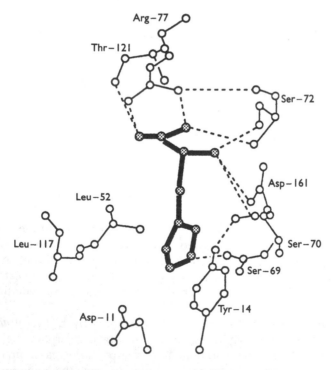

Figure 9.4 Histidine adsorption site structure of HisJ. Adapted from Oh *et al.*, 1994.

Certain bacteria such as *Escherichia coli* or *Salmonella typhi murium* have a specific histidine binding protein (HisJ) involved in the transmembrane transport of this amino acid. The structure of HisJ complexed with histidine was recently resolved by X-Ray crystallography (Oh *et al.*, 1994).

As shown in Table 9.16 and in Fig. 9.4 the histidine binding site consists of charged amino acids (Arg 77; Asp 161) hydrophobic and aromatic residues (Leu 52; Tyr 14) and other hydrogen bonding residues with $^-$OH groups (Ser 69, Ser 70, Ser72 and Thr 121). This complex structure of the histidine binding site with multiple interactions (hydrophobic, aromatic, ionic and hydrogen bonding interactions) resulted in a high binding strengh ($K_D = 4 \times 10^{-8}$ M).

In the case of molecules studied with HLAC, particulary IgGs as discussed above, the retention is based on the same type of interactions, but may involve fewer residues as compared to the histidine binding site of the protein HisJ. This explains the weaker interaction ($K_D = 10^{-6}$ M).

The different data, indicated the involvement of charged residues, as elution was equally possible by both Lys, Arg and Asp, Glu and the involvement of Ser and Tyr residues, shown by the studies with model peptides.

In addition, the similar results with both histidine and histamine used as ligands for the adsorption of different proteins revealed the importance of hydrophobic environment of the protein surface residues in specific binding to imidazole.

Conclusion

In conclusion, one can observe that histidine or histamine can be successfully used as ligands in affinity chromatography. Proteins can be efficiently purified in a minimum number of steps, even from complex biological mixtures, such as total sera or crude extracts from culture media. HLAC is also useful for the fine separation of IgG subclasses or protein isoforms by fine tuning the adsorption and/desorption conditions, while maintaining gentle, non-denaturing chromatographic conditions.

References

Akoum, A., Vijayalakshmi, M. A. and Sigot, M. (1989) Scale-up of "Myxaline" purification by a pseudo-affinity method using a radial flow column. *Chromatographia*, **28**, 157–160.

Amourache, L. and Vijayalakshmi, M. A. (1984) Affinity chromatography of kid chymosin on histidyl-Sepharose. *J. Chromatogr.: Biomed. Appl.*, **303**, 285–289.

Blow, D. M., Birktoft, J. J. and Hartley, B. S. (1969) Role of a buried acid group in the mechanism of action of chymotrypsin. *Nature*, **221**, 337–340.

Buchner, J., Renner, M., Lilie, H., Hinz, H. J., Jaenicke, R., Kiefhabel, T. and Rudolph, R. (1991) Alternatively folded states of an immunoglobulin. *Biochemistry*, **30**, 6922–6929.

Bueno, S. M. A., Haupt, K. and Vijayalakshmi, M. A. (1995) Separation of Immunoglobulin G from human serum by pseudobioaffinity chromatrography using immobilized L-histidine in hollow fiber membranes. *J. Chromatogr.: Biomed. Appl.*, **667**, 57–67.

Cain, B. D. and Simoni, R. D. (1988) Interaction between Glu-219 and His-245 within the subunit of F1F0-ATPase *Escherichia coli*. *J. Biol. Chem.*, **263**, 6603–6612.

Chang, S. H., Gooding, K. M. and Regnier, F. E. (1976) Use of oxiranes in the preparation of bonded phase supports. *J. Chromatogr.*, **120**, 321–333.

Dev, I., Yates, B. B., Atashi, J. and Dallas, W. S. (1989) Catalytic role of Histidine 147 in *Escherichia coli* Thymidylate synthase. *J. Biol. Chem.*, **264**, 19132–19137.

El kak, A. and Vijayalakshmi, M. A. (1991) Study of the separation of mouse monoclonal antibodies by pseudobioaffinity chromatography using matrix-linked histidine or histamine. *J. Chromatogr.: Biomed. Appl.*, **570**, 29–41.

El kak, A. and Vijayalakshmi, M. A. (1992) Separation and purification of IgG1 and IgG2 from IgG-Cohn-II fraction of human plasma by pseudobioaffinity chromatography on histidyl-AH-Sepharose. *Bioseparation*, 47–53.

El kak, A., Manjini, S. and Vijayalakshmi, M. A. (1992) Interactions of Immunoglobulin G with immobilized Histidine: mechanistic and kinetic aspects. *J. Chromatogr.: Biomed. Appl.*, **604**, 29–37.

Emöd, I., Trocheris, I. and Keil, B. (1977) Separation of proteinases and in particular of clostripain and collagenase by affinity chromatography. In: *Affinity chromatography* (ed.), O. Hoffmann-Ostendorf, M. Breitenbach, F. Koller, D. Kraft and O. Scheiner. Pergamon Press, London, pp. 123–128.

Ezzedine, M., Lawny, F. and Vijayalakshmi, M. A. (1993) Purification and depyrogenation of antihemophilic F VIII:C from human plasma. In: *Biotechnology of blood proteins* (ed.), J. F. Stoltz and C. Rivat. INSERM/John Libbey, **227**, 115–123.

Fairbrother, W. J., Walker, P. A., Minard, P., Littechild, J. A., Watson, H. C. and Williams, R. J. P. (1989) NMR analysis of site-specific mutants of yeast/Phosphoglycerate kinase: An investigation of the triose-binding site. *Eur. J. Biochem.*, **183**, 57–67.

Harper, E. (1979) Mechanism of action of collagenase. Irreversible inhibition by cysteine; reversible inhibition by histidine or imidazole. *Fed. Proc.*, **25**, 790–795.

Haupt, K. and Vijayalakshmi, M. A. (1993) Interaction of catechol-2,3-dioxygenase of *Pseudomonas putida* with immobilized histidine and histamine. *J. Chromatogr.: Biomed. Appl.*, **644**, 289–297.

Haupt, K., Bueno, S. M. A. and Vijayalakshmi, M. A. (1995) Interaction of human immunoglobulin G with L-Histidine immobilized onto poly(ethylene vinyl alcohol) hollow fiber membranes. *J. Chromatogr.: Biomed. Appl.*, **674**, 13–21.

Hjalmarsson, S. and Akesson, R. (1983) Modern Kjeldahl procedure. *Int. Lab.*, 70–76.

Kanoun, S., Amourache, L., Krishnan, S. and Vijayalakshmi, M. A. (1986) A new support for the large scale purification of proteins. *J. Chromatogr.: Biomed. Appl.*, **376**, 259–267.

Klapper, M. H. (1977) The independent distribution of amino acid near neighbor pairs into polypeptides. *Biochem. Biophys. Res. Communi.*, **78**, 1018–1023.

Legallais, C., Anspach, F. B., Bueno, S. M. A., Haupt, K. and Vijayalakshmi, M. A. (1997) Strategies for the depyrogenation of contaminated immunoglobulin G solutions by histidine-immobilized hollow fiber membrane. *J. Chromatogr.: Biomed. Appl.*, **691**, 33–41.

Mandjini, S. and Vijayalakshmi, M. A. (1993) Membrane based pseudobioaffinity chromatography of placental IgG using immobilized L-Histidine. In *Biotechnology of blood proteins* (ed.), J. F. Stoltz and C. Rivat. INSERM/John Libbey, **227**, 189–195..

Mbida, A., Kanoun, S. and Vijayalakshmi, M. A.(1989) Purification of IgG1-subclass from human placenta by pseudobioaffinity chromatography. In *Biotechnology of blood proteins* (ed.), J. F. Stoltz and C. Rivat. Colloque INSERM, **175**, 237–244.

Minobe, S., Watanabe, T., Sato, T., Tosa, T. and Chibata, I. (1982) Preparation of adsorbents for pyrogen adsorption. *J. Chromatogr.*, **248**, 401–408.

Minobe, S., Sato, T., Tosa, T. and Chibata, I. (1983) Characteristics of immobilized histamine for pyrogen adsorption. *J. Chromatogr.: Biomed. Appl.*, **262**, 193–198.

Nishikawa, S., Morioka, H., Kim, H. J., Fuchimura, K., Tanaka T., Uesugi, S., Hakoshima, T., Tomita, K. I., Ohtsuka, E. and Ikehara, M. (1987) Two histidine residues are essential for Ribonuclease T1 activity as is the case for Ribonuclease A. *Biochemistry*, **26**, 8620–8624.

Oh, B. H., Ames, G. F. and Kim, S. H. (1994) Structural basis for multiple ligand specificity of the periplasmic lysine-, arginine-, ornithine-binding protein. *J. Biol. Chem.*, **269**, 26323–26330.

Papini, E., Schiavo, G., Sandona, D., Rappuoli, R. and Montecucco, C. (1989) Histidine 21 is at the NAD+ binding site of Diphteria toxin. *J. Biol. Chem.*, **264**, 12385–12388.

Ruttyn, Y., Brandin, M. P. and Vijayalakshmi, M. A. (1989) Chromatography of human plasma on aminohexyl Sepharose: separation of Factor VIII/VWf and behaviour of Factors II, VII, IX, X and antithrombin III. *J. Chromatogr.*, **491**, 299–308.

Sada, E., Katoh, S., Kiyokawa, A. and Kodo, A. (1988) Effect of histidine residues in antigenic sites on pH dependence of immuno-adsorption equilibrium. *Appl. Microb. Biotech.*, **27**, 528–532.

Schellenberger, A. (1990) In *Enzymkatalyse*, Edition Gustav Fischer, Jena, 152–165.

Steyaert, J., Hallenga, K., Wyns, L. and Stanssens, P. (1990) Histidine 40 of Ribonuclease T1 acts as base catalyst when the true catalytic base, glutamic acid 58, is replaced by alanine. *Biochemistry*, **29**, 9064–9067.

Sulkowski, E, Davey, W. M. and Carter, A. W. (1976) Interaction of human interferon with immobilized hydrophobic amino acids and dipeptides. *J. Biol. Chem.*, 5381–5385.

Torsten, E., Hurley, T. D., Edenberg, H. J. and Borson, W. F. (1991) General base catalysis in a glutamine for histidine mutant at position 51 of human liver alcohol dehydrogenase. *Biochemistry*, **30**, 1062–1068.

Van loghen, E., Frangione, P., Recht, B. and Franklin, E. C. (1982) Staphylococcal protein A and human IgG subclasses and allotypes. *Scand. J. Immunol.*, **15**, 275–280..

Vijayalakshmi, M. A. (1989) Pseudobiospecific ligand affinity chromatography, *Tibtech.*, **7**, 71–76.

Vijayalakshmi, M. A. (1993) Pseudobiospecific addinity ligand chromatography: the case of immobilized Histidine as a Universal ligand. In *Molecular Interactions in Bioseperation*, T. T. Ngo, (ed.), Plenum, New York and London, 257–276.

Wu, X., Haupt, K. and Vijayalakshmi, M. A. (1992) Separation of IgG by high performance pseudobioaffinity chromatography with immobilized Histidine. A preliminary report on influence of the silica support and the coupling mode. *J. Chromatogr.: Biomed. Appl.*, **584**, 35–41.

Chapter 10

Immobilized metal-ion affinity chromatography

From phenomenological hallmarks to structure-based molecular insights

Nadir T. Mrabet and Mookambeswaran A. Vijayalakshmi

Introduction

Affinity chromatography is the most selective and the most rapid technique for the purification of proteins, and it has been utilized successfully for purifiying a great number of different proteins, including antibodies, antigens, enzymes, hormones, receptors, etc. (Cuatrecasas *et al.*, 1968; Porath and Kristiansen, 1975; Wilchek *et al.*, 1984; Scopes, 1987a). The success of affinity chromatography is essentially due to its high efficiency which originates from the specific or pseudospecific recognition between a solid phase-immobilized ligand and the molecule to be separated. Affinity purification methods can be divided into two large classes depending on whether the mechanism of protein/ligand recognition is biospecific or pseudobiospecific (Vijayalakshmi, 1989). Proteins usually bind biospecific ligands with high affinity (10^{-7} to 10^{-15} M). As a consequence, protein desorption in biospecific ligand affinity chromatography often requires drastic conditions which are likely to result in ligand and/or protein denaturation. In contrast, pseudobiospecific ligand affinity chromatography involves interactions of medium affinity (Cuatrecasas *et al.*, 1968; Scopes, 1987b).

Yet methods have been devised to provide for a fairly high selectivity (Corradini, 1988; Mrabet, 1992a). As a result, this has led to the development of gentle protocols for the purification of a large panel of proteins (Vijayalakshmi, 1989; Porath, 1992). It is the purpose of this chapter to present the state of the art in a distinct class of pseudobiospecific affinity chromatography.

A little more than 20 years have elapsed since Porath first introduced immobilized metal-ion affinity chromatography (IMAC),[1] a technique that takes advantage of the property of a few amino acids to bind chelated transition metals, as a purification method for biological molecules (Porath *et al.*, 1975).

---

1 Abbreviations: IMA, immobilized metal-ion affinity; IMAC, IMA chromatography; IDA, iminodiacetic acid; TED, tris(carboxymethyl)ethylenediamine; IDA-Me(II), chelate complex between IDA and any divalent first-group transition metal ion; IDA-Cu(II)-IMAC, IMAC with IDA-Cu(II) as affinity ligand; Im, imidazole; HPLC, high-performance liquid chromatography; FPLC, fast protein-liquid chromatography; XI, D-xylose isomerase; MOPS, 4-morpholinopropanesulfonic acid; MES, 4-morpholinoethanesulfonic acid; MMA, buffer solution of defined concentration containing equimolar amounts of MOPS, MES, and acetic acid; ASA, accessible surface area, defined as the area of the surface generated by the center of a spherical probe as it rolls over the van der Waals surface of a given molecule; Tris, tris(hydroxy-methyl)amino-methane; EDTA, ethylenediaminetetraacetic acid; SDS, sodium dodecyl sulfate; PAGE, polyacrylamide gel electrophoresis.

The forerunner of this very interesting approach is the "ligand exchange chromatography" widely studied by Davankov and Semechkin (1977), and others. This approach was mainly applied for the separation of small molecules such as amino acids, peptides etc. Due to the differential recognition of the specific chemical groups present on the molecules, separation of enantiomers was possible.

The ligand exchange chromatography, though similar to IMAC, differs from IMAC in many aspects. This brings out the necessity for some basic consideration on the metal-biomolecule/protein interaction. Taking a few steps back, we should consider the important differences between the free metals and the chelated metals in terms of their interactions with biomolecules. Further the nature of the chelating group will itself influence the interaction.

In IMAC, metal ions are immobilized by complex formation with a metal-chelating agent which is, itself, covalently attached to a hydrophilic support. When a protein mixture is percolated through an IMAC column, some proteins, which carry on their external surface amino acid residues with electron-donating character, can bind to the chelated metal through the available coordination sites, and are hence adsorbed, while others elute from the column unretarded.

In terms of purification of biological molecules, the harvest has been quite munificent. Applications of IMAC range from the separation of small molecules such as amino acids (Hemdan and Porath, 1985), nucleotides (Hubert and Porath, 1981; Fanou-ayi and Vijayalakshmi, 1983) or aromatic amines (Liu and Yu, 1990), to the purification of a variety of proteins (Sulkowski, 1985), including membrane glycoproteins (Corradini et al., 1988) and engineered proteins bearing synthetic metal-affinity sites on their surface (for a review, see Arnold, 1991), and even further extend to the separation of intact cells (Goubran-Botros and Vijayalaksmi, 1989; Nanak et al., 1995; Laboureau and Vijayalakshmi, 1997). Moreover, the potential for high resolution of metal-based affinity purification has been elegantly demonstrated by the separation in a single run of 19 peptide hormones, some of which differ in their primary sequence only by the configuration (L or D) of a single amino acid (Nakagawa et al., 1988).

How to do IMAC

The three major parameters, adsorption, desorption and regeneration are the criteria to be considered for any adsorption-based/affinity chromatographic operations which includes IMAC. These three parameters depend on (1) the ligand structure, (2) protein/polypeptide structure, which are the solute for chromatography, (3) physico-chemical interaction involved, (4) the thermodynamic and kinetic parameters of ligand-protein association/dissociation, (5) stability and sturdiness of the adsorbent and ligand.

Support matrices

As in any other affinity chromatographic methods the choice of the support matrix is based on:

- mechanical, physical and chemical robustness
- easy derivatization for coupling the ligand

- good porosity with high capacity of coupled ligand. This in fact is a trade off between porosity and polymer density of the support matrix
- stable bed volume
- easy regeneration and cleaning up possibilities

Beaded agarose under different commercial trade names (Sepharose 4B, 6B, chelating Fast Flow Sepharose, Superose, Novarose, etc.) is the most widely used. In fact, the seminal work of Porath *et al.* (1975) used the Sepharose 4B coupled with iminodiacetic acid (IDA) by the bisoxirane method. Other matrices such as silica, both for preparative and analytical HPLC (5 μm), hydrophylized resins and membranes have been used with iminodiacetate chelated metal ions (Hutchens *et al.*, 1988, 1989; Hutchens and Yip, 1990a,b; Dandeu *et al.*, 1990; Mrabet, 1992b; Chaga *et al.*, 1997; Reif *et al.*, 1994)

The coupling chemistry used is invariably based on the oxirane activation of the matrix followed by coupling of the chelator through its −NH−, −NH₂ or −SH groups, by nucleophilic attack, at alkaline pHs. Though in some cases other chemical activation methods such as succinyl, glutaraldehyde, etc. can be used.

Choice of the chelating groups

The metal is immobilized through coordination to a chelating group. In order for the metal to be stably bound while still disposing free coordination groups available for protein/peptide binding, at least a tridentate ligand, the IDA type is needed. The binding energy for commonly used transition metal ions is 15–25 kcal/mol. This rules out the use of common ion exchangers which are monodentate and have a rather low binding energy of 2–3 kcal/mol for the transition metal cation. As a general consideration, by varying the number and ratio of the coordinating atoms (O, N and S) and the overall structure of the chelator, one can produce a plethora of IMA adsorbents to meet specific demands. Carboxymethylated aliphatic amines with different number of NH₂ and COOH groups are reported (Porath, 1992).

Adsorbents based on IDA are the most frequently used (Fig. 10.1A). The other common chelator used for the immobilization of metal ions in IMAC is tris(carboxymethyl)ethylenediamine (TED). Since there is a single orbital left for ligand coordination in TED-Me(II), only coordination complexes can be formed with eventual

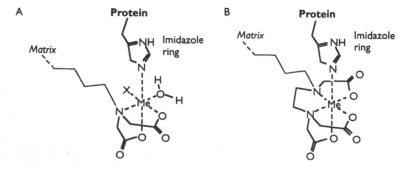

Figure 10.1 Interaction scheme between metal chelate and imidazole ring (Histidine) of protein. A with iminodiacetic acid (IDA) as chelating agent. B with tris(carboxymethyl)ethylenediamine (TED) as chelating agent.

ligands (Fig. 10.1B). In contrast, up to three coordination sites can be made available on IDA-Me(II); hence, genuine chelate structures may also be formed with proteins binding to this ligand. Furthermore, the metal is much more buried in TED-Me(II) than in IDA-Me(II) which is likely to contribute to the weaker retention of proteins in TED-based gels (Porath and Olin, 1983). Among the other different chelator, particular mention should be given to Tris(2-amino-ethyl)amine (TREN). Theoretically this chelator is tetradentate, but in IMAC adsorbent whether it is a tri or tetradentate is an open question.

The CM-TREN adsorbent, obtained after exhaustive treatment with bromo or chloro acetate of the TREN coupled matrix is a very powerful chelator (nonadendate) and may find its specific use in scavenging trace metals in biological extracts and loosely bound metals in proteins (Porath, 1992; Boden et al., 1995).

However, the more recent works with high density macroporous agarose matrices (Novarose™) interlaced with PEI seem to have significant capacity for heavy metals (about 1500 μmol/ml bed). These matrices have the additional advantage of being diffusion free, convective media (Steinman et al., 1994).

Metal ions and adsorption center

According to Pearson (1990), the metals could be classified into three groups: hard, soft and intermediate/borderline. Each group recognizes more selectively the O, N and S atoms in the biomolecule. Table 10.1 gives the classification of the metals into these three groups and their preferred atomic and molecular ligands.

In his seminal work, Porath et al. (1975) proposed the following IDA chelated transition metal ions: Cu(II), Ni(II), Zn(II) and Co(II). This can be extended to hard metals like Ca(II), Mg(II) which are of high biological relevance. At present, the soft metal, particularly Au, Pd are gaining much interest. Porath, the founder of the IMAC concept, in collaboration with our group, is now focusing on Au and Pd for the specific recognition of sulfur containing and aromatic amino acid residues in proteins and polypeptides.

The metals in the transition series viz Cu(II), Ni(II), Zn(II), Co(II) (particularly the metals of major interest in IMAC studies) and to some extent Fe(III) are known to be bound to specific peptide sequences in biological compounds which are either the transport sites or stabilizing sites in enzymes. The tripeptides Gly-Gly-His, N-methylamide

Table 10.1 Classification of metal ions and their ligands. From Chottard et al. (1984) and Glusker (1991)

Classification	Metal ions (Lewis acids)	Principal ligands (Lewis bases)
Hard	H^+, Li^+, Na^+, Mg^{2+}, Ca^{2+}, Mn^{2+}, Cr^{3+}, Co^{3+}, Al^{3+}, Ga^{3+}, La^{3+}, Nd^{3+}, Eu^{3+}	H_2O, ROH, OH^-, RO^-, NH_3, RNH_2, CO_3^-, $RCOO^-$ (essentially oxygen ligands)
Soft	Cu^+, Ag^+, Au^+, Ti^+, Pd^{2+}, Pt^{2+}, Cd^{2+}, Hg^+, Hg^{2+}	RSH, RS, R_2S, CN^-, H^-, I^- (essentially sulfur ligands)
Borderline	Zn^{2+}, Cu^{2+}, Fe^{2+}, Ni^{2+}, Co^{3+}, Sn^{2+}, Pb^{2+}, Rh^{3+}, Ir^{3+}, In^{3+}, Ru^{3+}	Imidazole, Pyridine, N_2, NO_2^-, N_3^-, Br^- (essentially nitrogen ligands)

derivatives and Gly-His-Lys have a copper binding site, simulating the human serum albumin Cu(II) transport/fixation site.

According to Vallee and Auld (1990) who have extensively studied the Zn containing proteins and their biological implications,

- The Zn(II) is amphoteric and exists in the hydrated form or as a hydroxide at near neutral pHs.
- The coordination sphere is flexible.
- The coordination complexes of Zn are characterized by their stereochemical adaptability.
- The multiplicity of coordination numbers and the geometry that the Zn atom can adopt, shows that the Zn atom adapts itself to the demands of the coordinating ligands.

In general, a combination of 3 amino acid residues, selected from His, Glu, Asp- and Cys- form the tridentate Zn binding sites of Zn enzymes/proteins with histidine being the most frequent N donor amino acid characterized by a tetradentate structure (catalytic site) and with Cys- being the important coordinating residue for Zn in the structural sites.

The IMAC uses the metals immobilized to a solid matrix through a chelator. Hence, the interacting metal ligand is in the chelated form named generally the "adsorption center". Particular attention is needed to understand and distinguish their interactions, with peptide/protein molecules in comparison to free metals interaction, as considered above in the case of metalloproteins; though the same type of amino acid residues viz His, Asp, Glu exposed on the protein surface can be expected to be involved in the recognition mechanism.

But, the exact structure of the immobilized chelated metal ion – the adsorption center- is yet a matter of debate. Firstly, the structure will depend on, (1) the nature of the metal ion and the chelating function, (2) the solvent conditions – buffers and salts used. These factors also determine the available sites for the protein interaction and association. According to Davankov and Semechkin (1977) Zn(II) and Cu(II) will leave one and Ni(II) three sites for solvent or buffer molecules when the tridentate IDA is used. Other chelating groups seem to assume coordination numbers higher than 4 for Zn(II) and Cu(II) ions.

Porath has proposed the following hypothetical structures for IDA, TED and other chelating groups immobilized onto conventional Sepharose gels and coordinated to Cu(II), Ni(II) or Zn(II) (Fig. 10.1). Thus, IDA-M(II) leaves three coordination sites free and TED-M(II) leaves only one coordination site available for solvent or buffer. Consequently, TED-M(II) ligands show weaker binding of proteins than the corresponding IDA-M(II) sorbents. Hochuli *et al.* (1987) have claimed that Ni(II) chelated with immobilized nitriloacetate (NTA) has a high specificity for proteins containing adjacent and multiple histidines. But the IDA-M(II) ligands do not bind in a specific manner the His-His sites in a protein (Berna *et al.*, 1996). These data should be considered in more details with regards to the spatial orientation of imidazole groups, hence the potential chelating sites of $N\delta$ and $N\varepsilon$ groups, as already discussed by Chakrabarti (1990) in his structure-based modelling studies of transition metal binding to His containing proteins.

Peptide/protein structure

Binding to chelated metal ions occurs by formation of a coordination bond between the metal and one or more electron-donor groups on the surface of the protein. From the foregoing discussion of free metal binding to peptides, one may expect at least in the beginning to have the same amino acids involved in the recognition of proteins by the immobilized chelated metal ions. Thus, in his seminal work, Porath *et al.* (1975) proposed that cysteine, histidine and tryptophan are the residues involved in the selective retention of serum proteins on the Sepharose-IDA-Cu(II) and Sepharose-IDA-Ni(II). However, the direct involvement of Cys residues is not yet demonstrated. On one hand, mostly the Cys residues are involved in disulphide bonds and hence the "S" group is not available. Further, the SH-containing thiol proteins, undergo quick oxidation, particularly in the presence of chelated copper.

A large number of papers since 1975 have discussed the involvement of different amino acid residues in the adsorption of proteins onto the widely used metal ions (Cu(II), Ni(II), Zn(II)) under different buffer conditions and ionic strength. Smith *et al.* (1988) have thus shown the involvement of acidic amino acid (Asp and Glu) in the interaction between the IDA-Cu(II) and the proteins. Similarly, Sulkowski (1987), Gauthier *et al.* (1990) and Mrabet (1992a), have evaluated and exploited the interference of charged residues due to electrostatic interactions under low ionic strength adsorption conditions. This was explained by the net negative residual charge of the IDA-chelated first series transition metals like Cu(II). Recently, Hearn's group has shown the involvement of charged residues (Asp, Glu, Arg, Lys) in the protein retention on IMAC columns using chelators of the type Tacn (Jiang *et al.*, 1998). As a result of several studies with model proteins, however, data has been accumulated to support the view that, near neutral pH, histidine is the 'preferred' protein ligand in IMAC (Sulkowski, 1987; Zhao *et al.*, 1991; Mrabet, 1992a).

Metal ions used in IMAC are first-group transition ions with a partially filled shell of d electrons and hence, they can engage in coordination bond formation. A general observation is that the equilibrium constants for complex formation with ligands that contain nitrogen as the donor atom fall in the following order of the metal ions: $Mn^{2+} < Fe^{2+} < Co^{2+} < Ni^{2+} < Cu^{2+} < Zn^{2+}$ (Cotton and Wilkinson, 1972). A rather similar behavior is encountered in the IMAC of proteins, the order being Cu(II) > Zn(II) > Ni(II) > Mn(II) or Cu(II) > Ni(II) > Zn(II) (Belew *et al.*, 1987). In this context, the influence of surface histidine topography on protein/metal-chelate interactions has been the subject of a sustained investigation by Sulkowski and colleagues (Sulkowski, 1985, 1987; Hemdan *et al.*, 1989; Zhao *et al.*, 1991) who were able to provide evidence to support the following ground rules for the interactions at near neutral pH and in the presence of added salt concentration to suppress the electrostatic interactions (Table 10.2): (1) A single surface-accessible histidine is sufficient to retain a protein on a IDA-Cu(II) column; (2) more than one histidine residue is required for protein binding to IDA-Ni(II); and (3) the presence of two surface-clustered histidine residues is mandatory for retention on IDA-Zn(II) or IDA-Co(II). These seminal data have led to the wide use of multiple histidine residues as "affinity tags" introduced into the sequence of recombinant proteins to facilitate direct purification from culture broths. Thus, Smith M. C. *et al.* (1988) used His-Trp added to the N-terminal of luteinising hormone releasing hormone (LHRH), and to proinsulin to purify these hormones.

Similarly, Hochuli, E. *et al.* (1987), used 6-histidine residues attached to different proteins for their easy purification. This approach is now very widely used (Table 10.3). Nevertheless, in less than 20% of cases, due to modification(s) in their 3D structures of the fusion proteins, induced by this additional peptide sequence -histidine tag-, the high affinity site for the metal chelate ligand, becomes inaccessible and the "affinity tag" does not serve its intended purpose (Trchtenberg, M.; Faye, L. personal communications).

Fe(III)-based adsorbents have also been described for the isolation of phosphoproteins (Andersson and Porath, 1986; Muszynska *et al.*, 1986). As their binding specificity is different from that of the more classical metal ions used in IMAC and as their ligand recognition mechanism appears much more complex, they fall outside the scope of the present study. Nevertheless, several natural proteins, have been successfully purified using different chelated metal ions, including iron, as shown in Table 10.4.

Table 10.2 Influence of histidine (His) topography in IMAC

Ligand	Cu	Ni	Zn	Co
0 His ou non accessible	−	−	−	−
I His	+	−	−	−
His-$(X)_n$-His	++	+	−	−
His-$(X)_n$-His n = 2, 3; α helix	+++	+	+	+
His-X-His β strand	+++	+	+	+

Table 10.3 A few examples of recombinant proteins with affinity tags purified by IMAC

Recombinant protein/peptide affinity tag	Metal chelate	References
β-galactosidase, Protein A Ala-His-Gly-His-Arg-Pro	IDA-Zn(II)	Ljungquist et al., 1989
Virus proteins (His)6	NTA-Ni(II)	Janknecht et al., 1991
Tu elongation factor Ser-(His)6	NTA-Ni(II)	Boon et al., 1992
Antibody Fv Fragment (E. coli) (His)6	IDA-Zn(II)	Essen and Skerra, 1993
Lysozyme/T4 His-Gln-(His)3	IDA-Cu(II), Ni(II), Zn(II)	Sloane et al., 1996
Acetylcholine muscarinic receptor (His)6	IDA-Co(II)	Hayashi and Haga, 1996

Table 10.4 A few examples of native proteins, without any affinity tag, purified by IMAC

Proteins purified from crude extracts	Metal chelate	References
Carboxypeptidases (A. niger)	IDA-Cu(II)	Krishnan and Vijayalakshmi, 1986
α-fetoproteins, albumin	IDA-Ni(II)	Andersson et al., 1987a,b
α_2-macroglobulin	IDA-Zn(II)	Kurecki et al., 1979
Fibronectin (collagen binding domain)	IDA-Co(II)	Gmeiner et al., 1995
Lectins	IDA-Ca(II)	Borrebaeck et al., 1981
Muscle enzymes	IDA-Fe(III)	Change et al., 1989
Phophorylase (rat)	IDA-Al(III)	Andersson, 1991
Transferrin and ferritin	DPA-Ni(II)	Winzerling et al., 1995
Immunoglobulin (goat)	TREN-Cu(II)	Boden et al., 1995
Calmodulin	TED-Eu(III)	Chaga et al., 1996

The influence of solvent composition

It follows from the principles listed above that both the adsorption and the elution of a protein in IMAC will depend on pH and on ionic strength. The requirement for the availability of an electron-donor group on the surface of the protein that is at least partially unprotonated would dictate to apply the sample on chelating gels at alkaline pH. Review of the literature, however, reveals successful peptide or protein adsorption at pH values as low as 5 (Krishnan and Vijayalakshmi, 1986; Corradini *et al.*, 1988; Nakagawa *et al.*, 1988). Moreover, almost all of the papers published between 1975 and 1998 mention pHs below 7, giving a mean pH value of 5.9 (1 s.d. = 0.5). The solvated imidazolyl side chain of histidine has a pK_a of about 6 (Perrin and Dempsey, 1987), is half-unprotonated at pH 6, and hence able to establish coordination bonds to chelated metals. Since binding to the chelating matrix causes a shift in the equilibrium towards the formation of unprotonated species, complete protein adsorption is ultimately accomplished. Are other amino acid side chains potential candidates for metal-chelate bond formation at pH 6? The thiol group of cysteine has a pK_a of about 9, while a pK_a value of 15 can be predicted for the side chain of tryptophan based on the Hammett equation (see Perrin *et al.*, 1981). These high pK_a values preclude the participation of these last two residues, and further suggest that histidine is the predominant ligand in IMAC.

Elution of bound proteins in IMAC has traditionally involved either a decrease in pH or the introduction of a competitive ligand such as imidazole. When these two approaches fail, then one must have recourse to a strong chelator such as EDTA and to column flushing of proteins and metal altogether.

When imidazole is used as an affinity eluent, it is recommended, for the purpose of reproducibility, to first *equilibrate* the metal-chelate resin with an imidazole-containing buffer before applying the protein sample and developing the column (Sulkowski, 1985). This is based on the fact that imidazole can form with the chelated metal, stable complexes of the form {chelate − Me(II)(Im)$_n$}. Let us note that the number of imidazole molecules participating in complex formation can vary from 0 to 3 in the case of IDA-Me(II), if the metal-coordination geometry is octahedral (Fig. 10.1). As complex formation corresponds to an equilibrium reaction, it follows that n can take *non-integer* values between 0 and 3. It is to be noted that, the use of imidazole as an eluant under certain experimental conditions (e.g. abrupt increase in concentration without prior "taming" with low concentrations of imidazole) may result in a precarious drop of pH in the mobile phase. This is dealt with in much details by Sulkowski, under the name "proton pumps" (Sulkowski, 1996a,b).

Moreover, even though imidazole must be present in the equilibration buffer, as mentioned above, its initial concentration must be low enough in order not to compete with coordination bond formation between IDA-Me(II) and the protein of interest. The same reasoning applies to other potential ligands, e.g. Tris buffers (Berna *et al.*, 1997), also present in the equilibration solvent. Only those metal-coordination orbitals not stably captured by such ligands can become available for bond formation with the protein.

To quench undesired non-specific electrostatic interactions in IMAC, it is common practice to include salts in the buffers. Yet on occasions such electrostatic interactions can be used to modulate binding selectivity (Corradini *et al.*, 1988; Mrabet, 1992b). Review of the literature shows variations in both the nature (e.g. NaCl, KCl, Na$_2$SO$_4$, or K$_2$SO$_4$) and the concentration (0 to 3 M) of salts. One should then keep in mind the fact that at high enough concentrations (0.5–1 M), salts, especially sulfates, can significantly increase the surface tension of water. This in turn favors ligand/ligate short-range interactions due to the phenomenon of co-solvent exclusion (Arakawa and Timasheff, 1982, 1984) and thereby promotes the formation of coordination bonds (Porath and Olin, 1983). Eventually, high ionic strength may not only stabilize the electron donor-acceptor bond, but also generate new interactions of the hydrophobic type (Figueroa et al., 1986). Therefore, salts can provide another means to adjust selectivity in IMAC.

The inclusion of additional components in IMAC buffers, such as detergents and organic solvents, has been reported (Porath and Olin, 1983; Corradini et al., 1988), and may further serve the purpose of controlling selectivity.

Solvents preparation

As discussed above, the choice for solvents in IMAC will obviously depend on the protein to be separated. If surface histidine residues are present, we can predict that a pH value of 7 is high enough to insure protein retention. Since ligand binding is stronger at higher pH, we can expect, however, that protein desorption will require elution conditions that are more vigorous. According to the bond-length variation rules (Gutmann, 1978), binding energy increases as the donor/acceptor bond length decreases; this in turn eventually favors the formation of additional coordination bonds with other ligands in the protein that are now brought in close contact with the metal, the end result being that the coordination center becomes completely buried, and hence unaccessible to competing electron-donor solutes newly introduced in the solvent for the purpose of elution. Thus, it becomes clear that in order to be able to control protein elution – and also yields – binding must not be too strong; instead, it should be adjusted by appropriate pH reduction and/or by increasing the concentration of a competing ligand such as imidazole (Sulkowski, 1985) or Tris (Berna et al., 1997) in the equilibration buffer. If these approaches fail, choosing a different metal ion such as Ni^{++}, or Zn^{++} or Co^{++} (see Table 10.2) may become relevant (see e.g. Hemdan et al., 1989).

As mentioned above, the chromatographic elution of proteins in IMAC can in some instances be conveniently achieved by reducing the pH of the mobile phase. As histidine becomes protonated with decreasing pH, the binding of this group to the chelated metal ion weakens until the protein is ultimately released to the solvent. The proton is clearly the smallest, and hence likely the best chemical entity one can use as a competing agent, yet its effect turns out to be significantly enhanced with other displacers, such as ammonia or imidazole, present in the solvent (Figueroa et al., 1986; our unpublished observations). Meanwhile, one should bear in mind that the stability of metal chelates is maintained at least through pH 5 for IDA-Cu(II) and IDA-Ni(II) but not for IDA-Zn(II) or IDA-Co(II) (Sulkowski, 1985). This further suggests that special care must be taken in the selection and in the preparation of solvents for proper pH control. Especially, the buffering capacity must be maintained over the whole pH range of the gradient to prevent sudden pH fluctuations. The preparation of buffer mixtures containing equimolar amounts of HEPES ($pK_a = 7.48$ at 25°C and 0.1 M),[2] MES ($pK_a = 6.09$ at 25°C and

---

2 The pK values for hydrolysis of Cu^{++}, Co^{++}, Zn^{++}, and Ni^{++} are 8.0, 8.9, 9.0, and 9.9, respectively, but the onset of precipitation usually occurs about 2–3 pH units below a pK value (Perrin, 1969).

$0.1\,M)^2$, and acetic acid ($pK_a = 4.76$ at $25°C)^2$ was previously described by Figueroa, and have shown to yield a linear pH decrease from 7 to 5 as a result of high, constant, buffer capacity over the pH range 4–8 (Figueroa et al., 1986). More recently, similar buffer mixtures were introduced (Mrabet, 1992a), in which MOPS ($pK_a = 7.15$ at $25°C$ and $0.1\,M)^2$ is substituted for HEPES to prevent the occurrence of oxidative processes that can be produced in piperazine ring-containing Good's buffers (e.g. HEPES; Good et al., 1966) in the presence of copper ions (Hegetschweiler and Saltman, 1986; Grady et al., 1988).

For the purpose of reproducibility, it is a good practice to standardize the preparation of chromatographic solvents. These can be readily obtained by dilution of a concentrated stock solution followed by pH adjustment. The stock solution should be 10–50 times more concentrated and prepared in a volumetric flask containing Milli-Q grade water from correctly weighed amounts of the *acidic* form of high-grade buffers. The resulting solution must then be filter-sterilized through a $0.2\,\mu m$ filter, and can be stored for sufficiently long periods of time (> 1–2 months) in the refrigerator. Although less prone to microbial contamination than phosphate-based buffers, the solvent mixtures described above, however, had better be supplemented with antimicrobial agents such as sodium azide (0.02%, final; at this concentration NaN_3 appears not to exert any influence on coordination). Also micromolar amounts of metal ion can be added to eventually compensate for metal bleeding from the chelating gel during the chromatographic run. At such low concentrations, the presence of free Cu^{++} has previously been shown to have no influence on IMAC of several proteins and peptides (Figueroa et al., 1986; Hutchens and Yip, 1990; Mrabet, 1992b).

In parallel, one should prepare a stock solution (5–10 N) of sodium hydroxide which should be stored in a dark, tightly capped bottle. The final buffer solutions can then be prepared 'on the spot' by mixing precalculated volumes of buffer stock solution and sodium hydroxide to yield the desired pH, adding salt if required, bringing the mixture to the appropriate volume, and finally filter-sterilizing the final solution. A significant advantage of preparing buffers by mixing predetermined amounts of acid and base, as derived from the Henderson-Hasselbalch equation, is reproducibility in terms of buffer composition, including pH and final ionic strength, but also the convenience of bypassing the use – and attendant lengthy, often elaborate calibration – of a pH meter. A buffer mixture containing equimolar amounts (20 mM) of MOPS, MES, and acetic acid, $2\,\mu M\ CuSO_4$, and 0.02% NaN_3 (20 mM MMA) permits good, reproducible pH gradients over the range 5–7 by mixing predetermined amounts of 20 mM MMA, pH 7.0, and 20 mM MMA, pH 5.0 (Mrabet, 1992a).

The elution protocol may also involve using ligand exchange with imidazole. Apart from the comment made earlier concerning the prior equilibration of the gel with the displacer, one should keep in mind that the effective concentration of imidazole ($pK_a = 6.95$ at $25°C$) is that of the unprotonated form. Consequently, unless otherwise required for specific applications, the buffer containing imidazole should have a neutral to slightly alkaline pH. Since the pH of the equilibration buffer is instead likely to be neutral to slightly acidic, this requirement should further promote the use of high buffer-capacity mixtures of the kind just described above.

Column packing

The resin should ideally be packed in a glass column with an adjustable top plunger. After washing with water, the desired amount of gel must be resuspended in a solution of high ionic strength (>0.2 M NaCl) before packing. This follows from the fact that the IDA-gel is highly negatively charged and electrostatic quenching is required for adequate packing. After the gel settles, the column plunger is then gently adjusted and the column is connected to the chromatographic equipment. Packing is continued at a higher flow rate (e.g. 2 mL/min) than the one to be used for purification (e.g. 1 mL/min) with at least 5 column volumes of the high ionic-strength solution while further adjusting the plunger. The column should further be washed with the same volume of water, and finally brought to pH 5 with an appropriate buffer. Acidification of the IDA-gel is intended to prevent the formation of weak bonds with metal ions and to provide for a more homogeneous distribution of the metal-ligation states (see e.g. Porath and Olin, 1983). In addition, divalent metal ions are known to undergo hydrolysis leading to precipitation of insoluble metal hydroxide, and use of lower pH is, therefore, recommended. The column is then saturated with a 0.2 µm-filtered stock solution of the desired metal ion (e.g. 10 mg/mL $CuSO_4$ in H_2O, for which the pH is ~4). Excess and loosely-bound metal is then removed by flushing with (i) 5 column volumes of the pH-5 buffer, (ii) 5 column volumes of the imidazole-containing buffer, (iii) 5 more column volumes of the pH-5 buffer to eliminate imidazole, and finally (iv) 5–6 column volumes of the desired equilibration buffer.

After a chromatographic run that incorporates imidazole as an affinity eluent, it is important to bring the concentration of the displacer back to 'equilibration' values. This requires flushing the column with at least 5–6 volumes of the equilibration buffer. A good indication that equilibration has not been achieved is provided by the premature elution of a reference protein. Many proteins have been successfully purified using IMAC, with different metals. A few examples, covering a period of more than 15 years and from a variety of classes e.g. enzymes; lectins etc. are presented in Table 10.3.

Structural aspects of molecular recognition in IMAC

As biomolecules, proteins are solid objects which can be represented by three-dimensional geometrical bodies of defined volume, shape, and surface. At least from a functional point of view, the external surface is the most important hallmark of biomolecules. This is where the (inter)action takes place. Protein external surfaces are implicated in a variety of interactions with the 'outside world' which includes molecular recognition and assembly, enzymatic catalysis, biochemical regulation, etc. As a result, these interactions require that the protein surface recognizes other surfaces that have a variety of shapes, sizes, and physico-chemical properties. We can therefore state that a full understanding of molecular interactions can be best achieved given a knowledge of the three-dimensional structures of the molecules involved, and more specifically of their molecular surfaces. The first insights into providing an understanding of the relationship between molecular surface structure and protein recognition of immobilized metal ligands were contributed by Sulkowski and colleagues (Sulkowski, 1985, 1987, 1989; Hemdan et al., 1989; Zhao et al., 1991). Sulkowski coined the name "Porath's triad", in recognition of the pioneering work of Porath (Porath et al., 1975), to designate the amino acids most likely involved in IMAC, histidine, tryptophan, and cysteine (Sulkowski, 1985; but see also Sulkowski, 1989). Using model proteins, Sulkowski was able to correlate the availability of electron-donating amino acids on protein surface and chromatographic behavior in IMAC (Sulkowski, 1985, 1987, 1989). Sulkowski was also the first to document a mechanistic link between histidine topography and protein binding selectivity in IMAC (Sulkowski, 1985, 1987, 1989; Zhao *et al.*, 1991).

Clues to IMAC/selectivity

Clues to predicting the specific behavior of a protein in IMAC – using conventional first group transition metal ions complexed with iminodiacetic acid – and hence to engineering selectivity, are likely to be provided by the following observations (Sulkowski, 1987): (i) Protein binding to immobilized metal/chelate complexes requires *sine qua non* that an electron-donor group be both present and accessible; (ii) multiple electron-donating groups on the surface of a protein will enhance its affinity for immobilized metal/chelate complexes; (iii) the microenvironment of the electron donor within the protein affects its pK_a and, hence, by and large determines its electron-donating 'power' and binding avidity; (iv) ligand clustering on the surface of the protein leads to stronger binding to chelated metal ions due to chelate effect; (v) the overall net charge of chelate/metal complexes, e.g. IDA-Cu(II), is negative; this would therefore suggest that ligand binding can be under the influence of both *electrostatic* and *metal-coordination* interactions (see Mrabet, 1992a,b, for an illustration of selectivity engineering by rational manipulation of these two parameters).

Sulkowski's original insights in IMAC were made possible thanks to the use of evolutionay variants of proteins from well-characterized families where at least one protein structure was available for each, at high resolution: cytochromes c, lysozymes, myoglobins, interferons. Clearly, however, the principles that were postulated to govern molecular recognition in IMAC remained based on phenomenological observations. As suggested by this author (Sulkowski, 1989), a precise understanding and demonstration of the mechanism for molecular recognition in IMAC called for the collaboration of "a crystallographer, a cloner and a chromatographer". The following two subheads will, hence, concentrate on important structural aspects relevant to molecular recognition.

Molecular and accessible surfaces

An understanding of protein external surface requires a knowledge of its tridimensional structure at high resolution. Indeed, computation of molecular and accessible surface areas in proteins relies on the atomic coordinates of the molecule. These data are generally obtained with experimental methods such as X-ray crystallography (Bernstein *et al.*, 1977) or nuclear magnetic resonance spectroscopy (Wütrich, 1986), but also by means of theoretical approaches such as structure predictions methods (see Rost and Sander, 1996; Jones, 1997) and molecular dynamics simulations (Goodfellow and Williams, 1992).

In physical models of molecules, atoms are represented by spheres whose size is determined by the atomic van der Waals radii. Molecular models are thus commonly represented as systems of fused hard spheres with unequal radii. Knowledge of atoms radii and coordinates allows one to calculate the area of several types of surfaces which we will describe below.

The "accessible surface" was introduced by Lee and Richards (1971) and is defined as the locus of the center of a probe sphere that rolls onto the molecule surface. The "molecular surface" was later defined by Richards (1977); it is the envelope that is produced by the internal part of the rolling sphere while in contact with the molecule. These two surfaces are shown in Fig. 10.2 which provides a 2D schema, simple yet explicit enough to illustrate the difference between them.

Figure 10.2 shows that the molecular surface is composed of two parts. The first part is the surface of atoms which are in contact with the rolling sphere; the second part, designated as reentrant surface, is the internal surface of the rolling sphere when it is in contact with more that one molecule atom at a time. The molecular surface is essentially utilized for the graphical represention of the surface of macromolecules, and for the study of molecular docking and recognition. Although the accessible surface has no physical "existence", it has been currently used given the facts that, (1) it is easier to compute, (2) it is continuous in contrast to the contact surface, and (3) also because it has been shown to serve in a number of studies as a practical correlation parameter as in, e.g. free energy of transfer.

Defining the size of the spherical probe

It is clear from the above that surface areas will vary with the size of the rolling spherical probe used. In physical terms, the spherical probe represents a small molecule or an

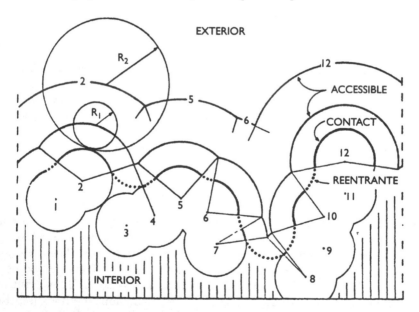

Figure 10.2 Molecular and accessible surfaces. Labeled spheres represent atoms. Two accessible surfaces are shown: One is generated with the sphere of radius, R_1, the other with a sphere of radius, R_2. The molecular surface is the sum of the CONTACT surface with the atoms, and of the REENTRANT surface (dotted line; see text). From Richards (1977; Fig. 1)

atom which explores the surface of the macromolecule. The most used spherical probe has a radius of 1.4 Å to model the water molecule and has served to define atoms in molecules which are either exposed, surface-accessible to solvent, or buried. The 1.4 Å probe, however, is not universal as ligands also vary in size. This feature is clearly illustrated in Fig. 10.2 by using a second spherical probe whose radius is larger than that of water. We readily see that with a change in probe size the accessible surface changes both quantitatively and qualitatively; in particular some "surface" atoms (labeled 1, 3, 4, 7, 8, 9, 10 and 11) which are accessible to the smaller probe (R1) become now buried to the larger probe with radius R2.

These considerations explain the challenge one faces in the process of establishing a reliable method to identify, by means of molecular modeling, atoms in a molecule which can serve as recognition sites to a given ligand. As explained earlier, ligands vary in size but also in shape. Moreover, while any ligand molecule is expected to gyrate in solution and hence behave as a sphere regardless of its actual shape, the effective contact within the encounter complex may require only a small subset of the total surface of the ligand, along with a fixed geometry.

The occurence of such a situation is illustrated below in the identification process of molecular recognition mechanisms that are involved in IMAC. To identify macro-molecular sites accessible to the "elongated" IDA-Cu(II) ligand, the basic molecular modeling rational used is to build a model of a spherical probe whose size is intended to mimic best the metal/chelate complex while in interaction with the macromolecule. Let us consider the copper ion-bound affinity ligand used in Chelating Sepharose Fast Flow, N-[(3'-methoxy-2'-hydroxypropyloxy)-2-hydroxypropyl]-IDA-Cu(II) (des-ignated below as R-IDA-Cu(II); Fig. 10.3). A three-dimensional model of R-IDA-Cu(II) has been built with the modeling tools present in BRUGEL (Delhaise *et al.*, 1985) using standard bond lengths, angles, and energy parameters. The IDA-ligands to the copper atom in R-IDA-Cu(II) were assumed to adopt the octahedral disposition previously described by Porath and Olin (Porath and Olin, 1983) in which the nitrogen atom and the oxygen in one of the carboxylate groups (designated O21 in Fig. 10.3A) are equato-rial ligands, while the oxygen from the other carboxylate (designated O22 in Fig. 10.3A) exists as an axial ligand. In this configuration, lines drawn from the copper atom to each of the coordination ligands are orthogonal. This starting structure was optimized by steepest descent minimization (Fletcher and Reeves, 1964; see Mrabet, 1992a).

Figure 10.3B shows that the molecule is slightly kinked at carbon C1 so that a "minimal" contact surface of the ligand to the protein is expected to include the cop-per atom and its two coordinating oxygens as well as the nearby protruding aliphatic hydrogens designated as H11 and H12 in Fig. 10.3A. On this basis, the probe sphere is centered on the geometric center of the group of atoms that constitute such contact surface. The sphere is then built to also enclose the copper atom and be tangent to its van der Waals surface. This yields a radius of 1.93 Å. In Fig. 10.3B, this spherical probe is represented by the large "open" polyhedron surrounding the copper atom shown as a black sphere (see Mrabet, 1992a).

The spherical probe with radius of 1.93 Å has since then been used in a number of studies to define amino acid residues in proteins as potential ligands to IDA-Cu(II). The first such study was performed in 1992 based on the then recently solved crystal struc-ture of *Actinoplanes missouriensis* D-xylose isomerase (Rey *et al.*, 1988). This led to the

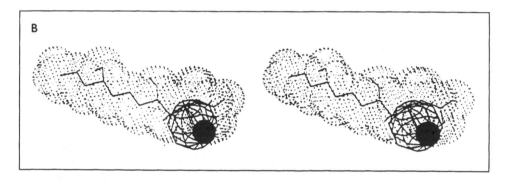

Figure 10.3 Modeled structure of N-[(3'-methoxy-2'-hydroxypropyloxy)-2-hydroxypropyl]- IDA-Cu(II). Panel A shows the chemical structure of R-IDA-Cu(II). Only atoms of interest are labeled. Panel B is a stereo representation of the modeled structure of the probe sphere used in this study to analyze the accessibility of amino acyl residues of R-IDA-Cu(II). The van der Waals surface of the "desolvated" R-IDA-Cu(II) molecule is shown as a Connoly surface in dots (Connoly, 1983) and was generated by using a solvent probe sphere with radius 0. The 1.93 Å probe sphere is represented by an "open" polyhedron surrounding the copper atom shown as a black sphere. In this side view, both the oxygenand the hydrogen pairs, O21 and O22 and H11 and H12, are being juxtaposed perpendicularly to the plane of the figure so that a plane of the contact surface – represented by atom Cu, O21, O22, H11, and H12 – between R-IDA-Cu(II) and the protein would be horizontal and perpendicular to the figure. For the sake of simplicity, the only hydrogens shown in the wire structure are those of the "contact surface", H11 and H12. From Mrabet (1992a, Fig.12.7).

identification of a single surface histidine at position 41 as a candidate to binding to IDA-Cu(II) (Mrabet, 1992a). Replacement of this single residue into either lysine or arginine by site-directed mutagenesis was, indeed, shown to completely abolish such binding, while yielding mutated enzymes with near wild-type properties, hence providing the first direct demonstration for the implication of histidines in IMAC (Mrabet, 1992a).

A more recent study, in 1997, also using the 1.93 Å probe sphere, was concerned with the IMA recognition mechanism of bovine chymotrypsin. This protein model appears ideal and simple as it only contains two surfaces histidines, at positions 40 and

57. Histidine 57 is a member of the catalytic triad (Blow *et al.*, 1970), while histidine 40 lies right at the entrance of the enzyme active site.

ASA computation indicated that only His-57 displayed sufficient accessibility to serve as a ligand to IDA-Cu(II) immobilized onto Novarose. Instead, His-40 was found buried, its side chain pointing toward the protein core. The participation of the catalytic histidine could, however, be clearly ruled out by means of site-specific chemical modification with either N-tosyl-L-phenylalanine chloromethyl ketone (TPCK; Schoellmann and Shaw, 1963) or methyl-4-nitrobenzene sulfonate (MNBS; Nakagawa and Bender, 1970). This apparent conflict between histidine accessibility and its lack of participation in an IMA event could be rationalized on the basis of the existence of a strong hydrogen bonding network around this residue thereby precluding its interaction with the metal/chelate complex.

A second major finding of this study concerns the "buried" His-40 whose implication as an electron donor to IDA-Cu(II) is strongly supported by binding and pH titration data in the same study. Therefore, such an occurence constitues a warning against the elimination of surface residues based on static accessibility calculation alone.

Similar studies were carried out using other serine proteases: bovine and porcine Trypsins, Subtilisins, Thrombin, etc. Contrary to the case of chymotrypsin, all the other serine proteases studied showed at least a partial involvement of the catalytic triad histidine in the protein retention on the IDA-Cu(II)-Novarose matrix (Boden *et al.*, 1998). This can be correlated to the "less strong" hydrogen bonding of the catalytic histidine residue in these serine proteases as opposed to the His 57 of the catalytic triad in chymotrypsin.

Micro analytical methods using the IMA concept

IMA in the Electrokinetic Chromatographic mode

The high potential of IMA-protein recognition as a complementary tool for protein surface/structure studies has prompted some authors to look for microanalytical methods based on IMA-protein recognition (Goubran-Botros and Vijayalakshmi 1991; Nanak *et al.*, 1992; Holmes *et al.*, 1992; Haupt *et al.*, 1996).

The two electrophoretic methods, viz. gel electrophoresis and capillary electrophoresis, using the IMA affinity ligand (soluble polymer coupled IMA-Metal (II)) incorporated with the systems have been worked out with success.

Within the context of this book we will consider the capillary electrophoresis, also known as "electrokinetic chromatography" integrated with IMA concept.

High performance capillary electrophoresis is a rapidly developping method for the analysis of protein and peptides (Lander, 1993). Integration of the affinity concept into the electrokinetic chromatography approach is already used for the study of interaction between proteins and ligands e.g. antigen–antibody complexes (Grossman *et al.*, 1989) monovalent mode protein–sugar interaction (Honda *et al.*, 1992); molecular recognition between proteins and small molecular weight receptor (Chu *et al.*, 1992). In these applications separation is based on different charge to mass characteristics for the protein–ligand complexes, compared to those of the unbound protein. This results in the differential migration in the electrokinetic chromatographic separation. With fast on-off kinetics, the ligand–protein complex equilibrium is quickly attained and one will observe only one peak at a given concentration of ligand. The affinity of the protein for the ligand could thus be calculated using the correlation between the ligand concentration and the differential migration of the protein in the absence and the presence of the ligand (Heegard *et al.*, 1994).

In the case of IMA-electrokinetic chromatographic mode which is named as IMACE (Immobilized Metal ion Affinity Capillary Electrophoresis) the well known metal chelate ligand [IDA-M(II); where M(II) is a bivalent transition metal ion such as Cu^{2+}, Zn^{2+}, Ni^{2+} etc.] is coupled to a soluble polymer and used in the dynamic mode by adding specific amount of the soluble polymer supported metal chelate into the buffer system (Haupt *et al.*, 1996).

By using the following equation

$$\Delta t_N = \frac{\Delta t_N \max C}{K_D + C}$$

where $\Delta t_N = t_N - t_{N0}$; t_N and t_{N0} = normalized retention times in the presence and in the absence of ligand, respectively; one can trace the adsorption isotherms and calculate the dissociation constants. The normalized retention time is used in order to eliminate the influence of electro "endosmosis flow" (EOF) on the migration by dividing the protein/protein–ligand complex migration times by the EOF marker, dimethyl formamide. "C" is the ligand concentration and k_D the ligand–protein dissociation constant.

Dissociation constants for the well established model protein could be determined as shown in Table 10.5.

The k_D values of the tested model proteins are in excellent qualitative agreement with the affinities already reported by the IMAC approach (Sulkowski, 1987), though the absolute values are different. The order of affinities does show a correlation with the number of surface accessible histidine residues in the homologous series of proteins e.g. cytochrome C (Zhao *et al.*, 1991).

Thus the electrokinetics mode of using IMAC could be validated for the quantitative analysis of protein–metal chelate interactions as already elucidated with the conventional column chromatographic approach as shown in the previous pages. This feature could be exploited for probing the histidine containing protein surfaces in terms of

Table 10.5 Dissociation constants of the different model proteins for binding of m-PEG 5000-IDA-Cu(II)

Protein	Dissociation constant K_D (mM)
RNase A (bovine pancreas)	1.31 ± 0.07
RNase B (bovine pancreas)	1.80 ± 0.20
Cytochrome c (Candida krusei)	0.55 ± 0.03
Cytochrome c (horse heart)	29.0 ± 10
Cytochrome c (tuna heart)	B.T.[a]
Kallikrein (porcine pancreas)	2.96 ± 0.10[b]

a Affinity too low.
b Using eCAP neutral capillary.
Source: Adapted with permission from Haupt et al., 1996.

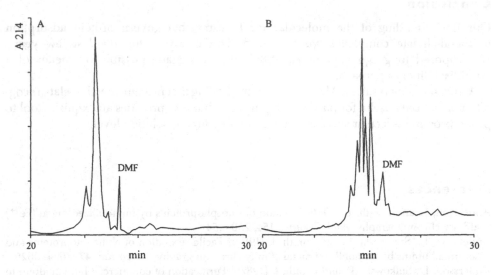

Figure 10.4 Microheterogeneity detection of histidine containing proteins (α-chymotrypsin sub-
species). Capillary electrophoresis separation of a 1 : 1 mixure of native and DIFP-modified
chymotrypsin in absence (a) and in presence of 4 mM (b) m-PEG 5000-IDA-Cu(II). Electrophoretic conditions: fused silica capillary, 27 cm × 20 μm ID. Voltage separation; after
10 min the run was continued with low pressure assistance. From Haupt *et al.* (1996).

structural modifications, albeit, with micro or nanomolar quantities of the sample and
in shorter analysis times.

A few examples of such studies are summarized below:

1. The microheterogeneity of a given histidine containing protein (e.g. chymotrypsin
    subsets) could be detected in Fig. 10.4. (Haupt *et al.*, 1996). As we have already
    seen with IMAC, the resolution of the zymogen and the different subsets of alpha
    chymotrypsin showed a similar pattern, which could be attributed to the differential
    accessibility of their conserved residue, Histidine 40.
2. The modification of histidine surface topography due to chemical modification of
    enzymes e.g. bovine pancreatic ribonuclease A and chymotrypsin and their relation
    to the functional properties could be studied (Baek Won-Ok and Vijayalakshmi,
    1997; Jiang *et al.*, 1999). In the case of bovine pancreatic ribonuclease, chemically
    coupled with amino sugars, through its aspartic or glutamic residues, a tremen-
    dous increase in thermal stability of the active form, could be correlated to the
    increased affinity to the metal chelate ligand, reflecting modification of the active
    site protonation.

    More interestingly, in the case of chemically glycosylated chymotrypsin, the
    affinity data seemed to indicate the generation of a new type of serine protease
    with less strong hydrogen bonds with the catalytic residue histidine 57, as opposed
    to the unmodified enzyme described by Berna *et al.* (1997).
3. The different quarternary structures of a given oligomeric enzyme (e.g. dimeric
    ribonuclease) either produced naturally or by physicochemical means could be
    distinguished and correlated to their functional properties, such as increased activity
    towards the double stranded RNA, cytotoxicity etc. (Varlamov *et al.*, 2001).

Conclusion

Our understanding of the molecular mechanisms that govern protein adsorption to metal-chelate complexes has increased significantly within the last few years. As proposed long ago (Sulkowski, 1989), this was made possible by means of a multidisciplinary approach.

An outstanding result in IMAC has been the finding that protein/metal-chelate recognition is not only useful for purification purposes, but also provides an exquisite tool to probe protein molecular surfaces at a remarkably high resolution level.

References

Andersson, L. and Porath, L. (1986) Isolation of phosphoproteins by immobilized metal (Fe^{3+}) affinity chromatography. *Anal. Biochem.*, **154**, 250–254.

Andersson, L., Sulkowski, E. and Porath, J. (1987a) Facile resolution of alpha-fetoproteins and serum albumins by immobilized metal affinity chromatography. *Cancer Res.*, **47**, 3624–3626.

Andersson, L., Sulkowski, E. and Porath, J. (1987b) Purification of commercial human albumin on immobilized IDA-Ni^{2+}. *J. Chromatogr.*, **421**, 141–146.

Arakawa, T. and Timasheff, S. N. (1982) Preferential interactions of proteins with salts in concentrated solutions. *Biochemistry*, **21**, 6545–6552.

Arakawa, T. and Timasheff, S. N. (1984) Mechanism of protein salting in and salting out by divalent cation salts: balance between hydration and salt binding. *Biochemistry*, **23**, 5912–5923.

Arnold, F. (1991) Metal-affinity separations: a new dimension in protein processing. *Bio/Technol.*, **9**, 151–156.

Baek, Won-Ok and Vijayalakshmi, M. A. (1997) Effect of chemical glycosylation of RNase A on the protein stability and surface histidines accessibility in immobilized metal ion affinity electrophoresis (IMAGE) system. *Biochim. Biophys. Acta.*, **1336**, 394–402.

Belew, M., Yip, T.-T., Andersson, L. and Ehrnström, R. (1987) High-performance analytical applications of immobilized metal ion affinity chromatography. *Anal. Biochem.*, **164**, 457–465.

Berna, P. P., Moraes, F. F., Barbotin, J. N., Thomas, D. and Vijayalakshmi, M. A. (1996) One step affinity purification of a recombinant cyclodextrin glycosyl transferase by Cu(II), Zn(II) tandem coloumn) immobilized metal ion affinity chromatography. *Adv. Mol. Cell Biol.*, **15**, 523–537.

Berna, P. P., Mrabet, N. T., Van Beumen, J., Devreese, B., Porath, J. and Vijayalakshmi, M. A. (1997) Residue accessibility, hydrogen bonding, and molecular recognition: metal-chelate probing of active site histidines in chrymotrypsins. *Biochemistry*, **36**, 6896–6905.

Bernstein, F. C., Koetzel, T. F., Williams, G. J. B., Meyer, E. F. Jr., Brice, M. D., Rodgers, J. R., Kennard, O., Shimanouchi, T., and Tasumi, M. (1977) The protein data bank: a computer-based archival file for macromolecular structures. *J. Mol. Biol.*, **112**, 535–542.

Blow, D. M., Birktoft, J. J. and Hartly, B. S. (1969) Role of a buried acid group in the mechanism of action of chymotrypsin. *Nature*, **221**, 337–340.

Boden, V., Winzerling, J. J., Vijayalakshmi, M. A. and Porath, J. (1995) Rapid one-step purification of goat immunoglobulins by immobilized metal ion affinity chromatography. *J. Immunol. Methods*, **181**, 225–232.

Boden, V., Rangeard, M. H., Mrabet, N. and Vijayalakshmi, M. A. (1998) Histidine mapping of serine protease: a synergic study by IMAC and molecular modelling. *J. Mol. Recogn.*, **11**, 32–39.

Boon, K., Vijgenboom, E., Madsen, L. V., Talens, A., Kraal, B. and Bosch, L. (1992) Isolation and functional analysis of histidine tagged elongation factor Tu. *Eur. J. Biochem.*, **210**, 177–183.

Borrebaeck, C. A. K., Lönnerdal, B. and Etzler, M. E. (1981) Metal ion content of dolichos biflorus lectin and effect of divalent cations on lectin activity. *Biochemistry*, 20, 4119–4122.

Chakrabarti, P. (1990) Geometry of interaction of metal ions with histidine residues in protein structures. *Prot. Eng.*, 4, 57–63.

Chaga, G., Andersson, L., Ersson, B. and Porath, J. (1989) Purification of two muscle enzymes by chromatography on immobilized ferric ions. *Biotechnol. Appl. Biochem.*, 11, 424–431.

Chaga, G. S., Guzman, R. and Porath, J. (1997). A new method of synthesizing biopolymeric affinity ligands. *Biotechnol. Appl. Biochem.*, 26, 7–14.

Chaga, G. S., Ersson, B. and Porath, J. (1996). Isolation of calcium-binding proteins on selective absorbents. Application to purification of bovine calmodulin. *J. Chromatogr. A*, 732, 261–269.

Chu, Y.-H., Avila, L. Z., Biebuyck, H. A. and Whitesides, G. M. (1992) Use of affinity capillary electrophoresis to measure binding constants of ligands to proteins. *J. Med. Chem.*, 35, 2915–2917.

Corradini, D., El Rassi, Z., Horvath, C., Guerra, G. and Horne, W. (1988) Combined lectin-affinity and metal-interaction chromatography for the separation of glycophorins by high-performance liquid chromatography. *J. Chromatogr.*, 458, 1–11.

Cotton, F. A. and Wilkinson, G. (1972) in *Advanced Inorganic Chemistry*, pp. 555–619, John Wiley and Sons, New York.

Cuatrecasas, P., Wilchek, M. and Anfinsen, C. B. (1968) Selective enzyme purification by affinity chromatography. *Proc. Natl. Acad. Sci. U.S.A.*, 61, 636–643.

Dandeu, J.-P., Rabillon, J., Beltrand, M.-J., Lux, M., Duval, R. and David, B. (1990) Immobilized metal ion affinity chromatography for the purification of *Fel dI*, a cat major allergen, from a house-dust extra. *J. Chromatogr.*, 512, 177–188.

Davenckov, V. A. and Semechkin, A. V. (1977) Ligand-exchange chromatography of racemates: Resolution of alpha-amino acids. *J. Chromatogr.*, 141, 313–353.

Delhaise, P., Bardiaux, M. and Wodak, S. J. (1985) Interactive Computer animation of macromolecules. *J. Mol. Graphics*, 2, 103–106. (see also http://www.algonomics.com)

Essen, L. O. and Skerra, A. (1993) Single-step purification of a bacterially expressed anti-body Fv fragment by immobilized metal affinity chromatography in the presence of betaine. *J. Chromatogr. A*, 657, 55–61.

Fanou-Ayi, L. and Vijayalakshmi, M. A. (1983) Metal-chelate affinity chromatography as a separation tool. *Ann. N. Y. Acad. Sci.*, 413, 300–306.

Figueroa, A., Corradini, C., Feibush, B. and Karger, B. L. (1986) High-performance immobilized-metal affinity chromatography of proteins on iminodiacetic acid silica-based bonded phases. *J. Chromatogr.*, 371, 335–352.

Gauthier, J., Amiot, J. and Vijayalakshmi, M. A. (1990) Preparative separation of small molecular weight peptides from casein hydrolysate using gel filtration and immobilized metal ion affinity chromatography. *Preparative Biochem.*, 20(1), 23–50.

Gmeiner, B., Leibl, H., Zerlauth, G. and Seelos, C. (1995). Affinity binding of distinct functional fibronectin domains to immobilized metal chelates. *Arch. Biochem. Biophys.*, 321, 40–42.

Good, N. E., Winget, G. W., Winter, W., Connolly, T. N., Izawa, S. and Singh, R. M. M. (1966) Hydrogen ion buffers for biological research. *Biochemistry*, 5, 467–477.

Goodfellow, J. M. and Williams, M. A. (1992) Molecular Dynamics. *Curr. Opin. Struct. Biol.*, 2, 211-216.

Goubran-Botros, H. G. and Vijayalaksmi, M. (1989) Cell surface interactions with metal chelates. *J. Chromatogr.*, 495, 113–122.

Goubran-Botros, H. and Vijayalakshmi, M. A. (1991) Immobilized metal ion affinity elec-trophoresis: A preliminary report. *Electrophoresis*, 12, 1028–1032.

Grady, J. K., Chasteen, N. D. and Harris, D. C. (1988) Radical from "Goods's" buffer. *Anal. Biochem.*, 173, 111–115.

Grossman, P. D., Colburn, J. C., Lauer, H. H., Nielson, R. G., Riggin, R. M., Sittampalam, G. S. and Rickard, E. C. (1989) Application of free-solution capillary electrophoresis to the analytical scale separation of proteins and peptides. *Anal. Chem.*, **61**, 1186–1194.

Gutmann, V. (1978) in *The Donor-Acceptor Approach to Molecular Interactions*, Plenum Press, New York.

Haupt, K., Roy, F. and Vijayalakshmi, M. A. (1996) Immobilized metal ion affinity capillary electrophoresis of proteins – a model for affinity capillary electrophoresis using soluble polymer-supported ligands. *Anal. Biochem.*, **234**, 149–154.

Hayashi, M. K. and Haga, T. (1996) Purification and functional reconstitution with GTP-binding regulatory proteins of hexahistidine-tagged muscarinic acetycholine receptors (m2 subtype). *J. Biochem.*, **120**, 1232–1238.

Heegard, N. H. H. and Robey, F. A. (1994) The emerging role of capillary electrophoresis as a tool for the study of biomolecular noncovalent interactions. *Int. Lab.*, **21**, 2–8.

Hemdan, E. S. and Porath, J. (1985) Development of immobilized metal affinity chromatography II. Interaction of aminoacids with immobilized nickel imino diacetate. *J. Chromatogr.*, **323**, 255–264.

Hemdan, E. S., Zhao, Y.-J., Sulkowski, E. and Porath, J. (1989) Surface topography of histidine residues: a facile probe by immobilized metal ion affinity chromatography. *Proc. Natl. Acad. Sci. U.S.A.*, **86**, 1811–1815.

Hochuli, E., Dobeli, H. and Schacher, A. (1987) New metal chelate absorbent selective for proteins and peptides containing neighbouring histidine residues. *J. Chromatogr.*, **411**, 177–184.

Hubert, P. and Porath, J. (1981) Metal chelate affinity chromatography. I. Influence of various parameters on the retention of nucleotides and related compounds. *J. Chromatogr.*, **206**, 164–168.

Holmes, L. D., Serag, A. A., Plunkett, S. D., Todd, R. J. and Arnold, F. H. (1992) Metal-affinity electrophroresis of histidine-containing peptides, in *Methods: A Companion to Methods in Enzymology*. (Arnold, ed.), vol 4, Academic Press Inc., New York, U.S.A., pp. 103–108.

Honda, S., Taga, A., Suzuki, S. and Kakehi, K. (1992) Determination of the association constant of monovalent mode protein-sugar. *J. Chromatogr.*, **597**, 377–382.

Hutchens, T. W., Yip, T.-T. and Porath, J. (1988) Protein interaction with immobilized ligands: quantitative analyses of equilibrium partition data and comparaison with analytical chromatographic approaches using immobilized metal affinity absorbents. *Anal. Biochem.*, **170**, 168–182.

Hutchens, T. W., Li, C. M., Sato, Y. and Yip, T.-T. (1989) Multiple DNA-binding estrogen receptor forms resolved by interaction with immobilized metal ions. Identification of a metal-binding domain. *J. Biol. Chem.*, **264**, 17206–17212.

Hutchens, T. W. and Yip, T.-T. (1990a) Differential interaction of peptides and protein surface structures with free metal ions and surface-immobilized metal ions. *J. Chromatogr.*, **500**, 531–542.

Hutchens, T. W. and Yip, T.-T. (1990b) Protein interactions with immobilized transition metal ions: quantitative evaluations of variations in affinity and binding capacity. *Anal. Biochem.*, **191**, 160–168.

Janknecht, R., Martynoff, G., Lou, J., Hipskind, R. A., Norheim, A. and Stunnenberg, H. G. (1991) Rapid and efficient purification of native histidine tagged protein expressed by by recombinant vaccinia virus. *Proc. Natl. Acad. Sci. U.S.A.*, **88**, 8972–8976.

Jiang, K.-Y., Pitiot, O., Anissimova, M., Adenier, H. and Vijayalakshmi, M. A. (1999) Structure/function relationship in glycosylated Chymotrypsin as probed by IMAC and IMACE. *Biochim. Biophys. Acta.*, **1433**, 198–209.

Jiang, W., Graham, B., Spiccia, L. and Hearn, M. T. W. (1998) Protein selectivity with immobilized metal ion-tacn sorbents: chromatographic studies with human serum proteins and several other globular proteins. *Anal. Biochem.*, **255**, 47–58.

Jones, D. T. (1997) Successful ab initio prediction of the tertiary structure of NK-lysin using multiple sequences and recognized supersecondary structural motifs. *Proteins*, 1, 185–191.

Krishnan, S. and Vijayalakshmi, M. A. (1986) Purification and some properties of three serine carboxy peptidases from Aspergillus niger. *J. Chromatogr.*, 370, 315–326.

Kurecki, T., Kress, L. F. and Laskowski, M. Sr (1979) Purification of human plasma alpha 2 macroglobulin and alpha 1 proteinase inhibitor using zinc chelate chromatography. *Anal. Biochem.*, 99, 415–420.

Laboureau, E. and Vijayalakshmi, M. A. (1997) Concerning the separation of mammalian cells in immobilized metal ion affinity partitioning systems: a matter of selectivity. *J. Mol. Recognit.*, 10, 262–688.

Landers, J. P. (1993) Capillary electophoresis: pioneering new approaches for biomolecular analysis. *TIBS*, 18, 409–414

Lee, B. and Richards, F. M. (1971) The interpretation of protein structures: estimation of static accessibility. *J. Mol. Biol.*, 55, 379–400.

Liu, Y. and Yu, S. (1990) Copper(II)-iminodiacetic acid chelating resin as a stationary phase in the immobilized metal ion affinity chromatography of some aromatic amines. *J. Chromatogr.*, 515, 169–173.

Ljungquist, C., Bertholtz, A., Brink-Nilsson, H., Moks, T., Uhlen, M. and Nilsson, B. (1989) Immobilization and affinity purification of recombinant proteins using histidine peptide fusions. *Eur. J. Biochem.*, 186, 563–569.

Mrabet, N. T. (1992a) One-step purification of Actinoplanes missouriensis D-xylose isomerase by high-performance immobilized copper-affinity chromatography: functional analysis of surface histidine residues by site-directed mutagenesis. *Biochemistry*, 31, 2690–2702.

Mrabet, N. T. (1992b) Physicochemical and structural implications for molecular recognition in immobilized metal affinity chromatography, in *Methods: A Companion to Methods in Enzymology*. (Arnold, ed.), vol 4, Academic Press Inc., New York, USA, pp. 14–24.

Muszynska, G., Andersson, L. and Porath, J. (1986) Selective adsorption of phosphoproteins on gel-immobilized ferric chelate. *Biochemistry*, 25, 6850–6853.

Nakagawa, Y. and Bender, M. L. (1970) Methylation of histidine-57 in alpha-chymotrypsin by methyl p-nitrobenzenesulfonate. A new approach to enzyme modification. *Biochemistry*, 9, 259–264.

Nakagawa, Y., Yip, T.-T., Belew, M. and Porath J. (1988) High-performance immobilized metal ion affinity chromatography of peptides: analytical separation of biologically active synthetic peptides. *Anal. Biochem.*, 168, 75–81.

Nanak, E., Abdoul-Nour, J. and Vijayalakshmi, M. A. (1992) Metal affinity electrophoresis: an analytical tool, in *Methods: A Companion to Methods in Enzymology*. (Arnold, ed.), vol 4, pp. 97–102, Academic Press Inc., New York, USA.

Nanak, E., Vijayalakshmi, M. A. and Chadha, K. C. J. (1995) Segregation of normal and pathological human red blood cells, lymphocytes and fibroblasts by immobilized metal-ion affinity partitioning. *J. Mol. Recognit.*, 8, 77–84

Pearson, R. G. (1990) Hard and soft acids and bases – The evolution of a chemical concept. *Coord. Chem. Rev.*, 100, 403–425.

Perrin, D. D. (1969) Dissociation constants for inorganic acids and bases, Buttherworths, London.

Perrin, D. D., Dempsey, B. and Serjeant, E. P. (1981) pK_a Prediction for Organic Acids and Bases, p. 61, Chapmann and Hall, London.

Perrin, D. D. and Dempsey, B. (1987) Buffers for pH and Metal Ion Control, p. 159, Chapman and Hall, London.

Porath, J. and Kristiansen, T. (1975) In *The Proteins* (Neurath, H. and Hill, R. L. eds), Vol. 1, pp. 95–178, Academic Press, New York.

Porath, J., Carlsson, J., Olsson, I. and Belfrage, G. (1975) Metal chelate affinity chromatography, a new approach to protein fractionation. *Nature*, 258, 598–599.

Porath, J. and Olin, B. (1983) Immobilized metal ion affinity adsorption and immobilized metal ion affinity chromatography of biomaterials. Serum protein affinities for gel-immobilized iron and nickel ions. *Biochemistry*, **22**, 1621–1630.

Porath, J. (1992) Immobilized metal ion affinity chromatography. *Protein Expr. Purif.*, **3**, 263–281.

Reif, O. W., Nier, V., Bahr, U. and Freitag, R. (1994) Immobilized metal affinity adsorbers as stationary phase for metal interaction. *J. Chromatogr.*, **664**, 13–25.

Rey, F., Jenkins, J., Janin, J., Lasters, I., Alard, P., Claessens, M., Matthyssens, G. and Wodak, S. J. (1988) Structural analysis of the 2.8 A model of xylose isomerase from actinoplances missouriensis. *Proteins: Struct., Funct., Genet.*, **4**, 165–172.

Richards, F. M. (1977) Areas, volumes, packing and protein structure. *Ann. Rev. Biophys. Bioeng.*, **6**, 151–176.

Rost, B. and Sander, C. (1996) Bringing the protein sequence-structure gap by structure predictions. *Annu. Rev. Biophys. Biomol. Struct.*, **25**, 113–136.

Schoellmann, G. and Shaw, E. (1963), Direct evidence for the presence of histidine in the active site center of chymotrypsin. *Biochemistry*, **2**, 252–255.

Scopes, R. K. (1987a) *Protein Purification: Principles and Practice*, pp. 133–141, Springer-Verlag, New York.

Scopes, R. K. (1987b) *Protein Purification: Principles and Practice*, pp. 167–172, Springer-Verlag, New York.

Sloane, R. P., Ward, J. M., O'Brien, S. M., Thomas, O. R. T. and Dunnill, P. (1996) Expression and purification of a recombinant metal-binding T4 lysozyme fusion protein. *J. Biotechnol.*, **49**, 231–238.

Smith, M., Furman, T. C., Ingolia, T. D. and Pidgeon, C. (1988) Chelating peptide-immobilized metal ion affinity chromatography. A new concept in affinity chromatography for recombinant proteins. *J. Biol. Chem.*, **263**, 7211–7215.

Steinmann, L., Porath, J., Hashemi, P. and Olin, A. (1994) Preparation and some properties of a polyethyleneimine-agarose metal adsorbent. *Talanta*, **41**, 1707–1713

Sulkowski, E. (1985) Purification of proteins by IMAC. *Trends Biotechnol.*, **3**, 1–7.

Sulkowski, E. (1987) *Protein Purification – Micro to Macro(UCLA Symposia on Molecular and Cellular Biology, New Series* (R. Burgess, ed.) vol. 68, pp. 149–162, Alan R. Liss, New York.

Sulkowski, E. (1989) The saga of IMAC and MIT. *BioEssays*, **10**, 170–175.

Sulkowski, E. (1996a) Immobilized metal-ion affinity chromatography: imidazole proton pump and chromatographic sequelae. I. Proton pump. *J. Mol. Recognit.*, **9**(5–6), 389–393.

Sulkowski, E. (1996b) Immobilized metal-ion affinity chromatography: imidazole proton pump and chromatographic sequelae. II. Chromatographic sequelae. *J. Mol. Recognit.*, **9**(5–6), 494–498.

Vallee, B. L. and Auld, D. S. (1990) Active-site zinc ligands and activated H_2O of zinc enzymes. *Proc. Natl. Acad. Sci. U.S.A.*, **87**, 220–224.

Varlamov, V., Anissimova, M., Baek, W. O. and Vijayalakshmi, M. A. (2001) Immobilized Metal ion Affinity gel Electrophoresis of microbial Ribonucleases and Protein inhibitor Barstar. *Int. J. Bio. Chromatogr.*, (in press)

Vijayalakshmi, M. A. (1989) Pseudo-biospecific ligand affinity chromatography, Tibtech. *Trends in Biotechnol.*, **7**, 71–76

Wilchek, M., Miron, T. and Kohn, J. (1984) Affinity chromatography. *Methods Enzymol.*, **104**, 3–55.

Winzerling, J. J., Pham, D. Q., Kunz, S., Samaraweera, P., Law, J. H. and Porath, J. (1996) Purification of recombinant insect transferrin from large volumes of cell culture medium using high capacity Ni(2+)-dipicolylamine gel. *Protein. Expr. Purif.*, **7**, 137–142.

Wütrich, K. (1986) N.M.R. of proteins and nucleic acids, John Wiley and Sons.

Zhao, Y.-J., Sulkowski, E. and Porath, J. (1991) Surface topography of histidine residues in lysozymes. *Eur. J. Biochem.*, **202**, 1115–1119.

Chapter 11

Thiophilic interaction chromatography

Sven Oscarsson and Francisco Batista Viera

Introduction

Thiophilic adsorption chromatography was introduced by Porath and coworkers in 1985 (Porath *et al.*, 1985). The thiophilic adsorbent (T-gel) displays an immobilized ligand: an aliphatic chain having adjacent, ($-SO_3-CH_2-CH_2-S-$) sulphone and thioether constituents. Since adsorption of proteins on a T-gel is promoted by antichaotropic salts, it can be readily reversed by depleting those salts in the mobile phase. Such cosolvents have a strong influence on the protein adsorption selectivity (Oscarsson *et al.*, 1997, 1998).

During the initial phase of the investigation of the T-gel most of the interest was focused on the application of this adsorbent for purification of immunoglobulins and monoclonal antibodies from different types of biological samples. However, several other proteins such as α_2-macroglobulin (Porath *et al.*, 1985), lysozyme, trypsin (Hutchens *et al.*, 1987), and sweet potato β-amylase (Franco-Fraguas *et al.*, 1992) have been successfully purified by this method.

Later, studies have been concerned with the mechanism of the interactions. The mechanistic studies have primarily focused on the adsorbent by studying the effect on the interaction after exchanging or combining different atoms in the ligand. Especially the importance of sulphur in the low molecular substance in combination with neighbouring atoms has been studied at the atomic level. During investigations concerning the mechanism several researchers have focused on finding the interaction site or sites between immunoglobulins and the thiophilic adsorbents but no experimental evidence for the proposed interaction sites has yet been published.

Factors affecting thiophilic adsorption

Molecular structure of the thiophilic ligand and the effect of different matrixes

The importance of the sulphur atom and the sulphone group in the thiophilic adsorbents was shown by Porath and coworkers. (Porath *et al.*, 1985). By using the epoxy activation method in combination with mercaptopyridine instead of the DVS-activation method the original general structure could be replaced by $M-O-CH_2-CH(OH)-CH_2-S-Pyridin$ (M is the agarose matrix) (Porath *et al.*, 1988). Sulphur was confirmed to be essential even in this structure but in combination with a pyridine (Oscarsson *et al.*, 1990). Thus, thiophilic adsorbents can be classified into two categories, depending on the method chosen for solid phase activation:

(i) divinylsulfone-based adsorbents, to which aliphatic or heterocycles have been coupled;
(ii) epoxy-activated supports, to which heterocycles have been coupled.

The original T-gel was developed using agarose as a matrix. As an alternative to agarose, derivatized silica beads have been used with the purpose to develop the one-step purification of polyclonal and monoclonal antibodies on HPLC mode (Nopper *et al.*, 1989; Schwartz *et al.*, 1994). This new silica-based thiophilic adsorbent bears palindromic thioethers around the essential sulfone group, $-S-CH_2CH_2-SO_2-CH_2CH_2-S-$. It was successfully employed for the fast HPLC purification of immunoglobulins from ascites fluid and serum. Purification of antibodies from hybridoma culture supernatant is also possible, provided that the growth medium does not contain the indicator phenol red (which binds the adsorbent and competes with antibodies, reducing the binding capacity for them by almost 90%). The "3S-silica" thiophilic adsorbent exhibits high capacity and is suitable for the rapid and single-step purification of all subclasses of mouse or rat monoclonal immunoglobulins in a relatively short time (10 min) and can easily be adapted to a preparative scale. The effects of introducing more sulphur atoms on the properties of thiophilic adsorbents have been evaluated (Schwarz *et al.*, 1994). The 3S and 4S structures seem to be best suited for thiophilic adsorption chromatography of antibodies from ascites and serum; but the 5S and 6S structures do not seem to be useful for protein chromatography, since they bind all proteins loaded which are difficult to elute under normal conditions.

El Rassi (El Rassi, 1989) has proved that macroporous microparticulate silica-based stationary phases, appropriately bonded with sulfone-thioether functions, are suitable for high-performance thiophilic interaction chromatography of proteins.

Comparison of the chromatographic behaviour of model proteins on both silica-sulfone-thioether and silica-bound polyether (an hydrophobic interaction phase) columns suggested that the retention of proteins on the sulfone-thioether column is due to mixed thiophilic and hydrophobic interactions.

A number of aromatic and heteroaromatic compounds containing hydroxyl or amino groups have been coupled to divinyl sulfone-activated agarose (Knudsen *et al.*, 1992). The resulting sulfone-aromatic adsorbents have the general formula: $M-O-CH_2CH_2-SO_2-CH_2CH_2-X-Y$, where M is the agarose matrix, X is oxygen or nitrogen, and Y is an aromatic or heteroaromatic compound.

These sulfone/aromatic sorbents displayed thiophilic binding properties when tested for the selective binding of immunoglobulins from human serum. With the purpose of performing fast one-step purification of antibodies two other adsorbents were synthesized, by choosing mercapto-heterocycles (mercapto-pyrimidine, mercapto-thiazoline) with more than one heteroatom in the ring structure, as they provide higher hydrophilicity and a higher electron density (Schwartz *et al.*, 1995). The purification of antibodies from ascites fluids was excellent, ca. 90% pure and the biological activity was preserved as well. According to Noel and coworkers (Noel *et al.*, 1996), the divinylsulphone matrix itself is enough to get the same binding capacity and purity for IgG and IgA. Even the recovery is the same from blood serum. Berna and Porath (Berna, P. *et al.*,

1996) has recently published a new type of thiophilic adsorbent. It is constituted by tricyanoaminopropene covalently coupled to DVS-activated agarose. The protein capacity was found to be 9 mg/ml of gel when serum was loaded on the column of which 65% are immunoglobulines.

The effect of the ligand density on adsorption and desorption efficiency

The ligand density on the adsorbent is very important for the extent of adsorption as well as desorption of proteins. The degree of substitution will affect not only the efficiency of adsorption but also the selectivity. By increasing the substitution degree the capacity of sorbent to bind proteins increases but in parallel the selectivity decreases.

On the other hand lower salt concentrations can often be used which counteract the decreasing selectivity and at the same time preserve biological activity (Schwartz et al., 1995). The tendency for the thiophilic adsorbents to behave like hydrophobic ones is more pronounced when the ligand density increases. The pure thiophilic effect will gradually be replaced by a hydrophobic effect (Knudsen et al., 1992). Oscarsson and coworkers compared the degree of adsorption and desorption of proteins from a thiophilic gel with traditional hydrophobic ones at different substitution degrees. They found this type of thiophilic gel to be at least as efficient as the hydrophobic adsorbents for protein adsorption and more efficient to desorb proteins from, simply by deleting salt from the buffer. The traditional hydrophobic adsorbents were too hydrophobic with difficulties to desorb proteins. (Oscarsson et al., 1995).

Effects of cosolvents

Studies of thiophilic gels based on the divinylsulfone molecular structure

Thiophilic interactions and hydrophobic interactions are both salt promoted processes. High concentrations of the structure-forming salts in the Hofmeister series have different effects on the adsorption capacities of the thiophilic and hydrophobic gels towards the proteins they selectively adsorb. Thus, for the hydrophobic gel, high concentrations of phosphate, sulphate and chloride anions increase the adsorption of proteins according to the order in the series. In the case of the thiophilic gel, however, high concentrations of chloride anions markedly decrease its adsorption capacity (Porath et al., 1985; Hutchens et al., 1986).

Studies of thiophilic gels based on heterocycles

The conditions for a true thiophilic interaction must be optimized and probably for each type of biological sample used. Not only the substitution degree of the ligand but also the type of salt and salt concentration must be optimized. By using potassium sulphate or sodium chloride of a certain concentration in thiophilic adsorption of a human serum sample, the lowest amount of human serum albumin (less than 0.05% of the total amount of HSA in the sample) and the highest amount of IgG were obtained in the eluate from a mercaptopyrine derivatized agarose (Oscarsson et al., 1995). However, the type of proteins identified in the elute was drastically changed by changing salt. The salient features of thiophilic ligand are the presence of a nucleophile (thioether sulphur, which can be replaced by nitrogen), and a sulfone group in close proximity to each other. These two groups seem to react with counter ligands on a protein in a cooperative fashion to produce an adsorption complex, through an EDA (electron donor-acceptor) mechanism (Porath et al., 1987).

Most probably aromatic amino acid side-chains constitute the counter sites on the proteins which interact with the T-gel. That is strongly suggested by the studies performed with model peptides; dipeptides composed entirely of aromatic amino acids, were bound by T-gel. The extent to which they were bound to the T-gel was in the order: $(Trp)_2 \gg (Phe)_2 > (Tyr)_2$.

It is interesting to note that two chemically very different structures, one based on divinylsulfone, the other based on mercaptoheterocycles, show the same chromatographic behaviour towards proteins in general and towards antibodies in particular. Even the affinity constants for the divinylsulfone based ligands and for the heterocycle-based ligands are of the same order of magnitude of 10^{-7} M for antibodies.

One interesting finding concerning electron density in the heterocyclic ligands was obtained when the electron density for three different heterocycles were calculated (Oscarsson et al., 1990).

From these calculations mercaptopyridine was found to have a lower electron density in the ring compared with hydroxypyridine and amino pyridine (Oscarsson et al., 1990). These results show that a polarisation exists in the molecule which can be the main contributing factors.

The studies of Khamlichi (Khamlichi et al., 1995) and Noel (Noel et al., 1996) show that the sulphone group itself in the original T-gel without the thioether is enough to get selective adsorption of IgG from serum which shows that the polarisation in the sulfone group itself is enough to get the thiophilic effect. In the presence of ammonium acetate six out of seven proteins were identified in the eluate by immuno diffusion. By using ammonium chloride two out of seven proteins were found (Oscarsson, 1995). The effect of different salts on the type of proteins adsorbed to the heterocyclic thiophilic adsorbents clearly shows that the thiophilic effect is not only dependent on the ligand but also on the salt. Why there is adsorption of one protein to an adsorbent in the presence of one salt but not in the presence of another salt?

Since proteins in solution are known to oscillate between different conformations (Dill, 1990) some of these switches can be more frequent under different microenvironments, leading to exposure of certain regions in the protein molecule which interact with the surface (Oscarsson, 1995).

Effect of pH

The alkaline instability of sulfone-based adsorbents as well as of adsorbents where mercaptopyridine is coupled directly to the epoxyactivated matrix (Oscarsson et al., 1990) limits the use of 1 M NaOH as an often used method to regenerate the adsorbent after finishing the purification procedure. This step is especially important on a preparative process scale to avoid problems with bacteria, viruses and pyrogen contaminations during storage and for the elimination of macromolecules still adsorbed to the gel after the final desorption step. An alkaline stable adsorbent has been developed, mercaptomethylenepyridine-derivatized agarose gel (Berna, N. et al., 1996) which has been shown to be stable against 1 M NaOH (Oscarsson *et al.*, 1996) and which shows the same selectivity and capacity for IgG before and after prolonged contacts with sodium hydroxide.

Mechanisms of thiophilic interaction

Principles underlying adsorption on thiophilic and hydrophobic gels have been clearly demonstrated by Porath and coworkers to be different (Porath *et al.*, 1985). Elementary ligand in thiophilic gel bears a thioethylsulfone backbone which possesses neither a pronounced hydrophobicity nor any charge. According to Porath (1987) nucleophilic attack on an electron-deficient portion of the protein molecule (the counter-ligand) may lead to the transfer of a fraction of an electron unit from the nucleophile on the ligand (represented as X in Fig. 11.1) to the electron-acceptor on the protein which could be a localized atom of an indole group. This will lead to the formation of a weak bond. This complex might by strengthened by a concomitant interaction between the sulfone group and a site on the protein which is in close proximity to the previous interaction site resulting in a four-point contact between ligand and counter-ligand. The driving force could be derived from the disruption of the organized water structure surrounding the interactants. The sulfone group interacts by virtue of its dipole character or by accepting counter-ligand electrons in the 3-d orbitals of the sulfur atom.

If the counter-sites on the protein were contained in hydrophobic regions of the protein backbone, the aqueous phase in such a partially-enclosed cavity would be relatively less polar than in the bulk of the surrounding water. This would be accentuated by the presence of structure-forming salts which impose highly ordered water structures around the ligand and its interacting counter-site on the protein. In this situation "salting-out" would be favored, resulting in close contact between the ligand and the counter-site on the protein. In such a predominantly non-polar environment enclosed within a hydrophobic cavity, the methylene group of the ligand might be activated to

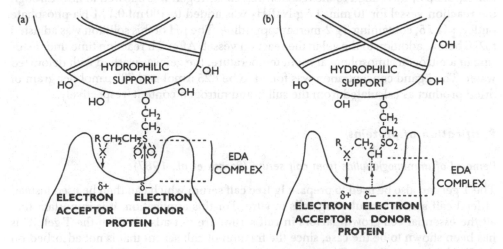

Figure 11.1 Schematic depiction of the mechanism of thiophilic interaction according to Porath *et al.* (a) Formation of the ligate–ligand complex, viz. an electron–acceptor complex (EDA-complex) or (b) formation of a hydrophobic "amphichelate".

form a "proton jump" due to its close proximity to a sulfone group. This "activated" hydrogen atom would tend to form a hydrogen bond with a π-electron system of an aromatic or heteroaromatic nucleus which is part of the interacting counter-site on the protein, thus forming an electron donor-acceptor (EDA) complex. The electron-deficiency in the aromatic nucleus would be counter balanced by the flow of electrons from the nucleophilic sulfur or nitrogen schematically illustrated in Fig 11.1.

Applications

The T-gel has proved to be a useful tool for the selective isolation of monoclonal antibodies from ascites fluid (Belew et al., 1987). It also has an affinity towards immunoglobulins in sera of several species (e.g. human, mouse, sheep, goat, bovine, pig, dog, hen, rabbit) and a high capacity (25 mg of immunoglobulin per ml packed gel) and allows for essentially one chromatographic purification step. The yield is generally high and up to 85–90% immunoglobulins are recovered from T-gels under low salt conditions.

Affinity for thiophilic ligands is not restricted to immunoglobulins, and T-gel could be employed also for purification of certain other proteins, such as α_1-macroglobulin (Porath et al., 1985), lysozyme, trypsin (Hutchens, 1987), and sweet potato β-amylase (Franco-Fraguas et al., 1992).

Synthesis of thiophilic sorbents

Thiophilic sorbents are commercially available from Sigma, Amersham Pharmacia Biotech and Pierce. However, their synthesis are easily performed and experimental protocols are available in the literature. (Porath et al., 1985, 1988; Hutchens et al., 1992; Nopper et al., 1989; Schwartz et al., 1994, 1995; Oscarsson et al., 1995; Berna et al., 1996).

Suction dried epoxy-activated agarose (25 g), prewashed with 0.1 M Na-phosphate buffer, pH 6.8, was added to the reaction vessel. Nitrogen was allowed to flow through the reaction vessel for 10 min. 1.5 g $NaBH_4$ was added to 100 ml 0.1 M Na-phosphate buffer, pH 7.5, containing 3 g 2-mercaptopyridine. The pH of this solution was adjusted to 6.6 before addition to the gel in the reaction vessel. After 3 h reaction time under stirring in a nitrogen atmosphere at room temperature, the gel was washed with deionized water. The ligand concentration was found to be 825 μmol and 793 μmol per gram of dried product as calculated from the sulfur and nitrogen content, respectively.

Purification of proteins

Removal of immunoglobulins from calf serum (Porath et al., 1987)

The T-gel can also be used to prepare Ig-free calf serum which can then be used instead of fetal calf serum for culturing cells in vitro. For this application, it is important that all the essential cell-growth factors in calf serum are not adsorbed on the T-gel. This has been shown to be the case, since the fraction of calf serum that is not adsorbed on the T-gel is essentially as effective as the control calf serum in maintaining the survival and growth of hybridoma cells in culture. In the same study, it was also shown that monoclonal antibodies produced in culture media using this Ig-free calf serum could be purified by a single-step chromatographic procedure on the thiophilic gel to yield a highly purified Mab preparation (see Fig. 11.2). Thus, the virtual absence of interfering Igs from serum obviates subsequent, often tedious purification of Mabs produced in cell culture media. This method will thus make it possible to replace the more expensive fetal-calf serum by Ig-free calf (or adult bovine) serum.

Secretory IgA, IgG and IgM immunoglobulins isolated simultaneously from colostral whey by selective thiophilic adsorption (Hutchens et al., 1989)

The major immunoglobulin classes typically present in colostrum were simultaneously removed from a porcine colostral whey model system using a single-step preparative scale procedure based on thiophilic interaction chromatography. The adsorption and recovery procedures operate efficiently under mild buffer conditions permitting the subsequent cooperative analyses of individual immunoglobulin classes for structural and functional heterogeneity. Thus, 1 litre columns of thiophilic adsorbent were employed to obtain pure, structurally intact immunoglobulins from 1 litre batches of porcine colostral whey.

Chromatographic purification of IgG from bovine milk whey (Konecny et al., 1994)

The purification of IgG from sweet cheese whey was accomplished on commercially available "classical" T-gels.

Preparation of samples for adsorption onto thiophilic gels requires only the addition of salt (potassium, ammonium or sodium sulphates). Sodium sulphate (at 0.5 M concentration) was found to be the most effective amongst the salts tested.

The thiophilic gel has proven to be useful in the isolation of IgG, giving a preparation with a purity comparable to that obtained by protein G chromatography (74% and 81%, respectively). Thus, this method may be suitable for large-scale whey IgG isolation. Although immunoglobulins are minor whey protein components, they have a high potential economic value.

Purification of monoclonal antibodies (Belew et al., 1987)

For many applications of monoclonal antibodies, it is desirable to have highly purified preparations free from the extraneous proteins present in ascites fluids or in cell culture media. Ideally, a purification method chosen should result in a homogeneous antibody preparation of a high yield. Conventional purification methods used include affinity chromatography on Protein A- or Protein G-Sepharose, ion-exchange chromatography on DEAE-Sepharose and chromatography on hydroxylapatite. Protein A or protein G-based adsorbents are expensive to operate due to the cost of the media. Furthermore, Protein A-Sepharose binds mouse IgG1 and IgM rather poorly and thus is quite unsuitable for their purification when produced by many hybridoma cell lines. Moreover, the low pH that is often used to elute the bound monoclonal antibodies from this adsorbent has adverse effects on the antibody activity of some monoclonals. Non-specific methods like hydroxyapatite or ion-exchange chromatography possess low capacity or yield antibodies contaminated with albumin and transferrin.

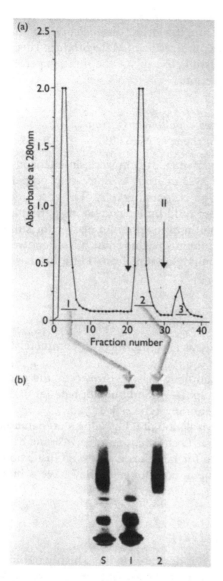

Figure 11.2 Thiophilic interaction chromatography of mouse ascites fluid. (a) Elution profile of mouse ascites fluid after fractionation on a column (16 × 35 mm., bed volume = 7 ml) of T-gel. The sample (7 ml) contains IgG2b monolconal antibodies. Equilibration buffer: 50 mM Tris–HCl, 0.5 M K_2SO_4. The sample also contains 0.5 M K_2SO_4 and was clarified by centrifugation prior to application onto column, (0–0), absorbance at 280 nm; x–x, distribution of anti-IgG2b activity. Pooled fractions (1–3) are shown by horizontal bars. (b) Gradient gel (4–30% polyacrylamide gel slabs) electrophoretic patterns of pooled fractions shown in, (a) and the unfractionated ascites fluid (S). With the exception of a minor impurity of low molecular weight, the purified MAbs (#3) are electrophoretically homogenous.

A one-step method for the purification of Mabs on a thiophilic adsorbent (T-gel) has been reported (Belew *et al.*, 1987). The use of "T-gel" allows the efficient purification of monoclonal antibodies from mouse ascites fluids and from the culture media of cloned cells . The recovery of the purified IgG is better than 90%, although for IgM is considerably lower. T-gel is well suited for purifying all the subclasses of mouse monoclonal IgG by a single chromatographic step and it has broad specificity towards immunoglobulins derived from several other species.

The degree of purification obtained is, in certain instances, comparable to that obtained by biospecific affinity chromatography based on antigen-antibody interactions. Since sample preparation requires only the addition of K_2SO_4 (0.5 M) to the ascites fluid or cell culture media, this purification method is also well suited for large-scale operations. The purified Igs are eluted by an essentially salt-free buffer at near neutral pH thus obviating the need for post-treatment of the sample before storage or use (see Fig. 11.3).

Procedure. The required amount of solid K_2SO_4 to give a final concentration of 0.5 M was added to the sample solution (cell culture medium or ascites fluid). The mixture was stirred gently until the added salt had dissolved and the solution was clarified by centrifugation. The T-gel was packed in a suitable column and equilibrated with 50 mM sodium phosphate buffer, containing 0.5 M K_2SO_4, pH 8.0 (adsorption buffer). After sample application, the column was washed with the adsorption buffer until unabsorbed material was washed out. The adsorbed Ig was then eluted with 50 mM sodium phosphate buffer, pH 8.0 (desorption buffer). The antibody activity in the fractions was determined and appropriate fractions were pooled and stored.

A thiophilic adsorbent for the high performance liquid chromatography purification of monoclonal antibodies (Nopper et al., 1989)

Thiophilic interaction chromatography developed for the conventional chromatography, was transformed to the HPLC mode upon preparation of new and improved thiophilic ligand containing silica beads. The new thiophilic adsorbent with basically the same molecular structure than the original T-gel was found to be of high capacity and is suitable for the rapid and single-step purification of all subclasses of monoclonal and polyclonal antibodies. Due to its broad specificity, the thiophilic silica column is an efficient, stable, and inexpensive substitute for protein A and G columns used to purify antibodies.

Purification of monoclonal antibodies on dextran coated silica support grafted by thiophilic ligands (Serres et al., 1995)

Dextran-coated porous silica beads grafted with mercaptoethanol by using divinyl-sulphone are promising supports for high-performance liquid chromatography of proteins. The affinity of monoclonal IgG subclasses from mouse ascitic fluids for the active phases has been analysed. These dextran-coated silica supports grafted with thiophilic ligands allow a one-step purification of these antibodies. Moreover, the chromatographic separation of two subclasses, IgG_1 and IgG_3, is observed and can be correlated to the high resolution of these new HPLC thiophilic supports.

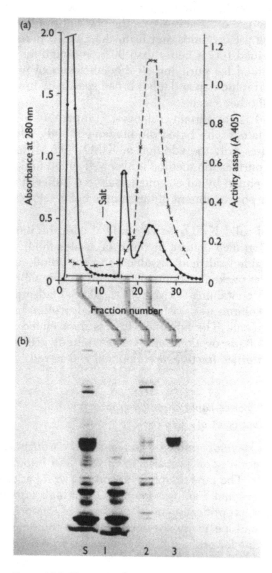

Figure 11.3 Thiophilic interaction chromatography of calf serum. (a) Elution profile of calf serum (2 ml) upon chromatography on a column (16 × 25 mm; bed volume = 5 ml) of T-gel. For experimental details, see legend to Fig. 11.2a. Arrows indicate the beginning of elution: I. 50 mM Tris–HCl, pH 7.6 and, II. 30% isopropanol in 50 mM Tris–HCl, pH 7.6. (b) Gradient gel electrophoretic patterns of the pooled fractions 1 and 2 shown in (a) and unfractioned calf serum (S). The position of calf Igs is indicated by the vertical arrow.

Purification of F(ab)₂ and Fc fragments of IgG1 antibodies from murine ascitic fluid (Yurov et al., 1994)

A thiophilic adsorption method has also been developed for the rapid purification and separation of mouse F(ab)₂ and Fc fragments, obtained after proteolytic digestion of

IgG1 monoclonal antibodies. Partially purified Mabs were digested with preactivated thiol-free papain. Thiophilic adsorption chromatography was performed in 20 mM Hepes pH 7.5, starting with 15% (w/v) ammonium sulphate, followed by stepwise elution with decreasing concentrations of the salt: 12.5, 10 and 0%, respectively. The bulk of contaminating proteins did not interact with the thiophilic adsorbent at 15% ammonium sulphate and was eluted in the pass through fraction.

Purified F(ab)$_2$ fragments were obtained after elution with 12.5% ammonium sulphate. They retained about 90% of the total antibody activity loaded onto the column, and were pure according to SDS-PAGE. Fc fragments (slightly contaminated with high-molecular weight proteins) were obtained after elution with 10% ammonium sulphate, while intact IgG1 was eluted with buffer containing no salt. Both flow rate and protein concentration proved to be critical factors affecting the efficiency of the chromatographic method.

Acknowledgements

I would like to thank the Swedish Ministry of Education and the Country Administration of Södermanland for financial support of my (S. O.) research. F. B. V. would like to thank the International Program in Chemical Sciences (IPICS), Uppsala University, for financial support.

References

Belew, M., Juntti, N., Larsson, A. and Porath, J. (1987) A one-step purification method for monoclonal antibodies based on salt-promoted adsorption chromatography on a thiophilic adsorbent. *J. Immunol. Meth.*, **102**, 173–182.

Berna, P. and Porath, J. (1996) Cyanocarbons as ligands for electron donor acceptor chromatography of human serum proteins. *J. Chromatogr. A*, **753**, 57–62.

Berna, N., Berna, P. and Oscarsson, S. (1996) Cosolvent-Induced adsorption and desorption of serum proteins on an amphiphilic mercaptomethylene pyridine – derivatized agarose gel. *Archives Biochem. Bioph.*, **330**, 188–192.

Dill, K. A. (1990) The meaning of hydrophobicity. *Science*, **250**, 297.

El Rassi, Z. (1989) High performance liquid chromatography of proteins with silica-bound sulfone-thioether functions. *Biochromatography*, **4**, 184–150.

Franco-Fraguas, L. and Batista-Viera, F. (1992) Thiophilic interaction chromatography of sweet potato β-amylase. *J. Chromatogr.*, **604**, 103–107.

Hutchens, T. W. and Porath, J. (1986) Thiophilic adsorption of immunoglobulins. Analysis of conditions optimal for selective immobilization and purification. *Anal. Biochem.*, **159**, 217–226.

Hutchens, T. W. and Porath, J. (1987) Thiophilic adsorption: a comparison of model protein behavior. *Biochemistry*, **26**, 7199–7204.

Hutchens, T. W. (1992) In: *Methods in Molecular Biology*, Vol. 11 (ed.), A. Kenney and S. Fowell, The Humana Press, Totowa, NJ, pp. 1–15. Thiophilic adsorption chromatography. (Review article).

Hutchens, T. W., Magnuson, J. S. and Yip, T. T. (1990) Secretory IgA, IgG and IgM immunoglobulins isolated simultaneously from colostral whey by selective thiophilic adsorption. *J. Immunol. Meth.*, **128**, 89–99.

Knudsen, K. L., Hansen, M. B., Henriksen, L. R., Andersen, B. K. and Lihme, A. (1992) Sulfone-aromatic ligands for thiophilic adsorption chromatography: purification of human and mouse immunoglobulins. *Anal. Biochem.*, **201**, 170–177.

Khamlichi, S., Serres, A., Muller, D., Jozefonviez, J. and Brash, J. L. (1995) Interaction of IgG and albumin with functionalized silicas. *Colloids and Surfaces B: Biointerfaces*, **4**, 165–172.

Konecny, P., Brown, R. J. and Scouten, W. H. (1994) Chromatographic purification of immunoglobulin G from bovine milk whey. *J. Chromatogr. A*, **673**, 45–53.

Noel, R. J., O'Hare, W. T. and Street, G. (1996) Thiophilic nature of divinyl-sulphone cross-linked agarose. *J. Chromatogr. A*, **734**, 241–246.

Nopper, B., Kohen, F. and Wilchek, M. (1989) A thiophilic adsorbent for the one-step high-performance liquid chromatography purification of monoclonal antibodies. *Anal. Biochem.*, **180**, 66–71.

Oscarsson, S. and Porath, J. (1990) Protein chromatography with pyridine and alkylthioether-based agarose adsorbents. *J. Chromatogr.*, **499**, 235–247.

Oscarsson, S., Angulo-Tatis, D., Chaga, G. and Porath, J. (1995) Amphiphilic agarose-based adsorbents for chromatography. Comparative study of adsorption capacities and desorption efficiencies. *J. Chromatogr. A*, **689**, 3–12.

Oscarsson, S. (1995). Influence of salts on protein interactions at interfaces of amphiphilic polymers and adsorbents. *J. Chromatogr. B.*, **666**, 21–31.

Oscarsson, S. and Porath, J. (1997) Alkaliresistant Protein Adsorbent. European Patent Bulletin, March 26. Publication nr. 0 764 049.

Porath, J. and Oscarsson, S. (1988) A new kind of thiophilic electron–donor–acceptor adsorbent. *Makromol. Chem. Macromol. Symp.*, **17**, 359–371.

Oscarsson, S. and Kårsnäs, P. (1998) Salt-promoted adsorption of proteins onto amphiphilic agarose based adsorbents. *J. Chromatogr. A*, **803**, 83–93.

Porath, J., Maisano, F. and Belew, M. (1985) Thiophilic adsorption, a new method for protein fractionation. *FEBS Lett.*, **185**, 306–310.

Porath, J. and Belew, M. (1987) Thiophilic interaction and the selective adsorption of proteins. *TIBTECH.*, **5**, 225–229.

Serres, A., Muller, D. and Jozefonvicz, J. (1995) Purification of monoclonal antibodies on dextran-coated silica support grafted by thiophilic ligand. *J. Chromatogr. A*, **711** 151–157.

Schwarz, A., Kohen, F. and Wilchek, M. (1994) Novel sulfone-based thiophilic ligands for the high-performance liquid chromatographic purification of antibodies. *Reactive Polymers*, **22**, 259–266.

Schwartz, A., Kohen, F. and Wilchek, M. (1995) Novel heterocyclic ligands for the thiophilic purification of antibodies. *J. Chromatogr. B*, **664**, 83–88.

Yurov, G. K., Neugodova, G. L., Verkhovsky, O. A. and Naroditsky, B. S. (1994) Thiophilic adsorption: rapid purification of F(ab)$_2$ and Fc fragments of IgG1 antibodies from murine ascitic fluid. *J. Immunol. Methods*, **177**, 29–33.

Miscellaneous methods in affinity chromatography

Part 1: Boronic acids as selective ligands for affinity chromatography

Xiao-Chuan Liu and William H. Scouten

Introduction

The interaction between borate and cis-diols was first noticed in 1874 when Vignon and Bouchardat attempted to titrate boric acid. They found that it was impossible to titrate boric acid unless glycerol was added. Subsequent studies indicated that the titration depended on a covalent interaction between borate and cis-diols. By the 1940s, this property had been employed as a tool in the analysis of carbohydrates (Boeseken, 1949). In the 1950s, the borate/cis-diol interaction was used for zone electrophoresis in borate buffers (Foster, 1957). In the 1960s, the borate/cis-diol interaction was used for ion exchange chromatography in borate buffers (Mattok and Wilson, 1965). However, the breakthrough came in 1970s when researchers developed immobilized boronate chromatography systems.

The use of boronate affinity chromatography for separation of nucleic acid components and carbohydrates was first reported by Weith *et al.* in 1970 (Weith *et al.*, 1970). Since then, the specificity of boronate ligand has been exploited for the separation of a wide variety of cis-diol-containing compounds, including catechols, nucleosides, nucleotides, nucleic acids, carbohydrates, glycoproteins and enzymes (Bergold and Scouten, 1983). A few examples of these applications in recent years include: affinity chromatography of serine proteinases using peptide boronic acids as ligands (Zembower *et al.*, 1996), selective isolation of target cells by monoclonal antibodies immobilized on magnetic beads coupled with boronic acid (Ugelstad *et al.*, 1996), binding of low-molecular-mass cis-diols and glycated hemoglobin using protein–boronic acid conjugates (Frantzen *et al.*, 1995). Selective extraction of quercetrin in vegetable drugs and urine by boronic acid affinity chromatography and HPLC (Bongartz and Hesse, 1995), separation and characterization of DNA adducts of stereoisomers of benzo[α]pyrene-7,8-diol-9,10-epoxide (Lau and Baird, 1994), robotic chromatography for assay of glycohemoglobin (Herold *et al.*, 1993), selective adsorption of immunoglobulins and glucosylated proteins (Brena *et al.*, 1992), high performance affinity chromatography for the rapid, efficient assay of glycated albumin (Yasukawa *et al.*, 1992), chromatography of glycated hemoglobin (Bisse and Wieland, 1992).

The interactions between boronate ligands and analytes

The interaction between boronate and cis-diol

The basic interaction in boronate chromatography is the esterification between boronate ligands and cis-diols. The major structural requirement for boronate\cis-diol esterification is that the two hydroxyl groups of a diol should be on adjacent carbon atoms and in a approximately coplanar configuration, that is a 1,2-cis-diol. Although interaction with 1,3-cis-diol and trident interaction with cis-inositol or triethanolamine can also occur, 1,2-cis-diols give the strongest ester bonds (Angyal et al., 1974; Ferrier, 1978).

The mechanism of interaction between boronic acids and cis-diols is not fully understood. In aqueous solution, under basic conditions, the boronate is hydroxylated from its trigonal coplanar form, yielding a tetrahedral boronate anion, which can then form esters with cis-diols (Fig. 12.1). This mechanism is supported by a recent publication of Westmark et al. (Westmark et al., 1994). The resulting cyclic diester can be hydrolyzed under acidic conditions, reversing the reaction. It is unusual in that, although two covalent bonds are formed, the reaction is quite reversible in aqueous solution. The boronate diester bond strength has not been well studied and only a few dissociation constants of phenylboronic acid diesters have been reported. Those reported include: adonitol, 2.2×10^{-3} M; dulcitol, 1.1×10^{-3} M (Evans et al., 1979); mannitol, 3.3×10^{-3} M (Zittle, 1951); and NADH, 5.9×10^{-3} M (Fulton, 1981). The dissociation constant of 4-(N-methyl)carboxamido-benzeneboronic acid and D-fructose diester is 1.2×10^{-4} M (Soundararajan et al., 1989). These dissociation constants are relatively large compared to the constants of 10^{-4}–10^{-8} M observed in most affinity ligand\protein interactions.

In organic solvents, trigonal boronates can react directly with cis-diols, but the rate of esterification is several orders of magnitude lower than in aqueous solution (Wulff et al., 1982).

Secondary interactions

Although boronate\cis-diol ester formation is the basis for boronate affinity chromatography, there are some secondary interactions that can play an important role. Four major secondary interactions are described below.

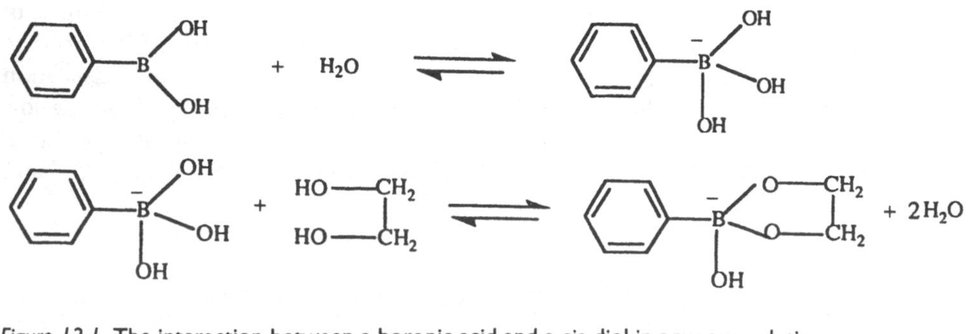

Figure 12.1 The interaction between a boronic acid and a cis-diol in aqueous solution.

Hydrophobic interactions

Because almost all boronate ligands used so far are aromatic boronate ligands, they can give rise to hydrophobic interactions. An aromatic $\pi-\pi$ interaction can also occur with phenyl groups. These can cause nonspecific adsorption of analytes, especially proteins. This is the major motivation for seeking aliphatic boronate ligands. On the other hand, hydrophobic interactions may, in certain cases, provide additional selectivity. To reduce the hydrophobic effect, ionic strength should be low, usually about 50 mM.

Ionic interactions

The negative charge of the active tetrahedral boronate can cause ionic attraction or repulsion. In general, this effect is weaker than boronate\cis-diol ester formation. In certain cases, ionic interactions can also provide additional selectivity. To decrease the ionic effect, the ionic strength should be high, but still should be lower than 500 mM to avoid hydrophobic interaction. A good compromise is between 50 and 500 mM.

Hydrogen bonding

Since a boronate acid has two hydroxyls (three in the active tetrahedral form), it offers sites for hydrogen bonding. Although this is usually small, under special circumstances hydrogen bonding is strong enough to be the basis for chromatographic separations, such as in the case of isolation of serine proteinase (Akparov and Stepanov, 1978).

Charge transfer interaction

Because in a trigonal uncharged boronate the boron atom has an empty orbital, it can serve as a electron acceptor for charge transfer interaction. Unprotonated amines are good electron donors and when an amine donates a pair of electrons to boron, the boron atom becomes tetrahedral, which explains why amines may serve to promote boronate\cis-diol esterification. However, if there is a hydroxyl group adjacent to the amine, this can block boronate\cis-diol esterification, therefore Tris and ethanolamines should be avoided in boronate chromatography buffers. Carboxyl groups can also serve as electron donors for charge transfer interaction. Together with α-hydroxyl groups, carboxyls can form stable complexes with boronates, as demonstrated by the esterification of lactic acid or salicylic acid with boronate (Higa and Kishimoto, 1986).

Boronate ligands

The earliest and still most widely used boronate ligand is 3-aminophenylboronic acid (3aPBA) (Fig. 12.2a). The anilino group is used to couple it to solid supports, and the meta-amino substitution also lowers its pKa. In all applications using 3aPBA, the pH must be basic, i.e. pH > 8. The pKa of 3aPBA is 8.8 (Boit, 1974), so that for optimum binding, the pH should be as high as reasonably possible. However, in many cases analytes may lose their biological activities at such high pH values. This is one major limitation to expanded use of this ligand.

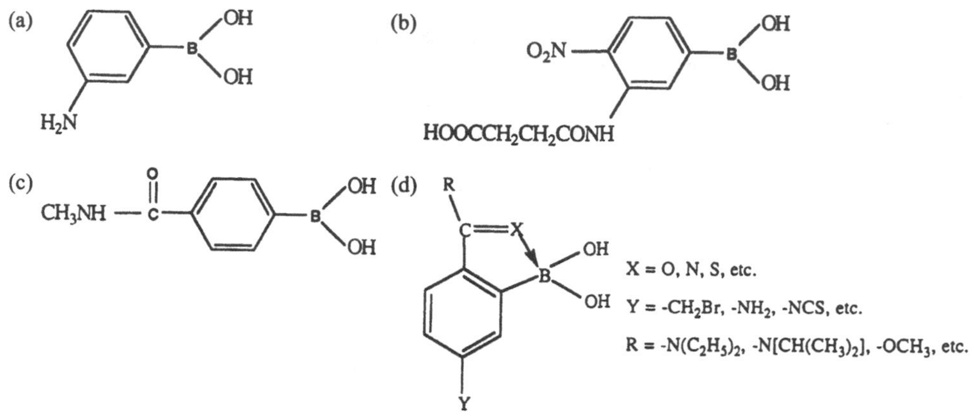

Figure 12.2 Various boronate ligands. (a) 3-aminophenylboronic acid, (b) N-(4-nitro-3-dihydroxy-borylphenyl)succinamic acid, (c) 4-(N-methyl) carboxamido-benzeneboronic acid, (d) a new type of boronate ligand with an internal coordination bond.

Several variants of boronate ligands have been prepared. In earlier studies, Yurkevich *et al.* (1975) prepared dextran and cellulose containing bipolar 2-[(4-boronophenyl)-methyl]-ethylammonio]ethyl and -diethylammonio]ethyl ligands and used them for separation of ribonucleosides, such as adenosine, cytidine, guanosine and uridine at pH 8.0. Even though this matrix bound adenosine in a nearly pH independent manner (from 2.5 to 8.2), the probable mechanism of this adsorption is not due to the boronate cis-diol esterification. Rather, it is very likely due to ionic interactions.

Akparov *et al.* (1978) coupled *p*-(*ω*-aminoethyl)phenyl-boronate to CH-Sepharose for biospecific chromatography of serine proteinases at pH 7.5. However, the binding is due to coordinated hydrogen bonding in the active site where the boronate serves as a transition state intermediate (Matthews *et al.*, 1975). A similar phenomenon was also observed with porcine pancreatic lipase (Garner, 1980).

Elliger *et al.* (1975) prepared poly(*p*-vinylbenzeneboronic acid)-coated porous polystyrene beads to separate vicinal diols near pH 8.

Wulff *et al.* (1982) and Wulff (1982) synthesized 2-dimethylaminomethylphenyl-boronic acid in which the intramolecular B-N bond was established by ^{11}B NMR. This ligand is highly specific for aliphatic cis-diols, but binds poorly to aromatic cis-diols, amines or monoalcohols. No data on its interaction with large molecules such as a glycoprotein or carbohydrate was reported.

A number of researchers have attempted to introduce a strong electron withdrawing group on the phenyl ring so that it can lower the pKa of ligands. Myohanen *et al.* (1981) coupled 3-nitro-4-carboxamidobenzeneboronic acid to Sepharose-CL6B and found the glycoprotein α-glucosidase bound to the support at pH 7.4. However, at pH 8.5 and 6.5, its chromatographic behavior was totally different. This disparity was apparently caused by the unstable amide linkage which is rapidly hydrolyzed at alkaline pH values (Soundararajan *et al.*, 1989).

Johnson (1981) coupled a mixture of 2-nitro-3-succinamido-benzeneboronic acid and 3-succinamido-4-nitro-benzeneboronic acid to aminoethyl polyacrylamide beads and used these to separate tRNA at pH 7. Unfortunately, it appears that 2-nitro-3-succinamido-benzeneboronic acid gradually hydrolyzes and the liberated amine functions give rise to strong ionic interactions.

Singhal *et al.* (1991) (Fig. 12.2b) chose a similar approach and coupled N-(4-nitro-3-dihydroxyborylphenyl)succinamic acid to a porous and semirigid spherical gel of vinyl polymer and found the matrix offers enhanced binding of many cis-diol-containing compounds.

Hageman *et al.* (Soundararajan *et al.*, 1989) (Fig. 12.2c) synthesized 4-(N-methyl)carboxamido-benzeneboronic acid and determined that it had a low pKa (7.86) and a high cis-diol ester formation constant with D-fructose of 8600. The authors suggest that it should provide sufficient acidity, binding capacity, and hydrolytic stability to make it an excellent boronate ligand for affinity supports. However, this boronate ligand has not been coupled to a support and no further publications have appeared concerning this ligand.

Liu and Scouten (1994) (Fig. 12.2d) recently reported another new type of boronate ligand with a general structure as shown in Fig. 12.2. Crystal structure shows an internal coordinate bond between X and B was indeed formed (Liu *et al.*, 1995). As a result, the boron is in a tetrahedral conformation, which is favorable for esterification between a boronate and a cis-diol. In solution, this type of ligand can esterify catechol at neutral pH as demonstrated by ^{11}B NMR studies. Sequentially, when this kind of ligand was immobilized onto a solid matrix, chromatography of catechol and horseradish peroxidase can be performed at neutral pH. In addition, aliphatic boronate ligands were also studied by this group (Adamek *et al.*, 1992), results indicate although these ligands can be used in chromatography for a short period of time, their insufficient stability is the main obstacle for prolonged applications.

Applications of boronate affinity chromatography

Boronate affinity chromatography has been employed for the separation of four major groups of biomolecules, as described below.

Carbohydrates

Carbohydrates containing cis-diols can bind to boronate affinity gels and the binding strength is proportional to the number of cis-diols. In the 1960s, Bourne *et al.* found that adding phenylboronic acid to developing solvents in paper chromatography can enhance the mobility of sugars that have cis-diols or cis-triols (Bourne *et al.*, 1963) because of boronate esters formed. This technique is also suitable for separation of free sugars that have cis-diols from their reduced polyol counterparts, since reduced sugars may not have the cis-diols needed to esterify with boronate. Boronate chromatography has been used for separation of monosaccharides and oligosaccharides, with compounds containing a cis-1,2-diol binding most strongly to boronate gels (Weith *et al.*, 1970; Schott, 1972; Glad *et al.*, 1980). Because of their strong binding, carbohydrates such as sorbitol or manitol are often used as competing diols for the elution of various analytes. In addition, isomeric pentose phosphates have been separated by Gascon *et al.* (1981) using boronate affinity chromatography. Resolution of D- and L-mannopyranoside racemates using boronate affinity chromatography was done by

Wulff *et al.* (1978). It should be mentioned that the matrix was synthesized by molecular imprinting (or templated polymerization) technology.

Polysaccharides are more constrained than their monosaccharide components, because the internal glycosidic linkages reduce the number of cis-diols, and because only the terminal residues are available for boronate esterification. This might be the reason why, many common polysaccharides such as starch, agarose, methylcellulose and inulin do not interact with boronate. Nonetheless, many gums and mucilages do react with borate (Zittle, 1951).

Nucleosides, nucleotides and nucleic acids

Ribose has 1,2-cis-diols at the $2', 3'$ position that give rise to strong interactions with boronate, therefore boronate affinity chromatography has been used successfully in separation of ribonucleosides, ribonucleotides, and RNA. Since there is no 3'-hydroxyl in DNA, it doesn't esterify with boronate matrices. Thus, boronate affinity chromatography can readily separate RNA from DNA (Schott, 1973; Ackerman, 1979). Since 3'-phosphorylated ribonucleotides don't bind to boronate gels for the same reason, these also can be separated from RNA (Rosenberg and Gilham, 1971). Oligonucleotides and large RNA molecules only have a cis-diol on the 3'-terminals, their binding to boronate gels is relatively weak, and the longer chain length correlates with weaker binding. mRNA can also be isolated using boronate affinity chromatography (Wilk *et al.*, 1982). Boronate affinity chromatography is also used for separating aminoacylated tRNA from non-aminoacylated tRNA (Rosenberg *et al.*, 1972). Unfortunately, the high pH required in boronate chromatography may hydrolyze the amino acid-tRNA bond (Schott *et al.*, 1973). Since dinucleotide cofactors, such as NAD(H), NADP(H) and FAD, have more than one accessible cis-diol, they bind more strongly to boronate chromatography gels than mononucleotides or oligonucleotides (Van Ness *et al.*, 1980).

Secondary interactions are also important in the interaction of the nucleic acid components with boronates. Negatively charged phosphate groups cause strong ionic repulsion that may weaken or prevent binding of cis-diols. To alleviate this, divalent cations such as Mg^{2+} are commonly used in boronate chromatography buffers. The nature of the base is also important, and purines, adenines, and guanines have stronger binding than other bases, probably due to hydrophobic and/or hydrogen bonding effects (Rosenberg *et al.*, 1972).

Glycoproteins and enzymes

One of the most important uses of boronate affinity chromatography is the separation of glycosylated hemoglobin from non-glycosylated hemoglobin (Herold *et al.*, 1993; Bisse and Wieland, 1992; Hjerten and Li, 1990; Klenk *et al.*, 1982; Gould *et al.*, 1982; Kluckiger *et al.*, 1984). In humans, glucose and other aldoses glycosylate hemoglobin at its amino terminal end as well as at certain lysine residues. The concentration of glycosylated hemoglobin reflects the blood glucose concentration over the past one or two months. Thus, measurement of the glycosylated hemoglobin level is an important indicator for the clinical management of diabetes (Benes *et al.*, 1993). Boronate affinity chromatography is a rapid, simple, and accurate method to assay diabetic hemoglobin. In addition, glycated albumin, which can also be used for evaluation of diabetic states, was also determined by boronate chromatography (Yasukawa et al., 1992).

Other glycosylated proteins have also been isolated by boronate affinity chromatography, including human immunoglobulins (Brena et al., 1992; Ugelstad et al., 1996); γ-glutamyltransferase (Yamamoto et al., 1991); human platelet glycocalicin (DeCristofaro et al., 1988), α-glucosidase from yeast (Myohanen et al., 1981); 3,4-dihydroxyphenylalanine-containing proteins (Hawkins et al., 1986); membrane glycoproteins from human lymphocytes (Williams et al., 1982); horseradish peroxidase and glucose oxidase (Fulton, 1981).

Since boronic acid derivatives are potent transition-state analogue inhibitors of serine proteinases (Matthews et al., 1975; Garner, 1980), they can be used as affinity ligands for the isolation and purification of serine proteinases, such as α-chymotrypsin, trypsin, and subtilisin (Akparov and Stepanov, 1978); human neutrophil elastase, human cathepsin G, porcine pancreatic elastase (Zembower et al., 1996).

In boronate affinity chromatography of glycoproteins , secondary interactions, especially hydrophobic and ionic interactions, are important. Since hydrophobic interactions can cause non-specific binding of adventitious proteins, detergents are sometimes added to buffers to lessen the hydrophobic binding (Williams et al., 1982). Ionic interactions can also be critical, and the negatively charged boronate can prevent anionic protein binding or cause nonspecific cationic protein binding. Divalent cations such as Mg^{2+} are often used at low concentration to reduce ionic interaction without causing hydrophobic interaction.

Proteins that don't normally interact with boronate may be isolated by "ligand-mediated" chromatography or "piggyback" chromatography. In this process, the boronate column is first saturated with a desired affinity ligand containing a cis-diol. Note that the affinity ligand in this case is not boronate but rather a ligand which has affinity for target proteins, and which is merely coupled to the matrix via a boronate cis-diol ester. The sample containing the target protein is then applied to the column. The target protein interacts with the affinity ligand and is thus either retained or retarded on the column, whereas all other proteins wash through the column. The bound protein can be then eluted by continued washing with buffers, soluble affinity ligands, or competing cis-diols. For example, concanavalin A has been isolated using methyl α-D-glucopyranoside as an affinity ligand (Fulton, 1981); glucose-6-phosphate dehydrogenase (yeast) has been isolated using $NADP^+$ as an affinity ligand (Bouriotis et al., 1981); hexokinase (yeast) has been isolated using ATP as an affinity ligand (Bouriotis et al., 1981); lactate dehydrogenase has been isolated using NAD^+ as an affinity ligand (Maestas et al., 1981); and UDP-glucose pyrophosphorylase has been isolated using UTP as an affinity ligand (Maestas et al., 1981). Affinity ligands that don't have diols may also be used if they can be derivatized to produce a cis-diol-containing product which is capable of binding to the enzyme (Ho et al., 1981).

Other small molecules

Some small biological molecules can also be isolated by boronate affinity chromatography. One major group of such compounds is the catechols which include catecholamines, D,L-dopa, 5-S-cysteinyldopa, dopamine, epinephrine, and nore-pinephrine (Hansson *et al.*, 1987; Elliger *et al.*, 1975; Higa *et al.*, 1977; Hansson *et al.*, 1978). Others include α-hydroxycarboxylic acids (lactic, etc., salicylic, etc.) (Higa and Kishimoto, 1986); pyridoxal (Maestas *et al.*, 1981); quercetrin (Bongartz and Hesse, 1995); and ecdysteroids (Pis and Harmatha, 1992). Typically the interaction between these molecules and boronate is due to boronate\cis-diol ester formation.

As described above, one can see that boronic acid and its derivatives are versatile ligands for the selective binding of a variety of biological molecules. Its unique, readily reversible esterification with cis-diols offers many advantages not only in affinity chromatography, but also in other areas such as oriented and reversible immobilization of enzymes (Liu and Scouten, 1996), and the new emerging technology of molecular imprinting (Wulff, 1995).

References

Ackerman, S., Cool, B. and Furth, J. (1979) Removal of DNA from RNA by chromatography on acetylated N-[N'-(*m*-dihydroxylborylphenyl)succinamyl]aminoethyl cellulose. *Anal. Biochem.*, **100**, 174–178.

Adamek, V., Liu, X.-C., Zhang, Y.-A., Adamkova, K. and Scouten, W. H. (1992) New aliphatic boronate ligands for affinity chromatography. *J. Chromatogr.*, **625**, 91–99.

Akparov, V. and Stepanov, V. (1978) Phenylboronic acid as a ligand for biospecific chromatography of serine proteinases. *J. Chromatogr.*, **155**, 329–336.

Angyal, S., Greeves, D. and Pickles, V. (1974) The stereochemistry of complex formation of polyols with borate and periodate anions, and with metal cations. *Carbohyd. Res.*, **35**, 165–173.

Benes, M. J., Stambergova, A. and Scouten, W. H. (1993) Affinity chromatography with immobilized benzeneboronates. In T. T. Ngo (ed.), *Molecular Interactions in Bioseparations*, Plenum Press, New York, pp. 313–322.

Bergold, A. and Scouten, W. H. (1983) Borate chromatography. In W. H. Scouten (ed.), *Solid Phase Biochemistry*, Wiley, New York, pp. 149–187.

Biedrzycki, M., Scouten, W. H. and Biedrzycka, Z. (1992) Derivatives of tetrahedral boronic acids. *J. Organomet. Chem.*, **431**, 255–270.

Bisse, E. and Wieland, H. (1992) Coupling of m-aminophenylboronic acid to s-triazine-activated Sephacryl: use in the affinity chromatography of glycated hemoglobins. *J. Chromatogr.*, **575**, 223–228.

Boeseken, J. (1949) The use of boric acid for the determination of the configuration of carbohydrates. *Adv. Carbohyd. Chem.*, **4**, 189–210.

Boit, H.-G. (1974) *Belstein*, **16**, Springer, Berlin, pp. 1284.

Bongartz, D. and Hesse, A. (1995) Selective extraction of quercetrin in vegetable drugs and urine by off-line coupling of boronic acid affinity chromatography and high-performance liquid chromatography. *J. Chromatogr. B*, **673**, 223–230.

Bouriotis, V., Galpin, I. J. and Dean, P. D. G. (1981) Applications of immobilized phenylboronic acids as supports for group-specific ligands in the affinity chromatography of enzymes. *J. Chromatogr.*, **210**, 267–278.

Bourne, E. J., Lees, E. M. and Weigel, H. (1963) Paper chromatography of carbohydrates and related compounds in the presence of benzeneboronic acid. *J. Chromatogr.*, **11**, 253–257.

Brena, B. M., Batista-Viera, F., Ryden, L. and Porath, J. (1992) Selective adsorption of immunoglobulins and glycosylated proteins on phenylboronate-agarose. *J. Chromatogr.*, **604**, 109–115.

De Cristofaro, R., Landolfi, R., Bizzi, B. and Castagnola, M. (1988) Human platelet glycocalicin purification by phenyl boronate affinity chromatography coupled to anion-exchange high-performance liquid chromatography. *J. Chromatogr.*, **426**, 376–380.

Elliger, C., Chan, B. and Stanley, W. (1975) *p*-Vinylbenzeneboronic acid polymers for separation of vicinal diols. *J. Chromatogr.*, **104**, 57–61.

Evans, W., McCourtney, E. and Carney, W. (1979) A comparative analysis of the interaction of borate ion with various polyols. *Anal. Biochem.*, **95**, 383–386.

Ferrier, R. J. (1978) Carbohydrate boronates. *Adv. Carb. Chem. Biochem.*, **35**, 31–80.

Foster, A. (1957) Zone electrophoresis of carbohydrates. *Adv. Carbohyd. Chem.*, **12**, 81–115.

Frantzen, F., Grimsrud, K., Heggli, D.-E. and Sundrehagen, E. (1995) Protein-boronic acid conjugates and their binding to low-molecular-mass cis-diols and glycated hemoglobin. *J. Chromatogr. B*, **670**, 37–45.

Fulton, S. (1981) *Boronate Ligands in Biochemical Separations*, Amicon Corp., Danvers, MA, USA.

Garner, C. W. (1980) Boronic acid inhibitors of porcine pancreatic lipase. *J. Biol. Chem.*, **255**, 5064–5068.

Gascon, A., Wood, T. and Chitemerese, L. (1981) The separation of isomeric pentose phosphates from each other and the preparation of D-xylulose 5-phosphate and D-ribulose 5-phosphate by column chromatography. *Anal. Biochem.*, **118**, 4–9.

Glad, M., Ohlson, S., Hansson, L., Mansson, M. and Mosbach, K. (1980) High-performance liquid affinity chromatography of nucleosides, nucleotides and carbohydrates with boronic acid-substituted microparticulate silica. *J. Chromatogr.*, **200**, 254–260.

Gould, B. J., Hall, P. M. and Cook, G. H. (1982) Measurement of glycosylated hemoglobins using an affinity chromatography method. *Clin. Chim. Acta.*, **125**, 41–48.

Hansson, C., Agrup, G., Rorsman, H., Rosengren, A. and Rosengren, E. (1978) Chromatographic separation of catecholic amino acids and catecholamines on immobilized phenylboronic acid. *J. Chromatogr.*, **161**, 352–355.

Hansson, C., Kaagedal, B. and Kaellgerg, M. (1987) Determination of 5-S-cysteinyldopa in human urine by direct injection in coupled-column high-performance liquid chromatography. *J. Chromatogr.*, **420**, 146–151.

Hawkins, C. J., Lavin, M. F., Parry, D. L. and Ross, I. L. (1986) Isolation of 3,4-dihydroxyphenylalanine-containing proteins using boronate affinity chromatography. *Anal. Biochem.*, **159**, 187–190.

Herold, C. D., Andree, K., Herold, D. A. and Felder, R. A. (1993) Robotic chromatography: development and evaluation of automated instrumentation for assay of glycohemoglobin. *Clin. Chem.*, **39**, 143–147.

Higa, S., Suzuki, T., Hayashi, A., Tsuge, I. and Yamamura, Y. (1977) Isolation of catecholamines in biological fluids by boric acid gel. *Anal. Biochem.*, **77**, 18–24.

Higa, S. and Kishimoto, S. (1986) Isolation of 2-hydroxy carboxylic acids with a boronate affinity gel. *Anal. Biochem.*, **154**, 71–74.

Hjerten, S. and Li, J.(1990) High-performance liquid chromatography of proteins on deformed non-porous agarose beads. *J. Chromatogr.*, **500**, 543–553.

Ho, N., Duncan, R. and Gilham, P. (1981) Esterification of terminal phosphate groups in nucleic acids with sorbitol and its application to the isolation of terminal polynucleotide fragments. *Biochemistry*, **20**, 64–67.

Johnson, B. J. B. (1981) Synthesis of a nitrobenzeneboronic acid substituted polyacrylamide and its use in purifying isoaccepting transfer ribonucleic acids. *Biochemistry*, **20**, 6103–6108.

Klenk, D. C., Hermanson, G. T., Krohn, R. I., Fujimoto, E. K., Malia, A. K., Smith, P. K., England, J. D., Wiedmeyer, H. M., Little, R. R. and Goldstein, D. E. (1982) Determination of glycosylated hemoglobin by affinity chromatography: comparison with colorimetric and ion-exchange methods, and effects of common interferences. *Clin. Chem.*, **28**, 2088–2094.

Kluckiger, R., Woodtli, T. and Berger, W. (1984) Quantitation of glycosylated hemoglobin by boronate affinity chromatography. *Diabetes*, 33, 73–76.

Lau, H. H. S. and Baird, W. M. (1994) Separation and characterization of post-labeled DNA adducts of stereoisomers of benzo[α]pyrene-7,8-diol-9,10-epoxide by immobilized boronate chromatography and HPLC analysis. *Carcinogenesis*, 15, 907–915.

Liu, X.-C. and Scouten, W. H. (1994) New ligands for boronate affinity chromatography. *J. Chromatogr. A*, 687, 61–69.

Liu, X.-C., Hubbard, J. L. and Scouten, W. H. (1995) Synthesis and structural investigation of two potential boronate affinity chromatography ligands catechol [2-(diisopropylamino)carbonyl]phenyl-boronate and catechol [2-(diethylamino)carbonyl,4-methyl]phenyl-boronate. *J. Organomet. Chem.*, 493, 91–94.

Liu, X.-C. and Scouten, W. H. (1996) Studies on oriented and reversible immobilization of glycoprotein using novel boronate affinity gel. *J. Mol. Recogn.*, 9, 462–467.

Maestas, R., Prieto, J., Duehn, G. and Hageman, J. (1980) Polyacrylamide-boronate beads saturated with biomolecules: a new general support for affinity chromatography of enzymes. *J. Chromatogr.*, 189, 225–231.

Matthews, D., Alden, R., Birktoft, J., Freer, S. and Kraut, J. (1975) X-ray crystallographic study of boronic acid adducts with subtilisin BPN' (Novo). *J. Biol. Chem.*, 250, 7120–7126.

Mattok, G. and Wilson, D. (1965) Separation of catecholamines and metanephrine and normetanephrine using a weak cation-exchange resin. *Anal. Biochem.*, 11, 575–579.

Myohanen, T. A., Bouriotis, V. and Dean, P. D. G. (1981) Affinity chromatography of yeast α-glucosidase using ligand-mediated chromatography on immobilized phenylboronic acids. *Biochem. J.*, 197, 683–688.

Pis, J. and Harmatha, J. (1992) Phenylboronic acid as a versatile derivatization agent for chromatography of ecdysteroids. *J. Chromatogr.*, 596, 271–275.

Rosenberg, M. and Gilham, P. T. (1971) Isolation of 3′-terminal polynucleotides from RNA molecules. *Biochem. Biophys. Acta*, 246, 337–340.

Rosenberg, M., Wiebers, J. and Gilham, P. T. (1972) Studies on the interactions of nucleotides, polynucleotides, and nucleic acids with dihydroxylboryl-substituted cellulose. *Biochemistry*, 11, 3623–3628.

Schott, H. (1972) New dihydroxyboryl-substituted polymers for column-chromatographic separation of ribonucleoside-deoxyribonucleoside mixtures. *Angew. Chem., Int. Ed. Engl.*, 11, 824–825.

Schott, H., Rudloff, E., Schmidt, P., Roychoudhury, R. and Kossel, H. (1973) A dihydroxyboryl-substituted methacrylic polymer for the column chromatographic separation of mononucleotides, oligonucleotides, and transfer ribonucleic acid. *Biochemistry*, 12, 932–938.

Singhal, R. P., Ramamurthy, B., Govindraj, N. and Sarwar, Y. (1991) New ligands for boronate affinity chromatography. Synthesis and properties. *J. Chromatogr.*, 543, 17–38.

Soundararajan, S., Badawi, M., Kohlrust, C. M. and Hageman, J. (1989) Boronic acids for affinity chromatography: spectral methods for determinations of ionization and diol-binding constants. *Anal. Biochem.*, 178, 125–134.

Ugelstad, J., Stenstad, P., Kilaas, L., Prestvik, W. S., Rian, A., Nustad, K., Herje, R. and Berge, A. (1996) Biochemical and biomedical application of monodisperse polymer particles. *Macromol. Symp.*, 101, 491–500.

Van Ness, B., Howard, J. and Bodley, J. (1980) ADP-ribosylation of elongation factor 2 by diphtheria toxin. *J. Biol. Chem.*, 255, 10717–10720.

Weith, H. L., Wiebers, J. L. and Gilham, P. T. (1970) Synthesis of cellulose derivatives containing the dihydroxyboryl group and a study of their capacity to form specific complexes with sugars and nucleic acid components. *Biochemistry*, 9, 4396–4401.

Westmark, P. R., Valencia, L. S. and Smith, B. D. (1994) Influence of eluent anions in boronate affinity chromatography. *J. Chromatogr.*, 664, 123–128.

Wilk, H. E., Kecskemethy, N. and Schaefer, K. P. (1982) m-Aminophenylboronate agarose specifically binds capped snRNA and mRNA. *Nucleic Acids Res.*, 10, 7621–7633.

Williams, G. T., Johnstone, A. P. and Dean, P. D. G. (1982) Fractionation of membrane proteins on phenylboronic acid-agarose. *Biochem. J.*, 205, 167–171.

Wulff, G. and Vesper, W. (1978) Preparation of chromatographic sorbents with chiral cavities for racemic resolution. *J. Chromatogr.*, 167, 171–186.

Wulff, G. (1982) Selective binding to polymers via covalent bonds. The construction of chiral cavities as specific receptor sites. *Pure Appl. Chem.*, 54, 2093–2102.

Wulff, G., Dederichs, R., Grotstollen, R. and Jupe, C. (1982) On the chemistry of binding sites. Part II. Specific binding of substances to polymers by fast and reversible covalent interactions. *Anal. Chem. Symp. Ser.*, 9 (Affinity Chromatogr. Relat. Tech.), 207–216.

Wulff, G. (1995) Molecular imprinting in cross-linked materials with the aid of molecular templates–A way towards artificial antibodies. *Angew. Chem., Int. Ed. Engl.*, 34, 1812–1832.

Yamamoto, T., Amuro, Y., Matsuda, Y., Nakaoka, H., Shimomura, S., Hada, T. and Higashino, K. (1991) Boronate affinity chromatography of .gamma.-glutamyltransferase in patients with hepatocellular carcinoma. *Am. J. Gastroenterol.*, 86, 495–499.

Yasukawa, K., Abe, F., Shida, N., Koizumi, Y., Uchida, T., Noguchi, K. and Shima, K. (1992) High-performance affinity chromatography system for the rapid, efficient assay of glycated albumin. *J. Chromatogr.*, 597, 271–275.

Yurkevich, A., Kolodkina, I., Ivanova, E. and Pichuzhkina, E. (1975) Study of the interaction of polyols with polymers containing N-substituted [(4-boronophenyl)methyl-ammonio groups. *Carb. Res.*, 43, 215–224.

Zembower, D. E., Neudauer, C. L., Wick, M. J. and Ames, M. M. (1996) Versatile synthetic ligands for affinity chromatography of serine proteinases. *Int. J. Pept. Protein Res.*, 47, 405–413.

Zittle, C. (1951) Reaction of borate with substances of biological interest. *Advan. Enzym.*, 12, 493–502.

Miscellaneous methods in affinity chromatography

Part 2: Shielded affinity chromatography in packed bed and expanded bed mode

Igor Yu. Galaev and Bo Mattiasson

Introduction

A critical element of modern process biotechnology is the separation and purification of the target product from a fermentation broth or cell rupture supernatant. As it represents the major manufacturing cost, competitive advantage in production will depend not only on innovations in molecular biology sciences but also on innovation and optimization of separation and down-stream processes. The recent trend in bioseparations is to use affinity technology in the initial steps of the purification process allowing overall reduction in working volumes and thereby processing costs (Sii and Sadana, 1991). Affinity ligand to be used at an early stage of the purification protocol must be resistant to chemical and biological degradation, since the conditions used in the initial stages are much harsher than those used in the later stages. Low molecular weight, group specific ligands, the reactive triazine dyes included, are highly stable and are, therefore, favoured in such applications (Kaul and Mattiasson, 1992).

The major drawback of using group-specific ligands is their low selectivity. A protein molecule can interact with a dye molecule in several ways. Specific interactions occur at the natural ligand binding site (specific interactions). Similar interactions (electrostatic, hydrophobic, hydrogen bonding and charge transfer), termed as nonspecific, can also take place at sites away from the natural ligand binding site (Guo *et al.*, 1994).

These nonspecific interactions with dye–ligands are very significant since the molecular structure of the dye offers multiple possibilities for interactions at many sites (Scopes, 1996). Although the individual nonspecific interactions are weak, their effects are additive or even synergistic; they can lead to a very strong retention of the target protein on the affinity matrix. Consequently the recovery of bound protein from the affinity column may be hampered. Nonspecific interactions can have also another negative effect on the purification process. Even in the presence of the eluent, weak nonspecific interactions between the protein and the matrix retard the protein as it moves down the column resulting in 'tailed' elution peaks. Elimination of these nonspecific interactions has been one of the major objectives in the development of new affinity supports.

Concept of polymer shielding

The idea of polymer shielding is to apply a solution of a polymer (such as poly(N-vinylpyrrolidone), PVP) to a dye-matrix whereby the polymer molecules would bind noncovalently to the matrix via multipoint attachment. When a crude protein extract

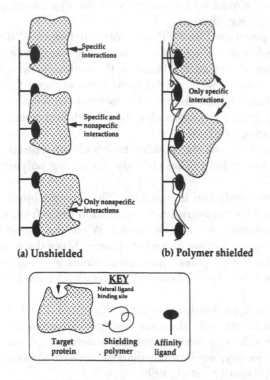

(a) Unshielded   (b) Polymer shielded

KEY

Natural ligand binding site

Target protein   Shielding polymer   Affinity ligand

Figure 12.1 Schematic representation of the concept of polymer shielded dye affinity chromatography. (a) On nonshielded column the target protein can be retained by both specific and nonspecific interactions with the immobilised dye ligands. (b) On a polymer shielded column, the nonspecific interactions of the target protein with the ligand are "blocked" due to the presence of the shielding polymer, the target protein interacts with the ligands mainly via the stronger specific interactions. Reproduced with permission from Mattiasson *et al.* (1996).

is introduced on such a polymer shielded column, a competition between the protein and the bound polymer for binding to the ligand takes place. If the interactions of the dye with the protein are stronger than those with the polymer, then the protein will bind to the column, resulting in a local displacement of the bound polymer. A schematic diagram of the shielding effect is shown in Fig. 12.1. In the ideal case the bound polymer should "shield" the nonspecific interactions of the protein with the immobilised dye molecules, without affecting its specific interactions.

The interactions between several polymers and the dye Cibacron Blue 3GA in solution were studied by difference spectroscopy and dye–polymer interactions were quantified by mathematical treatment of the data (Galaev *et al.*, 1994c; Galaev and Mattiasson, 1994b). Anionic polymers like poly(acrylic acid) had no pronounced interactions with the dye since the dye itself is anionic. Poly(ethylene imine), a polymer positively charged at neutral conditions, interacted extremely strongly with the dye, and has been used as a displacer for proteins bound to dye-affinity columns (Galaev *et al.*, 1995). Regeneration of the column was achieved by washing at highly basic conditions where net charge of the polymer was reduced and hence its binding to the column was weakened. Polysaccharides showed almost no interaction with the dye except in cases where they were positively charged e.g. chitosan.

Noncharged, weakly hydrophobic polymers like PVP and poly(vinyl alcohol) displayed moderate interactions with the free dye. Each polymer molecule was shown to interact simultaneously with several dye molecules. For instance, the molecular weight of the PVP segment responsible for interaction with one dye molecule was about 1 500 independently of molecular weight of the polymer. Hence, PVP molecule with molecular weight of 40 000 interacted with 25 dye–ligand molecules, the dissociation constant for each of the interactions was in the range 2–6 μM.

Polymer binding is reversible. Bound PVP was eluted either by a high concentration of mobile ligand i.e. free dye in solution or by a more strongly interacting polymer, poly(ethylene imine) (Garg et al., 1997)

Polymer shielding modulates the protein–ligand interactions. The enzyme binding capacity of the column is decreased but the recoveries are higher than those from an unshielded column since the overall retention force is decreased. When the eluent is introduced in the system, the protein begins to move down the column. Since the weak nonspecific interactions are masked by the polymer, the protein elutes in a narrow band. Thus sharper elution peaks have been obtained using columns which have been pretreated with polymer (Garg et al., 1997).

Specific interactions of proteins with dyes (binding constant, K_d about 1 μM) are approximately two orders of magnitude stronger than the nonspecific interactions (K_d about 100 μM) as judged by the values of binding constants determined using different techniques (difference spectroscopy, equilibrium dialysis, analytical affinity chromatography, inhibition analysis) (Mattiasson et al., 1996).

For a polymer shielding system to be useful, the strength of the polymer–dye interactions should be higher than the strength of protein–dye nonspecific interactions. This should ensure that the nonspecific interactions are masked. However, the polymer binding should not be excessively strong so that protein binding to the polymer shielded column is completely prevented i.e. the specific protein–dye interactions should be possible in the presence of the polymer. Therefore, the strength of the polymer–dye interactions should be lower than the strength of the protein–dye specific interactions. Thus, the optimal K_d value for the shielding polymer should be in the range of 10–20 μM.

Suitable polymers for shielding

The above presented discussion of the concept of polymer shielding confers certain requirements upon a suitable shielding polymer:

- The polymer should bind to the dye–ligand matrix via multipoint attachment to ensure that the polymer is not displaced by either the protein or the eluting agents used to recover the protein.
- The binding constant of polymer should be in between K_d values for specific and nonspecific binding of the protein of interest.
- The polymer should be inert towards proteins. This would ensure that no additional nonspecific interactions are introduced in the system.
- The polymer should be chemically stable, non-toxic and non-immunogenic.

- The polymer should be inexpensive and readily available since the idea of polymer shielding is to simplify separations, and this can be achieved only if the shielding agents are available as on-the-shelf chemicals.

Synthetic polymers like PVP and PVA meet these requirements with respect to triazine dyes and the proteins isolated using such ligands. They bind to the dye-matrix via multipoint interactions of an intermediate strength i.e. stronger than nonspecific protein–dye interactions but weaker than specific ones. Both these polymers are chemically stable and readily available. In addition, PVP, which is used as a plasma substitute, is practically non-immunogenic.

Strategy

A rational approach was required by which suitable shielding polymers could be selected for a given purification system. Therefore, a strategy for the design of polymer shielded dye-affinity chromatography systems was developed (Fig. 12.2). This involves selection of dyes making suitable interactions with the target protein. The protein–dye interactions can be measured using difference spectroscopy. With enzymes, activity

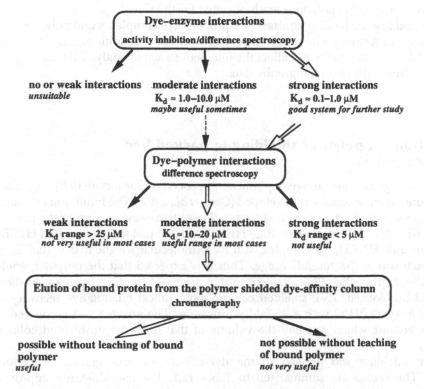

Figure 12.2 The proposed strategy for designing a polymer shielded dye-affinity chromatography system. The "useful system" is traced by the open arrows. Reproduced with permission from Mattiasson *et al.* (1996).

inhibition studies can also be used. The dissociation constant between an appropriate dye and the protein of interest should be in the range 0.1–1.0 μM. A higher binding strength (K_d < 0.1 μM) results in very tight binding of the protein to the column and consequent difficulties in elution. A lower binding strength (K_d > 1.0 μM) would result in very weak protein binding to the column.

This is followed by the selection of a polymer which interacts suitably with the chosen dye. The strength of this interaction may be estimated using difference spectroscopy. The binding constant for the polymer–dye complex should lie in the range 10–20 μM. Stronger polymer–dye interactions (K_d < 10 μM) prevent the binding of the target protein to the column, while a weaker interaction (K_d > 20 μM) may result in displacement of the polymer by the target protein i.e. leaching of the polymer from the column. The strength of the polymer–dye interactions can be modulated by altering the molecular weight and nature of the polymer. The data from difference spectroscopy indicate that with an increase in the polymer molecular weight, the number of dye molecules interacting with one polymer molecule (the "n" value) increases. This gives rise to an increased number of attachment points for the polymer molecule on the immobilised dye support resulting in a stronger polymer–dye complex (Mattiasson *et al.*, 1996).

The nature of the polymer will influence the strength of the complex, such that cationic and more hydrophobic polymers give stronger complexes whereas anionic and less hydrophobic polymers form weaker polymer–dye complexes. Nonionic, moderately hydrophobic polymers are best suited for the shielding.

It is essential that the binding constants for protein–dye complexes and polymer–dye complexes are measured under similar if not identical buffer conditions, since the ionic strength and pH of the buffer can affect the interactions significantly. This also applies to the collection of the chromatography data.

Applications of polymer shielding in packed bed chromatography

Using the strategy outlined above, a purification procedure for lactate dehydrogenase from porcine muscle extract was developed (Garg *et al.*, 1997). The inhibition constants of two of the seventeen dyes screened for binding to this enzyme were in the desired range (i.e. Ki = 0.27 μM for Procion Blue HERD and 0.15 μM for Procion Red HE3B). For Procion Blue HERD, the complex with PVP (molecular weight 10 000) had K_d = 10 μM which was in the "useful" range. Thus it is expected that the polymer would cover all the sites on the affinity matrix so that access of the target protein to these sites would be blocked. PVP shielded column gave almost quantitative recovery of the bound enzyme (94%) with a 30-fold purification. The enzyme was recovered in an elution volume which was half the volume of that from the unshielded column (Fig. 12.3).

Polymer shielding was applied to the dye-affinity chromatography of various enzymes. The results are summarised in Table 12.1. Polymer shielding improved the efficiency of the purification process (in terms of smaller elution volumes and higher recoveries) in all cases. It was also applied successfully in an expanded bed chromatography system.

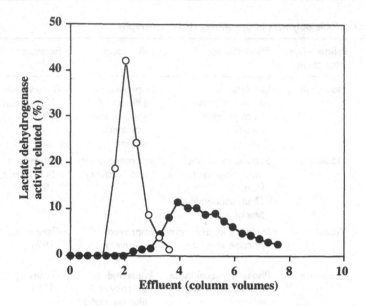

Figure 12.3 Elution profile of porcine muscle lactate dehydrogenase from Procion Blue HERD-Sepharose. (●) nonshielded; and (○) PVP-shielded. Conditions: column had an i.d. of 1.0 cm and a bed volume of 4.9 ml, chromatography was carried out at room temperature. Reproduced with permission from Garg *et al.* (1997).

Applications of polymer shielding in expanded bed chromatography

Expanded bed chromatography is a promising method for simplifying the downstream processing of particulate containing crude extracts (Chase, 1994). Basically, an upward flow of liquid is passed through an adsorbent bed which is not constrained by an upper adapter. As the flow rate is increased, the external voidage of the bed increases, as a result of which particulate matter can pass through the bed unhindered.

Polymer shielding looked especially promising for the application in the expanded bed mode where the problem of nonspecific interactions is even more pronounced than in the packed bed mode because of dealing with very crude extracts.

Streamline®-Cibacron Blue 3GA matrix was shielded with PVP (molecular weight 40 000) and the elution of lactate dehydrogenase from porcine muscle was optimised in a packed bed mode. Whereas the major part of the LDH activity eluted from an unshielded matrix at 0.6 M KCl, it was eluted at a lower concentration (0.12 M) from a PVP-shielded matrix. In general, an increase in enzyme recovery compromises the purification fold and vice versa. Therefore, the elution conditions are optimised so that high recoveries of an adequately purified enzyme in a reasonable elution volume is obtained. In order to obtain an idea of the purification fold during the different salt elution steps, the cumulative specific activity (calculated on the basis of the cumulative activity and cumulative OD 280 nm) of the fractions under each elution peak was determined (Fig. 12.4). The highest values of the cumulative specific activity from the polymer shielded column were obtained under the elution peaks with KCl concentration

Table 12.1 Effect of water soluble polymers in dye affinity chromatography

Dye ligand	Polymer	Polymer–Dye interactions	Protein/Source	Advantages	Reference
Cibacron Blue 3GA	PVP	Moderate	Lacatate dehydrogenase from porcine muscle	Improved effiency of specific and nonspecific elution	Galaev and Mattiasson, 1994a
Procion Scarlet H2G	PVP	Moderate	Secondary alcohol dehydrogenase from *Thermoanaerobium brockii*	Improved purity and recovery	Galaev and Mattiasson, 1994a
Procion Red HE3B	Poly(vinyl alcohol)	Weak	Pyruvate kinase from porcine muscle	Improved recovery	Garg et al., 1994
Cibacron Blue 3GA	PVP	Moderate	Phosphofructokinase from baker's yeast	Improved effiency of elution, higher yield	Galaev et al., 1994c
Procion Blue HERD	PVP	Moderate	Lactate dehydrogenase from porcine muscle	Improved effiency of elution, higher yield	Garg et al., 1997
Cibacron Blue 3GA	PVP	Moderate	Lactate dehydrogenase from porcine muscle	Improved purification and recovery in expanded bed mode	Garg et al., 1994
Cibacron Blue 3GA	Poly(N-vinylcapro-lactam)	Increased with temperature from moderate to strong	Lactate dehydrogenase from porcine muscle	Temperature induced elution	Galaev et al., 1994d
Cibacron Blue 3GA, Procion Red HE-3B	Poly-(ethylene imine)	Very strong	Lactate dehydrogenase from porcine muscle	Protein displacement	Galaev et al., 1995

increasing up to 0.06 M. On an unshielded column, the highest values were obtained under the elution peaks with KCl concentration increasing up to 0.15 M KCl. Therefore, 0.15 M KCl was chosen as the optimal eluent. For both unshielded and shielded columns, larger amounts of foreign proteins were eluted at higher ionic strengths.

In the expanded bed runs, sample loading and washing steps were carried out in the expanded bed mode but the elution was done in a packed bed mode. Figure 12.5 shows the chromatography profile from an unshielded Streamline-CB column during expanded bed operations. Both the recovery (calculated as a percentage of the bound

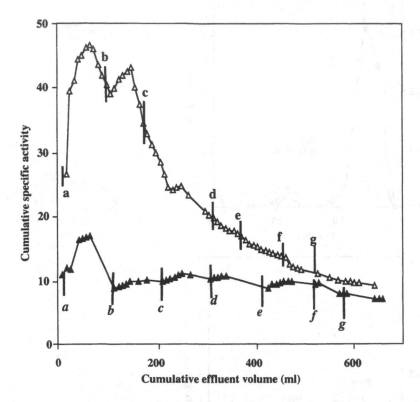

Figure 12.4 Cumulative specific activity profile (▲) untreated; (△) PVP-treated. The values were obtained by dividing the cumulative lactate dehydrogenase activity (Units) with the cumulative OD 280 nm (mg); The ionic strength of the KCl eluent was increased stepwise; a = 0.03 M, b = 0.06 M, c = 0.12 M, d = 0.15 M, e = 0.3 M, f = 0.6 M and g = 1.5 M. Untreated: The settled bed height was 2.6 cm and the column had an internal diameter of 1.6 cm. The linear flow rate was 119 cm/h. PVP treated: The column had a settled bed height 3.0 cm and an internal diameter of 1.6 cm. The linear flow rate was 122 cm/h. Reproduced with permission from Garg *et al.* (1996).

enzyme, 17%) and purification factor (1.8) were relatively low. PVP-shielding of the column increased significantly recovery up to acceptable level of 78%. The purification fold of 4.1 was also higher in the case of the polymer shielded column as compared to unshielded column (Garg *et al.*, 1996).

The reduced nonspecific interactions of the dye ligand with lactate dehydrogenase accounted for its higher recovery from a polymer shielded column. Incorporation of a washing step (with a high ionic strength buffer) which could remove some of the foreign proteins which co-elute with the target protein, is not possible here, since the target protein itself elutes from the PVP treated column at a very low ionic strength.

The concept of shielding reduces nonspecific interactions. This feature is attractive in all types of separations but especially so when crude preparations are processed. For that purpose, the combination of shielding with expanded bed chromatography is very attractive.

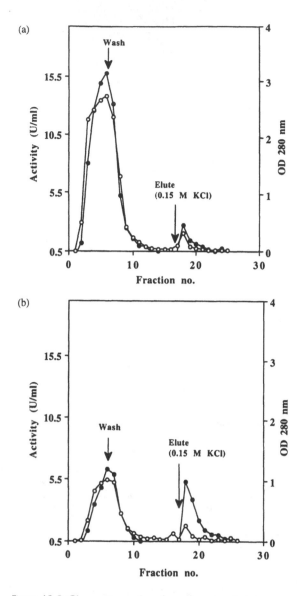

Figure 12.5 Chromatography of porcine muscle homogenate on Streamline-CB in an expanded bed system. (•) activity; (o) OD 280 nm. (a) Untreated: The settled bed height was 2.6 cm and the column had an internal diameter of 1.6 cm. The degree of expansion was 1.7 at a linear flow rate of 143 cm/h. Fifty milliliters of crude extract containing 1200 Units of lactate dehydrogenase activity and 113 mg of protein was introduced onto the column at the zero value on the X-axis. (b) PVP-treated: The settled bed height was 3.0 cm and the column had an internal diameter of 1.6 cm. The degree of expansion was 1.7 at a linear flowrate of 146 cm/h. Forty eight milliliters of crude extract containing 470 Units of lactate dehydrogenase activity and 50 mg of protein were introduced in the column at the zero value on the X-axis. Reproduced with permission from Garg *et al.* (1996).

Acknowledgement

The support of Swedish Center for Bioseparation is greatly acknowledged.

References

Chase H. A. (1994) Purification of proteins by adsorption chromatography in expanded beds. *Trends Biotechnol.*, 12, 296–303.

Galaev, I. Yu. and Mattiasson, B. (1994a) Poly(N-vinylpyrrolidone) shielding of matrices for dye-affinity chromatography. Improved elution of lactate dehydrogenase from Blue Sepharose and secondary alcohol dehydrogenase from Scatlet Sepharose. *J. Chromatogr. A*, 662, 27–35.

Galaev, I. Yu. and Mattiasson, B. (1994b) Polymer-shielded dye-affinity Chromatography. In: D. L. Pyle (ed.) *Separations for Biotechnology*, SCI, Cambridge, 179–185.

Galaev, I. Yu., Garg, N. and Mattiasson, B. (1994c) Interaction of Cibacron Blue with polymers: implications for polymer-shielded dye-affinity chromatography of phosphofructokinase from baker's yeast. *J. Chromatogr. A*, 684, 45–54.

Galaev, I. Yu., Warrol, C. and Mattiasson, B. (1994d) Temperature-induced displacement of proteins from dye/affinity columns using an immobilized polymeric displacer. *J. Chromatogr. A*, 684, 37–43.

Galaev, I. Yu., Arvidsson, P. and Mattiasson, B. (1995) Polymer displacement in dye-affinity chromatography. *J. Chromatogr.*, 710, 259–266.

Garg, N., Galaev, I. Yu. and Mattiasson, B. (1994) Effect of poly(vinyl alcohol) treatment of the dye/matrix on the chromatography of pyruvate kinase. *Biotechnol. Techn.*, 8, 645–650.

Garg, N., Galaev, I. Yu. and Mattiasson, B. (1996) Polymer shielded dye–ligand chromatography of lactate dehydrogenase from porcine muscle in an expanded bed system. *Bioseparation*, 6, 193–199.

Garg, N., Galaev, I. Yu. and Mattiasson, B. (1997) Chromatography of lactate dehydrogenase from porcine muscle on polymer shielded dye–ligand columns. An attempt for the rational choice of polymer/dye combination. *Isolation Purification*, 2, 301–318.

Guo, W., Shang, Z., Yu, Y. and Zhou, L. (1994) Membrane affinity chromatography of alkaline phosphatases. *J. Chromatogr.*, 685, 344–348.

Kaul, R. and Mattiasson, B. (1992) Secondary purification. *Bioseparation*, 3, 1–26.

Mattiasson, B., Garg, N. and Galaev, I. Yu. (1996) Polymer-shielded dye-affinity chromatography. *J. Mol. Recogn.*, 9, 509–514.

Scopes, R. K. (1986) Screening for protein purification: is there an optimum adsorbent for every protein? *J. Chromatogr.*, 376, 131–140.

Sii, D. and Sadana, A. (1991) Bioseparation using affinity techniques. *J. Biotechnol.*, 19, 83–98.

Chapter 13

Glycobiology and biochromatography

Henri Debray, Gérard Strecker and Jean Montreuil

Introduction

From biochemistry to glycobiology and glycotechnologies

Carbohydrates, together with proteins, lipids and nucleic acids are the fourth class of constituents of living matter. As far back as the middle of the nineteenth century scientists launched very active research because of their economic importance, and the industry of high polymers such as starch, cellulose, and pectins rapidly developed. In addition, at the end of the last century, the interest of scientists turned to a new class of complex carbohydrates, widely distributed, having various physiological activities, and playing an important role in the social life of cells: the glycoconjugates. These substances are constituents of numerous biological fluids and of all biomembranes. They are recognition signals and markers of cancer and are the underlying principles for numerous diseases. So were born two new words and domains, those of *Glycobiology* and of *Glycopathology*.

The present chapter is essentially devoted to glycoproteins but the described methods are of general application and could be applied to the study of glycolipid glycan structure.

Glycoproteins result from the classical processes of translation of the genomic message at the level of membrane bound polysomes leading to the synthesis of a peptide chain to which carbohydrate moieties, called *glycans*, are subsequently conjugated through covalent linkages. Most proteins are glycosylated and the glycoproteins are widely distributed in all organisms: animals, plants, yeasts, microorganisms, and viruses.

The biological importance of glycoconjugates in general, and of glycoproteins in particular, has been demonstrated through a series of crucial discoveries which pointed to the biological roles of glycans. As a result, the fundamental concept of *Glycobiology*, *i.e.* the molecular biology of glycoconjugates has emerged.

Biological role of glycans

During the last few decades, the chemical and biochemical characteristics of glycoproteins have acquired an importance as great as that of proteins and nucleic acids. Due to this, development of the methods for the isolation and primary structure determination, and the structure of thousands of glycans have been established. On these solid bases, numerous structure–function relationships have been defined leading to the establishment of the foundations for the genetics and molecular biological characteristics of glycoproteins and we know now that glycans:

  (i) increase the solubility of proteins,
 (ii) induce and maintain the secondary and tertiary structure of proteins in a biologically active form,
(iii) protect the peptide chain against proteolytic attack,
 (iv) control the proteolysis of pro- and polyproteins leading to active proteins or peptides,
  (v) control the membrane permeability due to their high hydrophilicity and to their chaotropic effect on water molecules, and thus powerfully regulate cell metabolism,
 (vi) are related to immune response through both glycoprotein antigenicity and immunogenicity,
(vii) control the life span of circulating glycoproteins and cells,
(viii) constitute recognition signals for carbohydrate receptors called membrane lectins or endogenous lectins which are present in all of the membranes of all living organisms and in the envelope of viruses. In this way, glycans are involved in cell–cell recognition and adhesion, in cell differentiation and development and in cell-contact inhibition, thereby intervening in the social life of cells,
 (ix) are specific receptors for viruses, bacteria, fungi and parasites, thus explaining the host cell specificity of these organisms.

Molecular pathology of glycoproteins

Research on normal and pathological metabolism of glycoconjugates was developed at the same time as the exploration of glycan structure. In fact, the first determination, in the early 1970s, of glycoprotein glycan primary structure, immediately spurred intensive research in the field of normal and pathological glycan biosynthesis and catabolism. The pathogenesis of numerous diseases called glycoproteinoses has been, in turn elucidated in relation to the observed misglycosylation, the latter related either to glycosyltransferases or to glycosidases. The most illustrative example is that of a series of diseases that are due to genetic lack or deficit in lysosomal glycosidases. In fact, in the 1970s, research of clinicians and biochemists began on a type of genetic and lethal disease characterized by the same symptoms: facial dismorphy, mental retardation and accumulation of carbohydrate materials in tissues and urine. The elucidation of the structure of these carbohydrates led the investigators to the conclusion that they were confronted with a disease of glycoconjugates, due to deficits in lysosomal glycosidases and thus to cessation of recurrent degradation of glycans in lysosome with, as a consequence, the accumulation of the undegraded glycans in tissues, and ensuing pathological symptoms mentioned above.

Development of glycotechnology

Glycoconjugates have recently entered the industrial field of genetic engineering of human glycoproteins of therapeutic interest. This gives rise to a formidable problem, because the production of recombinant human glycoproteins in non-human eukaryotic cells or in prokaryotic cells which are devoid of the enzymic equipment for glycan biosynthesis leads to the expression of misglycosylated or non-glycosylated proteins. Since proteins may require proper glycosylation for therapeutic effectiveness and safety, eukaryotic cells have been engineered to produce recombinant glycoproteins which strictly conform to the native glycoprotein. In this regard, very few recombinant glycoproteins have been, up to now, commercialized and used for therapy since our present knowledge concerning the regulation of glycan biosynthesis is too limited to achieve reliable biosynthesis of the authentic glycans of recombinant glycoproteins. This leads, in many cases, to misglycosylation with dramatic consequences: increase of hydrophobicity, decrease or inhibition of secretion leading to decrease in yield, decrease of stability, shortening of *in vivo* life of molecules by increase in their clearance, decrease of affinity for specific receptors, and increase of immunogenicity. Moreover, the recombinant glycoproteins are not the exclusive interest of the Glyco-Industry. In fact, sugars or sugar derivatives are used in various developing therapies: (1) drug targeting by coupling adequate oligosaccharides to the active drugs, in order to direct the "drug missiles" to their target cells; (2) competitive inhibition of metastasis by using neoglycoconjugates; (3) competitive inhibition of bacterial adhesion on cells or mucus by sugars for preventing or treating pulmonary infections or diarrhea of children; (4) preparation of synthetic vaccines; (5) cancer immunodiagnosis and immunotherapy using antigenized "tumor associated antigens" (TAAs) of a carbohydrate nature.

Primary structure of glycoprotein glycans

Monosaccharide constituents

For a long time, the list of "classical" monosaccharides constituting the glycans were D-galactose (Gal), D-glucose (Glc), D-mannose (Man), L-fucose (Fuc), D-xylose (Xyl), L-arabinofuranose (Ara), *N*-acetyl-D-glucosamine (GlcNAc) and -D-galactosamine (GalNAc), D-glucuronic acid (GlcA), L-iduronic acid (IduA), *N*-acetyl-D-neuraminic (NeuAc) and *N*-glycolyl-D-neuraminic (NeuGc) acids. However, improvements of the analytical methods and extension of research from higher animals to all of the other living organisms led to the identification of numerous new monosaccharides.

Among the monosaccharides, sialic acid must be especially mentioned since their number now is close to 40. They differ in the substituent of the amino group (acetyl, glycolyl or *O*-acetylated *N*-glycolyl) and also in the number (0–3), position (4, 7, 8, or 9), and nature (acetyl, lactyl, methyl) of substituents of the hydroxyl groups of neuraminic acid. Two recent additions are (1) the 4,6-anhydro-*N*-acetylneuraminic acid found in the edible bird's nest mucin, which is a hydrolysis artefact, and (2) the 3-deoxy-D-galactononulosonic acid or 2-keto-3-deoxynonulosonic acid (Kdn or KDN) abundant in fish and batracian glycoproteins, in which the amino group of neuraminic acid is replaced by a hydroxyl group.

Types of glycan–protein linkages

Glycans are conjugated to peptide chains through two types of primary covalent linkages (*N*-glycosyl and *O*-glycosyl) leading to the definition of three classes of glycoproteins: *N*-glycosylproteins, *O*-glycosylproteins, and *N,O*-glycosylproteins.

The most distributed N-glycosidic bond presently found in glycoproteins is N-acetylglucosaminyl-asparagine: GlcNAc(β1–N)Asn. In contrast, the O-glycosidic bond presents a wide variety of linkages, the most common being the following ones:

(a) Mucin-type: alkali-labile linkage between N-acetyl-D-galactosamine and L-serine or L-threonine: GalNAc(α1–3)Ser/Thr.
(b) Proteoglycan-type: alkali-labile linkage between D-xylose and L-serine: Xyl(β1–3)Ser.
(c) Collagen-type: alkali-stable linkage between D-galactose and 5-hydroxy-L-lysine: Gal(β1–5)OH-Lys.
(d) Extensin-type: alkali-stable linkage between L-arabinofuranose and 4-hydroxyl-L-proline: L-Araf(β1–4)OH-Pro identified in plant glycoproteins.
(e) Glycogenin-type: alkali-stable linkage between α-D-glucose and tyrosine in glycogen.

Concepts and rules

THE CONCEPT OF THE COMMON "INNER-CORE"

The glycans of N- and O-glycosylproteins are derived from the substitution of oligosaccharide structures common to numerous glycans, which are consequently nonspecific. These structures are conjugated to the peptide chain and constitute the most internal part of glycans. They are designated as core or innercore (Fig. 13.1). Core A exists in all the O-glycosylproteins of the mucin type. Core B constitutes the terminal sequence of almost all the glycosaminoglycans of proteoglycans. Core C is common to all N-glycosylproteins in which the glycan–protein linkage is the glycosylamine linkage GlcNAc(β1–N)Asn.

THE CONCEPT OF THE ANTENNA

The glycan structures are derived from the substitution of inner-cores by a very wide variety of glycosidic structures that confer specificity to the glycans. On the basis of the spatial conformation of the glycans, of their mobility in space and of their role as recognition signals the outer branches embellishing the inner cores are called "antennae".

Gal(β1–3)GalNAc(α1–0)Ser/Thr A

Gal(β1–3)Gal(β1–4)Xyl(β1–0)Ser B

Man(α1–6)
                \
        Man(β1–4)GlcNAc(β1–4)GlcNAc(β1–N)Asn C
                /
Man(α1–3)

Figure 13.1 Oligosaccharide inner-cores of some glycoprotein glycans.

MICROHETEROGENEITY OF GLYCANS – THE GLYCOFORMS

In addition to genetically determined variants expressed as variations in their polypeptide chains, almost all glycoproteins reveal another form of polymorphism associated with their carbohydrate residues. In fact, a given glycan located at a given amino acid in a glycoprotein often presents a structural heterogeneity, termed "microheterogeneity" because it involves the number and position of the most external monosaccharides in the glycan moieties (Schmid *et al.*, 1962). These variants are called "glycoforms". An illustrative example is given by the human Tamm-Horsfall glycoprotein, in which 30 different glycans have been described at the level of the three potential sites of glycosylation (Hård *et al.*, 1992). Looking at Fig. 13.2 one can realize that the microheterogeneity of glycoprotein glycans is one of the most formidable problems encountered by the glycobiologist. In fact, we totally ignore the significance of this phenomenon. In addition, the isolation of each glycoform represents an analytical achievement which is of

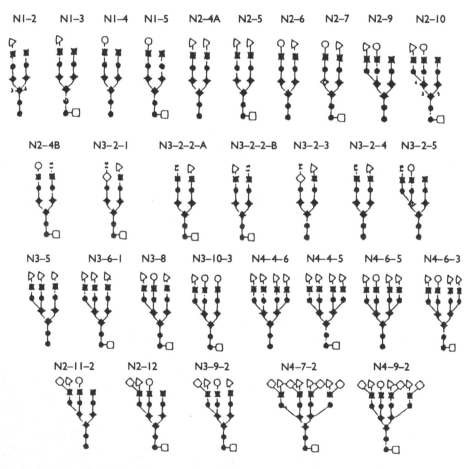

Figure 13.2 Structure of the 30 glycans isolated from the Tamm-Horsfall glycoprotein after treatment of the peptide by *N*-glycanase F. ●: GlcNAc; ◇: Man; ■: Gal; △: α-2,3-NeuAc; ○: α-2,6-NeuAc; ⊏: GalNAc; ☐: Fuc. In addition, SO_3-GalNAc-Gal and GalNAc[NeuAc(α2-3)]Gal are present.

fundamental interest to the field of recombinant glycoproteins, which present the same microheterogeneity.

General features of the primary structure of glycoprotein glycans

N-GLYCOSYLPROTEIN GLYCANS (N-GLYCANS)

The inner core C of Fig. 13.1 can be substituted by different chains, leading to the formation of the antennae and to three families of glycans.

In the first family, the inner-core is substituted uniquely by mannose residues; these glycans are said to be of the oligomannosidic or high mannose type (Fig. 13.3). In animals and plants, the number of additional mannose residues varies from 0 to 6, leading to the formation of the so-called M_3 to M_9 glycans.

In the second family, the inner-core is substituted by a variable number of N-acetyllactosamine $Gal(\beta 1-4)GlcNAc$ residues. These glycans are of the N-acetyllactosaminic or complex type (Fig. 13.4).

In the third family, glycans simultaneously present both oligomannosidic and N-acetyllactosaminic structure and thus belong to the hybrid type (Fig. 13.5).

The family of N-acetyllactosaminic glycans presents a tremendous diversity of structures related (1) to the number of antennae, which varies from one to five (Fig. 13.4), and (2) to the number of additional monosaccharides and to their position in the antennary basic structures: sialic acids, fucose, N-acetylgalactosamine replacing galactose residue(s), methylated, phosphorylated, sulfated monosaccharides, etc. Consequently, the number of possible glycan structures is limitless so that the glycans of the N-acetyllactosaminic type are considered to function virtually, as specific recognition signals.

```
Man(α1–2)Man(α1–6)
                   \
                     Man(α1–6)
                   /          \
Man(α1–2)Man(α1–3)              Man(β1–4)GlcNAc(β1–4)GlcNAc(β1–N)Asn   1
                              /
Man(α1–2) Man(α1–2)Man(α1–3)


      Man(α1–6)
             \
               Man(α1–6)
             /          \
Man(α1–3)                Man(β1–4)GlcNAc(β1–4)GlcNAc(β1–N)Asn   2
                        /
      Man(α1–3)
```

Figure 13.3 Structure of glycans of the oligomannosidic-type. 1: This structure, conventionally assigned as M9, is present in calf thyroglobulin unit A, human IgD and myeloma IgM, Chinese hamster ovary cell glycoproteins, bovine lactotransferrin, soybean agglutinin, Newcastle virus, and scorpion haemocyanin. 2: This structure, conventionally assigned as M5, has been found in Taka-amylase, hen ovalbumin, and human myeloma IgM.

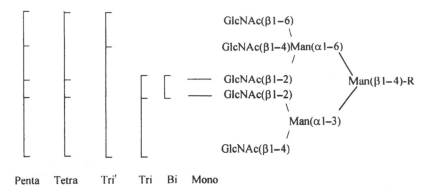

Figure 13.4 Definition of the various types of antennae found in N-glycans of the N-acetyllactosaminic type from mono- to pentaantennary structures. R : GlcNAc(β1–4) [Fuc(α1 – 6)]$_{0-1}$ GlcNAc (β1–N)Asn.

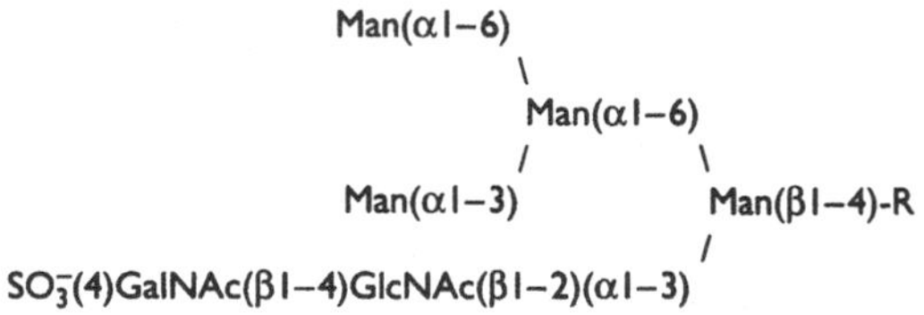

Man(α1–6)
\
    Man(α1–6)
    /   \
Man(α1–3)   Man(β1–4)-R
                        /
SO$_3^-$(4)GalNAc(β1–4)GlcNAc(β1–2)(α1–3)

Figure 13.5 Glycan of the hybrid type of a pituitary hormone. R: GlcNAc(β1–4) GlcNAc (β1–N)Asn.

An example of each type of glycan of the *N*-acetyllactosaminic type, from the bi- to the tetra-antennary structures, is given in Fig. 13.6.

O-GLYCOSYLPROTEIN GLYCANS (O-GLYCANS)

Classification of *O*-glycosylproteins is based on the nature of the carbohydrate–protein linkages.

1. *N-acetylgalactosamine–Serine/Threonine Linkage.* This group comprises glycans designated as "mucin-type" structures, even if they are present in plasma cell membranes and in glycoproteins from biological fluids. As shown in Fig. 13.7, in which some *O*-glycan structures are described, the main observation which can be made concerning these structures is the lack of structural specificity, except for glycans carrying tissular or blood group epitopes, such as T, Tn, and O epitopes. It is postulated that these glycans, often located in strategic domains of the peptide chain, like the hinge region of IgA$_1$, play a role in the maintenance of the protein in a biologically active conformation.

2. *Xylose–Serine Linkage.* This type of linkage in which xylose takes part of the trisaccharidic inner core Xyl(β1–0)Ser is found in the well-defined and homogeneous family of glycosaminoglycans. Conjugated to proteins, they constitute the important class of *proteoglycans.* They are high molecular weight carbohydrates which constitute the major part of the ground substance of connective tissue, also called the extracellular matrix,

NeuAc(α2–6)Gal(β1–4)GlcNAc(β1–2)Man(α1–6)

                     \

                        Man(β1–4)GlcNAc(β1–4)GlcNAc(β1–N)Asn **1**

                     /

NeuAc(α2–6)Gal(β1–4)GlcNAc(β1–2)Man(α1–3)

       Gal(β1–4)GlcNAc(β1–2)Man(α1–6)

       | (α1–3)   \

         Fuc   Man(β1–4)GlcNAc(β1–4)GlcNAc(β1–N)Asn **2**

                      /

NeuAc(α2–6)Gal(β1–4)GlcNAc(β1–2)Man(α1–3)

NeuAc(α2–6)Gal(β1–4)GlcNAc(β1–2)Man(α1–6)

                     \

NeuAc(α2–6)Gal(β1–4)GlcNAc(β1–4)   Man(β1–4)GlcNAc(β1–4)GlcNAc(β1–N)Asn **3**

                    \   / | (α1–6)

                Man(α1–3)   Fuc

              /

NeuAc(α2–6)Gal(β1–4)GlcNAc(β1–2)

NeuAc(α2–6)Gal(β1–4)GlcNAc(β1–6)

                     \

                Man(α1–6)

              /   \

NeuAc(α2–6)Gal(β1–4)GlcNAc(β1–2)

                         Man(β1–4)GlcNAc(β1–4)GlcNAc(β1–N)Asn **4**

NeuAc(α2–6)Gal(β1–4)GlcNAc(β1–4)   /

                    \

                Man(α1–3)

              /

NeuAc(α2–6)Gal(β1–4)GlcNAc(β1–2)

Figure 13.6 Structure of glycans of the *N*-acetyllactosaminic type (complex type). 1: biantennary glycan of human serum transferrin; 2: difucosylated biantennary glycan of human lactotransferrin; 3: triantennary glycan of human serum transferrin; 4: tetraantennary glycan of human α_1-acid glycoprotein

                GalNAc(α1–0)Ser/Thr **A**

       NeuAc(α2–6)GalNAc(α1–0)Ser/Thr **B**

          Gal(β1–3)GalNAc(α1–0)Ser/Thr **C**

NeuAc(α2–3)Gal(β1–3)GalNAc(α1–0)Ser/Thr **D**

                /

          NeuAc(α2–6)

Fuc(α1–2)Gal(β1–3)GalNAc(α1–0)Ser/Thr **E**

Figure 13.7 Structure of some O-glycans of the "mucin type". A: epitope of Tn group; B: human and ovine submaxillary mucin; C: antifreeze glycoprotein from antarctic fish, porcine submaxillary mucin, human chorionic gonadotropin, human IgA, T-reactive erythrocytes, rat brain glycoproteins, intestinal mucin; D: human glycophorin, fetuin, bovine kappa casein, human gonadotropin, lymphocyte membranes; E: human erythrocyte of O group, IgA: immunoglobulin A.

GlcNAc(β1–4)GlcA(β1–3)[GlcNAc(β1–4)GlcA(β1–3)]n GlcNAc(β1–4)GlcA **A**

[GalNAc(β1–4)GlcA(β1–3)]$_n$ GalNAc(β1–4)GlcA(β1–3)Gal(β1–3)Gal(β1–4)Xyl(β1–0)Ser **B**

| 4 or 6 | 4 or 6

SO$_3$H   SO$_3$H

[L – Idu(α1–4)GlcNSO$_3$H(α1–4)GlcA(β1–4)]$_n$ Gal(β1–3)Gal(β1–4)Xyl(β1–0)Ser **C**

Figure 13.8 Primary structure of some proteoglycans. A: hyaluronic acid (MM, 4–8 · 10^6 Da); B: SO$_3$H in C-4 position: chondroitin sulfate A (MM, 5–50· 10^3 Da) of bones, cartilages, cornea, umbilical cord; SO$_3$H in C-6 position: chondroitin sulfate C of cartilage, heart valves, saliva, skin, tendon; C: heparan sulfate (MM, 2–10 · 10^3 Da) of arterial wall, lung, cell surface.

in which the fibroblasts are embedded. They are also constituents of cell membranes and of the extracellular cement.

All are linear polymers made up of disaccharide repeating units consisting of a repeating sequence of uronic acid (D-glucuronic or/and L-iduronic acid) residue or of galactose residue linked to a hexosamine, either glucosamine or galactosamine, generally *N*-acetylated. Moreover, sulfate groups are present either as *O*-sulfate groups substituting the *N*-acetylhexosamine and galactose residues on C-4 or C-6 position, or as *N*-sulfate groups substituting the amino group of hexosamine.

In Fig. 13.8 are shown some structures of glycosaminoglycans restricted to hyaluronic acid, which is a free polysaccharide, and to chondroitin sulfates and heparin, which are proteoglycans.

It should be mentioned that heparan sulfate I from cornea is an *N*-glycan conjugated to asparagine and containing the pentasaccharidic inner-core of the *N*-glycosylproteins.

3. *Galactose–Hydroxylysine Linkage.* This linkage is widely distributed in collagens and tropocollagens of numerous animals. In all of these glycoproteins, the sugar moiety is present either as β-galactose only or as disaccharide Glc(α1–2)Gal(β1–0)OH-Lys.

4. *Arabinofuranose–Hydroxyproline Linkage.* Until now this type of glycan has been found only in plants and has been called "extensin type". The classical example is that of glycans isolated from tobacco cell wall: [L-Ara$f$ (β1–3)]$_{0-1}$L-Ara$f$ (β1–2)L-Araff (β1–0)OH-Pro]$_{0-1}$.

GLYCOSYLPHOSPHATIDYLINOSITOL (GPI) MEMBRANE ANCHORS

Glycosylphosphatidylinositol (GPI) membrane anchors are complex glycophospholipids constituted of two parts. The first is firmly integrated in the external lipid monolayer of the cell membrane through two fatty acid chains. It supports the second part, which comprises, in an external position, a protein or a glycoprotein. In this way, the active (glyco)protein is not directly integrated in the lipid bilayer of the membrane but is supported by a long and flexible arm. The GPIs are found in many eukaryotic cells, from protozoa, yeast, and slime mold to *Drosophila* and higher animals. All of the GPI anchors have a conserved basic core structure: ethanolamine-PO$_4$-(6)Man(α1–2)Man(α1–6)Man(α1–4)GlcNH$_2$(α1–6)-myo-inositol-1-

PO_4-diglyceride Species, and tissue-specific variations depend (1) on the nature of fatty acids, (2) on the substituents of the core tetrasaccharides, and (3) on the presence of an extra phosphoethanolamine residue. The GPI is linked to the (glyco)protein through an amide bond between the C-terminal amino acid-α-carboxyl group and the amine group of ethanolamine.

Overview of the methodology of glycan isolation and primary structure determination

The problem of the determination of glycan primary structure can be considered as virtually solved due to the development of efficient methods for the isolation of glycoprotein variants and of their glycan residues, mainly by using HPLC and affinity chromatography on immobilized lectins, and also the progress in chemical, enzymatic, and physical methodologies. In this regard, the collaboration between our laboratory and the one of J. F. G. Vliegenthart led to the introduction of a very efficient and sensitive method for determining the complete primary structure of glycans by associating the permethylation procedure with 360–600 MHz ^{1}H-NMR spectroscopy, which requires 25–100 µg of total sugars, is of a general application and is described under the subhead "Isolation of Glycans". Developments in mass spectrometry, particulary the "fast atom bombardment" method (FAB), and "matrix assisted laser desorption-time of flight mass spectrometry" (MALDI-TOF), have resulted in considerable progress. The description of the excellent, but not yet widely applied method of Yamashita et al. (1982) which combines gel filtration analysis and the stepwise degradation of glycans by glycosidases, has also been omitted due to lack of space.

In what follows next, we aim to describe the chromatographic methods currently used in our laboratory and elsewhere, for isolating oligosaccharides, glycopeptides and glycoproteins, by using affinity chromatography on immobilized lectins.

Lectin affinity chromatography of glycoconjugates

Specificity of lectins

Problems of lectin specificity

Lectins are sugar-binding proteins or glycoproteins of non-immune origin which agglutinate cells and/or precipitate glycoconjugates (Goldstein et al., 1980). They possess at least two sugar binding sites, the presence of which explains the ability of lectins to precipitate polysaccharides, glycoproteins or glycolipids and why they agglutinate cells.

Lectins have now been isolated from virus, bacteria, plants and from a variety of animal tissues and species. However, only plant lectins are now commonly used in research and in clinical laboratories for the detection and fractionation of soluble and membrane glycoproteins as well as glycopeptides or glycans derived from these glycoproteins (for reviews on plant lectins, see Goldstein and Hayes, 1978; Sharon and Lis, 1989; Goldstein et al., 1997).

Very often, lectins are still classified according to the monosaccharide which inhibits the interaction between a lectin and a cell or which allows the specific elution of a

Table 13.1 Lectins commonly used for glycoprotein study and classified according to their monosaccharide specificity

α-D-mannose, α-D-glucose	
Canavalia ensiformis	Con A
Lens culinaris	LCA
β-D-galactose, N-acetyl-β-D-galactosamine	
Ricinus communis	RCA$_I$
	RCA$_{II}$
Glycine max (Soybean)	SBA
Arachis hypogaea (Peanut)	PNA
α-D-Galactose, N-acetyl-α-D-galactosamine	
Griffonia simplicifolia I	GSA$_I$
Dolichos biflorus	DBA
N-acetyl-β-D-glucosamine	
Triticum vulgare (Wheat germ)	WGA
α-L-fucose	
Aleuria aurantia	AAA
Lotus tetragonolobus	LTA
Ulex europeus I	UEA$_I$
α-N-acetylneuraminic acid	
Limulus polyphemus (Limulin)	

bound glycoconjugate from an immobilized lectin column. Table 13.1 presents such a classification of some commonly used lectins in terms of monosaccharide specificity.

The structural basis of selective monosaccharide recognition by plant lectins investigated by X-ray crystallography is now well documented (Rini, 1995; Weis and Drickamer, 1996), explaining in terms of hydrogen bonds the low affinity (K_d in the 0.1–10 mM range) found in the interaction between a monosaccharide and a given lectin. However, it is well known that in most cases, complex oligosaccharides are several thousand-fold more potent inhibitors of lectins than monosaccharides (Kornfeld and Ferris, 1975; Debray et al., 1981). These high selectivities of binding towards complex oligosaccharides, first determined by biochemists, are now also explained by X-ray crystallography studies in terms of extended binding sites on a lectin. In addition to some amino acid residues forming the monosaccharide-binding site, other amino acid residues are involved in additional direct and water-mediated contacts between oligosaccharides and the lectin surface (Bourne et al., 1994; Weis and Drickamer, 1996; Weis, 1997).

It is very important to know this complex specificity before using a lectin as a probe in the exploration of cell surface glycoconjugates or as a tool to fractionate various glycoconjugates by affinity chromatography.

Determination of the "complex" specificity of lectins

The specificity of lectins towards monosaccharides or oligosaccharidic sequences belonging to glycoproteins or glycolipids can be determined by inhibition experiments in which monosaccharides or oligosaccharides of known structures are tested for their ability to inhibit either hemagglutination (Debray *et al.*, 1981) or precipitation of polysaccharides (Wu *et al.*, 1988). However, a major drawback of these methods is that they need large quantities of oligosaccharides often available only in limited amounts.

A second approach to determine the complex specificity of a lectin is to study the affinity of the immobilized lectin towards complex oligosaccharides (Baenziger and Fiete, 1979a; Debray and Montreuil, 1983; Cummings and Kornfeld, 1982; Debray *et al.*, 1983). In this approach, lectins are first immobilized onto insoluble matrices. Small columns containing 2–10 ml of the immobilized lectins are then prepared and equilibrated in an appropriate buffer and the behaviour of radiolabelled oligosaccharides or glycopeptides of known structure applied on these columns is examined.

Oligosaccharides are reduced at their terminal reducing monosaccharides with tritiated sodium borohydride according to Takasaki and Kobata (1974) and glycopeptides can be N-[^{14}C]-acetylated with [^{14}C]-acetic anhydride according to the procedure of Koide and Muramatsu (1974).

Table 13.2 shows the structures of N-glycosylpeptides which can be used for studying the specificities of immobilized lectins.

In a typical experiment, radiolabelled oligosaccharides or glycopeptides (2–30×10^3 DPM; 0.1–10 nmoles) are applied to a column (2–10 ml) of lectin immobilized on Sepharose 4B equilibrated in the appropriate buffer at room temperature. Elution is performed first with the starting buffer at a flow rate of 9 ml/h and then with the buffer containing 0.005 to 0.5 M of the monosaccharide recognized by the lectin. Fractions of 1.5 ml are collected and the radioactivity is counted in aliquots by liquid scintillation spectrometry.

Four elution profiles can be obtained:

- The elution of oligosaccharides or glycopeptides at the void volume of the column reflects a lack of affinity of the immobilized lectin towards the saccharides.
- Other saccharides, weakly recognized by the immobilized lectin, are eluted from the column by the equilibration buffer as retarded fractions.
- A sharp elution profile, obtained with the running buffer containing the competitive monosaccharide, reflects a strong interaction between the lectin and the applied oligosaccharides with association constants greater than 4×10^6 M^{-1}.
- A broad, trailing peak obtained also with the equilibration buffer containing the competitive monosaccharide indicates a very strong affinity between the saccharide and the immobilized lectin.

This second approach to determine the fine specificity of an immobilized lectin is of particular interest because it calls for only small amounts of oligosaccharides, and also because once the precise specificity of an immobilized lectin is established, it becomes possible to predict the primary structure of glycopeptides or oligosaccharides displaying similar elution profiles on the same lectin column.

Specificity of lectins towards complex oligosaccharides

From the inhibition methods or from the studies of the affinity of immobilized lectins towards complex oligosaccharides, important conclusions can be drawn on the carbohydrate-binding specificity of plant lectins.

Table 13.2 Structure of *N*-glycosylpeptides used to study immobilized lectin specificity

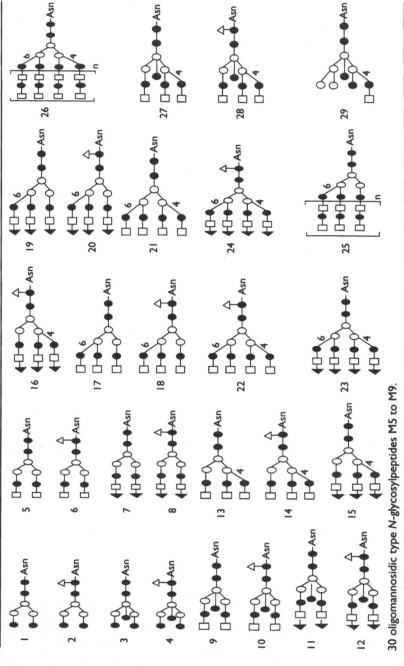

30 oligomannosidic type *N*-glycosylpeptides M5 to M9.

Numbers given in the schemes refer to glycosidic linkages 4: $\beta 1$–4; 6: $\beta 1$–6. In all schemes, the antennae linked to the $\alpha 1,3$ and $\alpha 1$–6-mannose residues are the lower and the upper ones, respectively.

●: GlcNAc; ☐: Gal; ○: Man; ▲: NeuAc; ▽: Fuc.

Table 13.3 Specificity of commonly used lectins towards oligosaccharide sequences belonging to N-glycosylproteins

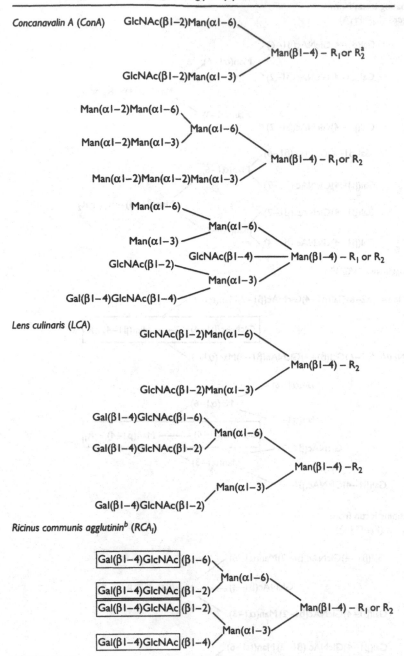

Concanavalin A (ConA)

$\text{GlcNAc}(\beta 1-2)\text{Man}(\alpha 1-6)$
$\text{GlcNAc}(\beta 1-2)\text{Man}(\alpha 1-3)$
$\text{Man}(\beta 1-4) - R_1 \text{ or } R_2^a$

$\text{Man}(\alpha 1-2)\text{Man}(\alpha 1-6)$
$\text{Man}(\alpha 1-2)\text{Man}(\alpha 1-3)$
$\text{Man}(\alpha 1-6)$
$\text{Man}(\alpha 1-2)\text{Man}(\alpha 1-2)\text{Man}(\alpha 1-3)$
$\text{Man}(\beta 1-4) - R_1 \text{ or } R_2$

$\text{Man}(\alpha 1-6)$
$\text{Man}(\alpha 1-3)$
$\text{Man}(\alpha 1-6)$
$\text{GlcNAc}(\beta 1-2)$
$\text{GlcNAc}(\beta 1-4)$
$\text{Man}(\alpha 1-3)$
$\text{Man}(\beta 1-4) - R_1 \text{ or } R_2$
$\text{Gal}(\beta 1-4)\text{GlcNAc}(\beta 1-4)$

Lens culinaris (LCA)

$\text{GlcNAc}(\beta 1-2)\text{Man}(\alpha 1-6)$
$\text{GlcNAc}(\beta 1-2)\text{Man}(\alpha 1-3)$
$\text{Man}(\beta 1-4) - R_2$

$\text{Gal}(\beta 1-4)\text{GlcNAc}(\beta 1-6)$
$\text{Gal}(\beta 1-4)\text{GlcNAc}(\beta 1-2)$
$\text{Man}(\alpha 1-6)$
$\text{Man}(\beta 1-4) - R_2$
$\text{Man}(\alpha 1-3)$
$\text{Gal}(\beta 1-4)\text{GlcNAc}(\beta 1-2)$

Ricinus communis agglutinin[b] (RCA_I)

$\boxed{\text{Gal}(\beta 1-4)\text{GlcNAc}}(\beta 1-6)$
$\boxed{\text{Gal}(\beta 1-4)\text{GlcNAc}}(\beta 1-2)$
$\text{Man}(\alpha 1-6)$
$\boxed{\text{Gal}(\beta 1-4)\text{GlcNAc}}(\beta 1-2)$
$\text{Man}(\beta 1-4) - R_1 \text{ or } R_2$
$\boxed{\text{Gal}(\beta 1-4)\text{GlcNAc}}(\beta 1-4)$
$\text{Man}(\alpha 1-3)$

Table 13.3 (Continued)

Leukoagglutinating lectin from
Phaseolus vulgaris (L$_4$ – PHA)

Gal(β1–4)GlcNAc(β1–6)

Man(α1–6)

Gal(β1–4)GlcNAc(β1–2)

Man(β1–4) – R$_1$ or R$_2$

Gal(β1–4)GlcNAc(β1–2)

Man(α1–3)

Gal(β1–4)GlcNAc(β1–6)

Man(α1–6)

Gal(β1–4)GlcNAc (β1–2)

Man(β1–4) – R$_1$ or R$_2$

Gal(β1–4)GlcNAc (β1–2)

Man(α1–3)

Gal(β1–4)GlcNAc (β1–4)

Wheat germ agglutinin (WGA)[b]

NeuAc(α2–6)Gal(β1–4)GlcNAc(β1–2)Man(α1–6)

GlcNAc(β1–4) ——— Man(β1–4) – R$_1$

NeuAc(α2–6)Gal(β1–4)GlcNAc(β1–2)Man(α1–3)

Man(α1–6)

Man(α1–6)

Man(α1–3)

GlcNAc(β1–4) ——— Man(β1–4) – R$_1$

GlcNAc(β1–2)

Man(α1–3)

Gal(β1–4)GlcNAc(β1–4)

Erythroagglutining lectin from
Phaseolus vulgaris (E$_4$–PHA)

Gal(β1–4)GlcNAc(β1–2)Man(α1–6)

GlcNAc(β1–4)——— Man(β1–4) – R$_1$ or R$_2$

Gal(β1–4)GlcNAc(β1–2) Man(α1–3)

Gal(β1–4)GlcNAc (β1–2) Man(α1–6)

Gal(β1–4)GlcNAc (β1–2) GlcNAc(β1–4) ——Man(β1–4) – R$_1$ or R$_2$

Man(α1–3)

Gal(β1–4)GlcNAc (β1–4)

Table 13.3 (Continued)

Datura stramonium agglutinin
(DSA)

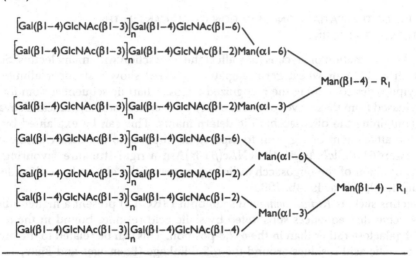

a R_1 : GlcNAc(β1–4)GlcNAc(β1–N)Asn; R_2: GlcNAc(β1–4)[Fuc(α1–6)]GlcNAc(β1–N)Asn.
b Sequences in boxes are the minimal oligosaccharide structure necessary for lectin recognition.

LECTINS CAN INTERACT WITH INTERNAL OLIGOSACCHARIDIC SEQUENCES OF A GLYCAN

Very few lectins recognize terminal non-reducing monosaccharides on a glycan, most of them recognize internal sequences of oligosaccharides.

LECTINS IDENTICAL IN TERMS OF MONOSACCHARIDE SPECIFICITY CAN PRESENT DIFFERENT COMPLEX SPECIFICITY

For example, both Con-A and *Lens culinaris* agglutinin (LCA) display the same monosaccharide specificity for α-D-mannose or α-D-glucose. However, as shown in Table 13.3, they present a higher affinity for different N-glycosylpeptides and related oligosaccharides. In particular, the presence of a fucose residue at the C-6 position of the GlcNAc residue involved in the N-glycosylamine linkage in a biantennary N-acetyllactosamine – type glycopeptide enhances the affinity of LCA for this glycan and is an important determinant for the glycan – binding specificity of the lectin (Debray *et al.*, 1981; Kornfeld *et al.*, 1981).

Moreover, a given lectin can recognize very different oligosaccharidic sequences. For example, ConA presents a strong affinity for oligomannosidic type as well as for some hybrid-type glycans and a weaker affinity for biantennary N-acetyllactosamine-type glycans (Table 13.3).

These complex glycan specificities of plant lectins result from the existence of extended carbohydrate-binding sites on the lectins.

It is also worth noting that different lectins can recognize different saccharidic sequences but belonging to a same glycan. As these sequences are common to numerous glycoproteins, results obtained with immobilized lectins during a fractionation of gly-coproteins or by western blot analysis of glycoproteins with lectins must be interpreted with caution.

IMPORTANCE OF THE SPATIAL CONFORMATION OF GLYCANS IN THE INTERACTION WITH LECTINS

The spatial conformation of glycans may affect the interaction with many lectins. Some lectins, such as LCA or wheat germ agglutinin (WGA) show a stronger affinity for *N*-glycosylpeptides containing the recognized oligosaccharidic sequences than for the glycans released from these glycopeptides either by chemical or enzymatical cleavages and still containing the oligosaccharidic determinants. This can be explained by the fact that the attachment of a glycan to asparagine imposes to the trisaccharidic core sequence Man(β1-4)GlcNAc(β1-4)GlcNAc(β1-N)Asn a rigid structure favouring the specific recognition of the oligosaccharidic sequences on the glycan by a given lectin (Montreuil, 1980, 1984a, 1984b, 1995).

Some lectins such as *Ricinus communis* agglutinin I (RCA I) present a higher affinity for oligosaccharidic sequences substituted by sialic acid residues bound in the α-2,6-position of galactose rather than in the α-2,3-position. This can be related to the higher mobility of sialic acid residues around the α-2,6-linkage (Baenziger and Fiete, 1979a; Debray *et al.*, 1981; Green *et al.*, 1987a.)

However, for other lectins such as isolectins E4- or L4-PHA (isolectins from *Phaseolus vulgaris* seeds with erythro-agglutinating or leuco-agglutinating activities), this higher mobility of the sialic acid residues around the α-2,6-linkage can mask the internal oligosaccharidic determinants recognized by the lectins. This can explain why sialy-lated glycans in the α-2,6-position of galactose are not recognized by these lectins while sialylated glycans but in the α-2,3-position of galactose interact with them (Green *et al.*, 1987b, 1988).

The concept of a larger mobility in space of oligosaccharidic sequences around an α-1,6-glycosidic linkage compared to the higher rigidity imposed by the α-1,3-linkage can explain the higher affinity of some lectins such as LCA or L4-PHA for tri'-antennary *N*-acetyllactosamine-type glycans (Table 13.3) in which one of the α-Man residues is substituted by the third antennae at the C-2 and C-6 positions, rather than for trianten-nary glycans containing another α-Man substituted at C-2 and C-4 positions (Kornfeld *et al.*, 1981; Cummings and Kornfeld, 1982; Green *et al.*, 1988).

In conclusion, due to their extended carbohydrate-binding sites, most lectins will display very precise specificity towards well-defined oligosaccharidic sequences belong-ing either to *N*- or O-glycosylproteins. Thus far, classifications of lectins according to monosaccharide specificity must be superseded by classifications taking into account the concept of "dominant-oligosaccharides" with either internal or peripheral positions on a glycan recognized by lectins. However, a few lectins will present a specificity directed towards terminal non-reducing dominant monosaccharides (for reviews, see Gallagher, 1984, 1989; Merkle and Cummings, 1987; Osawa and Tsuji, 1987; Debray and Montreuil, 1991, 1992; Tsuji *et al.*, 1993; Yamamoto *et al.*, 1993; Kobata and Yamashita, 1993; Cummings, 1994, 1997; Lakhtin, 1995; Debray, 1995).

Table 13.3 presents the specificity of some commonly used lectins towards oligosac-charidic determinants belonging to *N*-glycosylproteins.

Use of immobilized lectins for fractionation of glycoproteins

Immobilization of lectins

Numerous methods have been proposed for preparing immobilized lectins and many of them are now available from different suppliers (Pharmacia Biotech, E. Y. laboratories, Sigma Chemical Co., Vector laboratories). Lectins immobilized to CNBr-activated agarose are the most popular and can be easily prepared at a density of 2–10 mg of lectin/ml of settled gel (agarose, Sepharose or Ultrogel) activated with CNBr according to the procedures of March et al., 1974 or Kohn and Wilchek, 1982.

ACTIVATION OF SEPHAROSE 4B ACCORDING TO MARCH ET AL. (1974)

50 ml of wet Sepharose 4B beads (Pharmacia Biotech) are washed on a sintered glass funnel with 1 l of ice-cold distilled water and transferred into a beaker cooled in an ice-bath.

The Sepharose beads are mixed with 100 ml of ice-cold 2 M K_2CO_3 solution under gentle magnetic stirring. Activation is started by addition of 6.25 ml of freshly prepared CNBr solution in acetonitrile (2 g/ml) for 2 min at 0°C in a well ventilated hood.

After exactly 2 min, the entire reaction mixture is quickly poured into a sintered glass funnel and the activated Sepharose beads are washed extensively with ice-cold distilled water. The activated Sepharose is transferred into a 250 ml measuring cylinder and the ice-cold lectin solution to be coupled (0.25 g of lectin dissolved into coupling buffer: 0.5 M NaCl, 0.2 M $NaHCO_3$, 0.2 M competitive monosaccharide, pH 8.5) is added. The measuring cylinder is sealed with parafilm and gently mixed end-over-end for 24 h at 4°C.

The reaction mixture is filtered through a sintered glass funnel and the gel is washed extensively with 1 l each of ice-cold distilled water, coupling buffer without competitive monosaccharide and distilled water, successively.

The approximate amount of uncoupled lectin can be estimated by measuring the absorbance of the collected filtrate at 280 nm.

The unreacted iminocarbonate groups of the Sepharose beads are blocked by suspending the gel into 100 ml of a 1 M glycine solution under gentle stirring, for 3 h at room temperature. The glycine-blocked gel is washed extensively with ice-cold distilled water and then with the running buffer to be used containing 0.02% sodium azide. The immobilized lectins are then stored at 4°C in the equilibration buffer until use.

OTHER COUPLING METHODS FOR IMMOBILIZATION OF LECTINS

Lectins can also be immobilized to insoluble absorbents by other coupling methods. Immobilization of lectins with glutaraldehyde to polyacrylic-hydrazido-Sepharose according to Wilchek and Miron (1974) as described (Montreuil et al., 1994) does not introduce charged groups into the matrix, a major drawback found in lectin affinity gels prepared by activation of Sepharose with CNBr.

Immobilized lectins can be prepared with activated agarose containing N-hydroxysuccinimide esters which react with amino groups of lectins (Wilchek and Miron, 1987). These activated gels are available from Bio-Rad as Affi-Gel 10 or Affi-Gel 15.

All these gels can be used in low-pressure chromatography with flow rates of 5–20 ml/h. However, lectins can be also immobilized on activated supports compatible with high-performance liquid chromatography (flow rate of 1 ml/min). This technique combines the high speed and resolution characteristics of high performance liquid chromatography (HPLC) with the selectivity of biospecific interactions.

For example, Green et al. (1987b) have used columns of silica-bound lectins both to define the oligosaccharidic specificity of lectins and to fractionate glycopeptides or glycans. Asialooligosaccharides released from human IgG have been separated by HPLAC with a column of Ricinus communis agglutinin I bound on poly(acrylicester) gel (WG003) (Harada et al., 1987). As proposed for affinity chromatography using lectins immobilized on agarose, most of the N-glycosylpeptides or related glycans can be fractionated into homogeneous classes by serial affinity HPLC using different columns of silica-bound lectins.

GENERAL REMARKS ON THE IMMOBILIZATION OF LECTINS

1   During the coupling reactions, lectin binding sites must be protected by addition of the competitive monosaccharide (0.2 M) in the coupling buffer.
2   Between uses at room temperature, the immobilized lectins must be stored at 2–4°C in the equilibration buffer containing 0.02% sodium azide as a bacteriostatic agent, without loss of activity for several years.
3   Some lectins possess metal-binding sites and the presence of metal ions is important to induce a proper conformation of the lectin favouring carbohydrate binding. For example, ConA requires Mn^{2+}, Mg^{2+} and Ca^{2+} for full activity and the buffers used during affinity chromatography on this lectin must contain $MnCl_2$, $MgCl_2$ and $CaCl_2$ (1 mM of each).

Fractionation of glycoproteins on immobilized lectins

Affinity chromatography on immobilized lectins is now widely used to fractionate either soluble or membrane glycoproteins and many examples have been reviewed elsewhere (Dulaney, 1979; Lotan and Nicolson, 1979; Hedo, 1984; Lis and Sharon, 1984, 1986a,b; Debray and Montreuil, 1991). We highlight here some particular points which can be useful during such fractionations.

USE OF CROSSED AFFINOIMMUNOELECTROPHORESIS (CAIE) OF GLYCOPROTEINS AS A GUIDE FOR LECTIN AFFINITY CHROMATOGRAPHY

Crossed affinoimmunoelectrophoresis (CAIE) introduced by Bog-Hansen (1973) combines the interaction between a lectin and glycoproteins in the first dimension electrophoretic step with crossed electrophoresis into an antibody containing gel in the second dimension. This sensitive technique can give important information about the interaction between a given lectin and the glycoprotein to be purified because a good correlation is generally observed between results obtained by CAIE and by affinity chromatography on the immobilized lectin.

Above all, the method rapidly reveals the glycan microheterogeneity of the glycoprotein to be purified. This method can also be used for the characterization of membrane glycoproteins solubilized in non-ionic detergents because both lectin-membrane glycoproteins interactions and antigenicity of membrane glycoproteins are not affected by non-ionic detergents such as Triton X-100 (Bjerrum and Bog-Hansen, 1976; Hagen et al., 1979).

Last but not least, determination of glycan microheterogeneity of serum glycoproteins by CAIE can be used for a rapid and discriminating diagnosis of various pathological conditions (for a review, see Heegard et al., 1992).

BINDING CAPACITY OF THE IMMOBILIZED LECTINS AND PROBLEMS OF THE ELUTION

Variations in the amount, as well as in the quality of the lectin immobilized on a gel, represent important factors influencing the binding of glycoproteins. Examples of these factors include affinity differences often observed between different commercially available ConA preparations. This implies the calibration of the lectin column with well-known glycoproteins or glycopeptides before using a new batch of immobilized lectin.

Three fractions are generally obtained reflecting relative affinities of the immobilized lectins for the glycoproteins.

1   The non-reactive compounds are eluted at the void volume of the column with the equilibration buffer. This fraction, when the exact capacity of the immobilized lectin is not known, must be submitted to a new cycle of adsorption and elution on the same column, to be sure that the immobilized lectin was not saturated during the first run. In order to limit non-specific interactions between glycoproteins and immobilized lectins, equilibration buffers must possess a moderate ionic strength (0.1–1 M in NaCl for example).
2   The weakly reactive glycoproteins give fraction(s) which are recovered by elution in the equilibration buffer as retarded fraction(s). In this case, the separation of weakly interacting glycoproteins can be obtained by using a long and thin lectin column which is more efficient than a wider and a shorter column containing the same amount of immobilized lectin. The spatial conformations of the native glycoproteins or non-specific hydrophobic interactions may modulate the accessibility of some glycans to the lectin and can explain the presence of some artefactual weakly reactive fractions. These fractions often are absent when the glycoproteins are reduced and alkylated before fractionation on the immobilized lectin (Bayard et al., 1981). It is also worthy to note that, according to the origin of the immobilized lectin, a weakly reactive glycoprotein can be either bound and eluted with the lectin-reactive fraction or unbound and eluted with the lectin-non-reactive fraction.
3   Strongly reactive glycoproteins are specifically eluted after extensive washing with the equilibration buffer containing the competitive monosaccharide (0.1–0.5 M). The specific displacement of glycoproteins by a competitive sugar is reversible and after extensive washing with the equilibration buffer, the immobilized lectin can be used again with the same efficiency. However, stronger lectin–glycoprotein

interactions may result either of a very high affinity of the lectin for some oligosaccharidic determinants of the glycoprotein or of the multivalent interactions between the immobilized lectin and a very high density of a saccharidic determinant of the glycoprotein recognized by the lectin (avidity effect). In the particular case of immobilized ConA, the recovery of high affinity glycoproteins can be improved by raising the temperature of the 0.5 M methyl α-D-glucoside or α-D-mannoside solution to 37°C or even 60°C. However, very often these strong interactions could be displaced only with non-specific desorption processes which may cause the irreversible denaturation of the immobilized lectin. However, such non-specific elutions can be performed by pH changes with either 20 mM acetic acid or diaminopropane solutions or with 0.02–0.1 M borate buffers (pH 8.0), without denaturation of the lectin. High-yield recovery can also be obtained by heating the immobilized lectin–glycoprotein complex for 3 min at 100°C in buffer containing 5% (w/v) sodium dodecyl sulphate and 8 M urea, but with irreversible inactivation of the lectin.

SEQUENTIAL AFFINITY CHROMATOGRAPHY OF GLYCOPROTEINS ON DIFFERENT IMMOBILIZED LECTINS

The sequential use of immobilized lectins, with different and well-defined specificities towards saccharidic determinants, can be applied to fractionate complex mixtures of glycoproteins into classes depending on their affinities for the different lectins. Immobilized ConA, LCA and WGA are the most commonly used.

When lectin affinity chromatography is used to fractionate membrane glycoproteins, the most important problem is the stability of the immobilized lectin in the detergent solution utilized for membrane protein extraction. This detergent must be present during all further purification steps of the solubilized membrane glycoproteins. However, this detergent may dissociate the lectin into subunits or change their active conformation. As shown by Lotan *et al.* (1977), non-ionic detergents such as Triton X-100 at a 0.1% concentration in the running buffer remain the most compatible with lectin affinity chromatography of membrane glycoproteins.

Protocol for affinity chromatography of glycoproteins on immobilized ConA

1   The lectin column (ConA-Sepharose 4B, Pharmacia LKB Biotechnology, 30 × 2.0 cm i.d.) is equilibrated in 5 mM sodium acetate buffer (pH 5.2) containing 0.1 M NaCl, 1 mM MnCl$_2$, 1 mM CaCl$_2$ and 1 mM MgCl$_2$ at a flow-rate of 10 ml/h at room temperature. 0.02% sodium azide is present in all buffers.
2   The glycoprotein mixture (30–50 mg) is dissolved in 3 ml of the equilibration buffer and centrifuged in order to remove any insoluble material.
3   The clear glycoprotein solution is applied to the lectin column which is then irrigated with the equilibration buffer. The effluent absorbance is monitored at 280 nm and 2 ml fractions are collected. As some ConA-weakly reactive glycoproteins can be recovered as a retarded fraction(s) with the equilibration buffer, the ConA column must be eluted with at least five column volumes of the equilibration buffer.
4   The weakly retained glycoproteins are eluted with 0.01 M methyl α-D-glucoside in the equilibration buffer and the strongly ConA-reactive glycoproteins with 0.3–0.5 M methyl α-D-glucoside solution.

5   The ConA column is then regenerated by an extensive washing with the equilibration buffer.

6   The separated glycoprotein fractions are pooled and extensively dialysed against distilled water before freeze-drying. When the exact capacity of the used ConA column is not known, the unretained fraction should be submitted to a new fractionation cycle on the regenerated column.

Limitations of lectin affinity chromatography in purification of glycoproteins

Affinity chromatography on immobilized lectins rarely permits the purification of a given soluble or membrane glycoprotein from complex mixtures in a single step. Usually, this method fractionates glycoproteins into different classes containing similar glycans. As different lectins will be able to recognize different saccharidic sequences but belonging to the same glycan, sequential affinity chromatography on different immobilized lectins will not improve the fractionation significantly.

However, a few membrane or soluble glycoproteins have been isolated in one step from complex mixtures by lectin affinity chromatography. For example, immobilized WGA allows the purification of either glycophorin, the major human erythrocyte membrane glycoprotein (Kahane *et al.*, 1976) or of the insulin receptor (Hedo *et al.*, 1981) in a single step. Laminin, a major component of the basement membrane, can be purified in one step on an immobilized *Griffonia simplicifolia* I-B4 lectin column (Shibata *et al.*, 1982).

Human IgA1 and IgD can be isolated in one step from human sera on an immobilized *Artocarpus integrifolia* lectin (jacalin) column which strongly interacts with the O-glycosidically linked Gal(β1–3)GalNAc determinants present in the hinge region of these glycoproteins (Roque-Barreira and Campos-Neto, 1985; Kondoh *et al.*, 1987; Aucouturier *et al.*, 1987; Zehr and Litwin, 1987).

α-2 macroglobulin from human sera is the only glycoprotein with oligomannosidic glycans recognized and eluted with a 0.1 M methyl α-D-mannoside solution from an immobilized *Galanthus nivalis* mannose-specific lectin, isolated from the snowdrop bulb (Shibuya *et al.*, 1988a).

However, lectin affinity chromatography usually fractionates glycoproteins into different classes containing similar carbohydrate determinants. Nevertheless, when a given glycoprotein can be purified in a first step from other contaminating glycoproteins, either by conventional biochemical procedures or by immunoaffinity chromatography, lectin affinity chromatography represents a very powerful tool to unravel the glycan microheterogeneity inside this glycoprotein in a second step (for an example concerning the glycosylation of human α1-acid glycoprotein, see Bierhuizen *et al.*, 1988b).

Use of immobilized lectins for fractionation of glycopeptides and oligosaccharides

Even though the purification and fractionation of glycoproteins by lectin affinity chromatography is encumbered with some limitations, this method represents a powerful tool for the fractionation of glycopeptides and glycans. Non-specific interactions often observed between glycoproteins and immobilized lectins or strong interactions resulting from the presence on a glycoprotein of a high density of a particular saccharidic determinant otherwise individually weakly recognized by the lectin are absent or very rare in the case of glycans and glycopeptides These compounds are here fractionated on the basis of a true affinity chromatography. Consequently, this implies, even more so than in glycoprotein fractionations, a very precise knowledge of the exact specificities of the immobilized lectins to be used. In these conditions, it becomes often possible to predict the primary structure of lectin-reactive glycopeptides or glycans.

Many fractionation schemes of glycopeptides or glycans, obtained from soluble or membrane-bound glycoproteins, have been proposed (for reviews, see Finne et al., 1980; Montreuil et al., 1986, 1994; Merkle and Cummings, 1987; Osawa and Tsuji, 1987; Cummings et al., 1989; Debray and Montreuil, 1991, 1992; Kobata and Endo, 1992; Kobata and Yamashita, 1993; Yamamoto et al., 1993; Tsuji et al., 1993; Cummings, 1994, 1997; Debray, 1995).

General comments

1   Before using a new batch of immobilized lectin or after repeated use of a lectin column which may lead to a decrease in the binding capacity, calibration of the lectin column with well-defined glycopeptides or glycans should be performed. These glycopeptides or glycans can be prepared from commercially available glycoproteins such as human α1-acid glycoprotein, human serum and lactotransferrin, hen ovalbumin, calf fetuin as described (Finne and Krusius, 1982; Montreuil et al., 1986, 1994; Verbert et al., 1995, Section 2). Standard glycopeptides or mixtures of glycopeptides to be fractionated can be N-[^{14}C]- or [^{3}H]- acetylated according to Koide and Muramatsu (1974) to follow easily the lectin column calibration or the fractionation. Standard oligosaccharides or mixtures of glycans to be fractionated, released from glycoproteins or glycopeptides either by chemical or by enzymatic cleavages can be labelled at the terminal reducing GlcNAc residue by reduction with [^{3}H]-sodium or potassium borohydride according to Takasaki and Kobata (1974).

2   Most lectin columns equilibrated in PBS containing 0.02% sodium azide can be run at room temperature (20°C) but should be stored at 4°C between consecutive runs. Most lectins are less efficient at 37°C than at room temperature or even at 4°C (Lotan et al., 1977; Kobata and Yamashita, 1993). The degree of separation of weakly reactive glycopeptides or glycans may depend on the geometry of the lectin column. A better separation of these compounds will be generally obtained with a long and thin column rather than with a wider column containing the same amount of immobilized lectins. The recovery of strongly reactive oligosaccharides from the lectin column can be improved by raising the temperature of the monosaccharide elution solution to 60°C.

3   When the exact capacity of a lectin column is not known, the unretained fraction must be recycled on the regenerated column. For example, commercially available ConA-Sepharose 4B, from Pharmacia Biotech is able to bind 50–75 μg of biantennary N-glycosylpeptides prepared from human serotransferrin, per ml of gel.

4   Most immobilized lectins show the same affinity for N-glycosylpeptides as for glycans released from them either by chemical or enzymatic cleavages. However, N-N'-diacetylchitobiose-Asn inner core is an important determinant for binding to immobilized LCA or WGA and glycans without the asparagine residue or a small peptidic sequence do not interact with these immobilized lectins. This is an important point to consider in the fractionation procedure to be used because the

discriminating power of an immobilized LCA – or WGA – Sepharose column is considerable and cannot be neglected.

5   As previously described for glycoproteins, sequential use of immobilized lectins with different and well-defined specificities can fractionate complex mixtures of glycopeptides or glycans into homogeneous families. Generally, lectins with affinity for internal saccharidic sequences are used first in the fractionation whereas immobilized lectins with a specificity towards terminal dominant-oligosaccharidic sequences or terminal non-reducing monosaccharides are used later.

Fractionation of N-glycosylpeptides or related glycans on immobilized lectins with affinity for internal oligosaccharidic sequences

AFFINITY CHROMATOGRAPHY ON IMMOBILIZED CONCANAVALIN A (CON A)

1   The ConA-Sepharose column (10 × 1.0 cm i.d.) is equilibrated in 5 mM sodium acetate buffer (pH 5.2), containing 0.1 NaCl, 1 mM $CaCl_2$, 1 mM $MnCl_2$, 1 mM $MgCl_2$, at a flow-rate of 9 ml/h at room temperature. 0.02% sodium azide is added to all buffers.

2   The glycopeptides (or the oligosaccharides) are dissolved in 1 ml of equilibration buffer and the clear solution is applied onto the column.

3   The lectin column is eluted (1.5 ml fractions) successively with five column volumes of equilibration buffer, then with three column volumes of 0.01 M methyl α-D-glucoside and finally with five column volumes of 0.3 M methyl α-D-glucoside.

On a ConA-Sepharose column, a mixture of N-glycosylpeptides and/or related glycans can be fractionated into three classes (Fig. 13.9).

• Non-reactive glycopeptides (or oligosaccharides) eluted at the void volume of the column with the equilibration buffer
• Weakly reactive derivatives obtained by eluting with the equilibration buffer itself. However, depending on the amount of immobilized ConA/ml of Sepharose, the same type of compounds can be weakly retained or may be eluted as a sharp peak with low concentration of the competitive sugar derivative (0.01 M methyl α-D-glucoside)
• Strongly reactive components, eluted as a sharp or broad trailing peak with 0.3 M methyl α-D-glucoside, depending on the ConA concentration in the gel.

The fractions are purified from salts and competitive sugar by gel filtration on a Bio-Gel P2 column (50 × 2 cm i.d.) equilibrated with distilled water. After elution with the competitive monosaccharide solutions, the ConA column is regenerated by extensive washing with the equilibration buffer.

AFFINITY CHROMATOGRAPHY ON IMMOBILIZED LENS CULINARIS AGGLUTININ

LCA-Sepharose 4B can be purchased from different manufacturers or the lentil lectin can be easily purified from Lens culinaris seeds according to Toyoshima et al. (1970) and coupled to CNBr-activated Sepharose 4B, at a concentration of 5 mg/ml of gel.

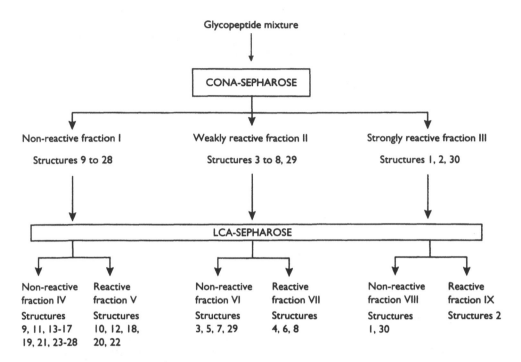

Figure 13.9 Scheme of fractionation of *N*-glycosylpeptides by combining affinity chromatography on immobilized Con-A and LCA Sepharose. Arabic numerals refer to glycopeptide structures of Table 13.2.

1   The lectin column (15 × 2.5 cm i.d.) is equilibrated in PBS (pH 7.4) containing 0.02% sodium azide (divalent cations such as Ca^{2+} or Mn^{2+} are not required), at a flow-rate of 9 ml/h at room temperature.

2   The glycopeptides are dissolved in 1 ml of PBS and the clear solution is applied to the column.

3   The non-reactive glycopeptides are eluted (1.5 ml fractions) with five column volumes of PBS and the lectin-reactive glycopeptides with five column volumes of PBS containing 0.15 M methyl α-D-glucoside.

4   The fractions containing glycopeptides are separated from salts and competitive sugar by gel filtration on a Bio-Gel P2 column (50 × 2 cm i.d.) equilibrated with distilled water.

5   The LCA column is regenerated by extensive washing with PBS.

The following comments apply to this procedure:

(a) The saccharidic structures found in each fraction are described in Fig. 13.9. From this figure, it clearly appears that the α-1,6-linked fucose residue is an important determinant for the binding of *N*-glycosylpeptides and that affinity chromatography on immobilized LCA is a valuable tool to fractionate glycopeptides into two classes: α-1,6-fucosylated and non-fucosylated.

(b) Only *N*-glycosylpeptides can be bound to immobilized LCA, not oligosaccharides. So, glycans released from *N*-glycosylpeptides either by hydrazinolysis, alkaline attack by 1 M NaOH–1 M NaBH4 for 6 h at 100°C or by enzymatic cleavage, do not interact with immobilized LCA and are eluted at the void volume of the lectin column.

(c) Immobilized *Vicia faba* and *Pisum sativum* lectins also interact with α-1,6-fucosylated *N*-glycosylpeptides. However, their affinity is weaker, so that the fractionation into the two classes is obtained with only the equilibration buffer.

AFFINITY CHROMATOGRAPHY ON OTHER LECTINS WITH A SPECIFICITY FOR INTERNAL SACCHARIDIC SEQUENCES

Other immobilized lectins presenting a specificity for internal saccharidic sequences can also be used to subfractionate *N*-glycosylpeptide families obtained by affinity chromatography on immobilized ConA and LCA.

1. *Immobilized Phaseolus vulgaris isolectin E4 (E4-PHA)*. As shown in Table 13.3, E4-PHA interacts with bisected bi- and tri-antennary *N*-acetyllactosamine type glycopeptides or related glycans. The Gal(β1–4)GlcNAc(β1–2)Man(α1–6)- branch is an important determinant in the lectin-oligosaccharide interaction; its sialylation by α-2,6-linked sialic acid residue abolishes the interaction.

Differences in the resolution of *N*-glycosylpeptides or oligosaccharides on immobilized E4-PHA depend on the amount of lectin per ml of gel. At a low coupling density of lectin (less than 1 mg/ml of gel), bisected biantennary glycopeptides are eluted as a retarded fraction with the equilibration buffer and in that case, a better resolution can be obtained with a long and thin column of the immobilized lectin. But, at higher coupling densities (3 mg/ml of gel), glycopeptides interact more strongly with the lectin and must be eluted either with 0.4 M *N*-acetylgalactosamine solution or with 0.05 M glycine–HCl buffer, pH 3.5 (Mellis and Baenziger, 1983).

The affinity of immobilized E4-PHA for free, reduced oligosaccharides released from *N*-glycosylproteins by a *N*-glycanase differs significantly from that of the lectin for *N*-glycosylpeptides. If desialylated bisected biantennary glycans still presents the stronger interaction with the immobilized lectin, desialylated non-bisected glycans containing one, two, tri or four *N*-acetyllactosamine antennae are retarded to varying extents by a E4-PHA column, in contrast to the *N*-glycosylpeptides containing these glycans which do not interact with the lectin (Green and Baenziger, 1987).

Immobilized E4-PHA presents also a stronger affinity at 2°C than at room temperature (20°C): non-bisected biantennary oligosaccharides which are not retained on a E4-PHA column at room temperature are retarded on the same column at 2°C (Kobata and Endo, 1992).

In conclusion, the specificity of E4-PHA is very complex and before use, E4-PHA columns must be carefully calibrated with standard oligosaccharides (free and non-reduced or free and reduced oligosaccharides, or *N*-glycosylpeptides) related to the oligosaccharides to be fractionated. Figure 13.10 shows the results obtained by subfractionating glycopeptide fractions IV and V isolated by sequential affinity chromatography on an immobilized ConA and LCA-Sepharose, on an immobilized E4-PHA column at 20°C.

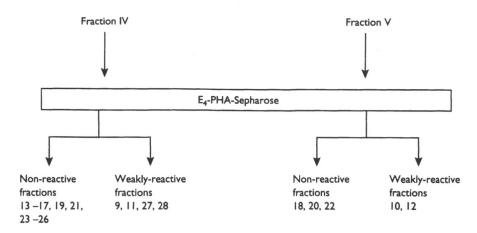

Figure 13.10 Scheme of subfractionation on immobilized E4-PHA of N-glycosylpeptide fractions IV and V from Fig. 13.9. Arabic numbers refer to glycopeptide structures in Table 13.2.

2. *Immobilized Phaseolus vulgaris isolectin L4 (L4-PHA)*. As shown in Table 13.3, L4-PHA interacts with asialotri'–and tetraantennary N-acetyllactosamine – type glycopeptides or related glycans, containing the dominant pentasaccharidic sequence Gal(β1–4)GlcNAc(β1–2)[Gal(β1–4)GlcNAc(β1–6)]Man.

Asialobi- and triantennary glycopeptides without the Gal(β1–4)GlcNAc(β1–6) branch as well as bisected biantennary glycopeptides show no interaction with the lectin. The interaction of tri'- and tetraantennary glycopeptides is completely abolished by the removal of Gal residues. The interaction with the lectin is also completely abolished when either α-2,6-linked NeuAc or α-1,3-linked fucose substitutes the galactose or the N-acetylglucosamine residue of the Gal(β1–4)GlcNAc(β1–2)Man(α1–6) antennae (Bierhuizen *et al.*, 1988).

However, if immobilized L4-PHA interacts with free, reduced asialotri'- and tetraantennary glycans released by N-glycanase, it also reacts to different extents with asialobi- and triantennary as well as with bisected asialobiantennary oligosaccharides (Green and Baenziger, 1987).

In conclusion and as previously emphasized for E4-PHA, the immobilized L4-PHA column to be used must be calibrated with the appropriate standards prepared in the same way as the oligosaccharidic structures to be analyzed.

Figure 13.11 shows the results obtained by subfractionating the fractions IV and V isolated on immobilized ConA and LCA-Sepharose on a L4-PHA column at 20°C.

3. *Immobilized Wheat germ agglutinin (WGA)*. As shown in Table 13.3, WGA interacts only with bisected hybrid-type N-glycosylpeptides which are bound on a WGA-Sepharose column, and to a lesser extent with bisected biantennary N-acetyllactosamine-type glycopeptides which are only retarded (Yamamoto *et al.*, 1981; Debray *et al.*, 1983).

N,N'-diacetylchitobiose-Asn inner core is an important determinant for the binding to immobilized WGA and bisected glycans released from N-glycosylpeptides by hydrazinolysis are no longer bound or retarded on an immobilized WGA column. Linear poly(N-acetyllactosamine)-type glycopeptides or glycans with repeating

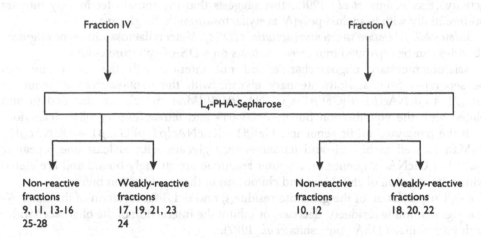

Figure 13.11 Scheme of subfractionation on immobilized L4-PHA of N-glycosylpeptide fractions IV and V from Fig. 13.9. Arabic numbers refer to glycopeptide structures in Table 13.2.

Gal(β1–4)GlcNAc units linked by β-1,3-linkages with blood group i activity and branched poly(N-acetyllactosamine)-type glycopeptides or glycans with additional repeating β-1,6-branched Gal(β1–4)GlcNAc(β1–3) sequences and I antigenic activity are also recognized with high affinity by immobilized WGA (Gallagher *et al.*, 1985; Ivatt *et al.*, 1986a,b).

Immobilized WGA interacts also with glycopeptides presenting a high density of O-glycosidically linked sialyloligosaccharides because of the similar configuration of the acetamido group of N-acetylneuraminic acid (Bhavanandan *et al.*, 1977; Furukawa *et al.*, 1986).

Fractionation of N-glycosylpeptides on immobilized lectins with a specificity directed towards terminal dominant-oligosaccharidic sequences

LECTINS WITH A SPECIFICITY FOR POLY(N-ACETYLLACTOSAMINE) TYPE GLYCANS

1. *Immobilized pokeweed mitogens (PWM)*. Five isolectins, Pa-1 to Pa-5, have been isolated from the roots of *Phytolacca americana* (Waxdal 1974, Yokoyama *et al.*, 1978). The immobilized isolectins Pa-1, Pa-2 and Pa-4 possess similar binding specificity towards branched poly(N-acetyllactosamine)-type glycopeptides with blood group I antigenic activity from human Band 3 glycoprotein which are retained on the lectin columns. In contrast, bi- and triantennary N-acetyllactosamine type N-glycopeptides do not interact with the lectins (Irimura and Nicolson, 1983).

2. *Immobilized Lycopersicon esculentum agglutinin (Tomato lectin)*. The immobilized tomato lectin interacts with high affinity with linear poly(N-acetyllactosamine)-type N-glycosylpeptides with blood group i activity and containing three or more Gal(β1–4)GlcNAc(β1–3) repeating sequences (Merkle and Cummings, 1987). However, as the immobilized lectin presents only affinity for oligosaccharides with repeating N-acetyllactosamine sequences and i-antigenic determinant and no affinity for oligosaccharides also with repeating N-acetyllactosamine sequences and i-antigenic

activity (Kawashima *et al.*, 1990), this suggests that the tomato lectin may interact preferentially with branched poly(*N*-acetyllactosamine)-type glycans.

3. *Immobilized Datura stramonium agglutinin (DSA)*. *N*-acetyllactosamine-type oligosaccharides can be separated into three fractions on a DSA-Sepharose column.

Asialobiantennary oligosaccharides do not interact with the lectin and can be separated from asialotriantennary glycans with the pentasaccharidic sequence Gal(β1–4)GlcNAc(β1–4)[Gal(β1–4)GlcNAc(β1–2)]Man, which are retarded in and eluted with the equilibration buffer. Asialotri'- and tetraantennary oligosaccharides with the pentasaccharidic sequence: Gal(β1–4)GlcNAc(β1–6)[Gal(β1–4)GlcNAc(β1–2)]Man as well as bi-, tri- and tetraantennary glycans with at least one repeating Gal(β1–4)GlcNAc sequence on an outer antennae are strongly bound and are eluted with a 1% solution of chitobiose and chitotriose in the equilibration buffer.

α-2,3/6 sialylation of the galactose residue(s) and α-1,3-fucosylation of the outer *N*-acetylglucosamine residue(s) decrease or inhibit the interaction of the oligosaccharides with immobilized DSA (Yamashita *et al.*, 1987).

After careful calibration with standard oligosaccharides, an immobilized DSA column represents another useful tool for the fractionation of *N*-acetyllactosamine-type glycans with or without repeating *N*-acetyllactosamine sequences.

LECTINS WITH A SPECIFICITY FOR TERMINAL N-ACETYLLACTOSAMINE SEQUENCES

1. *Immobilized Ricinus communis agglutinin I (RCA I)*. Interaction of *N*-glycosylpeptides or related glycans with immobilized RCA I has revealed that RCA I recognizes terminal *N*-acetyllactosamine residues and to a lesser extent β-1,3-linked Gal residues. Substitution of the *N*-acetyllactosamine sequences by NeuAc residues at the C-6 position of Gal decreases the affinity of RCA I, but substitution by NeuAc residues at the C-3 position of Gal inhibits glycan–RCA I interaction.

The strength of the interaction increases with the number of terminal *N*-acetyllactosamine sequences and *N*-glycosylpeptides or glycans with an increasing number of *N*-acetyllactosamine residues can be either differentially retarded or bound and eluted with 0.1 M lactose solution in the equilibration buffer. However, the separation depends upon the amount of immobilized RCA I/ml of gel as well as on the geometry of the lectin column. As many interacting glycans can only be more or less retarded, the use of long and thin columns of immobilized RCA I is recommended (Kornfeld *et al.*, 1981; Irimura *et al.*, 1981; Debray *et al.*, 1983; Narasimhan *et al.*, 1986; Green *et al.*, 1987; Harada *et al.*, 1987).

2. *Immobilized Ricinus communis agglutinin II (RCA II)*. RCA II agglutinin interacts with β-galactose residues of *N*-acetyllactosamine-type glycans and also with terminal *N*-acetylgalactosamine residues (Baenziger and Fiete, 1979b; Debray *et al.*, 1981).

As immobilized RCA I, immobilized RCA II strongly interacts with *N*-acetyllactosamine-type oligosaccharides possessing terminal β1,4-linked galactose residues. However, in contrast to RCA I, bound oligosaccharides can only be eluted with a 0.2 M GalNAc solution in 1% acetic acid. Immobilized RCA II can also strongly interact with *N*-acetyllactosamine-type oligosaccharides containing terminal non-reducing β-1,4-linked GalNAc residues.

Whereas immobilized RCA I presents weak affinity for *N*-acetyllactosamine-type oligosaccharides with one or two terminal β-1,3-linked galactose residues, immobilized RCA II strongly binds these glycans which can be eluted with a GalNAc solution.

All these results obtained by Green *et al.* (1987a) clearly demonstrate that immobilized RCA I and RCA II present distinct oligosaccharide specificities and that the combined use of these two lectins allows the fractionation of *N*-acetyllactosamine-type glycans according to the nature and the linkage of their terminal sugar moieties.

3. *Immobilized Erythrina agglutinins.* The carbohydrate-binding specificity of four *Erythrina* lectins (*(E. cristagalli, E. latissima, E. corallodendron, E. lysistemon)* is similar and is directed towards unmasked terminal *N*-acetyllactosamine sequences. The affinity of the immobilized lectins increases with the number of such sequences when accessible to the lectins. Substitution of the *N*-acetyllactosamine residues by sialic acid either at the C-3 or the C-6 position of galactose completely abolishes the affinity of the immobilized lectins for the glycans. As for immobilized RCA I, the interaction of immobilized *Erythrina* lectins with *N*-acetyllactosamine-type glycans depends on the lectin density and improvement in the separation of weakly reacting, retarded fractions can be obtained using long and thin lectin columns (Debray *et al.*, 1986).

LECTINS WITH A SPECIFICITY FOR SIALYLATED N-ACETYLLACTOSAMINE SEQUENCES

1. *Immobilized Allomyrina dichotoma agglutinins (Allo A).* Two β-galactose-binding isolectins, Allo A I and Allo A II, have been isolated from the hemolymph of the beetle *Allomyrina dichotoma* (Umetsu *et al.*, 1984).

Immobilized *Allomyrina* isolectins recognize Gal(β1–4)GlcNAc sequences in *N*-acetyllactosamine-type glycopeptides or glycans. The affinity of the isolectins increases with the number of such unmasked Gal(β1–4)GlcNAc sequences on a glycan. However, oligosaccharides containing unsubstituted Gal(β1–4)GlcNAc sequences are only more or less retarded on immobilized *Allomyrina* lectins, but substitution of these sequences by α-2,6-linked NeuAc residues strongly enhances the affinity of the immobilized lectins. Such *N*-glycosylpeptides or glycans bind very strongly to the immobilized lectins and can be eluted only with the equilibration buffer containing lactose. On the contrary, substitution of the Gal(β1–4)GlcNAc sequences by α-2,3-linked NeuAc residues inhibits the interaction with the lectins. The immobilized lectins do not interact with either asialo-agalactoglycans or with oligosaccharides containing terminal Gal(β1–3)GlcNAc sequences. They display no affinity for the Gal(β1–3)GalNAc core sequence found in mucin-type glycoproteins (Sueyoshi *et al.*, 1988; Yamashita *et al.*, 1988, 1989).

2. *Immobilized Sambucus nigra agglutinin I (SNA I).* The immobilized lectin SNA I, isolated from the bark of elder (Broekaert *et al.*, 1984), recognizes oligosaccharides, glycopeptides or glycoproteins with terminal NeuAc(α2–6)Gal/GalNAc sequences which are bound and must be eluted from the lectin column with 50–100 mM lactose solution.

Asialo derivatives of oligosaccharides, glycopeptides or glycoproteins, as well as those containing NeuAc(α2–3)Gal/GalNAc sequences, do not interact with immobilized SNA I (Shibuya *et al.*, 1987).

3. *Immobilized Maackia amurensis leukoagglutinin (MAL).* Immobilized *Maackia amurensis* leukoagglutinin interacts with high affinity with *N*-acetyllactosamine-type glycopeptides containing terminal NeuAc(α2–3)Gal(β1–4)GlcNAc sequences.

These glycopeptides are strongly retarded on the lectin column. On the contrary, asialoglycopeptides as well as glycans with terminal NeuAc(α2–6)Gal(β1–4)GlcNAc sequences do not interact with the immobilized leukoagglutinin (Wang and Cummings, 1988).

Therefore, immobilized *Maackia amurensis* leukoagglutinin (MAL) and *Sambucus nigra* agglutinin I (SNA I) represent two interesting lectins which can be sequentially used to fractionate sialylated glycans on the basis of their sialic acid linkages and according to the number of sialic acid residues they contain.

4. *Immobilized mistletoe (Viscum album) lectin I (MLI).* Three different lectins have been isolated from mistletoe (*Viscum album*) by affinity chromatography (Franz *et al.*, 1981). The three lectins have different molecular weights and monosaccharide specificities. The major mistletoe lectin I (MLI), composed of two different subunits, has a molecular weight of 115 000 and belongs to the D-galactose-specificity group whereas lectin II (Mr = 60 000) and lectin III (Mr = 50 000) are D-galactose/N-acetyl-D-galactosamine- and N-acetyl-D-galactosamine-specific lectins, respectively (Franz, 1986).

Recently, the behavior of N-acetyllactosamine-type oligosaccharides and glycopeptides on a column of immobilized mistletoe lectin I was examined (Debray *et al.*, 1994). Though MLI belongs to the D-galactose-specificity group, the immobilized lectin showed no affinity for asialo-N-glycosylpeptides or related oligosaccharides with one to four unmasked terminal non-reducing N-acetyllactosamine sequences.

Surprisingly, substitution of at least one of the N-acetyllactosamine sequences by a sialic acid residue either at C-3 or C-6 of galactose enhances the affinity of MLI. Such sialylated N-glycosylpeptides or oligosaccharides are eluted from the lectin column by the equilibration buffer as retarded fractions. In this respect, MLI is very similar to other lectins presenting also a specificity towards either α-2,3-sialylated N-acetyllactosamine residues such as *Maackia amurensis* leukoagglutinin or α-2,6-sialylated N-acetyllactosamine sequences such as the *Sambucus nigra* agglutinin I or the *Allomyrina dichotoma* lectins. Thus, immobilized MLI provides another valuable tool for the fractionation of asialo-N-glycosylpeptides or related glycans which do not interact with the lectin and oligosaccharides or glycopeptides with terminal NeuAcα2,3/α2,6 Gal(β1–4)GlcNAc sequences which are retarded on the lectin column.

Moreover, the affinity of the mistletoe lectin I is higher for pentaantennary N-acetyllactosamine type N-glycosylpeptides with P1 serological activity. These glycopeptides possess one N-acetyllactosamine sequence substituted at C-6 of galactose by an N-acetylneuraminic acid residue together with three other N-acetyllactosamine sequences substituted each at C-4 of galactose by an α-D-galactose residue and one unmasked N-acetyllactosamine sequence. These glycopeptides are strongly bound on the lectin column and are eluted with 0.15 M galactose in the equilibration buffer.

Tetraantennary N-acetyllactosamine type glycopeptides isolated from bovine thyroglobulin with two to three substitutions of the N-acetyllactosamine moiety by galactose in α-1,3-linkage are also strongly bound on the lectin column and are eluted with a 0.15 M galactose solution. Immobilized MLI can represent a valuable tool for the fractionation and structural analysis of oligosaccharides and glycopeptides containing terminal non-reducing Gal(α1–4)Gal or Gal(α1–3)Gal sequences (Debray *et al.*, 1994).

Subfractionation of N-glycosylpeptides on immobilized lectins with a specificity directed towards terminal non-reducing dominant monosaccharides

LECTINS RECOGNIZING NON-REDUCING MANNOSE RESIDUES

1. *Immobilized Galanthus nivalis (snowdrop) agglutinin (GNA).* A lectin with an exclusive specificity towards mannose can be isolated from snowdrop (*Galanthus nivalis*) bulbs by affinity chromatography on immobilized mannose (Van Damme *et al.*, 1987).

Immobilized GNA interacts rather weakly, only with oligomannosidic-type glycopeptides containing a terminal non-reducing Man(α1–3)Man sequence which are retarded on the lectin column. The interaction with the lectin also depends on the number of these disaccharide units. However, hybrid-type glycopeptides with this Man(α1–3)Man sequence, together with a bisecting GlcNAc residue do not interact with the immobilized lectin (Shibuya *et al.*, 1988a). It is worthy of note that murine IgM and human α2-macroglobulin, two glycoproteins containing oligomannosidic-type glycans, tightly bind to immobilized GNA and can be eluted with a 0.1 M methyl α-D-mannoside solution (Shibuya *et al.*, 1988b).

2. *Immobilized Narcissus pseudonarcissus (daffodil) agglutinin (NPA).* Another lectin with a strict specificity for mannose can be isolated from daffodil (*Narcissus pseudonarcissus*) bulbs by affinity chromatography on an immobilized mannose column. (Van Damme *et al.*, 1988).

In contrast to the *Galanthus nivalis* lectin, which specifically interacts with terminal non-reducing Man(α1–3)Man sequences, the daffodil lectin not only recognizes terminal but also internal α-D-mannosyl residues. Various oligomannosidic-type glycopeptides, containing internal Man(α1–6)Man sequence(s) are retarded to different extents on the lectin column. However, hybrid-type glycopeptides containing one or two Man(α1–6)Man sequence(s) together with a bisecting GlcNAc residues do not interact with the immobilized lectin (Kaku *et al.*, 1990).

3. *Immobilized Hippeastrum hybrida (amaryllis) agglutinin (HHA).* Amaryllis bulbs also contain a mannose-binding lectin which can be isolated by affinity chromatography on an immobilized mannose column (Van Damme *et al.*, 1988).

Various oligomannosidic-type glycopeptides containing either α-1,3- or α-1,6-linked mannose residues are retarded to different extents on an immobilized HHA column, depending on the accessibility of these mannosyl units on the glycans. A Man5GlcNAc2-Asn glycopeptide with two Man(α1–3)Man and one Man(α1–6)Man sequences is tightly bound by the immobilized HHA and can be eluted only with the equilibration buffer containing 0.5 M methyl α-D-mannoside. However, hybrid-type glycopeptides with these Man(α1–3)Man or Man(α1–6)Man sequences together with a bisecting GlcNAc residue do not interact with immobilized HHA (Kaku *et al.*, 1990).

4. *Immobilized Bowringia milbraedii agglutinin (BMA).* Another mannose-specific lectin can be purified from the seeds of the Nigerian legume *Bowringia milbraedii* (Animashaun and Hughes, 1989).

Immobilized BMA presents a higher affinity for oligosaccharides with a terminal non-reducing Man(α1–2)Man sequence. High affinity binding of glycans on immobilized BMA requires at least a terminal Man(α1–2)Man(α1–6)Man(α1–6)Man sequence which is present in a typical Man9GlcNAc oligomannosidic type glycan (Table 13.3).

This glycan, as well as the Man8GlcNAc and Man7GlcNAc oligosaccharides containing the tetrasaccharide sequence, are tightly bound by the immobilized BMA and their elution from the lectin column requires a 0.2 M methyl α-D-mannoside solution. On the contrary, other Man8GlcNAc and Man7GlcNAc isomers as well as Man6GlcNAc and Man5GlcNAc oligosaccharides lacking this tetrasaccharide sequence are only weakly bound and are eluted with a 0.01 M methyl α-D-mannoside solution (Animashaun and Hughes, 1989).

5. *Immobilized Crocus vernus agglutinin (CVA)*. Recently, another mannose-binding lectin, specific for terminal Man(α1-3)Man sequences was isolated from bulbs of *Crocus vernus* All (Misaki *et al.*, 1997). Glycoproteins with the Man(α1–3)Man terminal non-reducing sequence are tightly bound by this immobilized lectin which may represent another tool for the fractionation of oligomannosidic-type glycopeptides and glycans with this saccharidic determinant.

In summary, the five lectins described above with a strict specificity for mannose provide interesting tools for the analysis and fractionation of glycoproteins or glycopeptides containing oligomannosidic-type glycans. They represent a good alternative to Concanavalin A which, together with its specificity for oligomannosidic-type glycans, may also interact with glycoproteins, glycopeptides or oligosaccharides containing *N*-acetyllactosamine-type glycans or hybrid-type glycans.

LECTINS RECOGNIZING TERMINAL NON-REDUCING *N*-ACETYLGALACTOSAMINE AND GALACTOSE RESIDUES

1. *Immobilized Griffonia simplicifolia isolectins I (GSA I)*. The seeds of *Griffonia simplicifolia* contain five tetrameric isolectins composed of two subunits, A and B (Murphy and Goldstein, 1977).

The carbohydrate-binding specificity of the two subunits differs significantly. The A4 tetrameric isolectin (GSA I-A4) recognizes terminal non-reducing α-linked *N*-acetylgalactosamine residues, whereas the B4 isolectin (GSA I-B4) presents a strict specificity towards terminal non-reducing α-linked galactose residues.

Immobilized GSA I isolectins have been used to isolate either α-Gal containing glycopeptides from blood group B erythrocytes or α-GalNAc containing glycopeptides from blood group A erythrocytes (Finne *et al.*, 1978).

Immobilized GSA I isolectins allow the separation of glycopeptides containing a single terminal non-reducing α-Gal residue, weakly retarded on the lectin column, from glycopeptides containing multiple α-Gal residues which are firmly bound and eluted with a 0.01 M methyl α-D-galactose solution (Spiro and Bhoyroo, 1984).

2. *Immobilized Wisteria floribunda agglutinin (WFA)*. The immobilized WFA binds with high affinity to glycopeptides containing the GalNAc(β1-4)GlcNAc sequence in their outer branch moieties. These glycopeptides are eluted with a 5 mM GalNAc solution. On the contrary, the immobilized lectin does not interact with oligosaccharides containing either terminal non-reducing GalNAc(β1–3) or GalNAc(α1–3) residues (Torres *et al.*, 1988; Nyame *et al.*, 1989; Srivatsan *et al.*, 1992; Nakata *et al.*, 1993).

LECTINS RECOGNISING TERMINAL NON-REDUCING *N*-ACETYLGLUCOSAMINE RESIDUES

1. *Immobilized Griffonia simplicifolia agglutinin II (GSA II)*. Another lectin isolated from the seeds of *Griffonia simplicifolia* presents a strong affinity for glycoconjugates with

terminal, non-reducing α- or β-linked N-acetylglucosamine residues (Ebisu *et al.*, 1978).

The immobilized GSA II represents a useful tool for the fractionation of glycopeptides or oligosaccharides with terminal, non-reducing GlcNAc residues. The affinity between immobilized GSA II and oligosaccharides increases with the number of terminal, non-reducing GlcNAc residues. With a low coupling density of lectin (2 mg of lectin per ml of gel), at least one GlcNAc residue is necessary to obtain a weak interaction between glycans and the immobilized lectin, resulting in a retarded elution. The elution volume increases with the number of terminal, non-reducing GlcNAc residues. Oligosaccharides with four terminal GlcNAc are strongly bound and must be eluted with a 0.15 M N-acetylglucosamine solution (Debray *et al.*, 1983).

2. *Immobilized Psathyrella velutina agglutinin (PVA)*. A lectin recently isolated from the fruiting bodies of the mushroom *Psathyrella velutina* by affinity chromatography on a chitin column interacts with glycoproteins or oligosaccharides containing terminal non-reducing β-linked GlcNAc residues (Kochibe and Matta, 1989).

The immobilized PVA binds asialoagalactobi-, tri- and tri'-antennary N-acetyllactosamine-type glycans which are eluted with the equilibration buffer containing 1 mM N-acetylglucosamine.

However, asialoagalactotetraantennary glycans are only retarded on the lectin column (Endo *et al.*, 1992). These results show that immobilized PVA may represent another useful tool for the detection and the fractionation of glycoproteins, glycopeptides or glycans with terminal non-reducing GlcNAc residues.

FUCOSE-BINDING LECTINS

Fucose-binding lectins have been isolated from several sources including *Ulex europaeus, Lotus tetragonolobus* and *Griffonia simplicifolia* seeds as well as from eel serum *Anguilla anguilla* and from the mushroom *Aleuria aurantia* (For review see Goldstein and Poretz, 1986). The specificity of these lectins towards L-fucose containing oligosaccharides was determined either by inhibition of hemagglutination, by inhibition of quantitative precipitation of blood group substances or by analysis of the behaviour of fucosylated oligosaccharides on immobilized lectin columns.

1. *Immobilized Ulex europaeus agglutinin I (UEA I)*. Pereira *et al.* (1978), using various blood group and milk oligosaccharides have shown that the best inhibitor for the UEA I is a blood group H monofucosyl disaccharide of the "type 2 structure": Fuc(α1–2)Gal(β1–4)GlcNAc(β1–6)-R.

The addition of a second α-1,3-linked Fuc to the GlcNAc residue reduces the inhibitory power of the oligosaccharide and UEA I does not react with Le^a active blood group oligosaccharide Gal(β1–3)[Fuc(α1–4)]GlcNAc(β1–3)Gal(β1–4)Glc.

If the α-1,6-linked Fuc residue of either the glycopeptide Fuc(α1–6)GlcNAc(β1–N)Asn or the disaccharide Fuc(α1–6)GlcNAc is well recognized by UEA I (Debray *et al.*, 1981), immobilized UEA I has no affinity for N-acetyllactosamine-type glycopeptides or related oligosaccharides containing either an α-1,3- or α-1,6-linked fucose residues or both (Debray *et al.*, 1983). However, the affinity of immobilized UEA I toward glycopeptides or oligosaccharides containing α-1,2-linked fucose residue (blood group H determinant) has not yet been investigated.

2. *Immobilized Lotus tetragonolobus agglutinin (LTA)*. In contrast to UEA I, the best inhibitor found for the lectin isolated from the seeds of *Lotus tetragonolobus* is the

oligosaccharide containing two fucose residues on a "type 2 chain": $Fuc(\alpha 1-2)Gal(\beta 1-4)[Fuc(\alpha 1-3)]GlcNAc(\beta 1-6)R$ (Pereira and Kabat, 1974).

Immobilized LTA has a weak affinity for the glycopeptide $Fuc(\alpha 1-6)GlcNAc(\beta 1-N)Asn$ which is retarded on a LTA column (Susz and Dawson, 1979), but no affinity for N-acetyllactosamine-type glycopeptides or related glycans containing either one α-1,3- or one α-1,6-linked fucose residue or both (Debray et al., 1983) . However, immobilized LTA displays a strong affinity for poly-N-acetyllactosamine-type N-glycosylpeptides containing high amount of fucose linked α-1,3- to N-acetylglucosamine residues within the linear repeating disaccharide $(3-Gal(\beta 1-4)GlcNAc(\beta 1-)n$ (Lewis^x antigenic blood group). These glycopeptides are bound to an immobilized LTA column and can be eluted with a 0.4% fucose solution (Srivatsan et al., 1992).

3. *Immobilized Aleuria aurantia agglutinin (AAA)*. Another fucose-binding lectin can be purified by affinity chromatography from fruiting bodies of the mushroom *Aleuria aurantia* (Kochibe and Furukawa, 1980; Debray and Montreuil, 1989). Inhibition of hemagglutination by various fucosylated oligosaccharides shows that the lectin recognized fucose residues irrespective of the substituting position (Kochibe and Kurukawa, 1980).

The structural requirements for the interaction of fucosylated glycopeptides or oligosaccharides were also established by analysis of the elution behaviour of these fucosylated structures on an immobilized AAA column (Yamashita et al., 1985; Amano et al., 1985; Harada et al., 1987; Debray and Montreuil, 1989; Kobata and Endo, 1992).

These studies show that immobilized AAA strongly interacts with all N-glycosyl-peptides or related glycans containing a fucose residue in α-1,6-linkage to the innermost GlcNAc residue of the core. Immobilized AAA reacts weakly with glycans containing a fucose residue in α-1,3-linkage to one of the outer GlcNAc residue of the N-acetyllactosamine units. The presence of both α-1,6- and α-1,3-linked fucose residues enhances the affinity of the lectin for the glycan (Debray and Montreuil, 1989).

In addition, oligosaccharides isolated from human milk and from urine of patients with fucosidosis, containing either the $Fuc(\alpha 1-2)Gal(\beta 1-4)GlcNAc$ or $Gal(\beta 1-4)[Fuc(\alpha 1-3)]GlcNAc$ sequences, interact with the immobilized lectin, but to a lesser extent than N-acetyllactosamine type glycans possessing an α-1,6-linked fucose in the core. Oligosaccharides with the $Fuc(\alpha 1-2)Gal(\beta 1-3)GlcNAc$ or $Gal(\beta 1-4)GlcNAc(\beta 1-3)Gal(\beta 1-4)[Fuc(\alpha 1-3)]GlcNAc$ sequences are not recognized by the immobilized lectin (Yamashita et al., 1985).

In conclusion, immobilized AAA represents a very valuable tool for the resolution of microheterogeneity of glycopeptides and glycans due to the presence of different L-fucose substituents.

Fractionation of O-glycosylpeptides using immobilized lectins

A large panel of lectins with well-defined specificities towards oligosaccharidic sequences belonging to N-glycosylproteins is now available to study glycan micro-heterogeneity or for fractionation of N-glycosylproteins, glycopeptides or related glycans. However, very few applications can be found in the literature of similar studies using lectins specifically recognizing O-glycosidically-linked glycans.

Nonetheless, by inhibition of hemagglutination or by inhibition of quantitative pre-cipitation, many lectins were shown to bind to mucin-type oligosaccharides. These lectins have been reviewed in a classification according to their specificity towards Gal or GalNAc (Wu, 1984) and more recently, according to their uses as specific tools in study of O-linked glycans (Peumans and Van Damme, 1998).

However, the carbohydrate-binding specificity of five of these lectins: ABA I isolated from the mushroom *Agaricus bisporus* (Presant and Kornfeld, 1972; Sueyoshi *et al.*, 1985), PNA isolated from *Arachis hypogaea* (Lotan and Sharon, 1978), BPA isolated from *Bauhinia purpurea* (Osawa *et al.*, 1978), SBA isolated from *Glycine max* (Lis and Sharon, 1972), and VVA-B4 isolated from *Vicia villosa* seeds (Tollefsen and Kornfeld, 1983a,b) has been studied by affinity chromatography of mucin-type glycopeptides and related oligosaccharides of known structures (Sueyoshi *et al.*, 1988).

Another lectin, jacalin, isolated from jackfruit (*Artocarpus integrifolia*) (Azevedo-Moreira and Ainouz, 1981) with a high affinity for the T-antigen Gal(β1-3)GalNAc (Sastry *et al.*, 1986) represents a new promising tool for the analysis and fractionation of glycoproteins containing O-glycosidically-linked glycans (Hortin and Trimpe, 1990).

Human plasminogen with a simple O-linked glycan, human chorionic gonadropin with four O-linked glycans on its β-subunit and bovine fetuin with three O-linked glycans and N-glycosidically-linked glycans are bound on a jacalin-agarose column and are specifically eluted by α-galactopyranosides such as melibiose or α-methylgalactopyranoside.

The immobilized lectin shows a higher affinity for the asialoglycoproteins than for the fully sialylated glycoproteins (Hortin and Trimpe, 1990).

Immobilized jacalin binds serum and secretory human IgA which are eluted from the lectin column with a 0.8 M galactose solution. IgM or IgG do not interact with the immobilized lectin (Roque-Barreira and Campos-Neto, 1985). Moreover, human secretory IgA, purified by conventional procedures including ion-exchange and gel-filtration can be fractionated, by affinity chromatography on immobilized jacalin, into s IgA of IgA2 subclass which are not retained on the lectin column and s IgA of IgA1 subclass which are eluted from the lectin column with a 0.5 M galactose solution (Kondoh *et al.*, 1987; Hagiwara *et al.*, 1988).

IgA1 has five serine O-linked glycans in its hinge region which can be recognized by the immobilized jacalin whereas IgA of IgA2 subclass lacks these O-glycosidically linked glycans (Baenziger and Kornfeld, 1974; Pierce-Cretel *et al.*, 1981).

Immobilized jacalin can also be used for isolating O-glycosylpeptides. A jacalin-agarose column binds specifically tryptic peptides from human plasminogen and bovine protein Z which contain O-linked glycans; they are eluted from the lectin column with a 20 mM α-methylgalactopyranoside solution (Hortin, 1990).

O-glycosylpeptides prepared from leukosialin by pronase digestion can be fractionated on immobilized jacalin into unbound glycopeptides eluted with the equilibration buffer and bound glycopeptides eluted with a 0.1 M melibiose solution (Maemura and Fukuda, 1992). Immobilized jacalin binds to sialylated small oligosaccharides such as NeuAc(α2-3)Gal(β1-3)[NeuAc(α2-6)]GalNAc but not to larger disialylhexasaccharide NeuAc(α2-3)Gal(β1-3)[NeuAc(α2-3)Gal(β1-4)GlcNAc(β1-6)]GalNAc. Moreover, sialylated O-glycosylpeptides containing N-acetyllactosamine repeats are also bound to immobilized jacalin (Maemura and Fukuda, 1992).

In conclusion, immobilized jacalin represents a new tool for the fractionation of O-glycosylpeptides or related oligosaccharide-alditols.

Isolation of glycans

Release of glycans from the glycopeptides

CHEMICAL CLEAVAGE OF O- AND N-GLYCOSIDIC LINKAGES

The structure analysis of the carbohydrate chains requires their release from the glyco proteins, which can be achieved in different ways. The action of alkali in the presence of sodium borohydride cleaves *O*-glycosidic linkages giving rise to oligosaccharide-alditols, accompanied with a simultaneous release of *N*-glycans in 10–30% yields, due to reductive cleavage of the *N*-glycosylamide bond with sodium borohydride. To prevent this side reaction, the addition of 5–10 mM cadmium acetate and 5–10 mM EDTA. Na$_4$ was proposed. These reagents prevent the reductive cleavage of the peptide chain and the formation of 2-amino-1,3-propanediol and 2-amino-1,3-butanediol from serine and threonine residues. Indeed, the presence of these amino-alcohols leads to a decrease in the yield of released *O*-glycans.

The liberation of *N*-glycans is obtained by hydrazinolysis, which results in a substantial degradation of *O*-glycans. Consequently, *N,O*-glycoproteins (*i.e.* fetuin) should retain our attention in the choice of the strategy. In this case, an enzymatic deglycosylation (peptide-*N*-glycosidase, also called glycanase) must precede the β-elimination.

1. *Reductive cleavage of O-glycosidic linkages (β-elimination)* The proposed method is a modification of the original one described by Likhosherstov *et al.* (1990).

Reagent: A mixture of solution of 0.1 M EDTA.Na$_2$ (4.5 ml) and cadmium acetate (23 mg ml^{-1}, 4.5 ml) is titrated with 0.5 M NaOH ($\sim$ 1.7 ml) to pH 7–7.5.
Protocol:

- Adjust the solution of *O*-glycosylprotein (10–20 mg/ml) to pH 10 with dilute NaOH and add immediately an equal volume of 0.1 M NaOH in 4 M NaBH$_4$.
- Add a volume of cadmium acetate solution to obtain a final concentration of 6 mM.
- Incubate at 37°C for 48 h.
- Stop the reaction by adding acetone, at + 4°C.
- Add Dowex 50 × 8 (mesh 25–50, H$^+$), until pH $\sim$ 6.5.
- After filtration, concentrate to dryness by rotary-evaporation.
- Eliminate boric acid by repeated evaporations in presence of anhydrous methanol (3 × 50 ml).
- Purify the material by gel-filtration on a Bio-Gel P2 column (2 × 75 cm).
- Detect the carbohydrate material on TLC plate (Silica gel) using orcinol reagent (200 mg orcinol in H$_2$SO$_4$ 20% in water).
- Eliminate peptidic material on a column (2 × 20 cm) of Dowex 50 × 2 (mesh 200–400, H$^+$)
- Purify the material on Bio-Gel P2. The material is ready for HPLC analyses.

2. *Hydrazinolysis of N-Glycosylproteins.*
Protocol: (Bendiak and Cumming, 1986)

- In a screw-capped tube with a teflon-silicone disc seal, introduce the freeze-dried glycopeptide or glycoprotein and the minimum amount of anhydrous hydrazine

(Pierce Chemical Co, Rockford, II, USA) to cover the sample. Heat at 100°C for 8–14 h.

- Eliminate the excess of hydrazine by repeated evaporations in presence of toluene under a stream of nitrogen.
- Remove the last traces of hydrazine in a vacuum dessicator over H_2SO_4
- Purify the material on a Bio-Gel P2 column (2 × 40 cm).

N-reacetylation:

- Dissolve the oligosaccharide fraction in 1 ml saturated $NaHCO_3$.
- Add 10 μl $(CH_3CO)_2O$ each 10 min (4–6 times)
- When the pH is under 7.5, add 1–2 ml of Dowex 50 × 8 (25–50 mesh, H^+). Filtrate and adjust the pH to 7, then dry to siccity.
- Dissolve the residue in 1 mM Copper (II) acetate, and incubate at 27°C for 30 min.
- Demineralize on Dowex 50 × 8 and rotary-evaporate to dryness.

Reduction of the carbohydrate:

- Dissolve the oligosaccharide fraction in 0.05 M NaOH (1 ml/mg), reduce with KBH_4 (5 mg/mg of sugar) for 16 h at 20°C and stop the reaction by adding Dowex 50 × 8 (25–50 mesh, H^+).
- Filtrate, wash the filter with water and concentrate the obtained solution under vacuum.
- Eliminate boric acid by repeated co-distillation in presence of methanol.
- Achieve the purification on Bio-Gel P2 column.

ENZYMATIC CLEAVAGE OF N-GLYCOSIDIC LINKAGES

Two types of endoglycosidases can release oligosaccharides from glycoproteins. In a first case, the enzyme splits the monosaccharide-peptide linkage, removing the complete glycan (aspartyl-N-acetylglucosaminidase or peptide-N-glycosidase, also called N-glycanase). Endo-N-acetylgalactosaminidases have been recently characterized which are only active towards disaccharide unit, and, therefore, have not been used for the the obtention of peptide-free glycans of the O-glycan type.

A second type of enzymes cleaves sugar-sugar glycosidic bonds, liberating part of the glycan (endo-N-acetyl-β-D-glucosaminidase and endo-β-D-galactosidase). The endo-β-D-galactosidase is mainly used for analyzing the peripheric moiety of O- and N-glycans of the poly-N-acetyllactosaminic type. Peptide-N-glycosidases present in almond emulsin (A) (Takashi and Nishibe, 1978) and the culture medium of *Flavobacterium meningosepticum* (F) (Plummer *et al.*, 1984) are of general use. N-glycanase F is able to hydrolyse all types of N-glycans, except when fucose residues are O-3 linked to the asparagine-linked N-acetylglucosamine. In this case, N-glycanase A should be used. Moreover, glycopeptides released by pronase digestion are poor substrates for these enzymes.

It is recommended to use denaturated glycoproteins or products of trypsin or pepsin digestion.

Protocols:
1. Use of peptide-*N*-glycosidase on glycopeptides (analytical scale):

- Dissolve 50 nmoles of glycopeptide in 50 mM Tris–HCl buffer pH 8.5 with 100 mU of enzyme. The final volume does not exceed 50 µl.
- Incubate the mixture at 37°C for 2–24 h.
- Denature the proteins by heating at 100°C for 3 min.
- After centrifugation, the supernatants can be used for fractionation or analysis (HPAE-PAD, HPLC, MS, PAGE, SDS-PAGE) without any further treatment. If the amount of salts is too high, the extracts are desalted on a mini-column containing AG50 × 2 and AG1 × 2 resins or gel filtered on TSK HW40 S.

2. Use of peptide-*N*-glycanase on denatured glycoproteins (analytical scale)

- SDS denaturation and heating the glycoprotein: dissolve 50 µg of glycoprotein in 10 µl of 1% SDS (w/v) and 0.5% of 2-mercaptoethanol (w/v) by heating for 3 min at 100°C
- Mix with 25 µl of 50 mM Tris–HCl buffer pH 8.5 containing 1% Nonidet P-40 (w/v)
- Add 100 mU of *N*-glycanase F and incubate at 37°C for 1 h (or more, depending on the conformation of the protein).

These procedures can be repeated on a preparative scale, by increasing proportionally the volumes and the reaction time. Carbohydrate material will be purified by gel-filtration before HPLC fractionation.

Preparative chromatography of glycans

General methods of preparative chromatography include Gel-filtration, paper chromatography, ion-exchange chromatography and High-Performance Liquid Chromatography (HPLC). HPLC has proved to be the most suitable procedure in oligosaccharide analysis and purification because of a wide range of methods as well as the quality of high resolved chromatograms. The number of methods and types of packing material have expanded so rapidly that it is impossible to survey all the technical approaches. We will consider the following:

1   The partition chromatography of neutral and acidic oligosaccharides on primary amino-bonded silica.
2   The reverse-phase (RP) chromatography of neutral oligosaccharides.
3   The anion-exchange chromatography of sialyl oligosaccharides.
4   The High pH Anion-Exchange Chromatography of oligosaccharides.

PARTITION HPLC OF NEUTRAL AND ACIDIC OLIGOSACCHARIDES ON PRIMARY AMINO-BONDED SILICA

Elution of oligosaccharides is accomplished by using acetonitrile-water-phosphate buffer. The gradients must be adapted to the nature of the material. Figure 13.12 illustrates the separation of neutral and acidic oligosaccharide-alditols obtained under

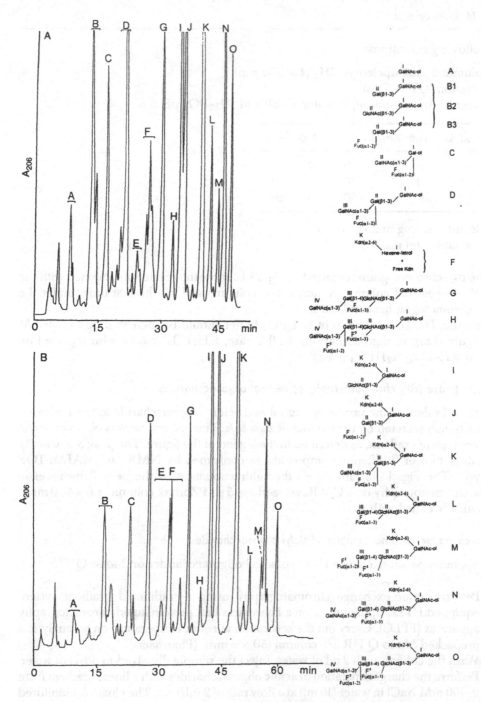

Figure 13.12 Separation of neutral and acidic oligosaccharide-alditols released by reductive
β-elimination from oviducal mucins of *Pleurodeles waltl* (Florea, D., Maes, E.,
Strecker G., personal observations). Experimental conditions: Supelcosyl LC – NH₂
column (Supelco); gradient: acetonitrile-water (80:20) to acetonitrile-KH₂PO₄ buffer
(50:50) in 1 h. (A): one year old column; (B): new column. Abbreviation: Kdn:
3-deoxy-D-glycero-D-galacto-nonulosonic acid, or deaminated sialic acid.

the following conditions:

Column: 5 μm Supelcosyl NH$_2$ (4 × 250 mm)
Detection: UV 206 nm
Solvents: A: acetonitrile, B: water, C: 30 mM KH$_2$PO$_4$ pH 5.8

Gradient	Time (min)	% A	% B	% C
	0	80	20	0
	60	50	0	50
	70	50	0	50

Injection: 1.5 mg in 25 μl water
Flow-rate: 1 ml min^{-1}

The two chromatograms depicted in Fig. 13.12 show the resolution obtained with the use of one-year-old column (A) and a new column used for the first time, under the same chromatographic conditions.

Remark: The concentration of KH$_2$PO$_4$ buffer should be increased up to 500 mM for highly charged oligosaccharides. In this case, KH$_2$PO$_4$ may be also replaced by 30 mM KH$_2$PO$_4$–K$_2$HPO$_4$ pH 7.0.

Reverse-phase (RP) chromatography of neutral oligosaccharides

Figure 13.13 depicts the profile of neutral and acidic oligosaccharide-alditols released from a mucin secreted by the oviduct of *Bufo bufo*. This separation was obtained using another type of gradient, as described in the legend of the figure. The peak 3 is actually a mixture of 5 or 6 different compounds, as confirmed by NMR and MALDI-TOF analysis. The Fig. 13.13 also shows the subfractionation of the peak 3 by reverse-phase chromatography on a C18 Reverse-phase 5 μM Zorbax column (4.6 × 250 mm), isocratically eluted with water.

Anion-exchange chromatography of sialyl oligosaccharides

1. Preparative anion-exchange HPLC of sialyl oligosaccharides on Mono-Q®

- Perform anion-exchange chromatography using a traditional gradient system equipped HPLC apparatus or on a Pharmacia Fast protein liquid chromatography apparatus (FPLC). Carry out the separation at room temperature on an analytical prepacked Mono Q HR 5/5 column (50 × 5 mm) (Pharmacia).
- Wash the column with 2 ml of water. Inject the sample dissolved in 50 μl of water.
- Perform the charge separation of acidic oligosaccharides with a linear gradient from 0–100 mM NaCl in water (10 ml) at a flow rate of 2 ml/min. The eluate is monitored at 214 nm. Wash the column with 2 ml of 100 mM NaCl.

Monosialyl oligosaccharides are eluted at a 15 mM NaCl concentration, disialyl at 40 mM, trisialyl at 50 mM and tetrasialyl at 70 mM.

2. Preparative anion-exchange HPLC of sialyl oligosaccharides on Micropack AX-10 anion-exchange column (Fig. 13.14).

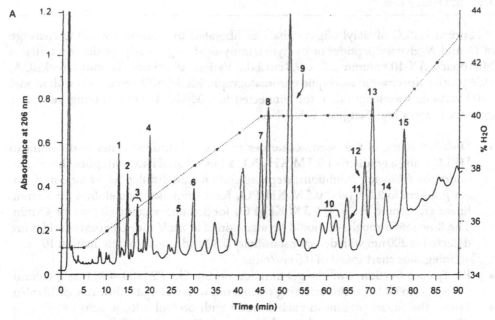

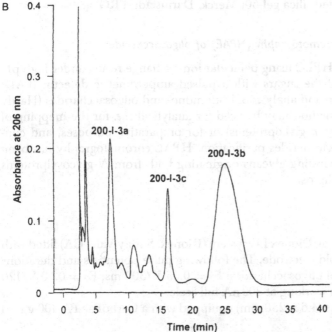

Figure 13.13 HPLC profiles of oligosaccharide-alditols released from the oviducal mucin of *Bufo bufo* (A) (Morelle and Strecker, 1997). Sample was chromatographed on a column (4.6 × 250 mm) of primary amine-bonded silica (Supelcosyl LC–NH₂; Supelco, Inc.) using gradient elution with acetonitrile/3 mM KH₂PO₄ as depicted on the profile. Flow rate was 1 ml/min. Absorbance was measured at 206 nm (B). Repurification of fraction A-3 on a C18 reverse-phase 5 μm Zorbax column (4.6 × 250 mm). Elution was performed isocratically by water at a flow rate of 0.5 ml/min.

Perform HPLC of sialyl oligosaccharides liberated by reductive alkaline cleavage of *O*- and *N*-glycosylpeptides or by hydrazinolysis of *N*-glycosylpeptides, on a 10 μm Micropack AX-10 column (50 × 0.8 cm i.d.; Varian Associates, Walnut Creek, CA, USA) with a Spectra-Physics liquid chromatograph (Model 8700) equipped with Model 8400 variable wavelength detector connected to a Model 4100 computing integrator (Spectra-Physics Inc., San Jose, CA, USA).

- Dissolve 20 mg of the oligosaccharides in 60 μl of distilled water and submit to HPLC using a gradient of 0.5 M KH_2PO_4 adjusted to pH 4.0 with phosphoric acid under the following conditions: stepwise elution with distilled water for 5 min, linear gradient to 2.5% (v/v) 0.5 M KH_2PO_4 for 15 min, isocratic elution for 25 min, linear gradient to 5% (v/v) 0.5 M KH_2PO_4 for 35 min, isocratic elution for 45 min. The flow rate throughout should be maintained at 2 ml/min. Oligosaccharides are detected at 200 nm with detector sensitivity 0.32 and integrator attenuation 16 using an integrator chart speed of 0.5 cm/min.
- Purify each fraction (4 ml) by gel filtration on Bio-Gel P2 (200–400 mesh) column (30 × 1.9 cm i.d.), the elution being carried out with water at a flow rate of 12 ml/h.
- Detect the sugars present in each fraction with orcinol-sulfuric acid reagent, on silica gel plates (precoated silica gel-60; Merck, Darmstadt, FRG).

High pH Anion-Exchange Chromatography (HPAE) of oligosaccharides

The recent introduction of HPLC using pellicular ion-exchange resins under high pH conditions and detection of the sugars with a pulsed amperometric detector (PAD) has simplified the separation and analysis of both mono- and oligosaccharides (Hardy and Towsend, 1988). The method may be used for analytical (*i.e.* for the mapping of oligosaccharides released from glycoproteins) or for preparative purposes, and constitutes a final step in oligosaccharides purification. HPAE chromatography has been successfully applied for separating glycans originating both from *N*-glycosylproteins and mucins and from glycolipids.

EQUIPMENT

- HPAE is realized using the Dionex LC system (Dionex, Sunny Vale, CA) fitted with a PAD detector with gold electrode. The following pulse potentials and durations are used for detection of oligosaccharides: $E_1 = 0.05$ V/300 ms; $E_2 = 0.60$ V/120 ms; $E_3 = 0.60$ V/60 ms working at 300 nA full scale.
- CarboPac PA-1 columns (4.6 × 250 mm) equipped with a CarboPac PA-100 guard column (Dionex).
- Elution is carried out at a flow rate of 1 ml/min at ambient temperature. Eluents are made by suitable dilutions of a 50% NaOH stock solution (Baker) and by increasing ionic strength with sodium acetate.

SEPARATION OF NEUTRAL OLIGOSACCHARIDES

- Separation of oligosaccharides from *N*-glycosylproteins: use the gradient described in Table 13.4.

Table 13.4 Elution gradient for fractionating neutral oligosaccharides by HPAE-Dionex chromatography

Time (min)	% Eluent 1 (0.1 M NaOH)	% Eluent 2 (0.15 M sodium acetate in 0.1 M NaOH)
0	100	0
10	100	0
60	40	60
65	40	60
125	100	0

Table 13.5 Low pH elution gradient for fractionating acidic oligosaccharides by HPAE-Dionex chromatography

Time (min)	% Eluent 1 (5 mM sodium acetate pH 4.65)	% Eluent 2 (0.2 M sodium acetate buffered to pH 4.65 with 0.165 M acetic acid)
0	100	0
5	100	0
30	95	5
60	70	30
70	70	30
80	100	0

Table 13.6 Alkaline pH elution gradient for fractionating acidic oligosaccharides by HPAE-Dionex chromatography

Time (min)	% Eluent 1 (0.1 M NaOH)	% Eluent 2 (0.1 M sodium acetate in 0.1 M NaOH)
0	95	5
25	95	5
85	91	9
95	85	15
102	95	5

• Separation of oligosaccharide-alditols released by reductive alkaline treatment of mucins. Due to the lower retention times of the alditols as compared to the native oligosaccharides, a very low base concentration (isocratic elution with 15 mM NaOH) is used for fractionated oligosaccharide-alditols.

SEPARATION OF ACIDIC OLIGOSACCHARIDES

Sialyloligosaccharides can be separated either at low pH (pH 4.0–6.0) or at pH 13 leading to very variable retention times (Tables 13.5 and 13.6).

The principle of the methods is based on the formation of sugar oxyanions under alkaline conditions. The contribution of the anomeric oxyanion to the retention time is dominant as demonstrated by the lower phase-interactions observed with oligosaccharide-alditols. Chromatographic selectivity for oligosaccharide oxyanions

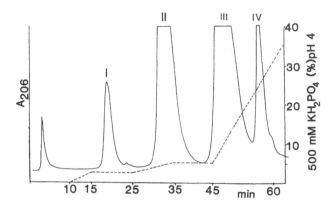

Figure 13.14 HPLC on 10 μm Micropak AX-10 column of sialoglycans liberated by hydrazinolysis of α_1-acid glycoprotein. I, II, III, IV: mono-, di-, tri-, and tetrasialylated glycans. The recovery was 91%.

is also related to the accessibility of the stationary phase of the readily ionizable hydroxyl groups. This phenomenon is observed with fucosylated compounds which are less retained as compared to their non-fucosylated counterparts. Although neutral oligosaccharides require alkaline conditions for separation by HPAE, acidic oligosaccharides can be separated both at low and high pH due to the ionization of acidic groups.

Conclusion

General strategy for the chromatographic separation of oligosaccharides

We described the more commonly used techniques, and we have to be precise that the examples given above do not represent universal procedures, applicable for each situation. In particular, the choice of the gradient acetonitrile-water-phosphate (for partition HPLC) is a function of the nature of the material. It can be modified by introducing plates of isocratic elutions for increasing the resolution. In some cases, neutral and sialic acid (or Kdn)-containing oligosaccharides can be fractionated in one step, as exemplified in Fig. 13.12. For more complex mixtures, a prior fractionation on an anion-exchanger will provide mono- di- tri- and tetra-sialyloligosaccharides, which will be more easily analyzed separately by partition chromatography. At last, the performances of the C18 column (reverse-phase chromatography) for the fine resolution of neutral compounds has to be not neglected.

References

For recent books and reviews see:

Allen, H. J. and Kisailus, E. C. (1992) *Glycoconjugates: Composition, Structure and Functions*, Marcel Dekker, New-York.

Amano, J., Messer, M. and Kobata, A. (1985) Structures of the oligosaccharides isolated from milk of the Platypus. *Glycoconjugate J.*, 2, 121–135.

Animashaun, T. and Hughes, R. C. (1989) *Bowringia milbraedii* agglutinin: specificity of binding to early processing intermediates of asparagine-linked oligosaccharide and use as a marker of endoplasmic reticulum glycoproteins. *J. Biol. Chem.*, **264**, 4657–4663.

Aucouturier, P., Mihaesco, E., Mihaesco, C. and Preud'homme, J. L. (1987) Characterization of Jacalin, the human IgA and IgD binding lectin from jackfruit. *Mol. Immunol.*, **24**, 503–511.

Azevedo-Moreira, R. and Ainouz, I. L. (1981) Lectins from the seeds of jackfruit (*Artocarpus integrifolia L.*) Isolation and purification of two isolectins from the albumin fraction. *Biol. Plant.*, **23**, 186–192.

Baenziger, J. and Kornfeld, S. (1974) Structure of the carbohydrate units of IgA1. II Structure of the O-glycosidically linked oligosaccharide units. *J. Biol. Chem.*, **249**, 7270–7281.

Baenziger, J. U. and Fiete, D. (1979a) Structural determinants of Concanavalin. A specificity for oligosaccharides. *J. Biol. Chem.*, **254**, 2400–2407.

Baenziger, J. U. and Fiete, D. (1979b) Structural determinants of *Ricinus communis* agglutinin and toxin specificity for oligosacharides. *J. Biol. Chem.*, **254**, 9795–9799.

Bayard, B. and Kerckaert, J. P. (1981) Uniformity of carbohydrate chains within molecular variants of rat α_1-Fetoprotein with distinct affinity for Concanavalin A. *Eur. J. Biochem.*, **113**, 405–414.

Bendiak, B. and Cumming, D. A. (1986) Purification of oligosaccharides having a free reducing end from glycopeptidic sources. *Carbohydr. Res.*, **151**, 89–103.

Bhavanandan, V. P., Umemoto, J., Banks, J. R. and Davidson, E. A. (1977) Isolation and partial characterization of sialoglycopeptides produced by a murine melanoma. *Biochemistry*, **16**, 4426–4437.

Bierhuizen, M. F. A., De Wit, M., Govers, C. A. R. L., Ferwerda, W., Koeleman, C., Pos, O. and Van Dijk, W. (1988) Glycosylation of three molecular forms of human α_1-acid glycoprotein having different interactions with concanavalin A. Variations in the occurrence of di-, tri-, tetraantennary glycans and the degree of sialylation. *Eur. J. Biochem.*, **175**, 387–394.

Bierhuizen, M. F. A., Edzes, H. T., Schiphorst, W. E. C. M., Van Den Eijnden, D. H. and Van Dijk, W. (1988) Effect of $\alpha(2-6)$-linked sialic acid and $\alpha(1-3)$-linked fucose on the interaction of *N*-linked glycopeptides and related oligosaccharides with immobilized *Phaseolus vulgaris* leukoagglutining lectin (L-PHA). *Glycoconjugate J.*, **5**, 85–97.

Bjerrum, O. J. and Bog-Hansen, T. C. (1976) The immunochemical approach to the characterization of membrane proteins. Human erythrocyte membrane proteins analyzed as a model system. *Biochim. Biophys. Acta.*, **455**, 66–89.

Bog-Hansen, T. C. (1973) Crossed immuno-affinoelectrophoresis. An analytical method to predict the result of affinity chromatography. *Anal. Biochem.*, **56**, 480–488.

Bourne, Y., Mazurier, J., Legrand, D., Rougé, P., Montreuil, J., Spik, G. and Cambillau, C. (1994) Structures of a legume lectin complexed with the human lactoferrin N2 fragment, and with an isolated biantennary glycopeptide: role of the fucose moiety. *Structure*, **2**, 209–219.

Broekaert, W. F., Nsimba-Lubaki, M., Peeters, B. and Peumans, W. J. (1984) A lectin from elder (*Sambucus nigra L.*) bark. *Biochem. J.*, **221**, 163–199.

Chaplin, M. F. and Kennedy, J. F. (1994) *Carbohydrate Analysis: A Practical Approach*, IRL Press, Oxford.

Cummings, R. D. (1994) Use of lectins in analysis of glycoconjugates. *Methods Enzymol.*, **230**, 66–86.

Cummings, R. D. (1997) Lectins as tools for glycoconjugate purification and characterization. In *Glycosciences*, Gabius, H. J., Gabius, S. (eds) Chapman and Hall, London, Glasgow, Weinheim, New York, Tokyo, Melbourne, Madras, pp. 191–199.

Cummings, R. D. and Kornfeld, S. (1982) Characterization of the structural determinants required for the high affinity interaction of asparagine-linked oligosaccharides with immobilized *Phaseolus vulgaris* leukoagglutinating and erythroagglutinating lectins. *J. Biol. Chem.*, **257**, 11230–11234.

Cummings, R. D., Merkle, R. K. and Stults, N. L. (1989) Separation and analysis of glycoprotein oligosaccharides. *Methods Cell Biol.*, **32**, 141–183.

Debray, H. (1995) Use of Lectins. In *Methods on Glycoconjugates. A Laboratory Manual*, Verbert, A. (ed.), Harwood Academic Publishers, Switzerland, pp. 103–133.

Debray, H., Decout, D., Strecker, G., Spik, G. and Montreuil, J. (1981) Specificity of twelve lectins toward oligosaccharides and glycopeptides related to N-glycosylproteins. *Eur. J. Biochem.*, **117**, 41–55.

Debray, H. and Montreuil, J. (1983) Structural basis for the affinity of four insolubilized lectins, with a specificity for α-D-mannose, towards various glycopeptides with the N-glycosylamine linkage and related oligosaccharides. *J. Biosci.*, **5**(1), 93–100.

Debray, H. and Montreuil, J. (1989) *Aleuria aurantia* agglutinin: a new isolation procedure and further study of its specificity towards various glycopeptides and oligosaccharides. *Carbohydr. Res.*, **185**, 15–26.

Debray, H. and Montreuil, J. (1991) Lectin affinity chromatography of glycoconjugates. *Adv. Lectin Res.*, **4**, 51–96.

Debray, H. and Montreuil, J. (1992) Specificity of lectins toward oligosaccharidic sequences belonging to N- and O-glycosylproteins. In *Affinity Electrophoresis: Principles & Application*, Breborowicz, J. and Mackiewicz, A. (eds) CRC Press, Boca Raton, pp. 23–57.

Debray, H., Montreuil, J. Lis, H. and Sharon, N. (1986) Affinity of four immobilized *Erythrina* lectins toward various N-linked glycopeptides and related oligosaccharides *Carbohydr. Res.*, **151**, 359–370.

Debray, H., Montreuil, J. and Franz, H. (1994) Fine sugar specificity of the mistletoe (*Viscum album*) lectin I. *Glycoconjugate J.*, **11**, 550–557.

Debray, H., Pierce-Cretel, A., Spik, G. and Montreuil, J. (1983) Affinity of ten insolubilized lectins towards various glycopeptides with the N-glycosylamine linkage and related oligosaccharides, In *Lectins: Biology, Biochemistry, Clinical Biochemistry*, Bog-Hansen, T. C. and Spengler, G. A. (eds), De Gruyter, Berlin, Vol. 3, 335–350.

Dulaney, J. T. (1979) Binding interactions of glycoproteins with lectins. *Mol. Cell. Biochem.*, **21**, 43–63.

Dumitru, S. (1992) *Polysaccharides in Medicinal Applications*, Marcel Dekker, New-York.

Ebisu, S., Iyer, P. N. and Goldstein, I. J. (1978) Equilibrium dialysis and carbohydrate-binding studies on the 2-acetamido-2-deoxy-D-glucopyranosyl-binding lectin from *Bandeiraea simplicifolia* seeds. *Carbohydr. Res.*, **61**, 129–138.

Endo, T., Ohbayashi, H., Kanazawa, K., Kochibe, N. and Kobata, A. (1992) Carbohydrate binding specificity of immobilized *Psathyrella velutina* lectin. *J. Biol. Chem.*, **267**, 707–713.

Finne, J. and Krusius, T. (1982) Preparation and fractionation of glycopeptides. *Methods Enzymol.*, **83**, 269–277.

Finne, J., Krusius, T. and Jarnefelt, J. (1980) Fractionation of glycopeptides In *27th Int. Congress of Pure and Applied Chemistry*, Varmavuory, A. (ed.) Pergamon Press, Oxford, New York, pp. 147–159.

Finne, J., Krusius, T., Rauvala, H., Kekomächi, R. and Myllylä, G. (1978) Alkali-stable blood group A- and B-active poly(glycosyl)-peptides from human erythrocyte membrane. *FEBS Lett.*, **89**, 111–115.

Franz, H. (1986) Mistletoe lectins and their A and B chains. *Oncology*, **43**(1), 23–43.

Franz, H. Ziska, P. and Kindt, A. (1981) Isolation and properties of three lectins from mitletoe (*Viscum album* L). *Biochem. J.*, **195**, 481–484.

Fukuda, M. and Hindsgaul, O. (2000) Molecular and Cellular Glycobiology, Oxford University Press, 289 p.

Fukuda, M. and Kobata, A. (1993) *Glycobiology: A Practical Approach*, IRL Press, Oxford.

Furukawa, K., Minor, J. E., Hegarty, J. D. and Bhavanandan, V. P. (1986) Interaction of sialo-glycoproteins with wheat germ agglutinin-Sepharose of varying ratio of lectins to Sepharose. Use for the purification of mucin glycoproteins from membrane extracts. *J. Biol. Chem.*, **261**, 7755–7761.

Gallagher, J. T. (1984) Carbohydrate-binding properties of lectins: a possible approach to lectin nomenclature and classification. *Biosci. Rep.*, **4**, 621–632.

Gallagher, J. T. (1989) Affinity chromatography of complex carbohydrates using lectins. In *HPLC of Macromolecules: A Practical Approach*, Oliver, R. W. A. (ed.) IRL Press, Oxford, New York, Tokyo, pp. 209–228.

Gallagher, J. T., Morris, A. and Dexter, T. M. (1985) Identification of two binding sites for wheat germ agglutinin on polylactosamine-type oligosaccharides. *Biochem. J.*, **231**, 115–122.

Goldstein, I. J. Winter, H. C. and Poretz, R. D. (1997) Plant lectins: tools for the study of complex carbohydrates. In *Glycoproteins II*, Montreuil, J., Vliegenthart, J. F. G., Schachter, H. (eds) Elsevier, Amsterdam, Lausanne, New York, Oxford, Shannon, Singapore, Tokyo, pp. 403–474.

Goldstein, I. J. and Hayes, C. E. (1978) The lectins: carbohydrate-binding proteins of plants and animals. *Adv. Carbohydr. Chem. Biochem.*, **35**, 127–340.

Goldstein, I. J., Hughes, R. C., Monsigny, M., Osawa, T. and Sharon, N. (1980) What should be called a lectin? *Nature* **285**, 66.

Goldstein, I. J. and Poretz, R.D. (1986) Isolation, physico-chemical characterization and carbohydrate-binding specificity of lectins In *The Lectins: Properties, Functions and Applications in Biology and Medicine*, Liener, I. E., Sharon, N., Goldstein, I. J. (eds) Academic Press, London, New York, pp. 33–247.

Green, E. D., Adelt, G., Baenziger, J. U., Wilson, S. and Van Halbeek, H. (1988) The asparagine-linked oligosaccharides on bovine fetuin. Structural analysis of *N*-glycanase-released oligosaccharides by 500-MHz ^{1}H-NMR spectroscopy. *J. Biol. Chem.*, **263**, 18253–18268.

Green, E. D. and Baenziger, J. U. (1987) Oligosaccharide specificities of *Phaseolus vulgaris* leukoagglutinating and erythroagglutinating phytohemagglutinins. Interactions with *N*-glycanase-released oligosaccharides. *J. Biol. Chem.*, **262**, 12018–12029.

Green, E.D., Brodbeck, R. M. and Baenziger, J. U. (1987a) Lectin affinity high-performance liquid chromatography. Interactions of *N*-glycanase-released oligosaccharides with *Ricinus communis* agglutinin I and *Ricinus communis* agglutinin II. *J. Biol. Chem.*, **262**, 12030–12039.

Green, E. D., Brodbeck, R. M. and Baenziger, J. U. (1987b) Lectin affinity high-performance liquid chromatography : interactions of *N*-glycanase-released oligosaccharides with leukoagglutinating phytohemagglutinin, Concanavalin A, *Datura stramonium* agglutinin and *Vicia villosa* agglutinin. *Anal. Biochem.*, **167**, 62–75.

Hagen, I., Bjerum, O. J. and Solum, N. O. (1979) Characterization of human platelet proteins solubilized with Triton X-100 and examined by crossed immunoelectrophoresis. *Eur. J. Biochem.*, **99**, 9–22.

Hagiwara, K., Collet-Cassart, D., Kobayashi, K. and Vaerman, J. P. (1988) Jacalin: Isolation, characterization and influence of various factors on its interaction with human IgA1, as assessed by precipitation and latex agglutination. *Molec. Immun.*, **25**, 69–83.

Harada, H., Kamei, M., Tokumoto, Y., Yui, S., Koyama, F., Kochibe, N. et al., (1987) Systematic fractionation of oligosaccharides of human immunoglobulin G by serial affinity chromatography on immobilized lectin columns. *Anal. Biochem.*, **164**, 374–381.

Hård, K., van Zadelhoff, H., Moonen, P., Kamerling, J. P. and Vliegenthart, J. F. G. (1992) The Asn-linked carbohydrate chains of human Tamm-Horofull glycoprotein of one male. Novel sulfated and novel *N*-acetylgalactosamine-containing *N*-linked carbohydrate chain. *Eur. J. Biochem.*, **209**, 295.

Hardy, M. R. and Towsend, R. R. (1988) Separation of positional isomers of oligosaccha-rides and glycopeptides by high performance anion-exchange chromatography with pulsed amperometric detection. *Proc. Natl. Acad. Sci. USA*, **85**, 3289–3293.

Hedo, J. A. (1984) Lectins as tools for the purification of membrane receptors, In *Receptor Purification Procedures*, Venter, C. and Harrison, L. (eds) Liss, New York, Vol. 2, pp. 45–60.

Hedo, J. A., Harrison, L. C. and Roth, J. (1981) Binding of insulin receptors to lectins: evidence for common carbohydrate determinants on several membrane receptors. *Biochemistry*, **20**, 3385–3393.

Heegard, P. M. H., Heegard, N. H. H. and Bog-Hansen, T. C. (1992) Affinity electrophoresis for the characterization of glycoproteins. The use of lectins in combination with immunoelec-trophoresis, in *Affinity electrophoresis: Principles & Applications*, Breborowicz, J. and Mackiewicz, A. (eds) CRC Press, Boca Raton, pp. 3–21.

Hortin, G. L. (1990) Isolation of glycopeptides containing O-linked oligosaccharides by lectin affinity chromatography on Jacalin-Agarose. *Anal. Biochem.*, **191**, 262–267.

Hortin, G. L. and Trimpe, B. L. (1990) Lectin affinity chromatography of proteins bearing O-linked oligosaccharides: application of jacalin-Sepharose. *Anal. Biochem.*, **188**, 271–277.

Hounsell, E. F. (1993) Glycoprotein analysis in biomedicine. *Meth. Mol. Biol.*, Humana Press, Totowa, N.J., **14**.

Irimura, T. and Nicolson, G. L. (1983) Interaction of pokeweed mitogen with poly-(*N*-acetyllactosamine)-type carbohydrate chains. *Carbohydr. Res.*, **120**, 187–195.

Irimura, T., Tsuji, T., Tagami, S., Yamamoto, K. and Osawa, T. (1981) Structure of a complex-type sugar chain of human glycophorin A. *Biochemistry*, **20**, 560–566.

Ivatt, R. J., Harnett, P. B. and Reeder, J. W. (1986a) Isolated erythroglycans have a high-affinity interaction with wheat germ agglutinin but are poorly accessible *in situ*. *Biochim. Biophys. Acta*, **884**, 124–134.

Ivatt, R. J., Reeder, J. W. and Clark, G. F. (1986b) Structural and conformational features that affect the interaction of polylactosamino-glycans with immobilized wheat germ agglutinin. *Biochim. Biophys. Acta*, **883**, 253–264.

Kahane, I., Furthmayr, H. and Marchesi, V. T. (1976) Isolation of membrane glycoproteins by affinity chromatography in the presence of detergents. *Biochim. Biophys. Acta*, **426**, 464–476.

Kaku, H., Van Damme, E. J. M., Peumans, W. J. and Goldstein, I. J. (1990) Carbohydrate-binding specificity of the daffodil (*Narcissus pseudonarcissus*) and Amaryllis (*Hippeastrum hyb.*) bulb lectins *Arch. Biochem. Biophys.*, **279**, 298–304.

Kawashima, H., Sueyoshi, S., Li, H., Yamamoto, K. and Osawa, T. (1990) Carbohydrate binding specificities of several poly-*N*-acetyllactosamine-binding lectins. *Glycoconjugate J.*, **7**, 323–334.

Kobata, A. and Endo, T. (1992) Immobilized lectin columns: useful tools for the fractionation and structural analysis of oligosaccharides. *J. Chromatogr.*, **597**, 111–122.

Kobata, A. and Yamashita, K. (1993) Fractionation of oligosaccharides by serial affinity chro-matography with use of immobilized lectin columns. In *Glycobiology: A Practical Approach*. Kobata, A. and Fukuda, M. (eds) IRL Press, Oxford, pp. 103–125.

Kochibe, N. and Furukawa, K. (1980) Purification and properties of a novel fucose-specific hemagglutinin of *Aleuria aurantia*. *Biochemistry*, **19**, 2841–2846.

Kochibe, N. and Matta, K.L. (1989) Purification and properties of an *N*-acetylglucosamine-specific lectin from *Psathyrella velutina* mushroom. *J. Biol. Chem.*, **264**, 173–177.

Kohn, J. and Wilchek, M. (1982) A new approach (cyano-transfer) for cyanogen bromide acti-vation of Sepharose at neutral pH, which yields activated resins, free of interfering nitrogen derivatives. *Biochem. Biophys. Res. Commun.*, **107**, 878–884.

Koide, N. and Muramatsu, T. (1974) Endo-β-D-acetylglucosaminidase acting on carbohydrate moieties of glycoproteins. Purification and properties of the enzyme from *Diplococcus pneumonia*. *J. Biol. Chem.*, **249**, 4897–4904.

Kondoh, H., Kobayashi, K. and Hagiwara, K. (1987) A simple procedure for the isolation of human secretory IgA of IgA$_1$ and IgA$_2$ subclass by a jackfruit lectin, jacalin, affinity chromatography. *Molec. Immun.*, 24, 1219–1222.

Kornfeld, K., Reitman, M. L. and Kornfeld, R. (1981) The carbohydrate-binding specificity of pea and lentil lectins. Fucose is an important determinant. *J. Biol. Chem.*, 256, 6633–6640.

Kornfeld, R. and Ferris, C. (1975) Interactions of immunoglobulin glycopeptides with con-canavalin A. *J. Biol. Chem.*, 250, 2614–2619.

Lakhtin, W. M. (1995) Use of lectins in the analysis of carbohydrate moieties of glycoproteins and other natural glycoconjugates. *Biochemistry* (Moscow), 60, 131–153.

Lennartz, W. K. and Hart, G. W. (1994) Guide to techniques in Glycobiology, *Meth. Enzymol.*, Academic Press, New York, 14 pp.

Likhoshertov, L. M., Novikova, O. S., Derevitskaya, V. A. and Kotchekov, N. K. (1990) A selective method for sequential splitting of O- and N-linked glycans from N,O-glycoproteins. *Carbohydr. Res.*, 199, 67–76.

Lis, H. and Sharon, N . (1986b) Lectins as molecules and as tools. *Ann. Rev. Biochem.*, 55, 35–67.

Lis, H. and Sharon, N. (1972) Soy bean (*Glycine max*) agglutinin. *Methods Enzymol.*, 28, 360–368.

Lis, H. and Sharon, N. (1984) Lectins: properties and applications to the study of complex carbohydrates in solution and on cell surfaces. In *Biology of Carbohydrates*, Ginsburg, V. and Robbins, P. W. (eds) Wiley, New York, Vol. 2, pp. 2–85.

Lis, H. and Sharon, N. (1986a) Applications of lectins In *The Lectins, Properties, Functions and Applications in Biology and Medicine*, Liener, I. E., Sharon. N., Goldstein, I. J. (eds) Academic Press, London, New York, pp. 265–291.

Lotan, R., Beattie, G., Hubbell, W. and Nicolson, G. L. (1977) Activities of lectins and their immobilized derivatives in detergent solutions. Implications on the use of lectin affinity chromatography for the purification of membrane glycoproteins. *Biochemistry*, 16, 1787–1794.

Lotan, R. and Nicolson, G. L. (1979) Purification of cell membrane glycoproteins by lectin affinity chromatography. *Biochim. Biophys. Acta.*, 559, 329–376.

Lotan, R. and Sharon, N. (1978) Peanut (*Arachis hypogaea*) agglutinin. *Methods Enzymol.*, 50, 361–367.

Maemura, K. and Fukuda, M. (1992) Poly-N-acetyllactosaminyl O-glycans attached to leukosialin. The presence of sialyl Le^x structures in O-glycans. *J. Biol. Chem.*, 267, 24379–24386.

March, S. C., Parikh, I. and Cuatrecasas, P. (1974) A simplified method for cyanogen bromide activation of Agarose for affinity chromatography. *Anal. Biochem.*, 60, 149–152.

Mellis, S. J. and Baenziger, J. U. (1983) Structures of the oligosaccharides present at the three asparagine-linked glycosylation sites of human IgD. *J. Biol. Chem.*, 258, 11546–11556.

Merkle, R. K. and Cummings, R. D. (1987) Lectin affinity chromatography of glycopeptides. *Methods Enzymol.*, 138, 232–259.

Merkle, R. K. and Cummings, R. D. (1987) Relationship of the terminal sequences to the length of poly-N-acetyllactosamine chains in asparagine-linked oligosaccharides from the mouse lymphoma cell line BW 5147. Immobilized tomato lectin interacts with high affinity with glycopeptides containing long poly-N-acetyllactosamine chains. *J. Biol. Chem.*, 262, 8179–8189.

Misaki, A., Kakuta , M., Meah, Y. and Goldstein, I. J. (1997) Purification and characterization of the α-1,3-mannosylmannose-recognizing lectin of *Crocus vernus* bulbs. *J. Biol. Chem.*, 272, 25455–25461.

Montreuil, J. (1980) Primary structure of glycoprotein glycans. Basis for the molecular biology of glycoproteins. *Adv. Carbohydr. Chem. Biochem.*, 37, 157–223.

Montreuil, J. (1984a) Spatial structures of glycan chains of glycoproteins in relation to metabolism and function. Survey of a decade of research. *Pure Appl. Chem.*, 56, 859–877.

Montreuil, J. (1984b) Spatial conformation of glycans and glycoproteins. *Biol. Cell.*, 51, 115–132.

Montreuil, J. (1995) Glycoprotein structure and conformation: an overview. In *Methods on Glycoconjugates: A Laboratory Manual,* Verbert, A. (ed.) Harwood Academic Publishers, Switzerland, pp. 1–23.

Montreuil, J. (1996) Glycobiology: general aspects. In Dimitru, S. (ed.) *Polysaccharides in Medical Applications,* Marcel Dekker, New York, pp. 265–271.

Montreuil, J. (1996) Structure biosynthesis of glycoproteins. In Dimitru, S. (ed.) *Polysaccharides in Medical Applications,* Marcel Dekker, New York, pp. 273–327.

Montreuil, J., Bouquelet, S., Debray, H., Lemoine, J., Michalski, J. C., Spik, G. and Strecker, G. (1994) Glycoproteins. In Chaplin, M. F. and Kennedy, M. F. (eds) *Carbohydrate Analysis: A Practical Approach,* IRL Press, Oxford, pp. 181–293.

Montreuil, J., Vliegenthart, J. F. G. and Schachter, H. (1995) Glycoproteins. In Neuberger, A. and van Deenen, L. L. M. (eds) *New Comprehensive Biochemistry,* 29A Elsevier, Amsterdam.

Montreuil, J., Vliegenthart, J. F. G. and Schachter, H. (1997) Glycoproteins. In Neuberger, A. and van Deenen, L. L. M. (eds) *New Comprehensive Biochemistry,* 29B Elsevier, Amsterdam.

Montreuil, J., Vliegenthart, J. F. G. and Schachter, H. (1996) Glycoproteins and Disease. In Neuberger, A. and van Deenen, L. L. M. (eds) *New Comprehensive Biochemistry,* Elsevier, Amsterdam.

Montreuil, J. and Verbert, A. (1997) *Analyse des glucides et des glycoprotéines,* Techniques de l'Ingénieur, Paris, P 3320, 1–24.

Morelle, W. and Strecker, G. (1997) Structural analysis of hexa to dodecaoligosaccharide-alditols released by reductive β-elimination from oviducal mucins of *Bufo bufo. Glycobiology,* 7, 1129–1151.

Murphy, L. A. and Goldstein, I. J. (1977) Five α-D-galactopyranosyl-binding isolectins from *Bandeiraea simplicifolia* seeds. *J. Biol. Chem.*, 252, 4739–4742.

Nakata, N., Furukawa, K., Greenwalt, D. E., Sato, T. and Kobata, A. (1993) Structural study of the sugar chains of CD 36 purified from bovine mammary epithelial cells: occurrence of novel hybrid-type sugar chains containing the Neu5Ac α2->6GalNAcβ1->4GlcNAc and the Manα1->2Manα1->3Manα1->6Man groups. *Biochemistry,* 32, 4369–4383.

Narasimhan, S., Freed, J. C. and Schachter, H. (1986) The effect of a "bisecting" N-acetylglucosaminyl group on the binding of biantennary, complex oligosaccharides to Concanavalin A, *Phaseolus vulgaris* erythroagglutinin (E-PHA) and *Ricinus communis* agglutinin (RCA-120) immobilized on Agarose. *Carbohydr. Res.*, 149, 65–83.

Nyame, K., Smith, D. F., Damian, R. T. and Cummings, R. D. (1989) Complex-type asparagine-linked oligosaccharides in glycoproteins synthetized by *Schistosoma mansoni* adult males contain terminal β-linked N-acetylgalactosamine. *J. Biol. Chem.*, 264, 3235–3243.

Osawa, T., Irimura, T. and Kawaguchi, T. (1978) *Bauhinia purpurea* agglutinin. *Methods Enzymol.*, 50, 367–372.

Osawa, T. and Tushi, T. (1978) Fractionation and structural assessment of oligosaccharides and glycopeptides by use of immobilized lectins. *Ann. Rev. Biochem.*, 56, 21–42.

Pereira, M. E. A. and Kabat, E. A. (1974) Specificity of the purified hemagglutinin (lectin) from *Lotus tetragonolobus. Biochemistry,* 13, 3184–3192.

Pereira, M. E. A., Kisailus, E. C., Gruezo, F. and Kabat, E. A. (1978) Immunochemical studies on the combining site of the blood group H-specific lectin 1 from *Ulex europeus* seeds. *Arch. Biochem. Biophys.*, 185, 108–115.

Peumans, W. J. and Van Damme, E. J. M. (1998) Plant lectins: specific tools for the identification, isolation and charaterization of O-linked glycans. *Crit. Rev. Biochem. Mol. Biol.*, 33, 209–258.

Pierce-Cretel, A., Pamblanco, M., Strecker, G., Montreuil, J. and Spik, G. (1981) Heterogeneity of the glycans O-glycosidically linked to the hinge region of secretory immunoglobulins from human milk. *Eur. J. Biochem.*, 114, 169–178.

Plummer, T. H., Elder, J. H., Alexander, S., Phelan, A. W. and Tarentino, A. L. (1984) Demonstration of peptide: N-glycosidase F activity in endo-β-N-acetyl-glucosaminidase F preparations. *J. Biol. Chem.*, **259**, 10700–10704.

Presant, C. A. and Kornfeld, S. (1972) Characterization of the cell surface receptor for the *Agaricus bisporus* hemagglutinin. *J. Biol. Chem.*, **247**, 6937–6945.

Rini, J. M. (1995) Lectin structure. *Ann. Rev. Biophys. Biomol. Struct.*, **24**, 551–577.

Roque-Barreira, M. C. and Campos-Neto, A. (1985) Jacalin: An IgA-binding lectin. *J. Immunol.*, **134**, 1740–1743.

Sastry, M. V. K., Banarjee, P., Patanjali, S. R., Swamy, M. J., Swarnalatha, G. V. and Surolia, A. (1986) Analysis of saccharide binding to *Artocarpus integrifolia* lectin reveals specific recognition of T-antigen (β-D-Gal1->3D-GalNAc). *J. Biol. Chem.*, **261**, 11726–11733.

Schmid, K., Binette, J. P., Kamiyama, S., Pfister, V. and Takahashi, S. (1962) Studies on the structure of α_1-acid glycoprotein III. Polymorphism of α_1-acid glycoprotein and the partial resolution and characterization of its variants. *Biochemistry*, **1**, 959–966.

Sharon, N. and Lis, H. (1989) *Lectins*, Chapman and Hall, London.

Shibata, S., Peters, B. P., Roberts, D. D., Goldstein, I. J. and Liotta, L. A. (1982) Isolation of laminin by affinity chromatography on immobilized *Griffonia simplicifolia* I lectin. *FEBS Lett.*, **142**, 194–198.

Shibuya, N., Berry, J. E. and Goldstein, I. J. (1988b) One-step purification of murine IgM and human α_2-macroglobulin by affinity chromatography on immobilized snowdrop bulb lectin. *Arch. Biochem. Biophys.*, **267**, 676–680.

Shibuya, N., Goldstein, I. J., Broekaert, W. F., Nsimba-Lubaki, M., Peeters, B. and Peumans, W. J. (1987) Fractionation of sialylated oligosaccharides, glycopeptides and glycoproteins on immobilized elderberry (*Sambucus nigra* L.) bark lectin *Arch. Biochem. Biophys.*, **254**, 1–8.

Shibuya, N., Goldstein, I. J., Van Damme, E. J. M. and Peumans, W. J. (1988a) Binding properties of a mannose-specific lectin from the snowdrop (*Galanthus nivalis*) bulb. *J. Biol. Chem.*, **263**, 728–734.

Spiro, R. G. and Bhoyroo, V. D. (1984) Occurrence of α-D-galactosyl residues in the thyroglobulins from several species. Localization in the saccharide chains of the complex carbohydrate units. *J. Biol. Chem.*, **259**, 9858–9866.

Srivatsan, J., Smith, D. F. and Cummings, R. D. (1992) *Schistosoma mansoni* synthesizes novel biantennary Asn-linked oligosaccharides containing terminal β-linked N-acetylgalactosamine. *Glycobiology*, **2**, 445–452.

Srivatsan, T., Smith, D. F. and Cummings, R. D. (1992) The human blood fluke *Schistosoma mansoni* synthesizes glycoproteins containing the Lewis X antigen. *J. Biol. Chem.*, **267**, 20196–20203.

Sueyoshi, S., Tsuji, T. and Osawa, T. (1985) Purification and characterization of four isolectins of mushroom *Agaricus bisporus*. *Biol. Chem. Hoppe-Seyler*, **366**, 213–221.

Sueyoshi, S., Tsuji, T. and Osawa, T. (1988) Carbohydrate-binding specificities of five lectins that bind to O-glycosyl-linked carbohydrate chains. Quantitative analysis by frontal-affinity chromatography. *Carbohydr. Res.*, **178**, 213–224.

Sueyoshi, S., Yamamoto, K. and Osawa, T. (1988) Carbohydrate binding specificity of a beetle (*Allomyrina dichotoma*) lectin. *J. Biochem.* (Tokyo), **103**, 894–899.

Susz, J. P. and Dawson, G. (1979) The affinity of the fucose-binding lectin from *Lotus tetragonolobus* for glycopeptides and oligosaccharides accumulating in fucosidosis. *J. Neurochem.*, **32**, 1009–1013.

Takasaki, S. and Kobata, A. (1974) Microdetermination of individual neutral and amino sugars and N-acetylneuraminic acid in complex saccharides. *J. Biochem.* (Tokyo), **76**, 783–789.

Takashi, N. and Nishibe, H. (1978) Some characteristics of a new glycopeptidase acting on aspartylglycosylamine linkages. *J. Biochem*, **84**, 1467–1473.

Tollefsen, S. E. and Kornfeld, R. (1983a) Isolation and characterization of lectins from *Vicia villosa*. two distinct carbohydrate binding activities are present in seed extracts. *J. Biol. Chem.*, **258**, 5165–5171.

Tollefsen, S. E. and Kornfeld, R. (1983b) The B4 lectin from *Vicia villosa* seeds interacts with *N*-acetylgalactosamine residues α-linked to serine or threonine residues in cell surface glycoproteins. *J. Biol. Chem.*, **258**, 5172–5176.

Torres, B. V., Mc Crumb, D. K. and Smith, D. F. (1988) Glycolipid-lectin interactions: reactivity of lectins from *Helix pomatia, Wisteria floribunda* and *Dolichos biflorus* with glycolipids containing *N*-acetylgalactosamine. *Arch. Biochem. Biophys.*, **262**, 1–11.

Toyoshima, S., Osawa, T. and Tonomura, A. (1970) Some properties of purified phytohemagglutinin from *Lens culinaris* seeds. *Biochim. Biophys. Acta.*, **221**, 514–521.

Tsuji, T., Yamamoto, K. and Osawa, T. (1993) Affinity chromatography of oligosaccharides and glycopeptides with immobilized lectins. In *Molecular Interactions in Bioseparations*, Ngo, T. T. (ed.) Plenum Press, New York, pp. 113–126.

Umetsu, K., Kosaka, S. and Suzuki, T. (1984) Purification and characterization of a lectin from the beetle *Allomyrina dichotoma*. *J. Biochem.* (Tokyo), **95**, 239–245.

Van Damme, E. J. M., Allen, A. K. and Peumans, W. J. (1987) Isolation and characterization of a lectin with exclusive specificity towards mannose from snowdrop (*Galanthus nivalis*) bulbs. *FEBS Lett.*, **215**, 140–144.

Van Damme, E. J. M., Allen, A. K. and Peumans, W. J. (1988) Related mannose specific lectins from different species of the family *Amaryllidaceae*. *Physiol. Plant.*, **73**, 52–57.

Varki, A. et al. (1999) Essentials of Glycobiology, Cold Spring Harbour, Laboratory Press, 652 p.

Verbert, A. (1995) *Methods on glycoconjugates: A laboratory manual*, Harwood Academic Publishers, Switzerland, Amsterdam.

Wang, W. C. and Cummings, R. D. (1988) The immobilized leukoagglutinin from the seeds of *Maackia amurensis* binds with high affinity to complex-type Asn-linked oligosaccharides containing terminal sialic acid-linked α-2,3 to penultimate galactose residues. *J. Biol. Chem.*, **263**, 4576–4585.

Waxdal, M. J. (1974) Isolation, characterization and biological activities of five mitogens from pokeweed. *Biochemistry*, **13**, 3671–3677.

Weis, W. I. (1997) Cell surface carbohydrate recognition by animal and viral lectins. *Curr. Opin. Struct. Biol.*, **7**, 624–630.

Weis, W. I. and Drickamer, K. (1996) Structural basis of lectin-carbohydrate recognition. *Annu. Rev. Biochem.*, **65**, 441–473.

Wilcheck, M. and Miron, T. (1974) Stable, high capacity and non charged agarose derivatives for immobilization of biologically active compounds and for affinity chromatography. *Mol. Cell. Biochem.*, **4**, 181–187.

Wilcheck, M. and Miron, T. (1987) Limitations of *N*-hydroxy-succinimide esters in affinity chromatography and protein immobilization. *Biochemistry*, **26**, 2155–2161.

Wu, A. M. (1984) Differential binding characteritics and applications of D-Galβ1,3D-GalNAc specific lectins. *Mol. Cell. Biochem.*, **61**, 131–141.

Wu, A. M., Sugii, S. and Herp, A. (1988) A guide for carbohydrate specificities of lectins. *Adv. Exp. Med. Biol.*, **228**, 819–847.

Yamamoto, K., Tsuji, T., Matsumoto, I. and Osawa, T. (1981) Structural requirements for the binding of oligosaccharides and glycopeptides to immobilized Wheat germ agglutinin. *Biochemistry*, **20**, 5894–5899.

Yamamoto, K., Tsuji, T. and Osawa, T. (1993) Analysis of asparagine-linked oligosaccharides by sequential lectin-affinity chromatography. In *Glycoprotein Analysis in Biomedicine, Methods in Molecular Biology* 14, Hounsell, E. F. (ed.) Humana Press, Totowa, New Jersey, pp. 17–34.

Yamashita, A. Mizuochi, T. and Kobata, A. (1982) Analysis of oligosaccharides by gel filtration. In V. Ginsburg (ed.) *Methods in Enzymology*, Academic Press, New York, **83**, 105–126.

Yamashita, K., Kobata, A., Suzuki, T. and Umetsu, K. (1989) *Allomyrina dichotoma* lectins *Methods Enzymol.*, **179**, 331–341.

Yamashita, K., Kochibe, N., Ohkura, T., Ueda, I. and Kobata, A. (1985) Fractionation of L-fucose-containing oligosaccharides on immobilized *Aleuria aurantia* lectin. *J. Biol. Chem.*, **260**, 4688–4693.

Yamashita, K., Totani, K., Ohkura, T., Takasaki, S., Goldstein, I. J. and Kobata, A. (1987) Carbohydrate binding properties of complex-type oligosaccharides on immobilized *Datura stramonium* lectin. *J. Biol. Chem.*, **262**, 1602–1607.

Yamashita, K., Umetsu, K., Suzuki, T., Iwaki, Y., Endo, T. and Kobata, A. (1988) Carbohydrate binding specificity of immobilized *Allomyrina dichotoma* lectin II. *J. Biol. Chem.*, **263**, 17482–17489.

Yokoyama, K., Terao, T. and Osawa, T. (1978) Carbohydrate-binding specificity of pokeweed mitogens. *Biochim. Biophys. Acta.*, **538**, 384–396.

Zehr, B. D. and Litwin, S. D. (1987) Human IgD and IgA$_1$ compete for D-galactose-related binding sites on the lectin Jacalin. *Scand. J. Immunol.*, **26**, 229–236.

Chapter 14

Capillary electrokinetic chromatography

Gargi Choudhary and Csaba Horváth

Introduction

High performance liquid chromatography and capillary zone electrophoresis are two high resolution separation processes based on the principle of differential migration and widely used for the analysis of non-volatile substances. HPLC employs pressure driven flow of the liquid mobile phase through a column packed with the stationary phase and the sample components are separated due to differences in their partitioning between the two phases. Following the trend towards miniaturization HPLC is increasingly carried out with packed fused silica capillary columns (μ-HPLC), mainly to facilitate applications involving its tandem use with the mass spectrometer.

Capillary zone electrophoresis (CZE) has gained considerable importance since mid 1980s [49]. It employs open fused silica capillaries filled with suitable electrophoretic medium and a steep voltage gradient to bring about separation of charged sample components. Sophisticated instruments for capillary electrophoresis have become available and this technique was the first to offer on a routine basis plate numbers over 1 00 000 for liquid phase analytical separations that can match the performance of gas chromatography (GC) in terms of efficiency. However, both GC and CZE have serious constraints on the nature of sample components that can be analyzed. Whereas, GC requires the sample components to be volatile, CZE separates only charged sample components.

Micellar electrokinetic chromatography (MEKC) and capillary electrochromatography (CEC) are microcolumn based techniques that harness the potential of an electric field in the separation of biomolecules. While CZE is a single phase system, MEKC and CEC are chromatographic techniques that employ electrosmotic force as well as electrophoretic migration besides partitioning between the two phases as the separation mechanism. In micellar electrokinetic chromatography and capillary electrochromatography, unlike in CZE, neutral species can also be separated. MEKC employs micelles of ionic surfactants as a pseudostationary phase that moves electrosmotically and if charged also electrophoretically under the influence of electric field. In contrast, CEC is a bona fide chromatographic technique and employs stationary phases that are very similar to those used in HPLC.

Micellar electrokinetic chromatography (MEKC)

Fundamentals

In 1984, Terabe *et al.* [116,118] introduced micellar electrokinetic chromatography (MEKC) as a new analytical technique that is also based on the differential migration principle of separation. Since then this technique has been employed in diverse analytical applications by using the same instrumentation developed for CZE. Thus, MEKC has expanded the scope of capillary electrophoresis to the separation of sample components that carry no electrical charges.

In MEKC, the micellar solution of an ionic surfactant is referred to as "pseudo stationary phase" since the separation is based in part on the differences in the partitioning of the analytes between the aqueous and the micellar phases. Thus, the latter plays a role which is similar to the function of a chromatographic stationary phase.

MEKC is most commonly performed with anionic surfactants, e.g., sodium dodecyl sulfate (SDS). The MEKC process with an anionic surfactant is schematically illustrated in Fig. 14.1. It is seen that the anionic micelles migrate electrophoretically towards the anode. On the other hand, due to the negatively charged inner surface of the fused silica capillary at pH >3, the electrosmotic flow, EOF, is towards the cathode. In practice the EOF velocity is greater than the electrophoretic migration velocity of the anionic SDS micelles so they move toward the cathode. Partitioning of neutral analytes between the moving micellar phase and the moving aqueous phase results in their apparent retention, the magnitude of which is determined by the hydrophobic properties of the analytes. An analyte that is not hydrophobic at all and hence doesn't interact with the micelle migrates with the EOF velocity (t_{eo}) whereas an extremely hydrophobic analyte which is taken up completely by the micelles moves with the

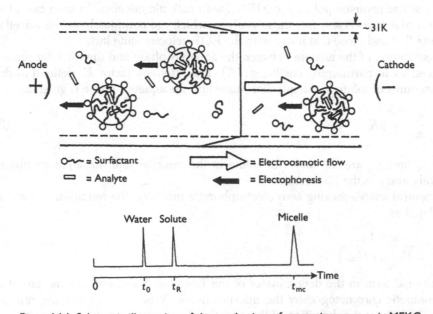

Figure 14.1 Schematic illustration of the mechanism of separation process in MEKC.

velocity of the micellar pseudo phase (t_{mc}). Migration time of all other neutral solutes falls in the migration time (or retention) window between t_{eo} and t_{mc} depending on their distribution coefficients. The existence of an elution window limits the peak capacity of MEKC as the migration time of all analytes to be separated has to lie between the migration times of the unretained and the fully retained analyte.

In view of the above discussion, the effective mobility of the micellar pseudo phase ($\mu_{eff,mc}$) is the vector sum of the electrosmotic mobility of the mobile phase and the electrophoretic mobility of the micelles

$$\mu_{eff,mc} = \mu_{eo} + \mu_{ep,mc} \tag{1}$$

where, μ_{eo} is the electrosmotic mobility that is responsible for the net convective flow and $\mu_{ep,mc}$ the electrophoretic mobility of the micelles.

In unmodified fused silica capillaries, which have a negatively charged surface, the direction of EOF is cathodic and the mobility of all species that migrate in this direction is taken as positive. Although, the electrophoretic mobility of an anionic micelles is negative their effective mobility is positive if the EOF is greater than the electrophoretic mobility of the micelle ($\mu_{eo} > -\mu_{ep}$). On the other hand, the effective mobility of the anionic micelles will be negative if their electrophoretic mobility is greater than the EOF ($\mu_{eo} < -\mu_{ep}$). This situation is usually observed when the EOF is too weak to carry the anionic micelles towards the cathode. The net mobility of the micelle becomes zero when the electrophoretic mobility of the anionic micelle is equal to the EOF mobility ($\mu_{eo} = -\mu_{ep}$). In this case the micelle is stationary and this typically occurs when SDS micelles are used at pH 5.0.

With cationic micelles the electrosmotic flow is usually reversed due to the adsorption of the micelle on the surface of the capillary and the direction of migration of both the cationic micelle and of the electrosmotic flow are towards the anode. Thus, it is necessary to use reversed polarity in MEKC with cationic micelles. In such cases the migration order is reversed, i.e., those analytes which are completely in the micellar phase elute first and those that move with the EOF velocity elute last.

The distribution of the analyte between the aqueous phase and the micellar phases is measured by its partitioning coefficient (K). The retention factor k', defined as the ratio of amounts of solute in the micellar phase and the aqueous phase is given as

$$k' = \frac{n_{mc}}{n_{aq}} = \varphi K \tag{2}$$

where, n_{mc} and n_{aq} are the moles of solute in the micellar and the aqueous phase, respectively and φ is the phase ratio.

For a neutral analyte having zero electrophoretic mobility, the retention factor can be calculated as

$$k' = \frac{t_R - t_{eo}}{t_{eo}[1 - (t_R/t_{mc})]} \tag{3}$$

The additional term in the denominator of the Equation 3 accounts for the fact that in electrokinetic chromatography the micelles move. When t_{mc} approaches infinity Equation 3 becomes the definition of the retention factor in liquid chromatography.

Migration behavior in MEKC can also be described in terms of electrophoretic mobility. Since, an uncharged analyte with zero electrophoretic mobility of its own usually partitions into the micelles and consequently, a fraction of time migrates with the micelles, its electrophoretic mobility is calculated by

$$\mu_{ep,a} = \frac{k'}{1+k'} \mu_{ep,mc} \tag{4}$$

$k'/1 + k'$ is the fraction of analyte in the micelles. The effective migration mobility of the analyte is represented by

$$\mu_{eff,a} = \mu_{ep,a} + \mu_{eo} \tag{5}$$

Thus, the retention factor k' can be expressed in terms of mobilities as

$$k' = \frac{\mu_{ep,a}}{\mu_{ep,mc} - \mu_{ep,a}} \tag{6}$$

In turn, the electrophoretic mobilities can be expressed in terms of experimentally measured parameters as

$$\mu_{ep,mc} = \frac{L_t L_a}{V} \left[\frac{1}{t_{mc}} - \frac{1}{t_{eo}} \right] \tag{7}$$

and

$$\mu_{ep,s} = \frac{L_t L_a}{V} \left[\frac{1}{t_R} - \frac{1}{t_{eo}} \right] \tag{8}$$

where, L_t and L_s are the respective total and separation lengths of the capillary, V is the applied voltage, t_R is the migration time of the solute and t_{mc} that of the micelle. Virtual migration distances have also been introduced to allow an uniform treatment of the migration parameters in chromatographic and electrophoretic separation domains [94].

Migration behavior of ionogenic analytes is more complicated than that of the neutral ones [117] since in addition to partitioning into the micelles and moving at the velocity of the micelles, they can also migrate according to their own electrophoretic mobilities that depend also on the fraction of the ionized form of the analyte. Therefore, the electrophoretic migration rate will depend on the pH. Figure 14.2 schematically illustrates the situation when both the ionized and the unionized forms of an acidic analyte may interact with anionic micelles. In this case, besides the electrosmotic flow mobility (μ_{eo}) and the electrophoretic mobility of the micelle ($\mu_{ep,mc}$), the electrophoretic mobility of the ionized analyte (μ_{A-}), the respective binding constants of the unionized and the ionized forms of the analyte with the micelle, $K_{mw,HA}$ and $K_{mw,A-}$ and the acid dissociation constant, K_a, of the analyte, are required to quantitatively describe the migration behavior of the charged analyte [54]. In MEKC with anionic micelles the migration behavior of cationic analytes is even more complex due to ion-pairing between the protonated form of the analyte and the micelle [105]. As a result the number of parameters that affects the migration behavior of the analytes and thus the selectivity of the separation are rather extensive. Nonetheless, these additional parameters if optimized effectively and efficiently, can provide additional means to manipulate selectivity and hence enhance the separation [54].

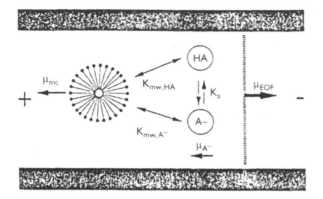

Figure 14.2 Schematic illustration of separation of an acidic analyte by MEKC with anionic micelles. The symbols are: μ_{EOF}, electrosmotic mobility; HA, acidic analyte; A^-, ionized form of the acidic analyte; K_a, acid dissociation constant; $K_{mw,HA}$, binding constant of the unionized analyte with the micelle; $K^-_{wa,A}$, binding constant of the ionized analyte with the micelle; μ_{mc}, electrophoretic mobility of the micelle; μ^-_A, electrophoretic mobility of the ionized analyte.

Resolution and efficiency

The resolution of neutral compounds in MEKC can be expressed as [25]

$$R = \left(\frac{N^{1/2}}{4}\right)\left(\frac{\alpha - 1}{\alpha}\right)\left(\frac{k'_2}{1 + k'_2}\right)\left[\frac{1 - (t_o/t_{mc})}{1 + (t_o/t_{mc})k'_1}\right] \tag{9}$$

where, R is the resolution between peaks 1 and 2, N is the plate efficiency, and α is the selectivity of the chromatographic system for the peak pair.

Just like in anyother chromatographic technique, the resolution in MEKC also depends on three parameters, i.e., efficiency, selectivity and retention. The last term in the resolution equation is unique to MEKC and reflects the limitations by the elution window. Again if the micelles were truly stationary ($t_{mc} \rightarrow \infty$), Equation 9 would be identical to that in HPLC. The size of elution window has significant impact on MEKC separations. In general better resolution is achieved with wider elution window (i.e., $t_{eo}/t_{mc} \rightarrow 0$). Another difference in MEKC and HPLC is the effect of the retention factor, k', on the resolution. In conventional LC the resolution rapidly increases with retention and eventually reaches a plateau. In MEKC, there is an optimum range of retention ($1 < k' < 5$). Outside this k' range, i.e., with poorly or strongly retained analytes, the resolution decreases rapidly due to the limitations by the elution window. As a result, strongly retained compounds are pushed to the end of the chromatogram and elute close to or at the t_{mc}. In MEKC, therefore the proper adjustment of parameters like the nature and concentration of the surfactant, as well as the pH and organic strength of the medium is of prime importance in optimizing the separation.

The influence of the plate efficiency on the resolution in MEKC is similar to that in chromatography and electrophoresis since resolution in all three cases is proportional to the square root of theoretical plates. The disadvantage of the limited elution window in MEKC can therefore be compensated by the large number of theoretical plates that are routinely achieved by this technique.

Yet, the use of micelles in the electrophoretic medium is the source of additional band broadening akin to MEKC. Besides band broadening due to longitudinal diffusion, mass transfer resistances and improper sample introduction, which are shared with other chromatographic techniques, there are additional sources of band broadening that are unique to MEKC. Generally, micelles are characterized by an aggregation number that is indicative of the average number of surfactant monomers contained by a micelle and it depends on both the nature of the surfactant and the chemical environment of the micelle. For example, SDS has an aggregation number of 62. However, this number does not reflect the size distribution of the micelles that can be quite polydisperse. In addition a given micellar system also manifests a charge and shape distribution of micelles. The polydispersity gives rise to a distribution of the electrophoretic mobility of the micelles that engenders additional band spreading [117]. Furthermore, temperature gradients generated due to Joule heating may also give rise to band broadening in MEKC.

Pseudo-stationary phases

Since the introduction of MEKC a host of pseudo-stationary phases has been employed. They fall into two categories; the first and most widely used pseudo-stationary phases are ionic micelles and the other type consists of covalently bound or polymerized charged molecular assemblies [53]. Despite the wide variety of surfactants available, only a limited number has been used for MEKC due to stringent requirements on their physicochemical properties and purity. Table 14.1 lists some of the widely used surfactants. A more exhaustive list of different micellar systems used in MEKC is provided by Terabe *et al.* [75] in a recent thematic issue of Journal of Chromatography dedicated to micelles as separation media in chromatography and electrophoresis. Micelles are spherical aggregates of the individual surfactant molecules present at concentrations above the critical micellar concentration (CMC) that are in dynamic equilibrium with the surfactant monomers. Their size, charge and shape are determined by the aggregation number (n). Kraft point is specific to each micelle and is described as the temperature above which the solubility of the surfactant molecules increases sharply and its concentration in solution exceeds the critical micellar concentration. In other words, micelles are formed only when the temperature is higher than the Kraft point. Variations in the hydrophobic moiety, the ionic head group and the type of counter ion alter the retention, the selectivity, and the size of the elution window and thus the overall separation efficiency in MEKC [53].

Ionic surfactants

Ionic surfactants have both ionic and hydrophobic groups and form spherical micelles having a hydrophobic core with the ionic groups at the surface. The analyte may be solubilized by the micelles in three modes: adsorption at the polar surface (polar analytes), incorporation into the hydrophobic core (nonpolar analytes) and incorporation into the micelle as a cosurfactant (analytes having both polar and nonpolar groups).

Table 14.1 Critical micellar concentration (CMC), aggregation number (*n*), and Kraft point (Kp) of some ionic surfactants

Surfactants	CMC [mM]	n	K_P
Anionic surfactants			
Sodium octyl sulfate	130–155	20	–
Sodium decyl sulfate	31–41	50	8
Sodium dodecyl sulfate (SDS)	8.1	62	16
Sodium tetradecyl sulfate (STS)	2.1 (50°C)	138 (0.1 M NaCl)	30
Sodium dodecanesulfonate	9.8	54	38
Sodium N-lauroyl-N-methyltaurate (LMT)	8.7		<0
Cationic surfactants			
Dodecyltrimethylammonium chloride (DTAC)	16 (30°C)		
Dodecyltrimethylammonium bromide (DTAB)	15	56	
Tetradecyltrimethylammonium bromide (TTAB)	3.5	75	
Cetyltrimethylammonium bromide (CTAB)	0.92	61	
Non-ionic surfactants			
N-octyl-β-D-glucoside	25	–	–
Polyoxyethylene sorbitan monolaurate (Tween 20)	0.059	–	–
Chiral surfactants			
Sodium N-dodecanoyl-L-valinate (SDVal)	5.7 (40°C)	–	–
Sodium cholate (SC)	13–15	2–4	
Sodium deoxycholate (SDC)	4–6	4–10	
Sodium taurocholate (STC)	10–15	5	
Sodium taurodeoxycholate (STDC)	2–6		

Reproduced with permission from Ref. [33].

The effect of surfactant on the selectivity depends on (i) the length of the hydrophobic alkyl chain (ii) the electric charge and the chemical nature of hydrophilic group and (iii) in enantiomeric separations, the chirality of the surfactant. Surfactants that have an alkyl chain length shorter than 10 generally have a high CMC and conductivity. They are therefore used mainly as additives to micelles to change selectivity. Surfactants that have long alkyl chains, carbon number >14, have such high Kraft points that they are seldom used in MEKC. Because the selectivity is only weakly dependent on the alkyl chain length surfactants with dodecyl group are widely employed. Surfactants with longer alkyl chains are used mainly when greater partition coefficient is required.

SDS is the most commonly used surfactant in MEKC. The popularity of SDS can be attributed to its high aqueous solubility, low CMC, low Kraft point, high transparency, its availability and modest price. SDS is stronger hydrogen bonding than most other surfactant systems such as bile salts, cationic (cetyltrimethylammonium bromide, CTAB) surfactants and methacrylate based polymeric surfactants. Since, the great majority of small solutes that are separated by MEKC contain hydrogen bonding functions, such as nitro, hydroxyl, cyano groups, the popularity of SDS is understandable. Figure 14.3 shows the separation of a mixture of 24 nitroaromatic compounds [76]. The efficiency, elution pattern, retention and the size of elution window in MEKC can also be affected by using a counter-ion other than sodium for the surfactant [1].

Most cationic surfactants have an alkyltrimethylammonium group and halides as their counter-ions. Cetyltrimethylammonium bromide (CTAB) is the most widely used

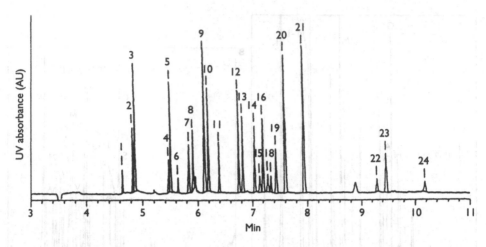

Figure 14.3 Chromatogram of 24 nitroaromatic compounds obtained by MEKC. 50 mM SDS micelles in borate buffer, applied voltage 25 kV, detection at 230 nm, total length 60 cm. (Reproduced with permission from [76].)

cationic surfactant. The cationic surfactants are adsorbed electrostatically on the inner-wall of a fused silica capillary so that it becomes positively charged thereby causing the direction of electrosmotic flow to be revered. Cationic surfactants exhibit selectivity different from the anionic surfactant and this is illustrated in Fig. 14.4 by the chromatograms of PTH-amino acid obtained in MEKC with SDS and DTAB [87].

Non-ionic surfactants

By themselves non-ionic surfactants as such are not useful as pseudostationary phases in MEKC because they have no electrophoretic mobility. However, they can be employed for the separation of charged amphophilic analytes such as peptides having closely related structures [70,71]. The combination of non-ionic surfactant with ionic co-surfactants can also be employed as pseudo-stationary phases in MEKC [67,93]. Most nonionic surfactants have a polyoxyethylene group as the polar function and it has been found that mixed micelles of the ionic and nonionic surfactants show remarkably different selectivity. As a rule of thumb, upon increasing the fraction of the nonionic surfactant in the mixed micelles, the surface charge of the micelles is reduced with concomitant lowering of the electrophoretic mobility of the micelles thereby narrowing the migration time window. Some natural chiral surfactants are uncharged and, therefore, they are used as mixed micelle with SDS [47,83,86].

Chiral surfactants

Bile salts are natural surfactants from biological sources. Both their non-conjugated and taurine conjugated forms are used in MEKC. Since carboxylic groups are the ionogenic functions in the non-conjugated form, they are employed with buffer systems having a pH higher than 5. Taurine conjugated forms have sulfonic acid groups and can therefore

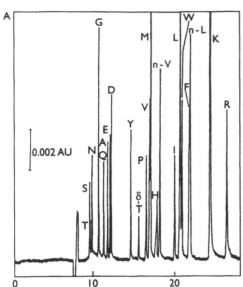
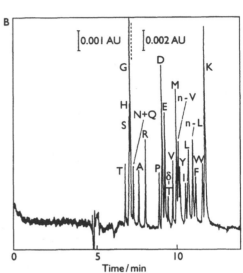

Figure 14.4 Comparison of chromatograms of PTH-amino acids obtained with different surfactants. Column, raw fused silica capillary, 50 μm × 50/65 cm; buffer, (A) 50 mM SDS in 100 mM borate-50 mM phosphate buffer, pH 7.0, (B) 50 mM DTAB in 100 mM Tris-HCl buffer, pH 7.0; applied voltage, (A) 10 kV, (B) 15 kV; detection, 260 nm. (Reproduced with permission from [87].)

be used even at pH as low as 3.0. Bile salts have relatively weak solubilizing power; hence they can be successfully employed to separate hydrophobic analytes that tend to be strongly taken up by micelles of long chain surfactants [20,79]. Synthetic chiral surfactants such as sodium N-dodecanoyl-L-valinate (SDVal) [30,31,84–86], sodium dodecanoyl-L-alaninate (SDAla) [30] and sodium N-dodecanoyl-L-glutamate (SDGlu) [83] have been employed for the separation of enantiomers by MEKC. Naturally occurring surfactants such as digitonin [85], and glycyrrhizic [47] have also been successfully used for the separation of optical isomers. Some ionic chiral surfactants show better chiral recognition when they are employed as mixed micelle with an achiral surfactant such as SDS [31,83,84]. Recently some new types of glucose [48] and tartaric acid [23,24] derived chiral surfactants have been described.

Macromolecular surfactants

Macromolecular surfactants, i.e. high molecular mass surfactants, have several advantages over conventional surfactants of low molecular mass, as their CMC is essentially zero, and hence the micellar concentration can be maintained precisely irrespective of slight changes in the temperature, buffer composition and additives. Furthermore, the size of the micelles is invariant over a wide range of organic modifier concentrations that is particularly important in MEKC.

Palmer *et al.* [90,91] synthesized undecylated oligomer by polymerizing 10-undecylenate forming the micelles in aqueous solution. The oligomer was successfully employed in a medium containing high concentration of acetonitrile for the separation of hydrophobic compounds. Terabe *et al.* [112] prepared copolymers of methacrylic acid, butyl acrylate and butyl methacrylate that with β-cyclodextrin as the mobile phase modifier provided better resolution than SDS for dansyl DL-aminoacids.

The very low or zero CMC is also of advantage in MEKC with the so called partial filling technique where a part of capillary is filled with SDS micellar solution. At the boundary between the micellar zone and the aqueous zone, the SDS micelles tend to break down into monomeric surfactant molecules resulting in excessive band broadening. By contrast, this does not occur with macromolecular surfactants because they retain their surfactant configuration even at low concentrations [77,78].

Another advantage of macromolecular surfactants is manifest in the stacking method of on-column sample concentration in MEKC [75]. The aqueous sample solution which has a very low salt concentration, is injected as a long plug. Upon application of voltage sample stacking occurs at the boundary between the micellar solution and the sample solution where the field strength is higher and therefore the micelles migrate faster. If the surfactant concentration is lower than the CMC in the sample zone, no stacking will occur. However, due to their low CMC and high partitioning coefficient of the sample components, macromolecular micelles can take up the sample components at even low concentrations. As a result, higher stacking efficiency is obtained with macromolecular surfactants than with SDS.

Certain novel types of polymers like dendimers [10,59,74,109,110] and resorcarenes [4] containing ionogenic functions have been also shown to work as pseudo-stationary phases in electrokinetic chromatography. One of the advantages of these polymer pseudo-stationary phases is their stability in buffers containing high concentration of organic solvent. Starbust dendrimers have completely symmetrical and highly branched monodisperse structures. Modification of the end groups of the dendrimers is used for altering the chromatographic selectivity [109]. Alkylated polyallylamines [75] which are easier to prepare than dendrimers showed high selectivity for aromatic compounds in buffers of high organic strength.

Aqueous phase modifiers

In order to modulate the retention factor in MEKC, different modifiers such as organic solvent, urea and cyclodextrins are frequently added to the aqueous buffer of MEKC. The main goal is to reduce the retention factors of the analytes that are strongly bound to the micelles, and thereby widen the elution window.

Organic solvents

Organic modifiers, such as methanol and acetonitrile have been extensively utilized for improving resolution in MEKC [2,6,8,11–14,26,50–52,55,58,82,97,99,103,108,120,126]. The main role of an organic modifier is to reduce the retention factor of highly hydrophobic solutes to, within, or near the optimum range. Addition of organic solvent to the micellar solution usually reduces the EOF velocity, widens the elution time window and enhances the resolution although at the expense of an increase in the time of analysis. Furthermore, it changes the CMC and the size of the micelles. When the organic solvent concentration is higher than 20% the micelles of standard surfactants may break down and this reduces the efficiency of separation. Thus, polymeric pseudo-stationary phases provide an opportunity to investigate the role of organic solvents in MEKC over a wide range of concentrations. Figure 14.5 shows the effect of organic modifier on the separation of ten estrogens [11]. Upon changing the organic modifier from 15% acetonitrile to 20% methanol all the ten estrogens could be completely resolved although the total separation time increased.

Glucose and urea

The use of urea and glucose as modifiers in MEKC has also been reported. Urea reduces the partitioning of hydrophobic compounds into the micellar pseudo-stationary phase by increasing their solubility in aqueous solutions [36,63,113,114]. This effect was utilized in MEKC to separate corticosteroids [114]. Migration times of eight corticosteroids

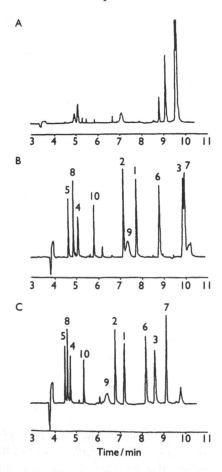

Figure 14.5 Effect of organic modifier on the separation of ten estrogens by MEKC. Column, raw fused silica capillary, 50 μm × 40/47 cm; buffer, 50 mM SDS in phosphate buffer, pH 7.0. (A) without organic solvent, (B) 15% acetonitrile, (C) 20% methanol. Sample (1) 17 β-estradiol, (2) 16-keto-17β-estradiol, (3) 2-methoxyestradiol, (4) 2-hydroxyestradiol, (5) 4-hydroxyestradiol, (6) estrone, (7) 2-methoxyestrone, (8) 4-hydroxyestrone, (9) 16α-hydroxyestrone, (10) estriol. (Reproduced with permission from [11].)

in 50 mM SDS solution were very close so that the separation of all components was not complete. However, upon addition of 6 M urea to the solution, the retention factor of these hydrophobic compounds was decreased and baseline separation of all eight corticosteroids was achieved as illustrated in Fig. 14.6. Chromatograms of PTH amino acids obtained in the presence and absence of urea illustrated in Fig. 14.7. Their comparison shows that addition of urea not only decreased the retention factors but also decreased the selectivity [114].

Kaneta *et al.* [51] have reported the use of glucose in the mobile phase to enhance the resolution of nine nucleosides in MEKC. Upon addition of 1 M glucose to the medium both the selectivity of the system and the electrophoretic mobility of the SDS micelles was enhanced. The latter effect yielded a wider elution window and in this particular case glucose was found to be more effective than methanol in improving the separation.

Cyclodextrins

In order to improve separations in MEKC cyclodextrins of different types have been employed as mobile phase additives [3,9,11,21,39,42,115]. In cyclodextrin modified micellar electrokinetic chromatography (CD-MEKC) [80,115] a non-ionic cyclodextrin, which is not taken up by the micellar phase is employed as an additive to the mobile phase for SDS–MEKC. The effect of a cyclodextrin is that it forms complexes with the hydrophobic analytes so that they are less retained and thus the selectivity of the MEKC

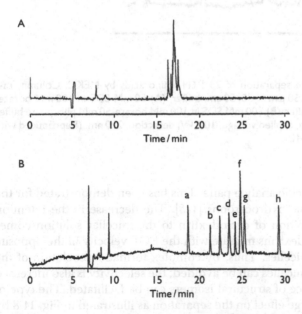

Figure 14.6 MEKC separation of eight corticosteroids. Column, raw fused silica capillary, 50 μm × 50/65 cm; buffer, (A) 50 mM SDS in 20 mM borate-20 mM phosphate, pH 9.0, (B) 50 mM SDS in 20 mM borate-20 mM phosphate buffer, pH 9.0 containing 6 M urea; applied voltage, 20 kV; detection, 220 nm. Sample, (a) hydrocortisone, (b) hydrocortisone acetate, (c) betamethasone, (d) cortisone acetate, (e) triamcinolone acetonide, (f) flucinolone acetonide, (g) dexamethasone acetate, (h) fluocinonide. (Reproduced with permission from [114].)

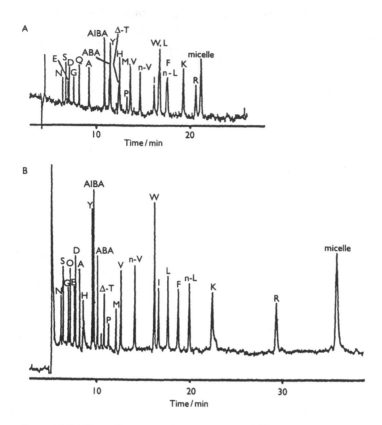

Figure 14.7 Effect of urea on the separation of 23 PTH-amino acids by MEKC. Column, raw fused silica capillary, 50 μm × 30/50 cm; buffer, (A) 50 mM SDS in 100 mM borate-50 mM phosphate buffer, (B) 100 mM SDS in 100 mM borate-50 mM phosphate buffer containing 4.3 M urea; applied voltage, 10.5 kV; detection, 220 nm. (Reproduced with permission from [114].)

system can be enhanced for specific analyte pairs. This has been demonstrated for the separation of polycyclic aromatic hydrocarbons [115]. The decrease in the retention factor of the analytes upon addition of cyclodextrin to the micellar solution comes about because uncharged cyclodextrins migrate with the EOF velocity in the opposite direction to the anionic SDS micelles. Thus, by complex formation coelution of the hydrophobic analytes with the micelles can be avoided; the selectivity is also increased so that the separation for instance of structural isomers can be facilitated. The type of cyclodextrin employed has a large effect on the separation as illustrated in Fig. 14.8 by the chromatograms of ten estrogens that were obtained by using β and γ cyclodextrins as additive [11]. It can be seen that γ-cyclodextrin than β cyclodextrin which has a larger cavity provides a better selectivity for these relatively large hydrophobic molecules.

Micelles of charged cyclodextrins have been used for the separation of neutral compounds. This approach was employed by Terabe *et al.* [116] to separate isomeric aromatic compounds by micellar carboxymethyl-β-cyclodextrin (β-CMCD).

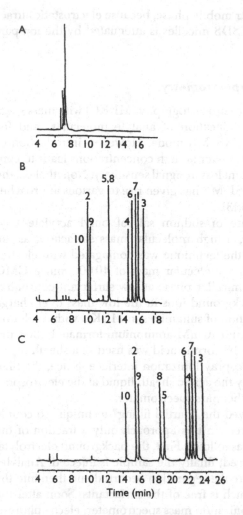

Figure 14.8 Effect of cyclodextrin on the separation of ten estrogens by MEKC. Buffer, 50 mM SDS in 10 mM sodium borate, pH 9.2. (A) no CD, (B) 20 mM β-CD, (C) 20 mM γ-CD. Other conditions and sample same as Fig. 14.5. (Reproduced with permission from [11].)

Ion-pairing reagents

The magnitude of retention and selectivity of ionized analytes in MEKC can also be modulated by ion-pairing with a suitable additive. As the magnitude of the partition coefficient of a charged analyte into the charged micelles is governed by electrostatic interactions, the addition of an ion-pairing agent alters this interaction and hence selectivity. For instance, negatively charged SDS micelles repel anionic analytes such as those containing carboxylate functions. When a tetra-alkylammonium salt is added to the micellar solution, it forms ion pairs with the negatively charged analytes and partly with SDS micelles and thus attenuates electrostatic repulsion between them. In turn, the partitioning coefficient and consequently the migration time of the analytes increases. In contradistinction, the migration time of cationic analytes decreases upon addition of tetra-alkylammonium salts to the micellar mobile phase, because electrostatic attraction between the cationic analyte and the SDS micelles is attenuated by the ion-pair formation [80].

Online coupling of MEKC with mass spectrometry

Tandem operation of micellar electrokinetic chromatography (MEKC) with mass spectrometry (MS) is attractive for direct identification of analyte molecules, and for the structure confirmation and analysis in MS–MS mode. However, introduction of nonvolatile surfactants into the mass spectrometer at high concentrations leads to contamination of the instrument with concomitant loss in signal sensitivity. Nonetheless, the need for online coupling of MEKC with ESI–MS has given rise to various approaches to overcome this problem [60,77,78,88,106,131].

Ozaki et al. [88] demonstrated the use of sodium salt of butyl acrylate-butyl methacrylate-methacrylic acid copolymer, a high molecular mass surfactant, as the pseudo stationary phase in MEKC when the technique was conjugated with electrospray ionization mass spectrometry. With a molecular mass of 40 000 and a CMC of near zero [89], the copolymer forms a micellar phase at low surfactant concentration that generates only a low level of background ions in the low mass over charge (m/z) region. Figure 14.9 shows the separation of sulfamides in MEKC with a solution containing 2% copolymer, 10% methanol and 10 mM ammonium formate buffer, pH 7.0. A water-methanol solution containing 1% formic acid was used as a sheath liquid to acidify the MEKC eluents in the electrospray ionization interface. Since, the high molecular mass surfactant is precipitated by the acidic sheath liquid at the electrospray interface it cannot enter and contaminate the mass spectrometer.

Nelson et al. [77,78] successfully employed the "partial filling" technique to couple MEKC to an electrospray ionization source. In this approach only a fraction of the capillary is filled with the MEKC solution as follows. First, the background electrolyte, and then the micellar solution are introduced; finally the sample is injected. Analytes first migrate into the micellar solution where the separation occurred and then into the electrophoresis background electrolyte which is free of the surfactants. Soon after the detection of analytes by the electrospray ionization mass spectrometer, electrophoresis was terminated to prevent the surfactant plug from entering the MS.

Yang et al. [131] demonstrated the use of anodically migrating micelles in coupling MEKC with the mass spectrometer. The net migration velocity of the micelles is given by the sum of their electrophoretic velocity and the velocity in the opposite direction of EOF. Thus, the effective micellar velocity can be directly manipulated by the adjustment of EOF rather than the electrophoretic mobility of the micelles. The magnitude of electrosmotic flow with respect to the electrophoretic velocity of the SDS micelles is adjusted by changing the pH of the background electrolyte solution in MEKC. For example, when the pH of the MEKC buffer is adjusted to 5.9, the SDS micelles migrate towards the inlet reservoir and non-volatile surfactants do not enter the ESI–MS. Figure 14.10 illustrates the result with online MEKC–ESI–MS in the analysis of chlorotriazine herbicides.

Lamoree et al. [60] used a two stage capillary system with buffer replenishment to preclude the MEKC surfactant from entering into the ESI–MS instrument. After the actual MEKC separation in the first capillary is completed the analyte zone is transferred

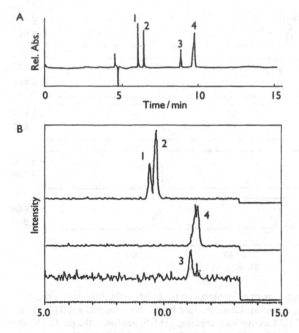

Figure 14.9 MEKC of a mixture of sulfamides monitored with (A) UV detection at 210 nm (B) ESI-MS. (A) Column, raw fused silica capillary, 50 μm × 40/48 cm; buffer, 1% sodium salt of butyl acrylate–butyl methacrylate–methacrylic acid copolymer in 10% methanol and 100 mM borate-50 mM phosphate buffer, pH 7.0; applied voltage, 20 kV; detection, 210 nm; (B) Column, raw fused silica capillary, 50 μm × 50 cm; buffer, 2% BBMA in 10% methanol and 100 mM ammonium formate, pH 7.0; applied voltage, 13 kV; sheath, water–methanol–formic acid (50:50:1, v/v/v), flow rate, 5 μl/min. Sample, (1) sulfamethazine, (2) sulfisomidine, (3) sulfadiazie, (4) sulfisoxazole. (Reproduced with permission from [88].)

into the second capillary where the analyte is separated from the SDS micelles by CZE before being introduced into the ESI–MS system. However, this approach is rather complicated, associated with considerable band spreading and allows only for a narrow separation window.

In a somewhat different approach Takeda *et al.* [106,107] constructed a microchemical ionization source for MEKC/ES/MS. In this interface, the solution was first electrosprayed and the droplets were then vaporized. Chemical ionization is known to be tolerant of non-volatile buffers and surfactants. With this design the authors were able to employ buffers containing phosphates and SDS for the separation with MS detection of a mixture of anilines.

Capillary electrochromatography

Introduction

Capillary electrochromatography (CEC) is a branch of liquid chromatography that employs capillary columns packed with stationary phase and electric field to propel the

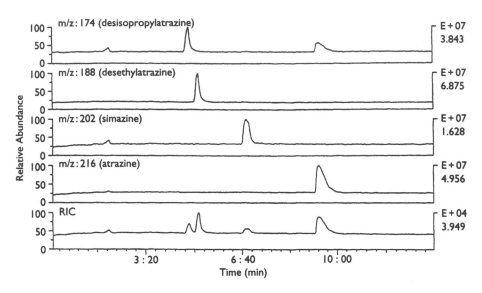

Figure 14.10 Selected ion electrophorograms of chlorotriazine herbicides obtained by MEKC–ESI–MS using anodically migrating micelles. Column, raw fused silica capillary, 50 μm × 25 cm; buffer, 10 mM SDS and 10 mM ammonium acetate, pH 5.9; applied voltage, 12 kV; sheath, water-methanol-acetic acid (50 : 49 : 1, v/v/v), flow rate, 5 μl/min. (Reproduced with permission from [131].)

liquid mobile phase through the column. In CEC the eluent flow is generated by elec-trosmosis upon application of high voltage and the separation of sample components takes place due to differences in their distribution between the mobile and stationary phases and, if charged, due to differences in their electrophoretic mobilities as well. Since, CEC has many features that are common to micro-HPLC and CZE it is relevent to compare it to these two analytical separation techniques. CEC is applicable to the analysis of both neutral and charged sample components and promises to offer much higher plate efficiencies than HPLC with packed capillary columns (micro-HPLC). Fur-thermore, it is expected to offer higher loading capacity and wider range of selectivity than CZE. A major advantage of CEC rests with the possibility of readily attaining rela-tively high flow rate in capillary columns packed with small particle that would require ultra high column inlet pressures in micro-HPLC due to their low permeabilities.

The practice of electrochromatography can be traced back to Mould and Synge [72,73] who used electrosmotic flow in the separation of polysaccharides with collodion membrane. In 1974 Pretorius *et al.* [92] suggested the use of EOF in both thin layer and in column liquid chromatography with narrow bore packed columns. In 1981 Jorgenson and Lukacs [49] demonstrated the feasibility of CEC with packed capillaries. Tsuda *et al.* [121,122] employed pressure driven flow and EOF together in liquid chromatography with packed capillary columns. Knox and Grant [56] showed that sufficient EOF can be generated with particles as small as 1.5 μm in diameter and separated aromatic hydrocarbons by CEC with plate efficiencies higher than those obtained in HPLC. More recently reports on experimental results in capillary electrochromatography were published from several laboratories [5,7,17,18,27–29,33,101,102,128–130].

Instrumentation

Most commercially available capillary electrophoresis units, with slight alteration to facilitate pressurization of both the inlet and outlet end of the packed capillary column, can be used for capillary electrochromatography. So far most applications of CEC were carried out by isocratic elution at applied voltages up to 30 kV. Nevertheless, the feasibility of a modular instrument designed with a dual 90 kV power supply was demonstrated [18]. The unit that is illustrated schematically in Fig. 14.11, can be operated at voltages up to 60 kV, which is twice as high as that available with commercially available units. EOF velocities as high as 6–7 mm/s could be realized at an applied voltage of 60 kV with a 50 μm × 23/32 cm fused silica capillary column packed with 6 μm Zorbax ODS particles as is shown in Fig. 14.12. The most striking observation is that the EOF velocity is not a linear function of voltage when the field strength exceeded 100 kV/m. The higher than expected EOF was not caused by decrease in viscosity due to Joule heating as seen from the linearity of the corresponding plots of the current versus applied voltage in Fig. 14.12. This effect may be advantageous for increasing the speed of separation even if in analytical applications a linear system generally offers greater reproducibility.

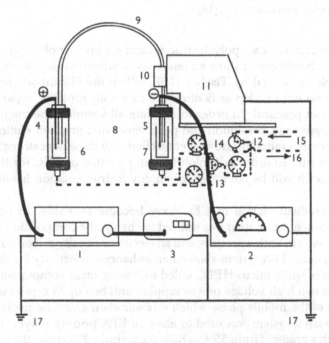

Figure 14.11 Schematic of the modular capillary electrochromatograph with a 90 kV dual power supply and pressurizable chambers for the column inlet and outlet. (1) 60 kV power supply, (2) 30 kV power supply, (3) digital electrometer (4,5) electrodes, (6,7) reservoir for mobile phase or the sample, (8), pressurizable chambers, (9) packed capillary column, (10) cell for on-column detection , (11) detector, (12) 4 port 2 way valve, (13) 4 port 3-way valves, (14) pressure gauges, (15) from nitrogen cylinder, (16) vent, (17) ground. (Reproduced with permission from [18].)

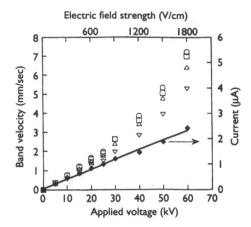

Figure 14.12 Plots of the migration velocities of acrylamide and small aromatic substances against the applied voltage up to 60 kV. Column, raw fused silica capillary, 50 μm × 23/32 cm packed with 6 μm Zorbax ODS having a mean pore diameter of 300 Å; eluent, 20% (v/v) 10 mM borate, pH 8.0 and 80% (v/v) ACN. Sample, (o) acrylamide, (□) benzylalcohol, (Δ) benzaldehyde, (∇) o-dichlorobenzene, injection for 2 s at 2 kV. (Reproduced with permission from [18].)

Most biological molecules of interest are polyelectrolytes and at a given mobile phase composition will either adsorb strongly or show no tendency to adsorb at all following the "all or nothing principle" espoused by Tiselius [119]. When the elution window of the sample components do not overlap as is often the case with proteins, separation by isocratic elution is not practical. In order to separate all sample components without compromising analysis time, resolution and peak sensitivity, gradient elution is employed in order to increase gradually and in a controlled way the eluent strength during the chromatographic run. In order to exploit the full potential of CEC for the analysis of complex mixtures it will be advisable to employ instrumentation having gradient elution capabilities.

Several approaches for gradient elution in CEC have become available. In one approach a conventional gradient LC system was utilized to change the composition of the mobile phase [5]. In this system both a pressure and an electrosmotically driven flow is generated through the system. This system showed an enhanced selectivity for the separation of oligonucleotides while micro-HPLC failed to resolve these components. Another approach employs two high voltage power supplies and two open capillaries to control the composition of the mobile phase which mix and then enter the packed separation column [129]. Such a system was used to elute 16 EPA priority polycyclic aromatic hydrocarbons with a gradient from 55% to 85% acetonitrile. Recently, the use of step gradient using a commercially available system has also been reported for CEC [32]. The separation of six diuretics of widely differing lipophilicity was carried out by elution with step gradient in a vastly reduced analysis time compared to that required by the use of isocratic elution.

In another scheme an LC gradient former consisting of two reciprocating displacement pumps was employed to control the composition of the eluent in the reservoir at the column inlet. The eluent of changing composition was then pulled into the column electrosmotically upon the application of electric field [44]. This system was used for the separation of 12 PTH-amino acids by RP-CEC in less than 15 min as shown in the chromatogram, Fig. 14.13. A similar system was employed by Taylor *et al.* (111) for the analysis of corticosteroids. Gradient elution was shown to facilitate trace enrichment at the head of the column in the analysis of biofluids by CEC [111].

Stationary phase

It has been customary to classify the various techniques of liquid chromatography according to the stationary phase employed. In HPLC, reversed phase chromatography with alkyl-silica bonded phases is used commonly. The stationary phase should have a large, readily accessible chromatographic surface with favorable retention thermodynamics and kinetics. In CEC, however, the stationary phase plays a dual role. First, it has to offer an appropriate surface to bring about the retention of the sample components

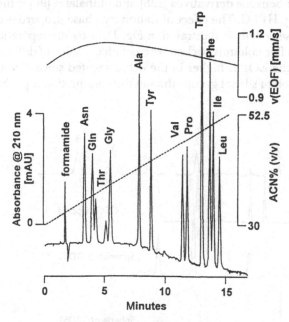

Figure 14.13 Chromatograms of PTH amino acids obtained by capillary electrochromatography with gradient elution. Column, 50 μm × 20.7/12.7 cm packed with 3.5 μm Zorbax ODS particles having a mean pore size of 80 Å. Starting eluent (A) 70% (v/v) 5 mM phosphate, pH 7.55, 30% (v/v) acetonitrile; gradient former (B) 40% (v/v) 5 mM phosphate, pH 7.55, 60% (v/v) acetonitrile; flow rate of mobile phase through inlet reservoir, 0.1 ml/min; gradient, 0–100% B in 20 min; voltage 10 kV; temperature, 25°C; UV detection at 210 nm; electrokinetic injection, 0.5 s, 1 kV; Peaks in order of elution: formamide, PTH-asparagine, PTH-glutamine, PTH-threonine, PTH-glycine, PTH-alanine, PTH-tyrosine, PTH-valine, PTH-proline, PTH-tryptophan, PTH-phenylalanine, PTH-isoleucine and PTH-leucine. The concentration of the PTH-amino acids dissolved in the mobile phase was 30–60 μg/ml. (Reproduced with permission from [44].)

with selectivity required for their separation and should have a structure that facilitates rapid mass transfer in order to minimize band spreading and thus make it possible to obtain high plate efficiency. Second, the stationary phase also has to have appropriate fixed charges at the surface to generate EOF in high electric field. Consequently, the retention factor of both charged and uncharged components may be different when a given column is operated in micro-HPLC and CEC mode under otherwise identical conditions [22].

Capillary electrochromatography is expected to have high separation efficiency and resolving power for environmental and pharmaceutical applications. So far CEC has been used for the analysis of neutral species having widely different molecular structures by reversed phase capillary electrochromatography. The employment of RP-CEC with alkyl silica stationary phases and neutral or alkaline hydroorganic mobile phases is possible because the silanol groups are dissociated under these conditions and the strongly negatively charged surface generates a high EOF while the alkyl chains provide the hydrophobic surface for retention by solvophobic interactions [43].

It has been shown that in CEC separation efficiency for polyaromatic hydrocarbons [18,28,95,96,129] polychlorinated benzene derivatives [128] and phthalates [96] is high in comparison to that provided by HPLC. The effect of stationary phase properties on the EOF velocity, retention and selectivity is illustrated in Fig. 14.14 by the separation of polyaromatic hydrocarbons on five columns packed with octadecyl-silica of different provenances [27]. It is seen that the EOF is higher in the octadecylated silica column having a high surface concentration of silanol groups than in the column that is packed

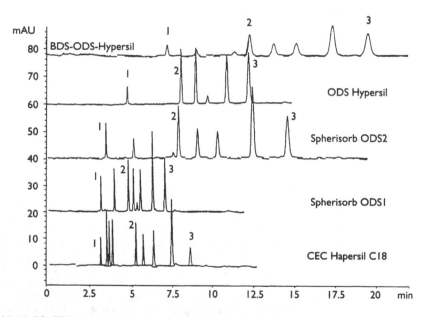

Figure 14.14 RP-CEC of PAHs by using columns packed with 3 μm octadecylated silicas of different provenances. Columns, 100 μm × 25/33.5 cm; eluent, 20% (v/v) 50 mM Tris–HCl, pH 8.0, 80% (v/v) ACN. The samples were not identical but all contained (1) thiourea, (2) napthalene, (3) fluoranthene. (Reproduced with permission from [27].)

with octadecylated silica having a low surface concentration of silanol groups (BDS-ODS-Hypersil).

In the area of pharmaceuticals, neutral compounds such as steroids [33,34,37,61,101, 102], diuretics [33,64,101], cephalosporin antibiotics [62,102], macrocyclic lactones [61], C- and N-protected peptides [33,100] nucleosides and purine bases [33], phthalates [96] and parabens [28] have been successfully separated by RP-CEC under conditions very similar to those employed in RP-HPLC except that for the driving force for the mobile phase. The analysis of diasterioisomers can particularly benefit from the high plate efficiency typical for CEC [33,34,102]. Analysis of triglycerides [98] was performed by RP-CEC with a mobile phase comprising of acetonitrile/isopropanol/n-hexane in the ratio of 57/38/5 and containing 50 mM ammonium acetate. Even with a primarily organic mobile phase CEC offered very good resolution for the analysis of triglycerides.

On the other hand, Smith and Evans (101) reported separation of strongly basic tricyclic antidepressants on a strong cation exchange column with apparent efficiencies of up to 8×10^6 plates per meter. Such staggering apparent plate efficiencies were also reported for certain charged analytes by other workers too. They can't be explained by classical chromatographic theory and they are most likely due to focussing effects (electrochromatofocussing) that comes into play with certain buffer and stationary phase combinations in the presence of an applied electric field [104].

The analysis of anionic analytes is hampered by their electrophoretic migration towards the anode that is counter directional to the usual cathodic EOF. Consequently, they may not be loaded onto the column or they do not reach the detector. It has been shown however, that acidic analytes can be separated at pH 2.5 [33] on a octadecylated silica by CEC at an applied voltage of 30 kV. At pH 2.5 the EOF velocity was 0.75 mm/s which is much lower than 1.5 mm/s at pH 7.8. Yet, even at such low EOF velocity efficient separations of acidic and neutral diuretics and anti-inflammatory arylpropionic acids are still possible [33].

Immobilized acid glycoprotein on a 5 μm silica support has been used to separate neutral and cationic enantiomers by CEC [66]. The separation efficiencies were higher than those obtained in HPLC but were nowhere close to those seen in RP-CEC of neutral sample components. The use of proteins in immobilized form in CEC instead of free solution as in CZE has the advantage that there is no loss of transparency due to the protein in the background electrolyte. A number of neutral and chiral benzodiazepines were resolved using human serum albumin immobilized a 7 μm silica support. The EOF was lower than in the acid glycoprotein column and the efficiencies were low [68]. Thus, so far CEC with proteinaceous stationary phases has not shown outstanding separation efficiencies. The enantiomeric separation of small drug molecules such as chlorthlidone and mainserin with hydroxyl-β-cyclodextrin (HPβCD) as the mobile phase additive or as a chiral stationary phase was examined in CEC [64]. The results were compared to those obtained in CE and HPLC. With HPβCD in the mobile phase baseline separation of the chlorthalidone enantiomers could be obtained but the time of analysis was rather long. By using a chiral stationary phase with HPβCD the analysis time could be reduced but not without compromising the separation efficiency. On the other hand chiral CE failed to resolve the enantiomers whereas chiral HPLC resulted in good separation. A major disadvantage of CEC with the chiral stationary phase was the required tedious column conditioning step.

In reversed phase CEC with siliceous bonded phases the EOF decreases as acidity of the mobile phase is increased since the dissociation of the silanol groups is suppressed. Therefore, for CEC with acidic eluents and cathodic EOF requires that stationary phase surface has to be covered with strong acidic functions that are negatively charged also at low pH. So far siliceous or polymeric supports with sulfonic acid groups have been employed for this purpose. The pore structure of the support is also important because EOF generated in wide pores by high electric field strength enhances intraparticulate mass transfer and hence column efficiency. Figure 14.15 shows an electrochromatogram of dipeptides that were rapidly separated by CEC with a column packed with gigaporous styrenic strong ion-exchanger with sulfonic acid groups at acidic pH. The column exhibited high efficiency as the reduced plate height values were around unity [18].

Another approach toward the separation of charged sample components is to functionalize the alkyl and sulfonic acid groups at the same chromatographic surface so that the sulfonic acid groups generate the EOF and the alkyl groups give rise to retention by hydrophobic interactions. Since the fixed sulfonic acid groups are ionized over the entire pH range the stationary phase can be used at low pH without compromising the magnitude of EOF velocity. Dittmann et al. [27] separated a test mixture of neutral solutes on a Spherisorb C6/SCX cation-exchanger stationary phase with alkyl ligate indicating that the alkyl groups play indeed a role in the separation of neutral molecules. The effect of pH on the separation of polyaromatic hydrocarbons on SCX/ODS Hypersil octadecylated cation-exchanger at three pH values is illustrated in Fig. 14.16. It is seen that both the EOF velocity and the efficiency were about the same at all pH values.

Stationary phases currently employed in CEC for the separation of small molecules have been primarily developed for HPLC. Indeed alkyl-silica stationary phases may serve as a paragon for the design of chromatographic surfaces that promise best results

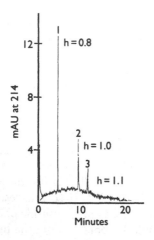

Figure 14.15 CEC of peptides with a strong cation exchanger column. Column, raw fused silica capillary, 180 μm × 28/37 cm, packed with 8 μm, gigaporous (1000 Å) PLSCX strong cation exchanger; eluent, 60% (v/v) 25 mM phosphate, pH 3.5 in ACN; applied voltage 15 kV. Sample, (1) acrylamide, (2) Trp-Gly-Gly-Phe-Met, (3) Trp-Met-Asp-Phe; injected for 2 s at 2 kV. (Reproduced with permission from [18].)

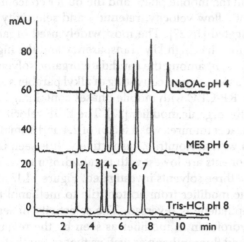

Figure 14.16 Effect of pH on the separation of PAHs by using 4 μm SCX/ODS Hypersil as the stationary phase. Column, raw fused silica capillary, 100 μm × 25/33.5 cm; eluent, 20% (v/v) 50 mM Tris-HCl, pH 8.0, 80% (v/v) ACN;. 20% (v/v) 50 mM MES, pH 6.0, 80% (v/v) ACN; 20% (v/v) 50 mM sodium acetate, pH 4.0, 80% (v/v) ACN; applied voltage 15kV. Samples (1) thiourea, (2) nitrobenzene, (3) napthalene, (4) biphenyl, (5) fluorene, (6) anthracene, (7) fluoranthene. (Reproduced with permission [27].)

in CEC. These are likely to be based on the dual functionality concept represented by a structure with the retentive functions constituting the top layer of the stratified surface and the fixed charges present at the support surface. The chemistry of the functional groups could be similar to that used for stationary phases in various branches of liquid chromatography. It appears to be important that the fixed charges are readily accessible only to small ions, which form the double layer and the mobile counterions upon imposing the electric field generate a sufficiently high EOF. In order to restrict access by the components of the sample to be analyzed to the fixed charges it may be necessary to have an intermediate screening layer between the fixed charges and the retentive functions. For instance, an appropriate uncharged hydrogel layer can be used for this purpose in the separation of proteins.

The history of chromatography teaches that the introduction of any new major technique was accompanied by the development of novel types of columns and stationary phases that are tailored to provide best results in terms of efficiency, speed and resolution. It is likely that the development of CEC will follow suit and we shall witness the introduction of new stationary phases specially designed for CEC.

Mobile phase

The most distinguishable feature of CEC is that it makes use of the phenomenon of electrosmosis to generate and sustain the flow of mobile phase through packed capillary columns. At present the major disadvantage of electrosmotic flow, which is considered parasitic in electrophoresis, is the lack of reliable control over the flow velocity of the eluent. This is in sharp contrast to HPLC where the flow is generated by high precision metering pumps. In CEC the electrosmotic flow depends on the nature of both the stationary and the mobile phases.

The influence of the organic modifier in the mobile phase and the buffer concentration on the magnitude of the electrosmotic flow velocity, retention and selectivity in RP-CEC has been systematically investigated [18,27]. The most widely used organic modifier in CEC has been acetonitrile which has high UV transparency and the highest ratio of dielectric constant to viscosity (ε/η) among the candidate organic solvents. Figure 14.17 shows the chromatograms of a test mixture consisting of alkyl parabens and poly aromatic hydrocarbons obtained by RP-CEC with mobile phases containing acetonitrile, methanol or tetrahydrofuran as the organic modifier [27]. The EOF velocity as measured by the elution time of the inert tracer thiourea was a factor of 2.4 and 3 smaller with methanol and tetrahydrofuran than with acetonitrile, respectively. It is seen that the retention factors of the sample components are lowest with tetrahydrofuran which has the highest eluent strength among the three solvents investigated. Figure 14.17 also illustrates that upon changing the organic modifier from acetonitrile to methanol the retention order of hexylparaben and napthalene is reversed. The selectivity of separation changes dramatically with tetrahydrofuran as modifier as seen by the reversal of elution order of fluorene, anthracene and fluoranthene as well as that of napthalene and heptylparaben. The changes in the selectivity upon changing the organic modifiers, however, are not unique to RP-CEC since they are observed in RP-HPLC also.

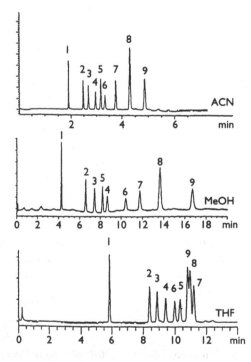

Figure 14.17 Effect of the organic modifier in CEC of neutral aromatics. Column, fused silica capillary, 100 µm × 25/33.5 cm, packed with 3 µm Hypersil C18. Eluent, 20% (v/v) 25 mM Tris-HCl, pH 8.0, 80% (v/v) ACN, applied voltage 15 kV. Samples (1) thiourea, (2) butylparaben, (3) pentylparaben, (4) hexylparaben, (5) naphthalene, (6) hexylparaben, (7) fluorene, (8) anthracene (9) fluoranthene. (Reproduced with permission from [27].)

With increasing organic strength of the electrophoretic media in CZE, the EOF velocity usually decreases, e.g., with increasing acetonitrile concentration, and this is attributed to a concomitant decrease in the zeta potential. In RP-CEC, however, the magnitude of EOF velocity increases with increasing acetonitrile concentration in capillary columns packed with octadecylated silica particles [18,27]. When methanol is used as an organic modifier in RP-CEC the EOF velocity first decreases with increasing methanol concentration in the range from 20% to 60% and increases thereafter [27].

The influence of the buffer concentration on the magnitude of EOF in CEC was investigated by varying the concentrations of Tris-HCl in the eluent [27]. Figure 14.18 shows that the EOF velocity decreases with increasing Tris-HCl concentration in the range from 5–100 mM. This is expected since the thickness of the diffuse double layer decreases with increasing ionic strength and this results in a decrease in EOF velocity [46].

Band Spreading in CEC

The most important expectation regarding CEC is that it yields plate numbers and isocratic peak capacities comparable to those obtained in CZE due to the use of electrosmotic flow of the mobile phase and thus facilitates fast separations which require plate numbers higher than 1 00 000. As the electrosmotic flow is generated at the surface of the stationary phase, band spreading should be significantly smaller in capillary electrochromatography than in conventional HPLC. Figure 14.19 illustrates the dependence of the reduced plate height on the reduced velocity for small neutral molecules in RP-CEC. It is seen that the reduced plate height is minimum (h ~ 1) at a reduced velocity of about 5 and at higher velocities reduced plate height plateaus at about 1.6 [18]. Silica based packing materials having pore sizes ranging from 60–4000 Å were employed to elucidate the role of pore size in CEC [65]. It was shown that in wide pore

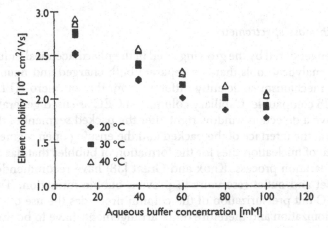

Figure 14.18 Effect of buffer concentration and temperature on EOF in CEC. Column, raw fused silica capillary, 100 μm × 25/33.5 cm packed with 3.0 μm Hypersil C18 particles; eluent, 20% (v/v) Tris–HCl of different concentrations, pH 8.0, 80% (v/v) ACN, applied voltage 20 kV. EOF marker thiourea. Buffer concentration given in the figure. (Reproduced with permission from [27].)

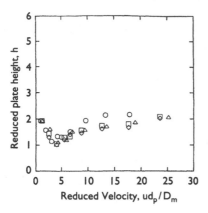

Figure 14.19 van-Deemter plot of data obtained with aromatic substances by RP-CEC at applied voltages up to 60 kV. Column, raw fused silica capillary, 50 μm × 23/32 cm packed with 6 μm Zorbax ODS having a mean pore diameter of 300 Å; eluent, 20% (v/v) 10 mM borate, pH 8.0 in ACN. Sample, (o) acrylamide, (□) benzylalcohol, (△) benzaldehyde, (▽) o-dichlorobenzene, injected for 2 s at 2 kV. (Reproduced with permission from [18].)

silica stationary phases intraparticulate electrosmotic transport increases intraparticulate mass transfer with concomitantly higher plate efficiencies. This is illustrated in Fig. 14.20 which shows plots of plate height against linear velocity for 7 μm Nucleosil C18 particles having different pore diameters. The electrosmotic enhancement of intraparticulate mass transport may lead to the use of stationary phases having relatively large particle size (5–10 μm) with large pore diameters. These are much easier to pack into capillary columns than the very small particles ($d_p < 2$ μm).

Online coupling of CEC with mass spectrometry

Recent interest in CEC is engendered by the growing need in the pharmaceutical industry for high performance analytical tools that can separate both charged and neutral sample components by a mechanism sufficiently different from that of micro-HPLC and CZE and is equally MS compatible. Capillary columns in CEC are used generally with UV detection and have a detection window right after the packed segment of the column. The retaining frit at the interface of the packed and the ensuing open segment is believed to be the source of nucleation sites for the formation of bubbles that has an untoward effect on the separation process. Knox and Grant [38] have recommended the use of pressurized inlet and outlet reservoirs to prevent bubble formation. This solves the problem in CEC but pressurization of the column precludes the use of the interface for electrospray ionization and therefore other arrangements have to be used for performing CEC–MS.

An electrochromatographic system with both pressure and voltage gradients across the packed capillary column was first coupled to a mass spectrometer by van der Greef *et al.* [124] and capillary columns with inner diameter of 220 μm were used to provide a flow rate required by the FAB interface. The same electrochromatographic system was

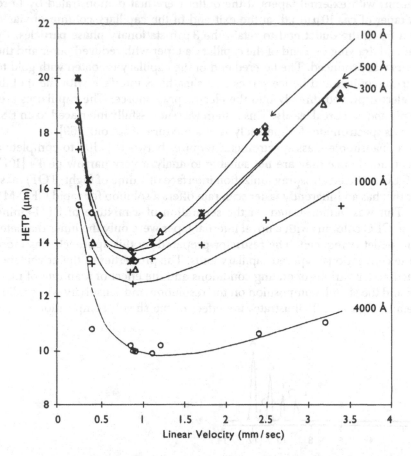

Figure 14.20 Plots of plate height versus linear flow velocity for columns packed with 7 µm
Nucleosil particles having different pore sizes. Column, raw fused silica capillary,
75 µm × 23/30 cm packed with 7 µm C18 Nucleosil particles having pore sizes of
100, 500, 300, 1000, and 4000 Å; 300 Å; eluent, 20% (v/v) 10 mM phosphate, pH 6.9
in ACN. Tracer, acetone. (Reproduced with permission from [65].)

also coupled to an electrospray-MS with a sheath flow interface [45]. A similar CEC
system was used to analyze a peptide mixture by CEC–MS [100].

An electrochromatographic system without applied pressure gradients was first coupled to an electrospray ionization mass spectrometer for the separation of steroid
hormones by Gordon *et al.* [37]. Unfortunately, the separation efficiency of this system was rather poor due to the long open segment of the capillary column. In other
early works the long separation column lengths led to poor separation efficiencies and
long elution times [62]. Since then great improvements have been made to reduce the
length of the capillary column from 90–45 cm [61].

The use of tapers as flow restrictors was first described in open tubular supercritical fluid chromatography to maintain supercritical conditions throughout the
column [15,16,35,40,81]. Later tapered capillaries with metallized tips were also used
in CE/ESI/MS with sheathless configuration [41,57,123,125,127]. In CEC/ESI–MS

capillary columns with external tapers at the outlet were first demonstrated by Lord *et al.* [69]. A taper of ca. 10 μm i.d. at the exit end of the capillary column obviated the need for a frit at the outlet end to retain the 3 μm stationary phase particles. By applying heat and drawing one end of the capillary a taper with reduced outer and the inner diameters was produced. The tapered end of the capillary is coated with gold to provide electrical contact and hence serves as a sheathless interface with the mobile phase being electrosprayed directly into the electrospray source. The capillaries are, however, fragile and can break easily. This system was successfully interfaced to an ESI quadrupole mass spectrometer for the analysis of a mixture of steroids [69].

At present a quadrupole mass spectrometer requires between 1–10 s to complete a single m/z scan and hence they are not suitable to analyze very narrow peaks [101]. Coupling of CEC to the electrospray ionization interface of a time of flight (TOF) mass spectrometer that has an inherently faster scan rate offers a solution for rapid CEC-MS applications. This was demonstrated for the separation of a mixture of PTH-amino acids [19] using CEC columns with a novel internal taper were only the inner diameter of the column outlet is reduced. The restrictor prepared by this approach was more robust than the conventional tapered capillary ends. The properties of the novel taper were examined under various operating conditions and the effect of scan rate of mass spectrometer and the sheath composition on the resolution and sensitivity was studied in greater details. Figure 14.21 illustrates the effect of the sheath composition on the

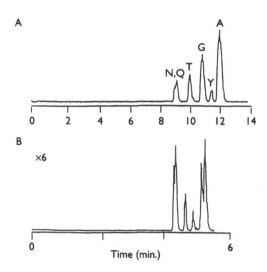

Figure 14.21 Effect of sheath composition on the separation of PTH-amino acids in CEC-MS. Column, raw fused silica capillary, 75 μm × 25 cm packed with 3.5 μm Zorbax ODS particles having a mean pore size of 80 Å; starting eluent (A) 2 mM ammonium acetate, pH 7.0; gradient former (B) 10% (v/v) 2 mM ammonium acetate, pH 7.0; 90% (v/v) acetonitrile; flow rate of mobile phase through inlet reservoir, 100 μL/min; gradient, 30% to 80% B in 5 min, 80% B for 5 min, 80% to 30% B in 1 min; applied voltage, 20 kV; electrokinetic injection, 2 kV, 2 s; integration time, 0.5 s/spectrum. Sheath, (a) methanol; (b) 10% (v/v) 0.2 mM ammonium acetate, pH 7.0, 90% (v/v) methanol; flow rate, 0.18 ml/h. Peaks in order of elution, PTH-asparagine; PTH-glutamine; PTH-threonine; PTH-glycine; PTH-tyrosine; PTH-alanine. (Reproduced with permission from [19].)

separation of six PTH-amino acids. It is seen that upon addition of ammonium acetate to pure methanol sheath decreases both the migration time as well as the signal intensity.

Acknowledgment

This work is supported by Grant No. GM 20993 from the National Institute of Health, US Public Health Service.

References

[1] Ahuja, E. S. and Foley, J. P. (1995) Influence of dodecyl sulfate counterion on efficiency, selectivity, retention, elution range and resolution in micellar electrokinetic chromatography. *Analytical Chemistry*, **67**, 2315–2324.

[2] Aiken, J. H. and Huie, C. W. (1993) Effects of 1-alkanols on separation performance in micellar electrokinetic capillary Chromatography. *Journal of Microcolumn Separations*, **5**, 95–99.

[3] Aumatell, A. and Wells, R. J. (1994) Enatiomeric differentiation of a wide range of pharmacologically active substances by cyclodextrin-modified micellar electrokinetic capillary chromatography using a bile salt. *Journal of Chromatography*, **688**, 329–337.

[4] Bachmann, K., Bazzanella, A., Haag, I., Han, K. Y., Arnecke, R., Bohmer, V. and Vogt, W. (1995) Resorcarenes as pseudostationary phases with selectivity for electrokinetic chromatography. *Analytical Chemistry*, **67**, 1722–1726.

[5] Behnke, B. and Bayer, E. (1994) Pressurized gradient electro-high-performance liquid chromatography. *Journal of Chromatography*, **680**, 93–98.

[6] Bjergegaard, C., Michaelsen, S., Mortensen, K. and Sorensen, H. (1993) Determination of flavonoids by micellar electrokinetic capillary chromatography. *Journal of Chromatography*, **652**, 477–485.

[7] Boughtflower, R. J., Underwood, T. and Paterson, C. J. (1995) Capillary electrochromatography – some important considerations in the preparation of packed capillaries and choice of mobile phase buffers. *Chromatographia*, **40**, 329–335.

[8] Bretnall, A. E. and Clarke, G. S. (1995) Investigation and optimization of the use of micellar electrokinetic chromatography for the analysis of six cardiovascular drugs. *Journal of Chromatography*, **700**, 173–178.

[9] Brumley, W. C. and Jones, W. J. (1994) Comparison of micellar electrokinetic chromatography (MEKC) with capillary gas chromatography in the separation of phenols, anilines and polynuclear aromatics: potential field-screening applications of MEKC. *Journal of Chromatography*, **680**, 163–173.

[10] Castagnola, M., Cassiano, L., Lupi, A., Messna, I., Patamia, M., Rabino, R., Rossetti, D. V. and Giardina, B. (1995) Ion-exchange electrokinetic capillary chromatography with Starburst (pamam) dendrimers: a route towards high-performance electrokinetic capillary chromatography. *Journal of Chromatography*, **694**, 463–469.

[11] Chan, K. C., Muschik, G. M., Issaq, H. J. and Siiteri, P. K. (1995) Separation of estrogens by micellar electrokinetic chromatography. *Journal of Chromatography*, **690**, 149–154.

[12] Chen, C. T. and Sheu, S. J. (1995) Separation of coumarins by micellar electrokinetic capillary chromatography. *Journal of Chromatography*, **710**, 323–329.

[13] Chen, N. and Terabe, S. (1995) A quantitative study on the effect of organic modifiers in micellar electrokinetic chromatography. *Electrophoresis*, **16**, 2100–2103.

[14] Chen, N., Terabe, S. and Nakagawa, T. (1995) Effect of organic modifier concentrations on electrokinetic migrations in micellar electrokinetic chromatography. *Electrophoresis*, **16**, 1457–1462.

[15] Chester, T. L. (1984) Capillary supercritical-fluid chromatography with flame-ionization detection: reduction of detection artifacts and extension of detectable molecular weight range. *Journal of Chromatography*, 299, 424–431.

[16] Chester, T. L., Innis, D. P. and Owens, G. D. (1985) Separation of sucrose polyesters by capillary supercritical chromatography/flame ionization detection with robot pulled capillary restrictors. *Analytical Chemistry*, 57, 2243–2246.

[17] Choudhary, G. (1998) Fundamentals of capillary electrochromatography and its coupling with mass spectrometry. *Ph. D. Thesis*, Yale University, New Haven, CT.

[18] Choudhary, G. and Horvath, Cs. (1997) Dynamics of capillary electrochromatography: experimental study on the electrosmotic flow and conductance in open and packed capillaries. *Journal of Chromatography*, 781, 161–183.

[19] Choudhary, G., Horváth, Cs. and Banks, F. (1998) Capillary electrochromatography of biomolecules with on-line electrospray ionization and time-of-flight mass spectrometry. *Journal of Chromatography*, 828, 469–480.

[20] Cole, R. O., Sepaniak, M. J., Hinze, W. L., Gorse, J. and Oldiges, K. (1991) Bile salt surfactants in micellar electrokinetic capillary chromatography: application to hydrophobic molecule separations. *Journal of Chromatography*, 557, 113–123.

[21] Copper, C. L. and Sepaniak, M. J. (1994) Cyclodextrin modified micellar electrokinetic capillary chromatography. *Analytical Chemistry*, 66, 147–154.

[22] Coufal, P., Claessens, H. A. and Cramers, C. A. (1993) The repeatability of quantitative analysis in electrochromatography. *Journal of Liquid Chromatography*, 16, 3623–3652.

[23] Dalton, D. D. and Taylor, D. R. (1995) Synthesis and use of a novel chiral surfactant based on (R,R)-tartaric acid and its application to chiral separations in micellar electrokinetic capillary chromatography (MECC). *Journal of Microcolumn Separations*, 7, 513–520.

[24] Dalton, D. D., Tylor, D. R. and Waters, D. G. (1995) Synthesis and use of novel chiral surfactants in micellar electrokinetic capillary chromatography. *Journal of Chromatography*, 712, 365–371.

[25] Davis, J. M. (1989) Random-walk theory of nonequilibrium plate height in micellar electrokinetic chromatography. *Analytical Chemistry*, 61, 2455–2461.

[26] Dinelli, G. and Bonetti, A. (1994) Micellar electrokinetic capillary chromatography analysis of water-soluble vitamins and multi-vitamin integrators. *Electrophoresis*, 15, 1147–1150.

[27] Dittmann, M. M. and Rozing, G. P. (1997) Capillary electrochromatography: investigation of the influence of mobile phase and stationary phase properties on electrosmotic velocity, retention, and selectivity. *Journal of Microcolumn Separations*, 9, 399–408.

[28] Dittmann, M. M. and Rozing, G. P. (1996) Capillary electrochromatography – a high efficiency separation technique. *Journal of Chromatography*, 744, 63–74.

[29] Dittmann, M. M., Wienand, K., Bek, F. and Rozing G. P. (1995) Theory and practice of capillary electrochromatography. *LC-GC*, 13, 800–814.

[30] Dobashi, A., Ono, T., Hara, S. and Yamaguchi, J. (1989) Enantioselective hydrophobic entanglement of enantiomeric solutes with chiral functionalized micelles by electrokinetic chromatography. *Journal of Chromatography*, 480, 413–420.

[31] Dobashi, A., Ono, T., Hara, S. and Yamaguchi, J. (1989) Optical resolution of enantiomers with chiral mixed micelles by electrokinetic chromatography. *Analytical Chemistry*, 61, 1984–1986.

[32] Euerby, M. R., Gilligan, D., Johnson, C. M. and Bartle, K. D. (1997) Step-gradient capillary electrochromatography. *Analyst*, 122, 1087–1088.

[33] Euerby, M. R., Gilligan, D., Johnson, C. M., Roulin, S. C. P., Myers, P. and Bartle, K. D. (1997) Analysis of capillary electrochromatography in pharmaceutical analysis. *Journal of Microcolumn Separations*, 9, 373–387.

[34] Euerby, M. R., Johnson, C. M., Bartle, K. D., Myers, P. and Roulin, S. C. P. (1996) Capillary electrochromatography in the pharamaceutical industry. Practical reality or fantasy? *Analytical Communications – Royal Society of Chemistry*, 33, 403–405.

[35] Fjeldsted, J. C., Kong, R. C. and Lee, M. L. (1983) Capillary supercritical-fluid chromatography with conventional flame detectors. *Journal of Chromatography*, 279, 449–455.

[36] Furuta, R. and Doi, T. (1994) Enantiomeric separation of diniconazole and uniconazole by cyclodextrin-modified micellar electrokinetic chromatography. *Journal of Chromatography*, 676, 431–436.

[37] Gordon, D. B., Lord, G. A. and Jones, D. S. (1994) Development of packed capillary column electrochromatography/mass spectrometry. *Rapid Communications in Mass Spectrometry*, 8, 544–548.

[38] Grant, I. H. and Knox, J. H. (1991) Electrochromatography in packed tubes using 1.5 to 50 μm silica gels and ODS bonded silica gels. *Chromatographia*, 32, 317–328.

[39] Greenaway, M., Okafo, G. N., Camilleri, P. and Dhanak, D. (1994) A sensitive and selective method for the analysis of complex mixtures of sugars and linear oligosaccharides. *Journal of Chemical Society Chemical Communications.*, 1691–1692.

[40] Guthrie, E. J. and Schwartz, H. E. (1986) Integral pressure restrictor for capillary SFC. *Journal of Chromatographic Science*, 24, 236–241.

[41] Hofstadler, S. A., Swanek, F. D., Gale, D. C., Ewing, A. G. and Smith, R. D. (1995) Capillary electrophoresis-electrospray ionization fourier ion cyclotron resonance mass spectrometry for direct analysis of cellular proteins. *Analytical Chemistry*, 67, 1477–1480.

[42] Holand, R. D. and Sepaniak, M. J. (1993) Qualitative analysis of mycotoxins using micellar electrokinetic capillary chromatography. *Analytical Chemistry*, 65, 1140–1146.

[43] Horváth, Cs., Melander, W. and Molnár, I. (1976) Solvophobic interactions in liquid chromatography with nonpolar stationary phases. *Journal of Chromatography*, 125, 129–156.

[44] Huber, C., Choudhary, G. and Horvath, Cs. (1997) Capillary electrochromatography with gradient elution. *Analytical Chemistry*, 69, 4429–4436.

[45] Hugener, M., Thinke, A. P., Tjaden, U. R., Niessen, W. M. A. and van der Greef, J. (1993) Pseudo-electrochromatography-negative-ion electrospray mass spectrometry of aromatic glucuronides and food colours. *Journal of Chromatography*, 647, 375–385.

[46] Hunter, R. J. (1981) *Zeta potential in colloid science: principles and applications*, Academic Press, London, pp. 27.

[47] Ishihama, Y. and Terabe, S. (1993) Enantiomeric separation by micellar electrokinetic chromatography using saponins. *Journal of Liquid Chromatography*, 16, 933–944.

[48] Jones, R. F. D., Camilleri, P., Kirby, A. and Okafo, G. N. (1994) The synthesis and micellar properties of a novel anionic surfactant. *Journal of Chemical Society Chemical Communications*, 11, 1311–1312.

[49] Jorgenson, J. W. and Lukacs, K. D. (1981) High-resolution separations based on electrophoresis and electroosmosis. *Journal of Chromatography*, 218, 209–216.

[50] Kaneta, T., Tanaka, S., Taga, M. and Yoshida, H. (1992) Effect of addition of glucose on micellar electrokinetic capillary chromatography with sodium dodecyl sulphate. *Journal of Chromatography*, 609, 369–374.

[51] Kaneta, T., Yamashita, T. and Imasaka, T. (1994) Effect of organic modifier on resolution of hydrophobic compounds by micellar electrokinetic chromatography. *Electrophoresis*, 15, 1276–1279.

[52] Katsuta, S., Tsumura, T., Saitoh, K. and Teramae, N. (1995) Control of selectivity in micellar electrokinetic chromatography by modification of sodium dodecyl sulfate micelles with organic hydroxy compounds. *Journal of Chromatography*, 705, 319–324.

[53] Khaledi, M. G. (1997) Micelles as separation media in high performance liquid chromatography and high-performance capillary electrophoresis: overview and perspective. *Journal of Chromatography*, 780, 3–40.

[54] Khaledi, M. G., Smith, S. C. and Strasters, J. K. (1991) Micellar electrokinetic chromatography of acidic solutes: migration behavior and optimization strategies. *Analytical Chemistry*, 63, 1820–1830.

[55] Kiyohara, C., Saitoh, K. and Suzuki, N. (1993) Micellar electrokinetic capillary chromatography of haematoporphyrin, protoporphyrin and their copper and zinc complexes. *Journal of Chromatography*, 646, 397–403.

[56] Knox, J. H. and Grant, I. H. (1991) Electrochromatography in packed tubes using 1.5 to 50 μm silica gels and ODS bonded silica gels. *Chromatographia*, 32, 317–328.

[57] Kriger, M. S., Cook, K. D. and Ramsey, R. S. (1995) Durable gold coated fused silica capillaries for use in electrospray mass spectrometry. *Analytical Chemistry*, 67, 385–389.

[58] Krogh, M., Brekke, S., Tonnesen, F. and Rasmussen, K. E. (1994) Analysis of drug seizures of heroin and amphetamine by capillary electrophoresis. *Journal of Chromatography*, 674, 235–240.

[59] Kuzdzal, S. A., Monnig, C. A., Newkome, G. R. and Moorefield, C. N. (1994) Dendrimer electrokinetic capillary chromatography: unimolecular micellar behaviour of carboxylic acid terminated cascade macromolecules. *Journal of Chemical Society Chemical Communications*, 13, 2139–2140.

[60] Lamoree, M. H., Tjaden, U. R. and van der Greef, J. (1995) On-line coupling of micellar electrokinetic chromatography to electrospray mass spectrometry. *Journal of Chromatography*, 712, 219–225.

[61] Lane, S. J., Boughtflower, R., Paterson, C. and Morris, M. (1996) Evaluation of a new capillary electrochromatography/mass spectrometry interface using short columns and high field strengths for rapid and efficient analyses. *Rapid Communications in Mass Spectrometry*, 10, 733–736.

[62] Lane, S. J., Boughtflower, R., Paterson, C. and Underwood, T. (1995) Capillary electrochromatography/mass spectrometry: principles and potential for application in the pharmaceutical industry. *Rapid Communications in Mass Spectrometry*, 9, 1283–1287.

[63] Lee, K. J., Lee, J. J. and Moon, D. C. (1994) Application of micellar electrokinetic capillary chromatography for monitoring of hippuric and methylhippuric acid in human urine. *Electrophoresis*, 15, 98–102.

[64] Lelièvre, F., Yan, C., Zare, R. N. and Gareil, P. (1996) Capillary electrochromatography: operating characteristics and enantiomeric separations. *Journal of Chromatography*, 723, 145–156.

[65] Li, D. and Remcho, V. T. (1997) Perfusive electrosmotic transport in packed capillary electrochromatography: mechanism and utility. *Journal of Microcolumn Separations*, 9, 389–397.

[66] Lis, S. and Lloyd, D. K. (1993) Direct chiral separations by capillary electrophoresis using capillaries packed with alpha(1)-acid glycoprotein chiral stationary phase. *Analytical Chemistry*, 65, 3684–3690.

[67] Little, E. L. and Foley, J. P. (1992) Optimization of the resolution of PTH-amino acids through control of surfactant concentration in micellar electrokinetic capillary chromatography: SDS vs. Brij 35/SDS micellar systems. *Journal of Microcolumn Separations*, 4, 145–164.

[68] Lloyd, D. K., Li, S. and Ryan, P. (1995) Protein chiral selectors in free-solution capillary electrophoresis and packed-capillary electrochromatography. *Journal of Chromatography*, 694, 285–296.

[69] Lord, G. A., Gordon, D. B., Tetler, I. W. and Carr, C. M. (1995) Electrochromatography-electrospray mass spectrometry of textile dyes. *Journal of Chromatography*, 700, 27–33.

[70] Matsubara, N., Koezuka, K. and Terabe, S. (1995) Separation of 11 Angiotensin-II analogs by capillary electrophoresis with nonionic surfactant in acidic media. *Electrophoresis*, 16, 580–583.

[71] Matsubara, N. and Terabe, S. (1992) Separation of closely related peptides by capillary electrophoresis with a nonionic surfactant. *Chromatographia*, 34, 493–496.

[72] Mould, D. L. and Synge, R. L. (1954) Separations of polysaccharides related to starch by electrokinetic ultrafiltration in collodion membranes. *Biochemical Journal*, 58, 571–585.

[73] Mould, D. L. and Synge, R. L. M. (1952) Electrokinetic ultrafiltration analysis of polysaccharides. A new approach to the chromatography of large molecules. *Analyst*, 77, 964–969.

[74] Muijselaar, P. G., Claesens, H. A., Cramers, C. A., Jansen, J. F. G. A., Meijer, E. W., De Brabander-van den Berg, E. M. M. and van der Wal, S. (1995) Dendrimers as Pseudo-stationary phases in electrokinetic chromatography. *Journal of High Resolution Chromatography*, 18, 121–123.

[75] Muijselaar, P. G., Otsuka, K. and Terabe, S. (1997) Micelles as pseuo-stationary phases in micellar electrokinetic chromatography. *Journal of Chromatography*, 780, 41–62.

[76] Mussenbrock, E. and Kleibohmer, W. (1995) Separation strategies for the determination of residues of explosives in soils using micellar electrokinetic capillary chromatography. *Journal of Microcolumn separations*, 7, 107–116.

[77] Nelson, W. M. and Lee, C. S. (1996) Mechanistic studies of partial-filling micellar electrokinetic chromatography. *Analytical Chemistry*, 68, 3265–3269.

[78] Nelson, W. M., Tang, Q., Harrata, A. K. and Lee, C. S. (1996) Online partial filling micellar electrokinetic chromatography electrospray-ionization mass-spectrometry. *Journal of Chromatography*, 749, 219–277.

[79] Nishi, H., Fukuyama, T., Matsuo, M. and Terabe, S. (1990) Separation and determination of lipophilic corticosteroids and benzothiazepin analogs by micellar electrokinetic chromatography using bile-salts. *Journal of Chromatography*, 513, 279–295.

[80] Nishi, H., Fukuyama, T. and Terabe, S. (1991) Chiral separation by cyclodextrin-modified micellar electrokinetic chromatography. *Journal of Chromatography*, 553, 503–516.

[81] Novotny, M., Springston, S. R., Peaden, P. A., Fjeldsted, J. C. and Lee, M. L. (1981) Capillary supercritical fluid chromatography. *Analytical Chemistry*, 53, 407A–414A.

[82] Otsuka, K., Higashimori, M., Koike, R., Karuhaka, K., Okada, Y. and Terabe, S. (1994) Separation of lipophilic compounds by micellar electrokinetic chromatography with organic modifiers. *Electrophoresis*, 15 1280–1283.

[83] Otsuka, K., Kashihara. M., Kawaguchi, Y., Koike, R., Hisamitsu, T. and Terabe, S. (1993) Optical resolution by high-performance capillary electrophoresis. Micellar electrokinetic chromatography with sodium N-dodecanoyl-L-glutamate and digitonin. *Journal of Chromatography*, 652, 253–257.

[84] Otsuka, K., Kawahara, J., Tatekawa, K. and Terabe, S. (1991) Chiral separations by micellar electrokinetic chromatography with sodium-N dodecanoyl-L-valinate. *Journal of Chromatography*, 559, 209–214.

[85] Otsuka, K. and Terabe, S. (1990) Effect of methanol and urea on optical resolution of phenylthiohydantoin-DL-amino acids by micellar electrokinetic chromatography with sodium N-dodecanoyl-L-valinate. *Electrophoresis*, 11, 982–984.

[86] Otsuka, K. and Terabe, S. (1990) Enantiomeric resolution by micellar electrokinetic chromatography with chiral surfactants. *Journal of Chromatography*, 515, 221–226.

[87] Otsuka, K., Terabe, S. and Ando, T. (1985) Electrokinetic chromatography with micellar solutions – separation of phenylthiohydantoin-amino acids. *Journal of Chromatography*, 332, 219–226.

[88] Ozaki, H., Itou, N., Terabe, S., Takada, Y., Sakairi, M. and Koizumi, H. (1995) Micellar electrokinetic chromatography-mass spectrometry using a high-molecular-mass surfactant on-line coupling with an electrospray ionization interface. *Journal of Chromatography*, 716, 69–79.

[89] Ozaki, H., Terabe, S. and Ichihara, A. (1994) Micellar electrokinetic chromatography using high-molecular surfactants. Use of butyl acrylate-butyl methacrylate-methacrylic acid copolymers sodium salts as pseudo-stationary phases. *Journal of Chromatography*, **680**, 117–124.

[90] Palmer, C. P. Khaled, M. Y. and McNair, H. M. (1992) A monomolecular pseudostationary phase for micellar electrokinetic chromatography. *Journal of High Resolution Chromatography*, **15**, 756–762.

[91] Palmer C. P. and McNair, H. M. (1992) Novel pseudostationary phase for micellar electrokinetic capillary chromatography. *Journal of Microcolumn Separations*, **4**, 509–514.

[92] Pretorius, V., Hopkins, B. J. and Schieke, J. D. (1974) Electroosmosis: a new concept for high-speed liquid chromatography. *Journal of Chromatography*, **99**, 23–30.

[93] Ramussen, H. T., Goebel, L. K. and McNair, H. M. (1991) Optimization of resolution in micellar electrokinetic chromatography, HRC. *Journal of High Resolution Chromatography*, **14**, 25–28.

[94] Rathore, A. S. and Horváth, Cs. (1996) Separation parameters via virtual migration distances in high-performance liquid chromatography, capillary zone electrophoresis and electrokinetic chromatography. *Journal of Chromatography*, **743**, 231–246.

[95] Rebscher, H. and Pyell, U. (1996) Instrumental developments in capillary electrochromatography. *Chromatographia*, **42**, 171–176.

[96] Ross, G., Dittmann, M., Bek, F. and Rozing, G. (1996) Capillary electrochromatography: enhancement of LC separation in packed capillary columns by means of electrically driven mobile phases. *American Laboratory*, **28**, 34–38.

[97] Saitoh, K., Kato, H. and Teramae, N. (1994) Separation of chlorophyll-cl and -c2 by micellar electrokinetic capillary chromatography. *Journal of Chromatography*, **687**, 149–153.

[98] Sandra, P., Dermux, A., Ferraz, V., Dittamma, M. and Rozing, G. (1997) Analysis of triglyceride by capillary electrochromatography. *Journal of Microcolumn Separations*, **9**, 409–419.

[99] Schafroth, M., Thormann, W. and Allemann, D. (1994) Micellar electrokinetic capillary chromatography of benzodiazepines in human urine. *Electrophoresis*, **15**, 72–78.

[100] Schmeer, K., Behnke, B. and Bayer, E. (1995) Capillary electrochromatography-electrospary mass spectrometry: a microanalysis technique. *Analytical Chemistry*, **67**, 3656–3658.

[101] Smith, N. W. and Evans, M. B. (1995) The efficient analysis of neutral and polar pharmaceutical compounds using reversed-phase and ion-exchange electrochromatography. *Chromatographia*, **41**, 197–203.

[102] Smith, N. W. and Evans, M. B. (1994) The analysis of pharmaceutical compounds using electrochromatography. *Chromatographia*, **38**, 649–657.

[103] Song, L. G., Zhang, S. M., Ou, Q. Y. and Yu, W. L. (1994) Studies of crude chloroform extract of roots of Podophyllum-Emoddil Var Chinesis Sprague by micellar electrokinetic chromatography. *Chromatographia*, **39**, 682–686.

[104] Ståhlberg, J. (1997) The theory of zone migration in electrochromatography. *Analytical Chemistry*, **69**, 3812–3821.

[105] Strasters, J. K. and Khaledi, M. G. (1991) Migration behavior of cationic solutes in micellar electrokinetic capillary chromatography. *Analytical Chemistry*, **63**, 2503–2508.

[106] Takada, Y. (1995) On-line combination of micellar electrokinetic chromatography and mass spectrometry using an electrospray-chemical ionization interface. *Rapid Communications in Mass Spectrometry*, **9**, 488–490.

[107] Takada, Y., Sakairi, M. and Koizumi, H. (1995) Atmospheric pressure chemical ionization interface for capillary electrophoresis/mass spectrometry. *Analytical Chemistry*, **67**, 1474–1476.

[108] Takeda, S., Wakida, S. I., Yamane, M., Kawahara, A. and Higashi, K. (1993) Migration behavior of phthalate esters in micellar electrokinetic chromatography with or without added methanol. *Analytical Chemistry*, 65, 2489–2492.

[109] Tanaka, N., Fukutome, T., Tanigaw, K., Hosoya, K., Kimata, K., Araki T. and Unger, K. K. (1995) Structural selectivity provided by starburst dendrimers as pseudostationary phase in electrokinetic chromatography. *Journal of Chromatography*, 699, 331–341.

[110] Tanaka, N., Tanigawa T., Hosoya, K., Kimata, K., Araki, T. and Terabe, S. (1992) Starburst dendrimers as carriers in electrokinetic chromatography. *Chemistry Letters*, 6, 959–962.

[111] Taylor, M. R., Teale, P. and Westwood, S. A. (1997) Analysis of corticosteroids in biofluids by capillary electrochromatography with gradient elution. *Analytical Chemistry*, 69, 2554–2558.

[112] Terabe, S., Chen, N. and Otsuka, K. (1994) Micellar electrokinetic chromatography, in *Advances in Electrophoresis*; Chrambach, A., Dunn, M. J. and Radola, B. J. (eds) VCH, Weinheim, Germany, Vol. 7, pp. 89–152.

[113] Terabe, S., Ishihama, Y., Nishi, H., Fukuyama, T. and Otsuka, K. (1994) Effect of urea addition in micellar electrokinetic chromatography. *Journal of Chromatography*, 545, 359–368.

[114] Terabe, S., Ishihama, Y., Nishi, N., Fukuyam, T. and Otsuka, K. (1991) Effect of urea addition in micellar electrokinetic chromatography. *Journal of Chromatography*, 545 359–368.

[115] Terabe, S., Miyashita, Y., Shibata, O., Branhart, E. R., Alexander, L. R., Patterson, D. G., Karger, B. L., Hosoya, K. and Tanaka, N. (1990) Separation of highly hydrophobic compounds by cyclodextrin-modified micellar electrokinetic chromatography. *Journal of Chromatography*, 516, 23–31.

[116] Terabe, S., Ostsuka, K. and Ando, T. (1985) Electrokinetic chromatography with micellar solution and open-tubular capillary. *Analytical Chemistry*, 57, 834–841.

[117] Terabe, S., Otsuka, K. and Ando, T. (1989) Band broadening in electrokinetic chromatography with micellar solutions and open capillaries. *Analytical Chemistry*, 61, 251–260.

[118] Terabe, S., Otsuka, K., Ichikwa, K., Tsuchiya, A. and Ando, T. (1984) Electrokinetic separations with micellar solutions and open tubular capillaries. *Analytical Chemistry*, 56, 111–113.

[119] Tiselius, A. (1955) Elektrophorese und chromatographie von eiweisskoerpern und polypeptiden. *Agnew. Chem.*, 67, 245.

[120] Tivesten, A. and Folestad, S. (1995) Separation of precolumn-labelled D- and L-amino acids by micellar electrokinetic chromatography with UV and fluorescence detection. *Journal of Chromatography*, 708, 323–337.

[121] Tsuda, T. (1998) Chromatographic behaviour in electrochromatography. *Analytical Chemistry*, 60, 1677–1680.

[122] Tsuda, T. (1987) Electrochromatography using high applied voltage. *Analytical Chemistry*, 59, 521–523.

[123] Valaskovic, G. A., Kelleher, N. L., Little, D. P., Aaserud, D. J. and McLafferty, F. W. (1995) Attomole-sensitivity electrospray source of large molecule mass spectrometry. *Analytical Chemistry*, 67, 3802–385.

[124] Verheij, E. R., Tjaden, U. R., Niessen, W. M. A. and van der Greef, J. (1991) Pseudo-electrochromatography-mass spectrometry: A new alternative. *Journal of Chromatography*, 554, 339–349.

[125] Wahl, J. H., Gale, D. C. and Smith, R. D. (1994) Sheathless capillary electrophoresis-electrospray ionization mass spectrometry using 10 μm I.D. capillaries: analyses of tryptic digests of cytochrome c. *Journal of Chromatography*, 659, 217–222.

[126] Weinberger, R. and Lurie, I. S. (1991) Micellar electrokinetic capillary electrochromatography of illicit drug substances. *Analytical Chemistry*, 63, 823–827.

[127] Wilm, M. S. and Mann, M. (1995) Analytical properties of the nanoelectrospray ion source. *Analytical Chemistry*, **68**, 1–8.
[128] Yamamoto, H., Baumann, J. and Erni, F. (1992) Electrokinetic reversed-phase chromatography with packed capillaries. *Journal of Chromatography*, **593**, 313–319.
[129] Yan, C., Dadoo, R., Zare, R. N., Rakestraw, D. J. and Annex, D. S. (1996) Gradient elution capillary electrochromatography. *Analytical Chemistry*, **68**, 2726–2730.
[130] Yan, C., Schaufelberger, D. and Erni, F. (1994) Electrochromatography and micro high-performance liquid with 320 μm I.D. packed columns. *Journal of Chromatography*, **670**, 15–23.
[131] Yang, L., Harrata, A. K. and Lee, C. S. (1997) Online micellar electrokinetic chromatography electrospray ionization mass spectrometry using anodically migrating micelles. *Analytical Chemistry*, **69**, 1820–1826.

Chapter 15

Imprinted polymers as tailor-made stationary phases for affinity separation

Karsten Haupt, Peter A. G. Cormack and Klaus Mosbach

Molecular imprinting has established itself as one of the most attractive and versatile methods for creating synthetic materials with specific molecular recognition properties. This is largely because molecular imprinting approaches can be readily applied to a broad spectrum of analytes, yielding chemically and physically robust materials that display strong and selective affinities for the analytes under investigation. Imprinted materials are thus ideally suited for numerous applications where molecular recognition events are of prime importance; they are currently attracting the greatest attention in the affinity separation area, where their utility in chromatographic applications, solid-phase extraction and membrane separations, *inter alia*, is being vigorously explored.

The principle of molecular imprinting

Molecular imprinting in organic polymers (Shea, 1994; Wulff, 1995; Mosbach *et al.*, 1998) occurs via a polymerisation process in which a rigid and insoluble, macroporous polymer network is formed around an analyte of interest (Fig. 15.1). In a typical imprinting experiment, the analyte is initially allowed to form, in solution, an assembly with one or more (usually vinylic or acrylic) functional monomers, that interact with the analyte via either covalent or non-covalent bonds. Once the assembly has been generated, copolymerisation with an excess of cross-linking monomer (usually >50 mol%) is initiated, and the insoluble polymeric product phase-separates from solution as the polymerisation proceeds. The analyte functions as a template during the polymerisation process, controlling the chemical functionality of the polymer network that forms around it. Since the polymer network is macroporous and the interactions between the analyte and the polymer are quite labile, the analyte can be subsequently extracted from the network, via either a simple solvent washing step or by relatively mild chemical treatment. Upon extraction of the analyte, binding sites are revealed within the polymeric network which are complementary to the analyte in terms of their size, shape and functionality. The polymer can, therefore, selectively rebind the analyte in these cavities. It is this ability that can be taken advantage of in affinity-based applications.

There are two distinct imprinting approaches which one can follow. One approach, which has been developed primarily by Wulff and co-workers (Wulff, 1995), is the so-called covalent or pre-organised approach in which the interactions between the analyte and the functional monomers in the pre-polymerisation assembly are covalent in nature. A polymerisable derivative of the analyte is prepared by forming covalent bonds with suitable monomers, and this is subsequently copolymerised with a cross

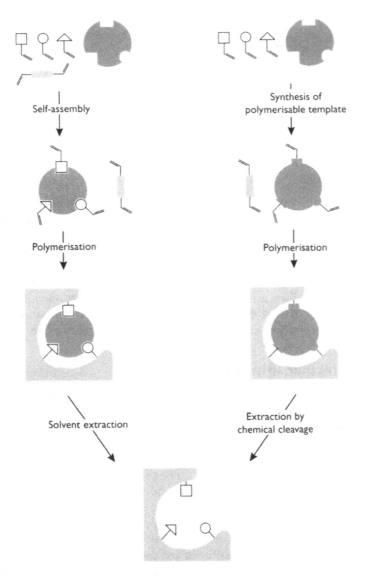

Figure 15.1 Schematic representation of the molecular imprinting principle: Non-covalent approach (left) and covalent approach (right).

linking monomer. Extraction of the analyte from the network requires these covalent bonds to be cleaved, and they are reformed upon subsequent analyte binding.

Another approach has been developed by Mosbach and co-workers (Mosbach *et al.*, 1998) who rely on the formation of a prepolymerisation complex between functional monomers and the template through non-covalent bonds such as ion pairs, hydrogen bonds or $\pi-\pi$ interactions. In this non-covalent or self-assembly approach, the template can be removed simply by solvent extraction. Rebinding of the analyte to the polymer is also non-covalent in nature.

The covalent and the non-covalent imprinting approaches each have their own merits and drawbacks. The covalent approach may yield binding sites which are better defined, however it requires chemical derivatisation of the analyte prior to polymerisation, which is not always easy or practical. The non-covalent approach, on the other hand, requires no chemical derivatisation step, and is therefore much more general in nature and applicable to a considerably wider range of analytes. Although the binding sites may be more heterogeneous, rebinding kinetics are more favourable. Indeed, because of its inherent simplicity, the non-covalent approach tends to be the method of choice.

Apart from synthetic organic polymers, inorganic matrices such as silicas have also been used for molecular imprinting (Wulff, 1995). Another related technique is the so-called bioimprinting, where an imprint of a small molecule is created in a biopolymer such as a protein (Ståhl et al., 1991). In the context of affinity separation, however, molecularly imprinted organic polymers represent the most extensively studied imprinted materials to date, and indeed have the most to offer to the affinity separation area, at least for the time being. The rest of this chapter will therefore deal exclusively with these organic polymers.

Characteristics of molecularly imprinted polymers

Analytes which can be imprinted

One of the many attractive features of the molecular imprinting method is that it can be applied to a diverse range of analytes (Mosbach and Ramström, 1996; Wulff, 1995). The imprinting of small, organic molecules (e.g. drugs, pesticides, amino acids, steroids and sugars) is now well established and considered almost routine. Metal ions and larger organic compounds (e.g. peptides) can be imprinted also. The imprinting of much larger analytes, e.g. proteins (Hjertén et al., 1997) and cells (Aherne et al., 1996), which are in principle, and in practice, more difficult to achieve, has also now been shown to be feasible. Various chemical and physical properties of an analyte to be imprinted are of considerable importance; besides being stable and inert under the polymerisation conditions employed, it must have a suitable chemical handle(s) for interaction with a functional monomer and be soluble in the solvent(s) used for imprinting.

Binding sites

The strength and the selectivity of analyte binding has been shown in some cases to be on a par with those of natural receptors such as antibodies, with dissociation constants in the nanomolar range having been recorded (Vlatakis et al., 1993; Andersson, 1996). In a typical imprinted polymer, however, there is usually a variety of binding sites with different affinities for the analyte, ranging from high (K_D in the nM range) to low (K_D in the μM–mM range) affinity. Most imprinted polymers can therefore be compared to polyclonal antibodies. There is considerable effort being made to prepare imprinted polymers with homogeneous binding sites that are more akin to monoclonal antibodies.

Physical properties

Besides their impressive molecular recognition properties, imprinted polymers have several other attractive features. They are exceedingly robust, and can be utilised under conditions where it would be impossible to use biomolecules. They are stable at elevated temperatures and pressures, and in many chemical environments, such as organic solvents, acids and bases. Furthermore, they are of low cost, have good shelf-lives and can be re-used repeatedly without significant deterioration in their performance.

Preparation and physical forms of molecularly imprinted polymers

A detailed description of all the relevant parameters that have to be considered when preparing molecularly imprinted polymers is far beyond the scope of this chapter. There are some general "rules of thumb" governing polymerisation conditions, choice of functional monomers, etc., which are outlined in the leading reviews cited earlier, however, imprinting conditions are frequently analyte dependent and demand careful optimisation. A good understanding of both the principles and the practical aspects behind the imprinting process is therefore essential for success. For a typical protocol, see Andersson (1996).

Polymer formulation

Functional monomers

Functional monomers are selected based on their ability to reversibly bind, via either covalent or non-covalent bonds, to the analyte. In covalent imprinting approaches, the covalent bonds linking the functional monomers to the analyte need to be labile to allow removal of the analyte from the polymer matrix under relatively mild conditions. This requirement is somewhat limiting, and only metal-chelates (Vidyasankar et al., 1997), boronic acid esters (Wulff and Poll, 1987) and Schiff bases (Wulff et al., 1986) have been developed to any great extent. The non-covalent approach is much less restrictive in this respect, and numerous vinylic and acrylic monomers have been successfully employed. A selection of currently used functional monomers is shown in Table 15.1.

In the non-covalent imprinting protocols, the analyte-functional monomer complex is dynamic in that the functional monomers exist in both free and complexed states, and indeed are free to move from one state to another. To drive the equilibrium towards assembly formation, an excess of functional monomer (typically two-fold or greater) is often used. This does have the side-effect of increasing the level of non-specific binding of the analyte to the polymer, but at the same time it increases the number of good quality binding sites, i.e., it is a compromise.

Cross-linking monomers

Copolymerisation of the functional monomers with an excess of cross-linking monomer (usually >50 mol%) yields an insoluble polymer matrix which phase separates from

Table 15.1 Examples of monomers commonly used in molecular imprinting

Monomer	Structure	Function
Acrylic acids	R = H, CH₃, CF₃	Acid, hydrogen bonding
Vinylpyridines		Basic, hydrogen bonding, π–π interactions
Acrylamide		Neutral, hydrogen bonding
Vinylbenzyliminodiacetic acid		Metal-chelation
Vinylphenylboronic acid		Covalent bond formation
Ethyleneglycol dimethacrylate		Cross-linking
Divinylbenzene		Cross-linking
Trimethylolpropane trimethacrylate		Cross-linking

solution as the polymerisation proceeds. High ratios of cross-linking monomers are generally required to give the polymer matrix the rigidity necessary to retain the integrity of the binding sites. Many different cross-linking monomers have been used, including several which act simultaneously as functional monomers, but the three following cross-linkers have been the most frequently used: ethyleneglycol dimethacrylate (EGDMA), divinylbenzene (DVB) and trimethylolpropane trimethacrylate (TRIM) (Table 15.1)

Porogenic solvents

The porogenic solvent has the function of dissolving all components of the imprinting mixture, and at the same time creating the pores in the polymer that allow access to the imprinted sites. A detailed investigation on the function of porogens has been reported by Sellergren and Shea (1993). Depending on the particular polymer system, there are porogens that are precipitants and others that are non-precipitants for the polymer matrix formed. Their effect is on the morphology of the polymer: precipitants yield large pores and small surface areas whereas non-precipitants yield small pores and large surface areas. Non-precipitating porogens are usually preferred for imprinted polymers. For non-covalent imprinting, non-polar solvents such as toluene or chloroform are more suitable because they promote complex formation between template and functional monomers, whereas polar, and in particular protic solvents, such as methanol, destabilise the analyte-functional monomer assembly by interacting with the functional monomers and the template. In some instances what is considered as a good porogen might be a poor solvent for the template and *vice versa.*

In both the covalent and the non-covalent approaches, the best recognition of the analyte is generally observed when the same solvent is used for imprinting and analyte rebinding, since the swelling of the polymer is similar in both cases. However, it has been demonstrated in many instances that imprinted polymers can be used in solvent systems different from the imprinting solvent, and even that polymers prepared in organic solvents can be used later in aqueous solvents (Andersson, 1996). Thus, it appears that once good binding sites have been created through molecular imprinting, the choice of the solvent for the application of the polymer is somewhat more flexible than for the imprinting process itself.

Initiators and polymerisation conditions

Classical free radical initiators such as 2,2'-azobisisobutyronitrile (AIBN) are commonly used to initiate the polymerisation under either thermal or photochemical conditions. Thermal conditions may be preferred in some cases due to limited analyte solubility, or if the analyte is light sensitive, but otherwise photochemical initiation at low temperatures has been shown to give better results in non-covalent imprinting (O'Shannessy *et al.*, 1989).

Physical forms of imprinted polymers

Molecularly imprinted polymers can be prepared in a variety of forms to suit the final desired application. The most common, and indeed the crudest, method for the preparation of molecularly imprinted polymers is via solution polymerisation, followed by mechanical or manual grinding of the monolithic block generated, to give small particles with a size in the micrometer range. If required, sizing of the particles through sieving and/or sedimentation can then be performed. Besides being time-consuming and wasteful, this method produces particles of irregular shape which are not ideal for chromatographic applications. Improved polymerisation methods which circumvent the need for grinding are therefore being developed.

One general method which overcomes the grinding problem entirely, involves the suspension polymerisation of imprinting mixtures in liquid perfluorocarbon continuous phases (Mayes and Mosbach, 1996). The perflurocarbon continuous phases do not disturb the pre-polymerisation assemblies between analytes and functional monomers, and the spherical beads of controlled, regular diameters (down to ca. 5 µm) that can be prepared reproducibly by this technique are isolated simply by filtration. Alternatively, imprinted spherical beads can also be obtained via either emulsion or seeded emulsion polymerisation methods (Hosoya *et al.*, 1994), although water has to be used as the continuous phase. A rather simple method for the preparation of imprinted supports not requiring processing is dispersion polymerisation (Sellergren, 1994).

Random aggregates or precipitates are obtained if no stabilisers are used; otherwise monodisperse beads are produced.

For chromatographic applications, another alternative to the grinding route is to perform the polymerisation directly inside the chromatography column, i.e. *in situ* polymerisation (Matsui, 1993). This approach is particularly attractive for capillary electrophoresis applications, where packing of the capillary with particles can often be problematic (Schweitz *et al.*, 1997).

One final format, which is attracting increasing interest, involves imprinted membranes. Generally, imprinted membranes are composed either of cross-linked polymers which have been prepared in the 'standard' way (Hedborg *et al.*, 1993), or of linear polymers, solutions of which have been precipitated in the presence of the analyte by a non-solvent (Wang *et al.*, 1996). They can be of two varieties: either free-standing or supported.

Applications for molecularly imprinted polymers in separation technology

There are several potential applications for imprinted polymers, e.g. as recognition elements in biomimetic sensors, as antibody binding mimetics or as catalysts (Mosbach *et al.*, 1998), but it is in the affinity separation area where they are attracting the greatest attention.

Chiral separations have been a major area of investigation, and indeed molecularly imprinted materials have been employed as chiral matrices in several separation techniques. A characteristic of imprinted chiral separation matrices is the pre-determined migration or elution order of the enantiomers, which depends only on which enantiomer is used as the template molecule. For instance, when the D-enantiomer is used as the template, it will be retained more strongly by the polymer than the L-enantiomer, and *vice versa* (Fig. 15.2). Highly selective, chirally discriminating recognition sites have been prepared using covalent or non-covalent imprinting protocols, and large separation factors between the enantiomers have been recorded (Wulff and Poll, 1987; Fischer *et al.*, 1991).

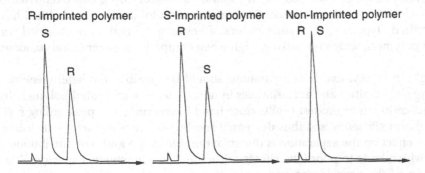

Figure 15.2 Schematic representation of the pre-determined elution order on an imprinted chiral stationary phase for HPLC. If the S-enantiomer was used as the template during imprinting, it will be retained longer than the R-enantiomer when the racemic mixture is administered, and *vice versa*. On a non-imprinted polymer prepared without a template, no enantioseparation is obtained.

For analytes containing two chiral centres, all four stereoisomers may be selectively recognised by the imprinted materials. For example, with a polymer imprinted against the dipeptide Ac-L-Phe-L-Trp-OMe, the LL-form can be distinguished from the DD-, the DL-, and the LD-isomers, with separation factors of 17.8, 14.2 and 5.21, respectively (Ramström *et al.*, 1994). In systems where more than two chiral centres are involved, such as carbohydrates, these properties of molecularly imprinted materials become even more significant. For example, in a study where polymers were imprinted against a glucose derivative, very high selectivities between the various stereoisomers and anomers were recorded (Mayes *et al.*, 1994).

Apart from the separation of enantiomers, imprinted polymers may also be useful for the separation of compounds with closely related structures. One application that is attracting increasing interest is the screening of libraries for new potential drugs, enzyme inhibitors etc. The first reported example involved a library of 12 closely related steroid structures (Ramström *et al.*, 1998a). Two of the library compounds were selected as targets and used to prepare imprinted polymers. It was then demonstrated chromatographically that the target compounds were specifically recognised by the respective polymers when the entire library was injected into the columns (Fig. 15.3).

The following is an overview of separation techniques in which molecularly imprinted polymers have been employed.

Liquid chromatography

The use of imprinted polymers as stationary phases for HPLC is by far the most prominent application. This is partly for historical reasons, because liquid chromatography has been a convenient method for assessing the quality of imprints, particularly during the optimisation of imprinting protocols.

Most research has focused on chiral resolution, and molecularly imprinted chiral stationary phases have been prepared for a wide range of compounds (Kempe and Mosbach, 1995; Wulff, 1995). Many of the early investigations employed amino acid derivatives as model substances. In recent years, however, a great deal of emphasis has been put on the chiral discrimination of drug compounds. The separation of physiologically active compounds, e.g. the anti-inflammatory drug naproxen (Kempe and Mosbach, 1994) or the β-adrenergic antagonist timolol (Fischer *et al.*, 1991) have been described. Typically, separation factors of between 1.5 and 5 are obtained with imprinted polymers, which is relatively high when compared to other chiral stationary phases.

Although, in theory, excellent separations should be possible, the heterogeneity in the binding site affinities and accessibilities in non-covalently imprinted polymers has led in practice to rather modest results since band broadening and peak tailing result in poor column efficiency and thus decreased resolution. Another factor which has a deleterious effect on the separation is the unfavourable shape and size distribution of particles, which leads to poor flow characteristics and low functional capacities. Thus optimisation of the particle size and shape, column packing and the mobile phase has resulted in an improved separation and resolution in many cases. Another important aspect is the capacity of the stationary phase, which can be increased by using a polymer formulation specifically adapted to separation materials. It has been shown that substituting TRIM for EGDMA as the cross-linker leads to higher load capacities,

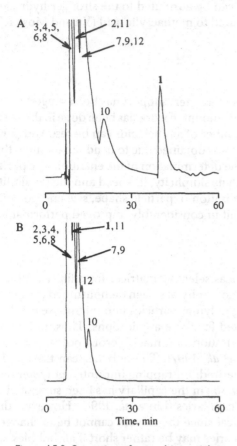

Figure 15.3 Screening of a combinatorial steroid library using HPLC on a molecularly imprinted
stationary phase. (A) Polymer imprinted with 11-α-hydroxyprogesterone. The template molecule is specifically recognised by the polymer and its elution retarded.
(B) Non-imprinted control polymer. Steroids: 11-α-hydroxyprogesterone (template molecule) (1); 11-β-hydroxyprogesterone (2); 17-α-hydroxyprogesterone (3);
progesterone (4); 4-androsten-3,17-dione (5); 1,4-androstadiene-3,17-dione (6); cor-
ticosterone (7); cortexone (8); 11-deoxycortisol (9); cortisone (10); cortisone
21-acetate (11); cortisol 21-acetate (12). Adapted from Ramström *et al.* (1998a),
with permission.

since a lower degree of cross-linking is necessary and more functional monomer can be
accommodated in the polymer, i.e. the number of theoretical binding sites is increased
(Kempe and Mosbach, 1995).

However, the most important issue is certainly the binding site heterogeneity. In order
to obtain a more homogeneous population of binding sites in an imprinted polymer,
the pre-polymerisation complex between the template and the functional monomers
has to be stabilised. Certainly, covalent bonds should give the best results in this
respect, but even strong or multiple non-covalent interactions between the monomer
and the template will afford a more stable complex. For example, acrylamide or triflu-
oromethacrylic acid can in some cases be substituted for methacrylic acid, resulting in

a considerably improved separation which can be attributed to the stronger hydrogen bonds formed by these monomers as compared to methacrylic acid (Yu and Mosbach, 1997; Matsui *et al.*, 1995).

Thin layer chromatography

Finely ground imprinted polymer coated onto an inert support has been suggested for use in chiral TLC. Even though only a limited amount of work has been done in this area, it has been shown that the racemates of a number of amino acids can be resolved (Kriz *et al.*, 1994). Although rather poor resolution was obtained due to band broadening, this method may nevertheless be attractive for the determination of the enantiomeric purity of compounds such as chiral drugs, owing to its simplicity, its speed and the possibility of running multiple parallel samples. Optimisation of particle shape, size and porosity as well as the binder used will certainly result in considerably improved performance.

Capillary electrochromatography

The feasibility of using imprinted polymers as selective matrices for affinity capillary electrophoresis and capillary electrochromatography has been demonstrated (Schweitz *et al.*, 1997). Due to the difficulty in packing polymer particles into microbore capillaries, *in situ* polymerisation seems better suited for these applications. Thus, imprinted capillaries have been prepared by polymerisation of a macroporous polymer monolith directly within the capillary (Schweitz *et al.*, 1997). The polymer can thereby be covalently attached to the capillary wall if desired. Entrapping imprinted polymer particles within a polyacrylamide gel formed *in situ* in the capillary has been suggested as an alternative way of preparing imprinted capillaries (Lin *et al.*, 1996). However, this approach seems to be somewhat less practical since the solvent cannot be exchanged easily and because the lifetime of such capillaries may be rather short if air bubbles are generated during operation.

Enantioselective imprinted columns for capillary electrochromatography could be very useful, especially because very high efficiencies can be obtained. Recently, the chiral separation of drugs such as the β-adrenergic antagonist propranolol has been reported, and an enantiomeric mixture containing as little as 1% S-enantiomer could be resolved in only three minutes (Schweitz *et al.*, 1997). Since imprinted capillaries can be prepared quickly and easily, and are normally very stable in use over a period of several months, this represents a highly promising development for analytical chiral separations.

Membrane-based separation

Molecularly imprinted polymeric membranes are particularly attractive for use as recognition elements in biomimetic sensors. They have also a great potential for applications in preparative separation, with the advantage that membranes can be used in continuous mode, as compared to the batch-wise operation in chromatography.

Imprinted membranes usually facilitate the diffusion of the compound which was imprinted relative to other closely related molecules. This was demonstrated by Mathew-Krotz and Shea (1996) who have observed facilitated transport of adenosine relative to guanosine across a free-standing membrane imprinted with 9-ethyladenine. Another group has cast a theophylline-imprinted polymer in the pores of a 500 nm thick alumina support membrane with a pore size of 20 nm (Hong *et al.*, 1998). The resulting imprinted membrane showed selective transport of theophylline which permeated faster than the structurally related caffeine.

Solid-phase extraction

The use of imprinted polymers for sample concentration and clean-up by solid-phase extraction is attractive due to their high specificity and stability, and also their compatibility with both aqueous and organic solvents. Often the work-up of samples in routine analysis involves a solvent extraction step or a solid-phase extraction step with a more general adsorbent, e.g. an ion exchange or hydrophobic resin. This could be replaced by solid-phase extraction with an imprinted polymer. The advantages are an increased selectivity of the extraction step, and a reduced solvent consumption.

The applicability of this method for analysis has been demonstrated with a number of model analytes such as drugs and herbicides, which can be selectively extracted even from complex samples like beef liver extract, blood serum, urine and bile. For example, polymers imprinted with atrazine were used to enrich the analyte atrazine in solvent extracts of beef liver. In this way, subsequent quantification of atrazine by HPLC or ELISA was facilitated (Muldoon and Stanker, 1997). The accuracy and precision were improved and the detection limit lowered *vis à vis* an assay of the crude solvent extract.

Apart from analytical applications, imprinted polymers may also be used for preparative separations, e.g. for product recovery or by-product removal during chemical and enzymatic syntheses, or from fermentation broths or production waste streams (Ye *et al.*, 1998; Ramström *et al.*, 1998b). It should also be mentioned here that imprinted polymer particles or beads can be made magnetic (Ansell and Mosbach, 1998), which can be advantageous in both analytical and preparative applications since it enables facile removal of the polymer from the extracted medium. However, at least for the time being, the rather low binding capacity of imprinted polymers might limit these applications.

Conclusions

In summary, molecularly imprinted polymers have much to offer in the area of affinity separation. Their attractive physico-chemical properties in conjunction with their impressive molecular recognition properties makes them particularly well suited for application in chromatography, solid-phase extraction, capillary electrophoresis and membrane separation. Although there are still many technical challenges to be overcome, the results presented to date are very promising, and one can be certain that molecularly imprinted polymers will have an important role to play in the future of affinity separation.

References

Aherne, A., Alexander, C., Payne, M. J., Perez, N. and Vulfson, E. N. (1996) Bacteria-mediated lithography of polymer surfaces. *J. Am. Chem. Soc.*, **118**, 8771–8772.

Andersson, L. I. (1996) Application of molecular imprinting to the development of aqueous buffer and organic solvent based radioligand binding assays for S-propranolol. *Anal. Chem.*, **68**, 111–117.

Ansell, R. J. and Mosbach, K. (1998) Magnetic molecular imprinted polymer beads for drug radioligand binding assay. *Analyst*, **123**, 1611–1616.

Fischer, L., Müller, R., Ekberg, B. and Mosbach, K. (1991) Direct enantioseparation of β-adrenergic blockers using a chiral stationary phase prepared by molecular imprinting. *J. Am. Chem. Soc.*, **113**, 9358–9360.

Hedborg, E., Winquist, F., Lundström, I., Andersson, L. I. and Mosbach, K. (1993) Some studies of molecularly imprinted polymer membranes in combination with field-effect devices. *Sens. Actuat. A*, **37–38**, 796–799.

Hjertén, S., Liao, J. L., Nakazato, K., Wang, Y., Zamaratskaia, G. and Zhang, H. X. (1997) Gels mimicking antibodies in their selective recognition of proteins. *Chromatographia*, **44**, 227–234.

Hong, J. M., Anderson, P. E., Qian, J. and Martin, C. E. (1998) Selectively-permeable ultrathin film composite membranes based on molecularly-imprinted polymers. *Chem. Mater.*, **10**, 1029–1033.

Hosoya, K., Yoshizako, K., Tanaka, N., Kimata, K., Araki, T. and Haginaka, J. (1994) Uniform-size macroporous polymer-based stationary-phase for HPLC prepared through molecular imprinting technique. *Chem. Lett.*, **8**, 1437–1438.

Hosoya, K., Yoshihako, K., Shirasu, Y., Kimata, K., Araki, T., Tanaka, N. and Haginaka, J. (1996) Molecularly imprinted uniform-size polymer-based stationary phase for high-performance liquid chromatography. Structural contribution of cross-linked polymer network on specific molecular recognition. *J. Chromatogr.*, **728**, 139–148.

Kempe, M. and Mosbach, K. (1994) Direct resolution of naproxen on a non-covalently molecularly imprinted chiral stationary phase. *J. Chromatogr.*, **664**, 276–279.

Kempe, M. and Mosbach, K. (1995) Receptor binding mimetics: a novel molecularly imprinted polymer. *Tetrahed. Lett.*, **36**, 3563–3566.

Kriz, D., Berggren-Kriz, C., Andersson, L. I. and Mosbach, K. (1994) Thin-layer chromatography based on the molecular imprinting technique. *Anal. Chem.*, **66**, 2636–2639.

Lin, J. M., Nakagama, T., Uchiyama, K. and Hobo T. (1996) Molecularly imprinted polymer as chiral selector for enantioseparation of amino acids by capillary gel electrophoresis. *Chromatographia*, **43**, 585–591.

Mathew-Krotz, J. and Shea, K. J. (1996) Imprinted polymer membranes for the selective transport of targeted neutral molecules. *J. Am. Chem. Soc.*, **118**, 8154–8155.

Matsui, J., Kato, T., Takeuchi, T., Suzuki, M., Yokoyama, K., Tamiya, E. and Karube, I. (1993) Molecular recognition in continuous polymer rods prepared by a molecular imprinting technique. *Anal. Chem.*, **65**, 2223–2224.

Matsui, J., Miyoshi, Y. and Takeuchi, T. (1995) Fluoro-functionalized molecularly imprinted polymers selective for herbicides. *Chem. Lett.*, **11**, 1007–1008.

Mayes, A. G., Andersson, L. I. and Mosbach, K. (1994) Sugar binding polymers showing high anomeric and epimeric discrimination obtained by non-covalent molecular imprinting. *Anal. Biochem.*, **222**, 483–488.

Mayes, A. G. and Mosbach, K. (1996) Molecularly imprinted polymer beads: Suspension polymerization using a liquid perfluorocarbon as the dispersing phase. *Anal. Chem.*, **68**, 3769–3774.

Mosbach, K. and Ramström, O. (1996) The emerging technique of molecular imprinting and its future impact on biotechnology. *Bio/Technology*, **14**, 163–170.

Mosbach, K., Haupt, K., Liu, X-C., Cormack, P. A. G. and Ramström, O. (1998) Molecular imprinting: *Status artis et quo vadere?* In Bartsch, R. A. and Maeda, M. (eds) "Molecular and ionic recognition with imprinted polymers". ACS Symposium Series 703, pp. 29–48, American Chemical Society, Washington DC.

Muldoon, M. T. and Stanker, L. H. (1997) Molecularly imprinted solid phase extraction of atrazine from beef liver extracts. *Anal. Chem.*, **69**, 803–808.

O'Shannessy, D. J., Ekberg, B. and Mosbach, K. (1989) Molecular imprinting of amino acid derivatives at low temperature using photolytic homolysis of azobisnitriles. *Anal. Biochem.*, **177**, 144–149.

Ramström, O., Nicholls, I. A. and Mosbach, K. (1994) Synthetic peptide receptor mimics: highly stereoselective recognition in non-covalent molecularly imprinted polymers. *Tetrahedr. Asymm.*, **5**, 649–656.

Ramström, O., Ye, L., Krook, M. and Mosbach, K. (1998a) Screening of a combinatorial steroid library using molecularly imprinted polymers. *Anal. Comm.*, **35**, 9–11.

Ramström, O., Ye, L., Krook, M. and Mosbach, K. (1998b) Applications of molecularly imprinted materials as selective adsorbents: emphasis on enzymatic equilibrium shifting and library screening. *Chromatographia*, **47**, 465–469.

Shea, K. J. (1994) Molecular imprinting of synthetic polymer networks: the *de novo* synthesis of macromolecular binding and catalytic sites. *Trends Polym. Sci.*, **2**, 166–173.

Schweitz, L., Andersson, L. I. and Nilsson, S. (1997) Capillary electrochromatography with predetermined selectivity obtained through molecular imprinting. *Anal. Chem.*, **69**, 1179–1183.

Sellergren, B. and Shea, K. J. (1993) Influence of polymer morphology on the ability of imprinted network polymers to resolve enantiomers. *J. Chromatogr.*, **635**, 31–49.

Sellergren, B. (1994) Imprinted dispersion polymers: a new class of easily accessible affinity stationary phases. *J. Chromatogr.*, **673**, 133–141.

Ståhl, M., Jeppsson-Wistrand, U., Månsson, M.-O. and Mosbach, K. (1991) Induced stereoselectivity and substrate selectivity of bio-imprinted α-chymotrypsin in anhydrous organic media. *J. Am. Chem. Soc.*, **113**, 9366–9368.

Vidyasankar, S., Ru, M. and Arnold, F. H. (1997) Molecularly imprinted ligand-exchange adsorbents for the chiral separation of underivatized amino acids. *J. Chromatogr. A.*, **775**, 51–63.

Vlatakis, G., Andersson, L. I., Müller, R. and Mosbach, K. (1993) Drug assay using antibody mimics made by molecular imprinting. *Nature*, **361**, 645–647.

Wang, H. Y., Kobayashi, T. and Fujii, N. (1996) Molecular imprint membranes prepared by the phase inversion precipitation technique. *Langmuir*, **12**, 4850–4856.

Wulff, G., Heide, B. and Helfmeier, B. (1986) Molecular recognition through the exact placement of functional groups on rigid matrices via a template approach. *J. Am. Chem. Soc.*, **108**, 1089–1091.

Wulff, G. and Poll, H. G. (1987) Enzyme-Analogue Built Polymers. 23) Influence of the structure of the binding sites on the selectivity for racemic resolution. *Makromol. Chem.*, **188**, 741–748.

Wulff, G. (1995) Molecular imprinting in cross-linked materials with the aid of molecular templates – A way towards artificial antibodies. *Angew. Chem. Int. Ed. Engl.*, **34**, 1812–1832.

Ye, L., Ramström, O. and Mosbach, K. (1998) Molecularly imprinted polymeric adsorbents for byproduct removal. *Anal. Chem.*, **70**, 2789–2795.

Yu, C. and Mosbach, K. (1997) Molecular imprinting utilizing an amide functional group for hydrogen bonding leading to highly efficient polymers. *J. Org. Chem.*, **62**, 4057–4064.

Chapter 16

Computer-aided simulation of biochromatography

Nicolas Voute

Introduction

The purification of biomolecules is an important challenge in the biopharmaceutical industry. In the recent past, liquid chromatography has emerged as a major technique not only in the laboratory but also at the manufacturing plant. The success of liquid chromatography lies in its ability to achieve high purification factors from complex mixtures while preserving the integrity of labile biomolecules. In addition, concomitant product separation and concentration are obtained under appropriate conditions. The resolving power of liquid chromatography is explained, on one hand, by the relatively vast choice of thermodynamic interactions that can be exploited to segregate the target component from its contaminants; and on the other hand, by the high efficiency of modern packing media. Moreover, the structure and activity of a biomolecule are preserved because of the mild operating conditions of biochromatography. Although it is used at the manufacturing scale, liquid chromatography still suffers from a low productivity compared to other biochemical processes. Further, some obstacles are still encountered with the scaling-up and optimization of liquid chromatography (Yamamoto, 1995). The need for high quality and cost effective bioprocesses has created incentives to establish rational process design and scale-up strategies.

The large number of operating parameters and thermodynamic variables, involved in liquid chromatography are partially responsible for the difficulties encountered when developing a new protocol. Moreover, the optimization goals may vary during the development of the separation method. While at the discovery stage the optimum separation conditions should lead to high purity, at the manufacturing stage recovery and high throughput are additionally required. Other criteria, such as robustness, reproducibility, cost effectiveness are also involved in the design of a large scale process (Wheelwright, 1991).

Hitherto, method development for chromatography separations has relied upon time intensive experimentation, based on a trial and error approach, or empirical approximation. These strategies, although successful, required the performance of a large number of experiments, using large amounts of target product, and traditionally had resulted in a long development time (Mao and Hearn, 1996).

Over the last forty years, the fundamental understanding of liquid chromatography substancially progressed. This knowledge is of paramount importance for process optimization. In the past, this information was rarely used for practical biotechnologic applications due to the complexity of the mathematical models. Today, with the availability of powerful desktop computer, simulation algorithms reform process optimization and scale-up approaches in liquid biochromatography (Jungbauer, 1996). The use of computer simulation, that have been the norm in other areas of process engineering is becoming more widespread in bioseparation. Starting from experimental data obtained in the lab, simulation allows the prediction of the performances of chromatographic column, and the identification of the critical variables prior to carrying out any real purification runs. This approach allows the chromatographer to focus on the most promising path and thus enabling to shorten the development time.

The complexity of biomolecules adsorption onto packing, and intraparticle transport should not, however, be overlooked. The accuracy of a simulation algorithm is strongly dependent on the pertinence of the mathematical model used to describe a given system, as well as on the accuracy of the model parameters.

In this chapter, an overview of theoretical models of biochromatographic purification, is discussed as well as the impact and opportunities of computer-aided simulation, made possible by the advent of fast microprocessors. Additionally, application examples of mathematical modeling in designing and scaling-up purification methods, are presented.

Definition and principle of liquid biochromatography

Definitions

The separation of a multicomponent liquid mixture by percolation through a column of particles is called liquid chromatography. The bed of particles is defined as stationary phase or solid phase. The liquid phase or mobile phase flows through the column within the interparticle space. If conditions are selected so that the components of the mixture carried by the flow have different equilibrium distribution coefficients with the stationary phase, their migration velocities will be different. The components will be separated in time over the length of the column and can be recovered at the column outlet. The solute with the higher affinity for the solid phase or higher equilibrium distribution coefficient will remain longer in the column than solutes of lower affinities, and thus they can be separated.

Depending on the type of interaction(s) between the solute and the stationary phase, the migration velocity of a component can range from zero to the fluid (liquid) phase velocity. For very favorable interaction – irreversible on the time scale of the separation – the solute binds very strongly to the stationary phase and its migration velocity is virtually zero. On the contrary the migration velocity of an unretained solute, totally excluded from the particle, is equal to the mobile phase velocity. When intermediate velocities are encountered, the quality of the separation relies on design parameters, and important among these are the mobile phase composition, the gradient profile of the mobile phase modifier, the length of the column and the flow velocity.

The optimal design of a liquid biochromatography purification procedure requires to relate the macroscopic performances of the column to the fundamental physico-chemical mechanisms controlling the separation. Thermodynamic equilibrium, fluid dynamics and mass transfer are the important physico-chemical phenomena governing liquid biochromatography.

The thermodynamic equilibrium simply relates the solute equilibrium concentrations between the stationary and the mobile phase. In most cases the equilibrium between the two phases is controlled by molecular interactions, such as electrostatic or hydrophobic interactions. Gel filtration is an exception as, essentially, there is no molecular interaction, but a steric exclusion of the solute from the pore network of the solid phase particle. The interphase distribution of solutes is controlled by the composition of the flowing solution. For example in ion-exchange chromatography, conditions are selected so that the molecule of interest binds to the charged particle surface (adsorption). The composition of the mobile phase is then changed in order to selectively repress the interaction, and allow the elution of the target solute. The thermodynamic equilibrium of the solutes is of the paramount importance as it determines the maximum performances of the column. For example, the selectivity between two components – defined as the ratio of their distribution coefficients – is only controlled by the sorption isotherm. Selectivity is of course a predominant factor of the resolution, and will depends on the mobile phase composition and the physico chemical structure of the resin. A second example of the importance of thermodynamic factors, is the maximum loading achievable in frontal chromatography or capture step. The equilibrium stationary phase concentration – or capacity – is defined by the adsorption isotherm. It depends on the solutes and the modulator concentrations in the feed, as well as the temperature the pH, ionic strength and the polarity of the mobile phase.

However, a chromatography separation is never operated in a state of ideal and perfect equilibrium between the stationary and moving phases. The deviation from the ideal equilibrium induces dispersive effects, that are responsible for loss of resolution in linear chromatography and spreading of breakthrough curve in frontal chromatography. The separation performances set by the isotherm of the sample components are systematically reduced by the mass transfer and flow dynamics at work in the column. Liquid chromatography involves interphase transport from the moving phase to a typically porous spherical bead. Therefore the kinetics of the equilibrium is not instantaneous, due to the boundary-layer mass transfer resistance, the finite diffusion inside the particles and the slow adsorption rate to the interaction sites or the inner particle surface.

The hydrodynamic dispersion resulting from the flow through the granular particle is also responsible for some level of mixing of the band that travel through the column. The relative importance of equilibrium and dispersive effects determine the overall quality of the separation, which is traditionally measured in term of resolution for the elution chromatography, or spreading of the breakthrough curve for the frontal chromatography. An overview of equilibrium and mass transfer theories is presented in the following sections.

Modes of operation

A biochromatographic separation is preferentially performed on a fixed-bed column, as this mode of operation maximizes the column efficiency. However other variants, such as fluidized-bed or stirred batch are implemented, when pressure drop, resin clogging or loading time are critical.

In essence, liquid chromatography is a batch process, involving sample loading and the subsequent elution of the solutes in the isocratic mode. More elaborated elution procedures also include washing out of the contaminant, regeneration, cleaning and reequilibration steps. Although possible, continuous modes of liquid biochromatography, such as annular chromatography and simulated moving bed chromatography (Wankat, 1986) are not popular for preparative biopurification.

The three typical modes of operation of a packed-bed column are elution chromatography, frontal chromatography and displacement chromatography.

In elution chromatography, the sample is first loaded onto the column, then a modulator with little affinity for the sorbent is introduced. The solute distribution between the stationary and mobile phases depends strongly on the concentration of the modulator. As a result, the solutes are eluted in the form of bands which travel through the column at velocities depending on the solute affinities for the sorbent, which is controlled by the composition of the mobile phase. Several types of elution are applicable for large scale operation: isocratic elution when the composition of the eluant phase remains constant, or gradient elution when it is varied over time. For the latter the variation is either linear (linear gradient elution) or discontinuous (step gradient elution).

Isocratic gradient elution always leads to a dilution of the solutes, in contrast to step and linear gradient elutions, when the operating conditions are carefully selected (Coffman *et al.*, 1994; Yamamoto *et al.*, 1992, 1993).

In frontal chromatography the sample is continuously fed to the column until the breakthrough of the target solute occurs. The less retained solute is eluted first, whereas the more retained is usually eluted by a drastic change in the equilibrium condition. This technique is best suited for a capture step using an affinity or an ion-exchange sorbent.

In displacement chromatography, the sample loading is followed by the injection of a modulator – also called displacer – characterized by a higher affinity for the sorbent than any of the solutes in the sample. The migration of the displacer through the column results in competitive desorption of the sample solutes which are readsorbed upstream of the modulator front. In this situation, the solutes are separated in the form of concentrated bands.

Thermodynamic equilibrium

Sorption may be defined as selective and reversible transfer of solutes from a liquid phase to a solid phase. The mathematical relationship describing the equilibrium distribution of solutes between the two phases is called thermodynamic equilibrium isotherm. Due to the complexity of the factors governing biomolecule sorption, the isotherm is often described by an empirical relationship, not necessarily based on a mechanistic description of the sorption phenomena. As an a priori prediction of the quantitative protein adsorption onto chromatographic media is still very difficult, only experimentally determined isotherms give reliable results. Moreover, an isotherm model fitting the experimental data with enough accuracy is sufficient for the prediction of the outcome in liquid biochromatography.

The sorption isotherm depends on numerous factors among them the temperature, the composition of the mobile phase (pH, ionic strength, polarity) and the chemical type of the resin and the concentrations of the solutes. For macromolecules like proteins, a small variation in the mobile composition can induce a shift from quasi irreversible adsorption, on the time scale of chromatography, to complete desorption. Therefore it is important to quantitatively determine the equilibrium distribution over the range of operating conditions that will be encountered for the column experiments, including the effect of the mobile phase composition. The mathematical model describing the isotherm must explicitly account for the target solute concentration, but also for the mobile phase modulator that will repress the solute binding. In this situation, adsorption and elution are represented by a unique equation and set of parameters, allowing the simulation of linear, and segmented gradient elution.

For a simple sample composition, where the target molecule is the predominant species, the equilibrium distribution may be described by a single component isotherm. Under these circumstances the influence of the contaminants on the adsorption of the target product can be neglected, yielding simple mathematical formulation of the isotherm. This situation is encountered in analytical separation, and also in preparative purification using a linear or a step gradient elution, in which the modulator concentration and the solute dilution are sufficiently large so that the solutes behave independently. It is also true when the packing media is operated under saturation condition, because enough interaction sites are available for the components of the sample to bind without recoursing to concomitant competition. However for a more complex sample, and when the sample load is high, a multicomponent isotherm is required. This type of isotherm, able to describe the competitive effects among the solutes is well adapted to the prediction of displacement and frontal chromatography, as well as elution chromatography with column overload.

Single component isotherms

As indicated in the following paragraphs, different classes of isotherm have been used to characterize biomolecule sorption onto specific types of chromatographic resins. Although different molecular interactions are exploited, the common profile of the adsorption model is convex upward, reflecting the finite capacity of the sorbent and the strong non-linearity of the isotherm.

Ion-exchange chromatography

Ion-exchangers are solid, generally porous, supports carrying covalently bound ion sites on their internal surface, that interact with mobile counterions of opposite charge. The counterions can be stochiometrically exchanged with other ions of the same charge present in the mobile phase, including biomolecules.

Several approaches have been used to depict the stochiometric exchange reaction.

(a) Stoichiometric displacement model (SDM)   The earliest model describing protein adsorption onto ion-exchange media is the Stoichiometric Displacement Model (Velayudhan and Horvath, 1988). The model assumes that when the protein binds to the adsorbent, it displaces an amount of salt counterion equivalent to the protein effective charge.

Therefore the protein adsorption–desorption process is represented by a stoichiometric exchange of protein resident in the mobile phase and salt counterions bound to the resin. The process of the ion-exchange equilibrium is represented by

$$\beta R_{esin} C_{ounterion} + P_{rotein} \rightleftarrows R_{esin\,\beta}\, P_{rotein} +_\beta C_{ounterion} \tag{1}$$

with $P_{protein}$ = protein molecule, $C_{ounterion}$ = counterion molecule, R_{esin} = ion-exchanger and β = characteristic charge of the protein.

For simplicity the equilibrium relation has been written for a monovalent salt counterion. In the case of a multivalent counterion, β would represent the ratio of the protein effective charge to the counterion valence.

The equilibrium constant of the ion-exchange process is defined as (Whitley *et al.*, 1989):

$$K_{eq} = \left(\frac{\overline{C}}{C}\right)\left(\frac{I}{\overline{I}}\right)^{\beta} \tag{2}$$

where C, I are the protein and counterion concentrations in the mobile phase, and $\overline{C}, \overline{I}$ the concentrations in the stationary phase.

The electroneutrality condition applied to the stationary phase yields:

$$\Lambda = \overline{I} + \beta\overline{C} \tag{3}$$

Λ is the ionic capacity of the resin (total number of charge/unit volume of resin). Combining (2) and (3) gives:

$$\overline{C} = K_{eq}C\left(\frac{\Lambda - \beta\overline{C}}{I}\right)^{\beta} \tag{4}$$

Equation (4) defines a single component isotherm, based on the law of mass action.

It should be pointed out that a numerical method is required to calculate the protein stationary phase concentration, given a mobile phase and a salt counterion concentration.

Note also that the effective charge is not necessarily an integer as it may account for some deviations from the ideal situation depicted by the model. For example the model neglects the possible coexistence of different preferential orientations of the adsorbed protein; the model also assumes a protein activity coefficient of 1 (Whitley *et al.*, 1989). Therefore β must be viewed as a pH dependent empirical parameter related to the protein surface charges and to the preferential binding orientation of the protein.

Two interesting limiting cases are derived from the SDM model.

1. At low protein concentration in the mobile phase:

$$\lim_{C \to 0} \overline{C} = 0. \tag{5}$$

Under linear conditions, the protein distribution coefficient (K), obtained from Equation (4) is:

$$K = \frac{\overline{C}}{C} = K_{eq}\left(\frac{\Lambda}{I}\right)^{\beta}. \tag{6}$$

Equation (6) is rearranged in the following form:

$$K = \frac{\overline{C}}{C} = \alpha I^{-\beta} \tag{7}$$

with α defined as:

$$\alpha = K_{eq}\Lambda^{\beta}. \tag{8}$$

One essential result, derived from Equation (7) is the linear dependency of the logarithm of the distribution coefficient on the logarithm of the salt counterion concentration with a negative slope given by the effective charge of the protein (Kopaciewicz $et\ al.$, 1983).

Since it defines the relation between distribution coefficient and column elution volume under isocratic condition, Equation (7) has been extensively used to characterize protein and peptide distribution coefficients, onto numerous ion-exchange resins (Bouhallab $et\ al.$, 1996; Gerstner $et\ al.$, 1994).

2. At high protein concentration in the mobile phase:

$$\underset{C \to \omega}{\mathrm{Lim}}\,\overline{I} = 0. \tag{9}$$

Under overloaded conditions, the maximum protein binding capacity, obtained from Equation (3) is:

$$\overline{C} = \overline{C}_{max} = \frac{\Lambda}{\beta}. \tag{10}$$

From Equation (10) it follows that the maximum protein uptake is independent of the mobile phase counterion concentration; however, experimental data indicate that only at very low mobile phase salt concentration does the isotherm reach the maximum value.

The potential of the stochiometric displacement model to depict protein sorption by high capacity cation exchangers has been evaluated by Fernandez and coworkers (Fernandez and Carta, 1996; Fernandez $et\ al.$, 1996). They have shown that bovine serum albumin, α lactalbumin and ovalbumin uptakes by Q HyperD™ F and Q HyperD™ M, at various salt concentrations are very well described, by the SDM model with single sets of parameters. An interesting study of ion-exchange equilibrium using the SDM model has been presented by Cysewski (Cysewski $et\ al.$, 1991). The influence of the protein effective charge as well as the influence of the counterion valence on the preparative elution profiles, obtained by isocratic and linear gradient elution, were reported. The effect of the protein dimerization on the isocratic elution profile under preparative conditions has been investigated by Vidal-Madjar (Vidal-Madjar $et\ al.$, 1992) using the SDM model.

A major limitation of the SDM model is its failure to account for the blocking of ion-exchange adsorption sites by adsorbed proteins, resulting in the reduction of the sorption capacity (Whitley $et\ al.$, 1989).

(b) Steric mass action law (SMA)   The basic idea of the SMA model is to include in the SDM model the steric hindrance of counterions by large adsorbed macromolecules (Brooks and Cramer, 1992).

The binding of the protein onto the resin results in the displacement of β monovalent counterions, but also in the blocking of some counterions hindered by the adsorbed large biomolecules.

The number of counterions sterically hindered by the adsorbed proteins per unit volume of stationary phase is given by:

$$\hat{I} = \sigma \overline{C} \tag{11}$$

with $\hat{I}$ = molarity of counterions sterically hindered by the adsorbed proteins, σ = steric factor of the protein, $\overline{C}$ = protein molarity in the stationary phase.

When the interphase equilibrium is reached the total number of counterions adsorbed to the support per unit volume is given by:

$$I_t = \hat{I} + \overline{I} \tag{12}$$

where I_t = total number of counterions adsorbed to the resin per unit volume, $\overline{I}$ = molarity of counterions adsorbed and available for exchange.

A consequence of the SMA model is that unbound proteins may only interact with unobstructed ion-exchange sites.

Electroneutrality condition on the resin requires:

$$\Lambda = \overline{I} + (\beta + \sigma)\overline{C}. \tag{13}$$

Substitution of Equation (13) into Equation (2), with $\overline{I}$ defined as molarity of counterions adsorbed and available for exchange yields the following isotherm:

$$\overline{C} = K_{eq} C \left(\frac{\Lambda - (\beta + \sigma)\overline{C}}{I} \right)^{\beta}. \tag{14}$$

As for the SDM model Equation (14) defines implicitly the protein stationary phase concentration for a given protein, and salt counterion concentrations. Galland (Galland *et al.*, 1995) claims that the inclusion of the steric hindrance factor to the isotherm equation leads to a superior description of the ion-exchange adsorption of biomolecule, compared to the SDM model.

At infinite solute dilution, the SMA model converges to the SDM model, Equation (7). At high solute concentration, the maximum capacity is given by

$$\overline{C} = \overline{C}_{max} = \frac{\Lambda}{\beta + \sigma}. \tag{15}$$

Both the SDM and SMA models are able to predict the stoichiometric exchange of counterion resulting from the binding of the biomolecules. The subsequent increase in the mobile phase salt counterion concentration, may induce perturbations in the salt profile that will propagate through the column and affect the binding of the biomolecules. An extensive study of the induced salt gradient effects on peak profiles was presented by Galland (Galland *et al.*, 1995).

(c) Modified Langmuir isotherm (MLI) A limitation of the SDM and SMA models is the requirement for a numerical method to solve the isotherm equation for the stationary phase concentration. Alternatively, explicit isotherm formalism can be employed to

avoid this pitfall. For example the MLI model, first described by Antia (Antia and Horvath, 1989) provides good agreement with experimental data. The MLI isotherm results from the incorporation of a linear dependency of the logarithm of the capacity factor on the logarithm of the modulator concentration, in the traditional Langmuir model.

Solute distribution coefficient derived from the MLI model is given by the following isotherm equation:

$$K = \frac{\overline{C}}{C} = \frac{\alpha I^{-\beta}}{1 + \alpha/\gamma I^{-\beta}C} \tag{16}$$

Limiting cases comparable to those of the SDM and SMA models are obtained with Equation (16):

- at low solute concentration Equation (16) reduces to Equation (7),
- at high solute concentration Equation (16) is similar to (10) and (15):

$$\overline{C} = \overline{C}_{max} = \gamma \tag{17}$$

Figure 16.1 shows the uptake of bovine serum albumin by the cationic resin Q HyperD™ F and the fit with the MLI equation. A good agreement between the data and the model is found, in particular, the model predicts the shift of the isotherm shape, from quasi-rectangular at low modulator concentration, to linear at high modulator concentration.

The MLI, SDM and MLA equations are identical in the linear part of the isotherm (low protein concentration and high salt concentration). The maximum capacities are also similar, however in the middle concentration range the profiles of the isotherms are different. The concept of MLI model has been revisited by Whitley (Whitley *et al.*,

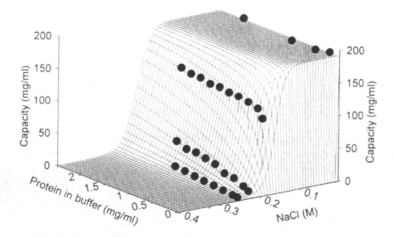

Figure 16.1 Equilibrium uptake of bovine serum albumin by Q HyperD™ F at different NaCl concentrations in a 50 mM Tris–HCl buffer pH 8.6. The lines are calculated with the modified Langmuir isotherm, Equation (16).

1991) to include a salt dependent maximum capacity. By adding another degree of freedom to the equation, this modification allows a better fit of experimental data.

(d) *Empirical equations* Empirical isotherm equations have also been used to depict protein adsorption onto ion-exchangers. For example, James (James and Do, 1991) has obtained an excellent fit of bovine serum albumin uptakes onto a DEAE ion-exchanger at pH 3 using the following Langmuir–Freunlich isotherm:

$$\overline{C} = \frac{\gamma \alpha C^\beta}{1 + \alpha C^\beta + \alpha' I^{\beta'}} \tag{18}$$

where α, β, γ, α', β' are empirical parameters.

It was also shown that the Langmuir–Freunlich isotherm could fit the uptake of phenylalanine and tyrosine onto a strong cation exchanger and at various chloride ion concentrations (James and Do, 1991).

The abilities of 56 equations derived from classical isotherms and including an explicit salt dependency have been investigated by Kaltenbrunner (Kaltenbrunner and Jungbauer 1996). It was concluded that the best models result from a combination of salt dependent maximum capacity with a classical nonlinear isotherm. However, it was also found that the curvature of the K vs C (distribution coefficient vs mobile phase concentration) curves is dependent on the salt concentration, and none of the equations was able to predict the shift in the isotherm bending.

To date, only a few investigations have been performed on the combined influence of modulator concentration, mobile phase composition and pH upon the uptake of macromolecules by ion-exchangers. These factors have a predominant impact on the performance of a separation procedure as they control the selectivity between sample components.

Reverse phase and hydrophobic interaction chromatography

Reverse phase and hydrophobic interaction chromatographies are based on the occurence of hydrophobic interactions between immobilized ligands and exposed hydrophobic sites/areas of the biomolecules.

Adsorption onto hydrophobic support is often described by the classical Langmuir isotherm:

$$\overline{C} = \frac{aC}{1 + bC} \tag{19}$$

yielding the two well known limiting cases.

1. At low solute concentration

$$\lim_{C \to 0} \frac{\overline{C}}{C} = a \tag{20}$$

a is dimensionless and represents the initial slope of the isotherm. In the limit of infinite solute dilution, the capacity factor is equal to Ha, where H is the phase ratio.

2. At high solute concentration

$$\lim_{C \to \omega} \overline{C} = \frac{a}{b} = \overline{C}_{max} \tag{21}$$

a/b is equivalent to the saturation capacity per unit volume of the sorbent.

The effect of the mobile phase modulator concentration on the initial slope of the isotherm has been described as follows (Snyder, 1980):

$$a = a_0 e^{-SI} \tag{22}$$

with a_0 = value of isotherm slope (a) at zero molar modulator concentration for reverse phase, and one molar for hydrophobic interaction chromatography; S = slope of a plot of logarithm of a vs logarithm of I.

The saturation capacity of the adsorbent is often assumed to be constant (Antia and Horvath, 1989; Guiochon *et al.*, 1994; Jacobson *et al.*, 1987) and independent of the modulator concentration.

Substituting Equations (22) and (21) into Equation (19) yields:

$$\overline{C} = \frac{a_0 e^{-SI} C}{1 + a_0/\overline{C}_{max} e^{-SI} C} \tag{23}$$

Using Equation (23), a theoretical study (Antia and Horvath, 1989) demonstrated the impact of the gradient slope and sample size on the band profiles in isocratic and linear gradient elution chromatography. At high loading, the large peak broadening of thermodynamic origin, observed in isocratic elution is offset, in linear gradient elution, by a peak compression effect due to the modulator concentration profile. Significant decreases of the peak asymmetry are observed for increasing gradient slopes.

Affinity chromatography

Affinity adsorption makes use of specific interactions between a biomolecule and a specific ligand. The binding of a single protein to a bioselective immobilized ligand, in the absence of inhibition effect is represented by the relation:

$$P_{rotein} + L_{igand} \underset{k_{des}}{\overset{k_{ads}}{\rightleftharpoons}} P_{rotein} L_{igand} \tag{24}$$

where P_{rotein} is the protein, L_{igand} the ligand, $P_{rotein} L_{igand}$ the complex and k_{ads}, k_{des} the association and dissociation rate constants, respectively.

A second-order kinetics is often assumed for the binding process:

$$\frac{d\overline{C}}{dt} = k_{ads} C(\overline{C}_{max} - \overline{C}) - k_{des} \overline{C} \tag{25}$$

where $\overline{C}$ and C are the protein concentrations in the stationary and mobile phases, respectively, and $\overline{C}_{max}$ the maximum protein binding capacity.

At equilibrium $d\overline{C}/dt = 0$ and thus Equation (25) yields the Langmuir isotherm:

$$\overline{C} = \frac{\overline{C}_{max} K_L}{1 + K_L C} \tag{26}$$

with $K_L = k_{ads}/k_{des}$ is dependent on the temperature, the pH and the composition of the mobile phase.

A review of chromatographic techniques employed for the determination of the affinity equilibrium binding constants as well as mass transfer parameters was presented by Arnold and coworkers (Arnold *et al.*, 1985a,b; Arnold *et al.*, 1986a,b).

Other special cases of adsorption chromatography

Two additional cases of adsorption chromatography are considered here: immmobilized metal ion affinity chromatography, also called IMAC, and hydroxyapatite chromatography.

IMAC adsorption is based on the coordination between immobilized metal ions (Cu, Zn, Ni) on the surface of an adsorbent and the electron donor groups (histidine, cysteine and tryptophane residue), resident on the protein surface. Using the SMA formalism Vunnun (Vunnum *et al.*, 1995) has developed an equilibrium model accounting for the multipoint attachment of the biomolecule and the steric hindrance of binding sites by adsorbed molecules. However, the masking effect is only significant for the large biomolecules, the small modulator is supposed to have access to all binding sites.

With these hypotheses the adsorption of the target molecule on the IMAC support is represented by the following implicit equation:

$$\overline{C} = K_{eq} C \frac{\left(\Lambda - (\beta + \sigma)\overline{C}\right)^{\beta}}{(1 + K_I I)^{\beta}} \tag{27}$$

where K_I is the adsorption equilibrium constant of the modulator (the other terms have been previously defined).

Equation (27) was used to depict the adsorption of ribonuclease A and myoglobulin on an iminodiacetic resin loaded with Cu^{2+} at various imidazole concentrations (Vunnum *et al.*, 1995). Excellent agreements were found between the experimental data and the model. Hydroxyapatite (HA) is a specific crystalline type of calcium phosphate with amorphous structure, on which proteins interact with anion and cation exchange sites present at the surface of the crystals. A general model of biomolecule adsorption on HA packing has been developed by Kawasaki (Kawasaki, 1991). The model accounts for the competition between the biomolecule and counterion for the adsorbing sites on the surface of the packed bed of HA crystals. It is thought that proteins can simultaneously be adsorbed on the two different ion-exchange sites of HA. On the basis of the competition model, the equilibrium distribution on the solute at infinite dilution can be written as (Kawasaki, 1991):

$$K = \lambda (\varphi I + 1)^{\nu} \tag{28}$$

where λ and φ are thermodynamic constants related to the strength of adsorption of the target molecule and the competing ion, respectively and ν is related to the number of adsorption sites hindered by adsorbed molecules.

Combining Equation (28) with the ideal model for linear gradient elution chromatography, Kawasaki (Kawasaki, 1991) has derived an equation predicting the modulator concentration at the peak maximum for any gradient slope and column length. Excellent agreement was found between data and the predictions of the model for the elution of chicken lysozyme using phosphate gradient as eluant.

Size exclusion chromatography

Size exclusion chromatography refers to the separation of solutes in solution based on their relative sizes and shapes with respect to those of a matrix pores. A large solute tends to be totally excluded from the pore network, whereas smaller solutes can penetrate the pore network to an extent depending on their Stoke radii. A simple empirical relation, also called calibration curve, is often used to describe the equilibrium distribution coefficient as a function of the solute molecular weight:

$$K = p - m \log MW \tag{29}$$

with m, p empirical constants and MW molecular weight.

However, biomolecules are generally flexible polymers of asymmetrical shape. Therefore, the accessibility of the media pore volume is not simply determined by the molecular weight, but depends on the hydrodynamic volume of the molecule. Factors such as mobile phase composition, pH, temperature and ionic strength are known to affect the hydrodynamic volume and, in consequence, the retention of the molecule in SEC (Gorbunov *et al.*, 1988). For many gel filtration media, Equation (29) is only valid within a limited range of molecular weight.

Multicomponent isotherms

Single component isotherms have been derived from different assumptions. However, all of them show a linear relation between mobile phase and stationary phase concentrations at infinite solute dilution, and a maximum solid phase concentration at high mobile phase concentration. They may differ however in the sensitivity of the isotherm parameters to the mobile phase modulator concentration.

The formulation of multicompoment isotherm as simple extension of the single component equilibrium is an important problem in biochromatogaphy, as the number of parameters and experiments required to determine these parameters increase significantly with the number of solutes.

Multicomponent isotherm equations derived from the SDM, SMA and MLI models are presented in Table 16.1 with appropriate references.

An interesting theoretical study of preparative ion-exchange chromatography using the SDM model was presented by Bellot (Bellot and Condoret, 1993). The dependency of the resin selectivity on the loading of the column, as well as displacement effects between proteins have been stressed.

The SMA model was used by Brooks (Brooks and Cramer, 1992) to calculate protein elution profiles and induced salt gradient in displacement chromatography. The chromatogram of α chymotrypsinogen and cytochrome c eluted by a DEAE-dextran displacer from a strong cation exchanger was comparable to the prediction of the model.

The impact of sample load on theoretical gradient elution profile of a binary mixture exhibiting competitive MLI isotherm was presented by Antia (Antia and Horvath, 1989). Theoretical production rate was also calculated under isocratic condition for numerous sample loadings.

Table 16.1 Multicomponent isotherm expressions for ion-exchange, reverse phase and hydrophobic interaction chromatography

Name	Expression		Equation	References
Stoichiometric Displacement Model	$\overline{C}_i = K_{eq,i} C_i \left(\dfrac{\Lambda - \sum\limits_{i=1}^{n} \beta_i \overline{C}_i}{\Lambda} \right)^{\beta_i}$	$i = 1, 2, \ldots n$	(1)	(Bellot and Condoret, 1993)
Steric Mass Action Model	$\overline{C}_i = K_{eq,i} C_i \left(\dfrac{\Lambda - \sum\limits_{i=1}^{n} (\beta_i + \sigma_i) \overline{C}_i}{\Lambda} \right)^{\beta_i}$	$i = 1, 2, \ldots n$	(2)	(Brooks and Cramer, 1992) (Galland et al., 1995)
Modified Langmuir isotherm for ion-exchange chromatography	$\overline{C}_i = \dfrac{\alpha_i I^{-\beta_i} C_i}{1 + \sum\limits_{j=1}^{n} \alpha_j / \gamma_j I^{-\beta_j} C_j}$	$i = 1, 2, \ldots n$	(3)	(Antia and Horvath, 1989) (Whitley et al., 1991)
Modified Langmuir isotherm for ion-exchange chromatography	$\overline{C}_i = \dfrac{\alpha_i I^{-\beta_i} C_i}{1 + \sum\limits_{j=1}^{n} \alpha_j / \gamma_j I^{-\beta'_j} C_j}$	$i = 1, 2, \ldots n$	(4)	(Whitley et al., 1991)
Modified Langmuir isotherm for reverse phase and hydrophobic interaction chromatography	$\overline{C}_i = \dfrac{a_{o,i} e^{-S_i I} C_i}{1 + \sum\limits_{j=1}^{n} a_{o,j} / \overline{C}_{max,j} e^{-S_j I} C_j}$	$i = 1, 2, \ldots n$	(5)	(Antia and Horvath, 1989)

Dynamics of chromatography

Modeling of liquid chromatography is a complex exercise that has to consider simultaneously, the thermodynamics of the phase equilibrium and the kinetics of the phase transfer. Predicting a column behavior requires to solve the model equations using the appropriate model parameters and operating conditions. The model equations include thermodynamic isotherms, mass balance equations, kinetic laws of mass transport and boundary conditions. The model parameters, namely the adsorption isotherm and mass transfer parameters need to be characterized by specific experiments, as *a priori* predictions of their values are still questionable. Specific column techniques have been described for ion-exchange chromatography (Jungbauer and Kaltenbrunner, 1996; Whitley *et al.*, 1991; Yamamoto, 1995, 1987) and reverse phase chromatography (Ford and Ko, 1996; Guiochon *et al.*, 1994).

Historically, three major theories have been developed for the modeling of liquid chromatography: the ideal theory, the plate theory and the rate theory. The ideal model neglects the influence of mass transfer resistances and fluid dynamics and focuses on the thermodynamics of the separation. Although, this theory is too simple to describe the actual operation, it provides an upper limit for the performances of the column. Dispersive effects due to finite rate of phase transfer and fluid dynamics are included in the plate and rate models. In contrast to the rate theory, the plate theory does not distinguish between different sources of dispersion (Li *et al.*, 1995). Accordingly, the rate model is the most complex and rigorous theory of liquid chromatography. The differential equations resulting from the rate theory cannot be solved analytically in closed form and thus numerical methods are invoked. This approach is often complex and requires long computational times. However, for practical applications, a method which offers mathematical simplicity and good predictability will be most useful for rapid parametric surveys of factors affecting process efficiency (Jungbauer, 1996; Mao and Hearn, 1996). Two major approaches have been explored to overcome the complexity of the rate theory (Lightfoot *et al.*, 1995). First, the different contributions to the band broadening can be lumped together into a single and constant apparent dispersion coefficient. Second, the numerical solution of the model can be simplified by assuming a major resistance either in the mobile phase flowing around the packing particles (equilibrium-dispersive model) or in the interphase exchange of solute (kinetic model).

The efficacies of various theoretical models with respect to simplicity of use, precision of the prediction, and validity range are reviewed in the next sections.

Ideal model

The simplest model of liquid chromatography, i.e. the ideal model, is based on the coupling of plug flow and isotherm equations. The ideal model neglects the contribution of mass transfer resistances and axial dispersion to the broadening of a band or a front (Wankat, 1986). Moreover interphase equilibrium is assumed to be instantaneous. Considerable simplifications result from these assumptions, however the ideal model is of limited interest for simulation of biochromatography, except for cases where broadenings of thermodynamic origin are preponderant (Guiochon *et al.*, 1994). Nonetheless, the ideal model is often used for the determination of the equilibrium parameters from column experiments generated under condition of low mass transfer resistance (Guiochon *et al.*, 1994; Yamamoto *et al.*, 1987). Table 16.2 summarizes analytical results derived from the ideal model of liquid chromatography for various modes of operation.

Plate model

In the plate or tank-in-series model, the flow of mobile phase passes through a series of mixing zones in which the solute is in equilibrium. An analytical solution was obtained first for a linear isotherm and an isocratic elution in the form of a Gaussian distribution. The plate model was more recently extended to account for non linear isotherm (Wankat, 1974), gradient elution (Yamamoto *et al.*, 1983), and non equilibrium effects (Mao and Hearn, 1996; Whitley *et al.*, 1991). For the latter the assumption of instantaneous equilibrium is relaxed to the profit of a linear driving force, consisting of a concentration gradient weighted by an overall mass transfer coefficient. The main limitation of the plate model is that mass transfer parameters are difficult to relate to operational variables (Whitley *et al.*, 1991). However the advantages of the plate models are their relative simplicity generating fast numerical solutions as there is no need to calculate the internal particle concentration profile.

Table 16.2 Analytical solutions derived from the ideal model of liquid chromatography

Type of isotherm	Type of elution	Expression	Equation	References
Linear	Isocratic elution	$t_e = t_o(1 + HK)$	(1)	(Wankat, 1986)
Linear ion exchange	Linear gradient elution	$t_e = \dfrac{(\alpha(\beta + 1)g(1 - \varepsilon)V_{column} + I_o{}^{\beta+1})^{\frac{1}{\beta+1}} - I_o}{gF} + t_o$	(2)	(Yamamoto et al., 1987)
Linear reverse phase	Linear gradient elution	$t_e = \dfrac{\ln(a_oSg(1 - \varepsilon)V_{column} + 1)}{SgF} + t_o$	(3)	(Snyder, 1980)
SMA ion exchange	Isocratic elution	Based on the equations of characteristic lines		(Galland et al., 1995)
Mono component Langmuir isotherm	Isocratic elution	$t_r = t_0 + (t_e - t_0)(1 - \sqrt{L_f})^2$ $L_f = (V_sC_o)/(V_{column}(1 - \varepsilon)a/b)$	(4) (5)	(Guiochon et al., 1994)
Two components Langmuir isotherm	Isocratic elution	Based on the shock velocity		(Guiochon et al., 1994)
Multivariant Langmuir	Displacement	Based on the h transform		(Jacobson et al., 1987)

Rate model

The rate model is based on the formulation of differential mass balance equations for the stationary and flowing mobile phases, with appropriate initial and boundary conditions. This theory takes into account the finite rate of mass transfer, the sorption kinetics and the continuous transport of the solute in the mobile phase. For packed-bed column the mass balance for the mobile phase can be written as:

$$\frac{\partial C}{\partial t} + v + u\frac{\partial C}{\partial z} = D_{ax}\frac{\partial^2 C}{\partial t^2},\tag{30}$$

where $\partial C/\partial t$ = accumulation in the mobile phase, v = rate of interface mass transfer, $u\partial C/\partial z$ = transport by convection in the mobile phase, $D_{ax}\partial^2 C/\partial t^2$ = transport by axial dispersion in the mobile phase, C = mobile phase concentration, t = time, u = superficial velocity, z = axial coordinate, D_{ax} = axial dispersion coefficient.

The rate of interface transport may be influenced by four fundamental mass transfer phenomena that occur in a packed-bed of particles. The individual transfer steps are listed below:

- mass transfer from the mobile phase to the external particle surface (boundary-layer resistance)
- intraparticle diffusion in the liquid filled pore (pore diffusion and convection enhanced diffusion)

- intraparticle diffusion in the sorbed state (solid diffusion and surface diffusion)
- adsorption kinetics (reaction kinetics).

In addition, mixing in the liquid phase due to axial diffusion and eddy diffusion is also responsible for slow broadening of eluting band.

All these mass transfer resistances can be explicitly included in the model (Arve and Liapis, 1987; Arve and Liapis, 1988; Berninger *et al.*, 1991), or alternatively a rate limiting step may be attributed to one or two of the resistances (Cowan *et al.*, 1989; Horstmann and Chase, 1989). A review of equations derived from the rate theory is given by Bellot (Bellot and Condoret, 1991) and Yang (Yang and Tsao, 1982).

Empirical and simplified models

The weakness of the rate model is the complexity of the mathematical equations, which are often responsible for intractable problems in the numerical solutions. The following sections present special cases where empirical or simplifed models are applicable.

Frontal chromatography

The rate equation is often simplified by assuming a homogeneous solid phase concentration and by lumping together all the sources of mass transfer resistances. This approximation, called linear driving force, is valid as long as the internal particle concentration profile is parabolic (Do and Rice, 1986; Yao and Tien, 1994).

For frontal chromatography the rate model has been further simplified with the assumption of a constant pattern profile. It is often observed in frontal chromatography with very favorable isotherm, that the profile of the wave front of a single solute reaches a constant profile after a short migration in the column. The constant profile arises because the self sharpening effect of the breakthrough curve, due to the curvature of the isotherm, is balanced by the spreading effects due to the non-equilibrium factors (Vermeulen *et al.*, 1984).

The constant pattern assumption allows considerable simplification of the rate model. Analytical solutions derived from the linear driving force or the constant pattern approximations are listed in Table 16.3.

Gradient-elution chromatography

For the modeling of gradient-elution chromatography with high efficiency packing media, the equilibrium-dispersive model is often used. It is derived from the ideal theory, with the inclusion of some levels of dispersive effects. More specifically, it is assumed that the column is operated under perfect equilibrium state. Therefore the interphase mass transfer kinetics is neglected, but an effective dispersion coefficient, incorporating mass transfer resistances is used in Equation (30) to compensate for this omission. The equilibrium model has been widely accepted for the simulation of non-linear chromatography for both reverse phase (Eble *et al.*, 1987; El Fallah and Guiochon, 1992) and ion-exchange interaction (Jungbauer and Kaltenbrunner, 1996; Yamamoto, 1995).

Table 16.3 Analytical solutions for breakthrough curves derived from constant pattern approximations and kinetic models

Limiting step	Assumption	Kinetic Law	Constant pattern profile	Equation	References
Liquid film	Constant pattern and linear driving force	$\dfrac{\partial \bar{C}}{\partial t} = k_f(C - C^*)$	$E - 1 = \dfrac{1}{N_f}\,\dfrac{\ln X - R\ln(1-X)+1}{1-R}$	(1)	(Vermeulen et al., 1984)
Solid film	Constant pattern and linear driving force	$\dfrac{\partial \bar{C}}{\partial t} = k_s(\bar{C}^* - \bar{C})$	$E - 1 = \dfrac{1}{N_s}\,\dfrac{R\ln X - \ln(1-X)-1}{1-R}$	(2)	(Vermeulen et al., 1984)
Solid film and liquid film	Irreversible isotherm and linear driving force	$\dfrac{\partial \bar{C}}{\partial t} = k_s(\bar{C}^* - \bar{C}) = k_f(C - C^*)$	depends upon residence time and equilibrium capacity	(3)	(Fernandez et al., 1996)
Reaction kinetics	Constant pattern	$\dfrac{\partial \bar{C}}{\partial t} = k_{ads}C(\bar{C}_{max} - \bar{C}) - k_{des}\bar{C}$	$E - 1 = \dfrac{1}{N_k}\,\dfrac{\ln X - \ln(1-X)}{1-R}$	(4)	(Vermeulen et al., 1984)
Reaction kinetics	Langmuir isotherm	$\dfrac{\partial \bar{C}}{\partial t} = k_{ads}C(\bar{C}_{max} - \bar{C}) - k_{des}\bar{C}$	Thomas solution		(Guiochon et al., 1994)
Pore diffusion and liquid film	Irreversible isotherm and fickian diffusion	$\dfrac{\partial \bar{C}}{\partial t} = \dfrac{D_e}{r^2}\dfrac{\partial}{\partial r}\left[r^2\dfrac{\partial \bar{C}}{\partial r}\right]$	$E - 1 = \left(\dfrac{1}{N_p} + \dfrac{1}{N_f}\right)\left\{\dfrac{\phi(X)+N_p/N_f(\ln X+1)}{(N_p/N_f)+1}\right\}$	(5)	(Vermeulen et al., 1984) (Arnold et al., 1985) (Yamamoto and Sano, 1992)

The one-dimensional continuity equation resulting from the equilibrium-dispersive model can be solved with a backward-forward finite difference technique. This implementation is exactly equivalent to the discontinuous flow plate theory, referred to as Craig model (Guiochon *et al.*, 1994).

The Craig model describes the column as a series of N plates in which a local equilibrium is achieved. After the equilibrium is reached in the nth plate the mobile phase is transferred to the next plate and replaced by the mobile phase coming from the previous plate. Therefore, the process is represented as a series of mobile phase transfer and equilibrium. The mass balance equations lead to the following recursive relations (one for the modulator and one for each protein) which can be solved iteratively in each stage.

Mass balance for a protein in stage I:

$$C_i^t = \frac{C_{i-1}^{t-1} + HK_i^{t-1}(C,I)\,C_i^{t-1}}{1 + HK_i^t(C,I)} \quad \text{for i = 1, N} \tag{31}$$

Mass balance for the modulator in stage I:

$$I_i^t = \frac{I_{i-1}^{t-1} + HK_{modulator}I_i^{t-1}}{1 + HK_{modulator}} \quad \text{for i = 1, N} \tag{32}$$

with C = protein concentration in the mobile phase, I = modulator concentration in the mobile phase, t = time increment, i = stage increment, H = phase ratio, K = component distribution coefficient.

With this model, peak spreading due to mass transfer resistances is accounted for by a lumped dispersion coefficient proportional to the column Hetp. Furthermore, the plate number of the continuous flow theory is related to the number of Craig stage and distribution coefficient as (Guiochon *et al.*, 1994):

$$N_{plate} = \frac{1 + HK}{HK} N_{Craig} \tag{33}$$

where N_{Craig} = number of Craig plate, N_{plate} = number of plate.

The mass balance equations are used in conjunction with an isotherm equation that relates the protein concentration in the stationary phase to the protein and salt concentrations in the mobile phase.

For example, substituting the MLI isotherm Equation (16) into Equation (31), one obtains an analytical solution describing the protein concentration in the column stage i. Note that when the loading is moderate, the elution curves show a geometrically similar profile indicating the absence of a shock front in the column.

Applications of computer-aided simulation of biochromatography

A successful route for rational process design and optimization includes four stages. First, mass transfer and thermodynamic parameters are extracted from simple small scale laboratory experiments, using fitting procedures. Second, the validity of the theoritical model and the numerical values of its parameters are assessed by comparing some simulation results with experimental chromatograms. Third, optimization is performed by investigating the influence of process variables with the model and validating the best configurations with experimental data. Last, predictive data on large-scale are investigated in terms of risks, performances and costs.

Experimental case studies

In the next sections application examples of theoretical models to practical optimization problems relative to ion-exchange and affinity chromatography are presented.

(a) Ion-exchange chromatography A challenge to the preparative ion-exchange chromatography optimization is to define the elution conditions that lead to the required purity and productivity, on a large-scale, with the maximum confidence in the process robustness. This challenge can be efficiently met with a simulation model. In the following example, the impact of gradient profile and composition on purity, productivity and dilution factor is assessed with the equilibrium-dispersive model. The sample protein employed in this study is bovine carbonic anhydrase. This sample is composed of at least two isozymes with a pI of 5.4 and 5.9. The enzyme concentration and the sample volume were respectively 1 mg/ml and 0.3 ml.

The sorbent, DEAE HyperD™ F from Biosepra (Cergy, France) was packed in a 10 cm (length) by 0.5 cm (diameter) column according to the manufacturer recommendation. The nominal particle diameter is 35 μm.

The mobile phase was a 50 mM Tris–HCl buffer solution (pH 8.7). Linear gradient elutions were performed by increasing sodium chloride concentration from 0 to 0.3 M. After each elution, the column was washed with 1 M sodium chloride followed by 0.5 M sodium hydroxide and reequilibrated with 50 mM Tris–HCl buffer (pH 8.7).

The experiments were controlled by an automatic chromatographic workstation, called PROSYS™ (Biosepra). The UV adsorption (280 nm) and the conductivity of the column effluent were monitored and saved on the PROSYS™ personnel computer. Data analysis, non linear regression, and simulation were performed with the appropriate PROSYS™ software.

The simulations are based on the dispersive-equilibrium model Equation (31) used in conjunction with the MLI isotherm Equation (16).

The isotherm parameters α and β are estimated with a procedure proposed by Yamamoto (Yamamoto *et al.*, 1983). Using the ideal model a simple relationship can be established between the gradient slope and the elution molarity (modulator concentration at the peak maximum):

$$\int_{I_0}^{I_r} \frac{dI}{\alpha I^{-\beta} - K_{modulator}} = g\,(1 - \varepsilon)\,V_{column} \tag{34}$$

with Ir = elution molarity, I_0 = starting modulator concentration, g = gradient slope, ε = packed-bed porosity, V_{column} = column volume.

A fitting of the experimental gradient slopes and elution molarities to Equation (34), allows the determination of the isotherm parameters α and β. The integral in Equation (34) is evaluated with a quadrature method.

The isotherm parameter γ is simply the maximum column capacity. It is determined by frontal analysis. The number of plates is determined by analyzing the isocratic elution curve of a pulse, under non binding conditions, using the moment method.

Based on Equation (34), the isotherm parameters α and β were determined from linear gradient elution curves. The fit of the data g vs Ir to Equation (34) is shown in Fig. 16.2a. Calculated isotherms are shown on Fig. 16.2b and fitted parameters are summarized in Table 16.4. In order to test the accuracy of the method, distribution coefficients were also determined from isocratic elution using the following equation derived from the ideal model:

$$K = \frac{V_{elution} - V_{column}}{V_o - V_{column}}, \tag{35}$$

where $V_{elution}$ = elution volume of the protein, V_{column} = column volume, V_o = column dead volume.

Data obtained from isocratic runs and linear gradient elutions are superimposed in Fig. 16.2b. A good agreement is found between the two methods.

The column capacity determined by frontal analysis, at 295 cm/h, was 67 mg/ml. Column hetp determined at 1, 2 and 4 ml/min were respectively 6, 8, and 10 mm. In the simulation runs, the hetp of the two isozymes was assumed to be equivalent. Figure 16.3 shows some typical experimental and simulated elution profiles. The parameters used in the simulations were those determined from the isotherm experiments together with the column HETP. No fitted data were used in the simulations. Agreements between the predicted and the experimental elution curves are excellent. For the steepest gradient

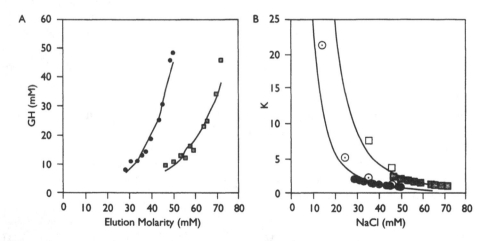

Figure 16.2 Determination of the isotherm parameters α and β for bovine carbonic anhydrase isozymes (resin = DEAE HyperD™ F, buffer = 50 mM Tris–HCl pH 8.7 + NaCl). (A) Dimensionless gradient slope GH = g(1 − ε) V column vs Elution Molarity (component 1: ○, component 2: □, line regression fit calculated from the ideal model – Equation 34). (B) Component distribution coefficients vs modulator concentration (⊙: data from isocratic elution for component 1, ●: data from linear gradient elution for component 1, □: data from isocratic elution for component 2, ▣: data from linear gradient elution for component 2, line calculated from the SDM model Equation 7).

Table 16.4 Isotherm parameters for bovine car-
bonic anhydrase isozymes on DEAE
HyperD™ F (buffer = 50 mM Tris–
HCl pH 8.7 + NaCl)

	α	β
Peak 1	4.74e-06	2.17
Peak 2	1.23e-06	2.61

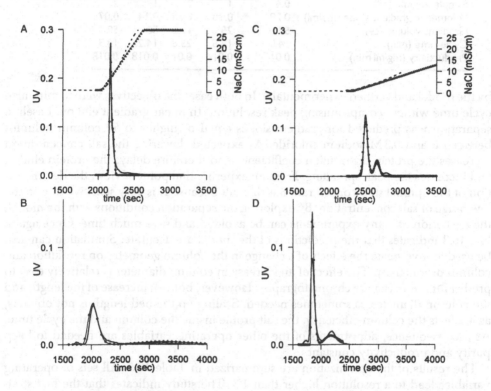

Figure 16.3 Linear and isocratic gradient elution of bovine carbonic anhydrase isozymes (resin = DEAE
HyperD™ F, buffer = 50 mM Tris–HCl pH 8.7+NaCl); comparison between experimental
data and simulations using the equilibrium dispersive model and the modified Langmuir
isotherm: Equations (31) and (16) (Actual UV: ——, actual conductivity: - - - -, predicted
UV: —●—, predicted conductivity: —▲—). (A) 10 min linear gradient elution using 50 mM
Tris–HCl pH 8.7 + 0–0.3 M NaCl at 1 ml/min. (B) 60 min linear gradient elution using
50 mM Tris–HCl pH 8.7 + 0–0.3 M NaCl at 1 ml/min. (C) Isocratic elution using 50 mM
Tris–HCl pH 8.7 + 2 mM NaCl at 1 ml/min. (D) Isocratic elution using 50 mM Tris–HCl
pH 8.7 + 3.4 mM NaCl at 1 ml/min.

slope, the separation between the two peaks is extremely poor. At the smallest gradient
slope, the resolution between the two peak is about 1.15.

Improvement of the separation between the two components was investigated with
the model. First, the steepest gradient slope leading to baseline separation was determined by simulation. Second, the change from gradient to step elution was investigated

Table 16.5 Comparison of two scale-up strategies for linear gradient ion exchange chromatography (strategy 1: constant volumetric gradient slope and constant flow rate, strategy 2: constant gradient volume relative to the column volume and constant residence time)

	Base case	Strategy 1		Strategy 2	
Column length (cm)	10	20	40	20	40
Column volume (ml)	1.96	3.93	7.85	3.93	7.85
Flow rate (ml/min)	1	1	1	2	4
Sample volume (ml)	0.4	1	2	1	2
Volumetric gradient slope (mS/ml)	0.28	0.28	0.28	0.14	0.07
Gradient volume (cv)	50	25	12.5	50	50
Cycle time (min)	14.0	18.5	25.8	14.2	14.3
Productivity (mg/ml min)	0.018	0.014	0.01	0.018	0.018

by the model and verified experimentally. In both cases the objectives were to minimize cycle time without compromising peak resolution. In linear gradient elution, baseline separation was predicted for gradient slopes equal or higher to 50 column volumes between 0 and 0.3 M sodium chloride. As expected, lowering the salt concentration increases the protein distribution coefficients, and therefore delays the protein elution and increases the peak spreading. From an experimental point of view, the determination of the optimal step concentration is difficult because K is very sensitive to I, in the low range of salt concentration. By exploring the separation conditions with the model, the execution of many experiments can be avoided and save much time. Once again, Fig. 16.3 indicates that the predictions of the model are accurate. Simulation can also be used to investigate the effects of a change in the column geometry on resolution and column productivity. The effect of an increase in column diameter is relatively easy to predict for ion-exchange chromatography. However, both an increase of the length and the column diameter, is sometimes needed. Scaling-up the bed length is not obvious, as it affects the column efficiency, the salt profile inside the column and the cycle time. As a consequence, adjustments of the other operating variables are needed to keep purity and productivity constant.

The results of the optimization are summarized in Table 16.5. All sets of operating variables lead to a resolution higher than 1.3. The study indicates that the first strategy, based on constant volumetric gradient slope, leads to a decrease of the column productivity. Optimum scale-up in column length can be achieved with the second strategy, where column loading, the residence time, and the gradient volume (defined in terms of column volume) are kept constant. One potential drawback of the second approach is the increase in the column pressure drop. However, modern media and LC instruments are designed to withstand high pressure.

(b) Optimization of a capture step using affinity chromatography The efficiency of a capture step based on strong affinity interaction, is predominally controlled by thermodynamic factors which are difficult to predict with a model. Most often the column selectivity is modulated by varying the adsorption, washing and elution conditions. However, the column performances, defined in term of protein weight or unit produced per unit of time and resin volume, can be readily optimized with the adequate model.

The sample protein used in this study in human polyclonal IgG dissolved at 10 mg/ml in a phosphate buffered saline solution at pH 7.4. The following columns and packing media were used: Protein A HyperD™ F (Biosepra, Cergy) packed in a 6.6 mm column of various lengths (50 to 230 mm). The columns were first equilibrated in the phosphate buffered saline solution pH 7.4, then the protein solutions were loaded onto the column. Next, the columns were washed by a 0.5 M sodium chloride in phosphate buffered saline solution pH 7.4 and eluted by 0.1 M citrate buffer pH 2.5.

Affinity chromatography is often used as a capture step for the selective concentration of a target molecule. Purification factors as high as 1000 are obtained with this technique, however cost constraints have offered serious incentives to optimize the operating conditions of preparative affinity chromatography. In particular column productivity, defined as the amount of target protein purify by unit of time and unit of column volume, must be increased by either increasing the column loading or decreasing the purification time (Yamamoto et al., 1992). This problem has become more stringent with the recent emergence of mechanically stable packing media, designed to withstand high pressure drop resulting from fast linear velocity. Rapid and efficient insight in the factors affecting the column productivity can be provided by the simulation of the chromatographic separation.

Affinity processes are performed in a frontal mode, with large loading of the column. The purification is primarily achieved by the high selectivity of the media for the target molecule. Most of the contaminants are eliminated during a washing step, followed by the selective elution of the target molecule achieved by a drastic change in the thermodynamic conditions. As affinity adsorption isotherms are very favorable, the loading phase has often been described with good approximation by the constant pattern approximation (Arnold et al., 1985a; Yamamoto and Sano, 1992).

For example, Fig. 16.4 shows the uptake of IgG onto a ProteinA HyperD™ F column at two linear velocities. The experimental curves are fitted with Equation (2) – Table 16.3, from which the number of transfer units and the equilibrium capacity can be determined. Note that other constant pattern models provide an equally good fit, and therefore the intrinsic mass transfer mechanism cannot be deduced from this experiment.

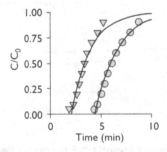

Figure 16.4 Human IgG breakthrough curve on ProteinA HyperD™ F (protein concentration = 10 mg/ml in phosphate buffered saline solution pH 7.4, column diameter = 1.13 cm, column volume = 5.05 ml, flow rate = 2.8 ml/min (◎), flow rate = 4.7 ml/min (▽). Lines calculated with the solid film constant pattern model (Equation (2), Table 16.3).

For preparative applications the loading of the column must be as high as possible, but should not lead to significant loss of the target protein. Typically column loading is stopped when the effluent concentration reaches 1 to 10% of the starting concentration. The amount of protein loaded to the column at this breakthrough point, called dynamic capacity is calculated from the following expression:

$$DBC_{x\%} = C_o \left(\frac{V_{x\%} - \varepsilon V_{column}}{V_{column}} \right) \tag{36}$$

with $DBC_{x\%}$ = dynamic capacity determined at x% breakthrough point, C_o = feed concentration, $V_{x\%}$ = breakthrough volume determined at x% breakthrough point, ε = packed-bed porosity, V_{column} = column volume.

Due to the increase in mass transfer resistances the dynamic binding capacity decreases with an increase in the linear velocity. The constant pattern approximation was used to describe the variation of experimental dynamic capacities at 10 and 50% with linear velocities for 3 bed heights. Figure 16.5 shows the experimental data and the calculated curves obtained by fitting all the experimental points to the model (Equation (2) Table 16.3).

Good agreement between the model and the data is found except for very high velocity and short column, where the assumption of constant pattern may not be

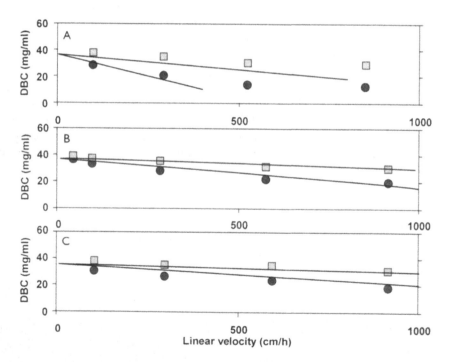

Figure 16.5 Dynamic human IgG binding capacity onto ProteinA HyperD™ F (capacities determined at 10% (●) and 50% (▨) breakthrough points, protein concentration = 10 mg/ml in phosphate buffered saline solution pH 7.4, column diameter = 0.66 cm, column length a = 5 cm, b = 15 cm, c = 23 cm). Lines calculated with the solid film constant pattern model (Equation (2), Table 16.3).

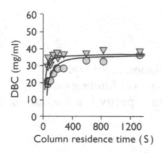

Figure 16.6 Effect of the column residence time on ProteinA HyperD™ F dynamic binding capacity (capacities determined at 10% (●) and 50% (▼) breakthrough points, protein concentration = 10 mg/ml in phosphate buffered saline solution pH 7.4, column diameter = 0.66 cm, column length = 5, 15 and 23 cm). Lines calculated with the solid film constant pattern model (Equation (2), Table 16.3).

valid. A validity criterion for constant pattern approximation has been proposed by Vermeulen (Vermeulen *et al.*, 1984). The data were consolidated in Fig. 16.6 that shows the experimental and calculated dynamic capacity vs the column residence time. Figure 16.6 indicates that to maintain a given dynamic capacity, linear velocity must be decreased with the concomitant decrease of the bed height. The column productivity is defined as the amount of protein eluted from the packing media divided by the media volume and the processing time. It is given by the following equation:

$$P = \frac{Q_{eluted}}{V_{column} \times T_{cycle}}, \tag{37}$$

where P is the column productivity, Q_{eluted} the amount of protein eluted from the column and T_{cycle} the processing time corresponding to a complete cycle.

Q_{eluted} is readily determined from:

$$Q_{eluted} = R_{elution} \left(Q_{load} - Q_{wasted} \right) \tag{38}$$

where $R_{elution}$ is the elution recovery, Q_{load}, the amount of protein loaded onto the column and Q_{wasted} the amount lost during the loading phase.

The elution recovery accounts for protein loss during the washing and elution step. The amount of protein loaded is simply the product of the dynamic binding capacity and the column volume. Similarly the amount lost during the loading phase can be defined as the product of a dynamic discarded quantity and the column volume, where the dynamic discarded quantity is:

$$DDQ_{x\%} = \frac{\int_0^{V_{x\%}} C\, dV}{V_{column}} \tag{39}$$

where $DDQ_{x\%}$ = dynamic discarded quantity determined at x% breakthrough point, C = effluent concentration, $V_{x\%}$ = breakthrough volume, V_{column} = column volume. The adsorption recovery ($R_{adsorption}^{X\%}$) can be calculated directly from Equations (36) and (39) as follows:

$$R_{\text{adsorption}}^{X\%} = 1 - \frac{DDQ_{X\%}}{DBC_{X\%}}. \tag{40}$$

The overall recovery is the product of adsorption and elution recovery.

Capture efficiency $(E_{X\%})$ defined as the ratio of the dynamic binding capacity determined at a given breakthrough point to the equilibrium capacity is a measure of the utilization of the media capacity.

$$E_{X\%} = \frac{DBC_{X\%}}{Qo}. \tag{41}$$

Dynamic binding capacity and dynamic discarded quantity are fully defined by the profile of the breakthrough curve which in turn depends on mass transfer and equilibrium parameters. The total processing time is the sum of the different steps that composed a cycle: loading, washing, elution and reequilibration time as indicated in Equation (42):

$$T_{\text{cycle}} = T_{\text{load}} + T_{\text{wash}} + T_{\text{elution}} + T_{\text{reequilibration}}. \tag{42}$$

It can be rearranged as follows:

$$T_{\text{cycle}} = t_{\text{res}} \left(\frac{DBC_{x\%}}{C_o} + \sum_{\text{step}} N_{\text{step}} A_{\text{step}} \right) \tag{43}$$

where t_{res} = column residence time, N_{step} = number of column volume needed to complete a given step, A_{step} = ratio of the step flow rate to the loading flow rate.

Although the loading time is dependent on the profile of the breakthrough curve, the other steps can be defined as dimensionless packed-bed volume weighted by a flow ratio. In other words it is assumed these steps are performed under an ideal equilibrium state.

Insertion of Equations (36), (38), (39) and (43) in Equation (37) yields:

$$P = \frac{R_{\text{elution}} \left(DBC_{x\%} - DDQ_{x\%} \right)}{t_{\text{res}} \left(DBC_{x\%}/C_o + \sum_{\text{step}} N_{\text{step}} A_{\text{step}} \right)} \tag{44}$$

As shown in Fig. 16.4, breakthrough curve of very favorable adsorption, such as IgG uptake on proteinA HyperD™, can be depicted with a constant pattern model. In consequence, dynamic binding capacity and dynamic discarded quantity are readily calculated from analytical solutions of constant pattern profiles (Table 16.3), for any operating variables including column length, column diameter, linear velocity, feed concentration and breakthrough point. The impact of the operating variables on the column productivity, and recovery are given by Equations (44) and (40), respectively.

Figure 16.7 shows the concomitant influence of linear velocity and breakthrough point ending column loading on productivity, recovery and capture efficiency using the solid diffusion model in conjunction with model parameters extracted from Fig. 16.6.

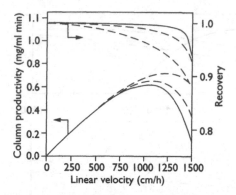

Figure 16.7 Productivity and adsorption recovery for a human IgG-ProteinA HyperD™ F column for various breakthrough point (——— 5%, · · · · 10% – – – – 20%, column length = 15, protein concentration = 1 mg/ml-buffer for wash elute and regenerate step = 10 cv. The productivity and the adsorption recovery are calculated with Equations (44), (40) and (2) from Table 16.3.

Clearly column productivity exhibits a maximum for a certain linear velocity value. This behavior was previously reported by Yamamoto (Yamamoto and Sano, 1992) and Mao (Mao and Hearn, 1996) for ion-exchange and affinity chromatographic processes. Moreover, the productivity increases with the increasing terminating effluent concentration, for velocities approaching or higher than the optimum velocity, but to the detriment of the overall recovery and capture efficiency.

As shown in Fig. 16.8 productivity is also a strong function of the protein concentration in the feed, as the time needed to saturate the column decreases with an increase of the protein in the feed solution.

It is also noteworthy that the model predicts an increase in the optimal linear velocity with increasing bed height, however their ratio is constant, as there is a unique optimum residence time. This concept may be of use for scaling-up a separation. However, it should be pointed-out that doubling the column length while preserving the residence time leads to four folds increase of the pressure drop.

Review of simulation software

Several simulation packages specifically developed for liquid chromatography have been available from commercial organizations or universities. Prosys™ (Biosepra) is an automatic liquid chromatographic system combined with software for automatic evaluation of model parameters, simulation of packed-bed elution chromatography, and scaling-up. The simulation software is based on the equilibrium-dispersive model and the modified Langmuir equation. The scale-up algorithm is based on the constant pattern approximation with pore diffusion as limiting step and includes user defined constaints such as pressure drop or batch duration. Alternative large-scale designs are compared in term of column performances and processing costs.

Dry Lab™ (LC Resources, USA) is intented for the optimization of analytical reverse phase separations, allowing rapid scouting of gradient profiles as well as of the processing temperature.

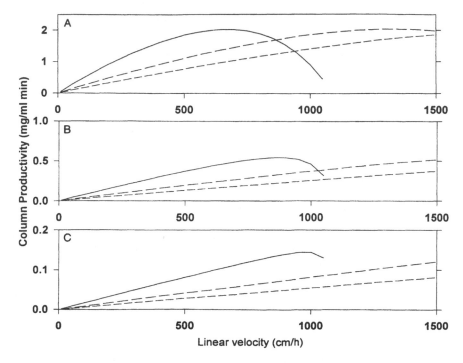

Figure 16.8 Impact of human IgG feed concentration, bed height and linear velocity on the productivity of ProteinA HyperD™ F column. Feed concentration: a = 5 mg/ml, b = 0.5 mg/ml, c = 0.1 mg/ml, column length: —— 10 cm, ···· = 20 cm, — — —— = 30 cm, breakthrough point = 10%, buffer for wash elute and regenerate step = 5 cv, the productivity is calculated with Equation (44). Lines calculated with the solid film constant pattern model (Equation (2), Table 16.3). The productivity is calculated with Equations (44) and (2) from Table 16.3.

Simulus (AEA Technology, UK) software package includes programs for the fitting of parameters and the simulation of batch, packed-bed and fluidized-bed adsorption column. Different algorithms are proposed including a rigourous pore diffusion rate model. Additionally, complex softwares are available from the academic experts. For example, the Versatile Reaction Separation model, also called Verse-LC (Berninger *et al.*, 1991) allows the addition of kinetics modules to a general rate model. PC software based on empirical and simplifed theories of preparative batch and column adsorption are also available from their authors (Mao and Hearn, 1996).

Concluding remarks

In this chapter, biopolymer adsorption/desorption behavior and mass-transport in liquid biochromatography supports have been examined. Significant developments have been achieved in chromatography theories from the equilibrium and mass transfer perspectives. Today, realistic and relatively fast predictions of column performances are attainable, opening the way for the robust and rational process optimization.

However, biopolymer adsorption has not yet received a definitive analysis and relatively sparse experimental information is available, rendering *a priori* prediction impossible. In this situation, simulation is completely dependent on the initial small-scale laboratory experiments. Given the projection that an increasing number of recombinant products will be developed from a limited number of expression systems, there is a need to improve our understanding of thermodynamics of adsorption and also to characterize the sorption behavior of the major contaminants resulting from each expression system.

Moreover the complexity of purification processes should not be overlooked. Stringent requirements relative to contaminant level, target molecule purity and activity, requisite multi-steps high resolution separation techniques that present tremendous challenges in term of modeling, simulation and overall process optimization.

Acknowledgments

The author thanks Dr L. Guerrier and Dr A. Schwarz for providing experimental data and also Dr E. Boschetti for his valuable comments during the preparation of this manuscript.

Notations

α'	Langmuir–Freunlich isotherm parameter
β'	Langmuir–Freunlich isotherm parameter
α	modified Langmuir isotherm parameter
γ	modified Langmuir isotherm parameter
ε	packed-bed porosity
β	isotherm parameter or characteristic charge of the protein
ν	related to the number of adsorption sites hindered by adsorbed molecules
σ	steric hindrance factor of the protein
Λ	ionic capacity of the resin (total number of charge/unit volume of resin)
φ	thermodynamic constants related to the strength of adsorption of the target molecule and the competing ion
$\phi(X)$	$2.44 + 3.66(1 - X)^{0.5}$
a	Langmuir isotherm parameter
$a_o = a_{I=0\,M}$	value of isotherm slope for $I = 0\,M$ for reverse phase
$a_{I=1\,M}$	value of isotherm slope for $I = 1\,M$ for hydrophobic interaction chromatography
A_{step}	ratio of the step flow rate to the loading flow rate
b	Langmuir isotherm parameter (equivalent to K_L)
$\overline{C}_{max}$	maximum protein binding capacity
$\overline{C}^*$	stationary phase concentration in equilibrium with C
$\overline{C}$	protein concentration in the stationary phase
C	protein concentration in the mobile phase
C^*	stationary phase concentration in equilibrium with $\overline{C}^*$
Co	feed concentration

$C_{ounterion}$	counterion molecule
D_e	effective diffusion coefficient
D_{ax}	axial dispersion coefficient
$DBC_{x\%}$	dynamic capacity at $X_\%$ breakthrough point
$DDQ_{x\%}$	dynamic discarded quantity at $X_\%$ breakthrough point
$E_{X\%}$	capture efficiency or dimensionless throughout volume
F	flow rate
g	gradient slope
$Hetp$	height equivalent to a theoretical plate
H	phase ratio
$\bar{I}$	modulator concentration in the stationary phase or number of counterions adsorbed and available for exchange
$\hat{I}$	number of counterions sterically hindered by the adsorbed proteins
I	modulator concentration in the mobile phase
i	stage increment
Io	starting modulator concentration
Ir	elution molarity
I_t	total number of counterions adsorbed to the resin
K	component distribution coefficient
k_f	liquid film mass transfer coefficient
k_s	solid film mass transfer coefficient
k_{ads}	association rate constant
k_{des}	dissociation rate constant
K_{eq}	equilibrium constant
K_I	modulator adsorption equilibrium constant
K_L	Langmuir isotherm parameter (equivalent to b)
L_{igand}	ligand
L_f	loading ratio
m	size exclusion chromatography isotherm parameter
MW	molecular weight
N_{Craig}	number of Craig plate
N_{plate}	number of plate
N_p, N_f, N_s, N_k	number of transfer unit for pore, fluid, particle and kinetics rate limiting steps
N_{step}	number of column volume needed to complete a given step
p	size exclusion chromatography isotherm constant
P	column productivity
P_{rotein}	protein molecule
$P_{rotein}L_{igand}$	protein ligand complex
Q_{eluted}	amount of protein eluted from the column
Q_{load}	amount of protein loaded onto the column
Q_{wasted}	amount lost during the loading phase
r	particle radius
R	separation factor
$R_{adsorption}$	adsorption recovery
$R_{elution}$	elution recovery

R_{esin}	ion-exchanger
S	isotherm parameter
t	time
t_e	elution time
t_o	holdup time
t_r	elution time of a front
T_{cycle}	cycle time
T_{elute}	elute time
T_{load}	load time
$T_{reequilibration}$	reequilibration time
t_{res}	column residence time
T_{wash}	wash time
u	superficial velocity
v	rate of interface mass transfer
V_{column}	column volume
$V_{elution}$	elution volume
V_S	sample volume
Vo	column dead volume
$V_{x\%}$	breakthrough volume at $X_\%$ breakthrough point
$X_\%$	dimensionless concentration (C/C_0)
z	axial coordinate

References

Antia, F. and Horvath, C. (1989) Gradient elution in non-linear preparative liquid chromatography. *J. Chromatogr.*, **484**, 1–27.

Arnold, F., Blanch, H. and Wilke, C. (1985a) Analysis of affinity separations I: predicting the performance of affinity adsorbers. *Chem. Eng. J.*, **30**, B9–B23.

Arnold, F., Blanch, H. and Wilke, C. (1985b) Analysis of affinity separations II: the characterization of affinity columns by pulse techiques. *Chem. Eng. J.*, **30**, B25–B36.

Arnold, F., Schofield, S. and Blanch, H. (1986a) Analytical affinity chromatography I: local equilibrium theory and the measurement of association and inhibition constants. *J. Chromatogr.*, **355**, 1–12.

Arnold, F., Schofield, S. and Blanch, H. (1986b) Analytical affinity chromatography II: rate theory and measurement of biological binding kinetics. *J. Chromatogr.*, **355**, 13–27.

Arve, B. and Liapis, A. (1987) The modeling and analysis of the elution stage of biospecific of biospecific adsorption in fixed beds. *Biotechnol. Bioeng.*, **30**, 638–649.

Arve, B. and Liapis, A. (1988) Adsorption in fixed bed and periodic countercurrent beds. *Biotechnol. Bioeng.*, **32**, 616–627.

Bellot, J. and Condoret, J. (1991) Liquid chromatography modelling: a review. *Process Biochem.*, **26**, 363–376.

Bellot, J. and Condoret, J. (1993) Theoretical study of the ion-exchange preparative chromatography of a two-protein mixture. *J. Chromatogr.*, **635**, 1–17.

Berninger, J., Whitley, R., Zhang, X. and Wang, N. (1991) A versatile model for simulation of reaction and nonlinear equilibrium dynamics in multicomponent fixed bed adsorption process. *Comput. Chem. Eng.*, **15**, 749–768.

Bouhallab, S., Henry, G. and Boschetti, E. (1996) Separation of small cationic bioactive peptides by strong ion exchange chromatography. *J. Chromatogr. A*, **724**, 137–145.

Brooks, C. A. and Cramer, S. (1992) Steric mass action ion exchange: displacement profiles and induced salt gradients. *AIChE J.*, **38(12)**, 1969–1978.

Coffman, J., Roper, K. and Lightfoot, E. (1994) High resolution chromatography of proteins in short columns and adsorptive membranes. *Bioseparations,* **4**, 183–200.

Cowan, G., Gosling, I. and Sweetenham, W. (1989) Modeling methods to aid the design and optimization of batch stirred tank and packed bed column adsorption and chromatography units. *J. Chromatogr.*, **484**, 187–210.

Cysewski, P., Jaulmes, A., Lemque, R., Sebille, B., Vidal-Madjar, C. and Jilge, C. (1991) Multivalent ion-exchange model of biopolymer chromatography for mass overload conditions. *J. Chromatogr.*, **548**, 61–79.

Do, D. and Rice, R. (1986) Validity of parabolic profile assumption in adsorption studies. *AIChE J.*, **32**, 149–154.

Eble, J., Grob, R., Antle, P. and Snyder, L. (1987) Simplified decription of HPLC separation under overload conditions based on the Craig distribution model. *J. Chromatogr.*, **384**, 25–44.

El Fallah, Z. and Guiochon, G. (1992) Prediction of protein band profile in preparative reversed-phase gradient elution chromatography. *Biotechnol. Bioeng.*, **39**, 877–885.

Fernandez, A. and Carta, G. (1996) Characterization of protein adsorption by composite silica-polyacrylamide gel anion-exchangers I: equilibrium and mass transfer in agitated contactors. *J. Chromatogr. A*, **746**, 169–183.

Fernandez, A., Laughinghouse, S. and Carta, G. (1996) Characterization of protein adsorption by composite silica-polyacrylamide gel anion-exchangers II: mass transfer in packed columns and predictability of breakthrough behavior. *J. Chromatogr. A*, **746**, 185–198.

Ford, J. and Ko, J. (1996) Comparison of methods for extracting linear solvent strength gradient parameters from gradient chromotagraphic data. *J. Chromatogr. A*, **727**, 1–11.

Galland, S., Kundu, A. and Cramer, S. (1995) Modeling non-linear elution of proteins in ion-exchange chromatography. *J. Chromatogr. A*, **702**, 125–142.

Gerstner, J., Bell, J. and Cramer, S. (1994) Gibbs free energy of adsorption for biomolecules in ion-exchange systems. *Biophys. Chem.*, **52**, 97–106.

Gorbunov, A., Solovyova, L. and Pasechnik, V. (1988) Fundamentals of the theory and pratice of polymer gel permeation chromatography as a method of chromatographic porosimetry. *J. Chromatogr.*, **448**, 307–332.

Guiochon, G., Golshan-Shirazi, S. and Katti, K. (1994) *Fundamentals of Preparative and Non Linear Chromatography*, Academic Press, New York.

Horstmann, B. and Chase, H. (1989) Modelling the affinity adsorption of immunoglobulin G to protein A immobilised to agarose matrices. *Chem. Eng. Res. Des.*, **67**, 243–254.

Jacobson, J., Frenz, J. and Horvath, C. (1987) Measurement of competitive adsorption isotherms by frontal chromatography. *Ind. Eng. Chem. Res.*, **26**, 43–50.

James, E. and Do, D. (1991) Equilibria of biomolecules on ion-exchange adsorbents. *J. Chromatogr.*, **542**, 19–28.

Jungbauer, A. (1996) Insights into the chromatography of proteins provided by mathematical modeling. *Current Opinion in Biotechnology*, **7**, 210–218.

Jungbauer, A. and Kaltenbrunner, O. (1996) Fundamental questions in optimizing ion-exchange chromatography of proteins using computer-aided process design. *Biotechnol. Bioeng.*, **52**, 223–236.

Kaltenbrunner, O. and Jungbauer, A. (1996) Adsorption isotherms in protein chromatography. Combined influence of protein and salt concentration on adsorption isotherm. *J. Chromatogr. A*, **734**, 183–194.

Kawasaki, T. (1991) Hydroxyapatite as a liquid chromatography packing. *J. Chromatogr.*, **544**, 147–184.

Kopaciewicz, W., Rounds, M., Fausnaugh, J. and Regnier, F. (1983) Retention model for high-performance ion exchange chromatography. *J. Chromatogr.*, **266**, 3–21.

Li, Q., Grandmaison, E., Hsu, C., Taylor, D. and Goosen, M. (1995) Interparticle and intraparticle mass–transfer in chromatographic separation. *Bioseparations.*, 5, 189–202.

Lightfoot, E., Athalye, A., Coffman, J., Roper, K. and Root, T. (1995) Nuclear magnetic resonance and the design of chromatographic separations. *J. Chromatogr. A*, 707, 45–55.

Mao, Q. and Hearn, M. (1996) Optimization of affinity and ion-exchange chromatographic processes for the purification of proteins. *Biotechnol. Bioeng.*, 52, 204–222.

Snyder, L. (1980) *High Performance Liquid Chromatography: Advances and Perspectives, Vol. I*, Academics Press, New York.

Velayudhan, A. and Horvath, C. (1988) Preparative chromatography of proteins analysis of the multivalent ion-exchange formalism. *J. Chromatogr.*, 443, 13–29.

Vermeulen, T., LeVan, M., Hiester, N. and Klein, G. (1984) Adsorption and ion exchange. Perry's chemical engineers' handbook, R. Perry (ed.) Mc Graw-Hill, New York.

Vidal-Madjar, C., Jaulmes, A., Sebille, B., Lemque, R., Piquion, J. and Daveine, L. (1992) Protein chromatographic separations on anion exchangers. Role of association in overloading conditions. *9th International Symposium on Preparative and Industrial Chromatography*, Nancy, France.

Vunnum, S., Gallant, S., Young, J. and Cramer, S. (1995) Immobilized metal affinity chromatography: modeling of non linear multicomponent equilibrium. *Chem. Eng. Sci.*, 50(11), 1785–1803.

Wankat, P. (1974) Theory of affinity chromatography separations. *Anal. Chem.*, 46(11), 1400–1408.

Wankat, P. (1986) *Large Scale Adsorption and Chromatography*, CRC Press, Boca Raton.

Wheelwright, S. (1991) *Protein Purification: Design and Scale up of Downstream Processing*, Hanser Publishers, Munich.

Whitley, R., Berninger, J., Rouhana, N. and Wang, L. (1991) Nonlinear gradient isotherm parameter estimation for proteins with consideration of salt competition and multiple forms. *Biotechnol. Prog.*, 7(6), 544–553.

Whitley, R., Wachter, R., Liu, F. and Wang, L. (1989) Ion-exchange equilibria of lysozyme, myoglobulin and bovine serum albumin. Effective valence and exchanger capacity. *J. Chromatogr.*, 465, 137–156.

Yamamoto, S. (1995) Plate height determination from gradient elution chromatography of proteins. *Biotechnol. Bioeng.*, 48, 444–451.

Yamamoto, S., Nakanishi, K., Matsuno, R. and Kamikubo, T. (1983) Ion exchange chromatography of proteins, prediction of elution curves and operating conditions. *Biotechnol. Bioeng.*, 25, 1465–1483.

Yamamoto, S., Nakanishi, K. and Matsusno, R. (1987) *Ion Exchange Chromatography of Proteins*, Marcel Dekker, New York.

Yamamoto, S., Nomura, M. and Sano, Y. (1992) Stepwise elution chromatography as a method for both purification and concentration of proteins. *Chemical Engineering Science*, 47(1), 185–188.

Yamamoto, S. and Sano, Y. (1992) Short-cut method for predicting the productivity of affinity chromatography. *J. Chromatogr.*, 597, 173–179.

Yamamoto, S., Suehisa, T. and Sano, Y. (1993) Preparative separation of proteins by gradient- and stepwise-elution chromatography: zone sharpening effect. *Chem. Eng. Comm.*, 119, 221–230.

Yang, C. and Tsao, G. (1982) Packed-bed adsorption theories and their applications to affinity chromatography. Advances in biochemical engineering, A. Fiechter (ed.), Springer-Verlag, Berlin.

Yao, C. and Tien, C. (1994) Approximate solution of intraparticle diffusion equations and their application to continuous-flow stirred tank and fixed-bed adsorption calculations. *Sep. Technol.*, 4, 67–80.

Chapter 17

Industrial biochromatography: engineering aspects

F. A. P. Garcia, D. M. F. Prazeres and J. M. S. Cabral

Introduction

Chromatography is unique in achieving the high standards of product purity dictated by the regulatory authorities for the commercial bioproducts. Apart from that, and in contrast to other separation techniques, there is no heat generation and the shear stresses are much less significant, therefore preserving the integrity of sensitive biomolecules. It is now well established either as an analytical tool or as a production scale unit operation in industrial processes of enzymes and drugs production. However, the design of a large scale chromatographic process is very complex and involves many factors which are not primarily "chromatographic" (e.g. economic considerations, process hygiene, fouling of the stationary phase, purity of the final product, integration with other up- and down-stream operations, productivity, etc.). Reviews of the existing knowledge have been published (Ruckenstein and Lesins (1988), Yang and Tsao (1982), Janson and Hedman (1982), Freitag and Horváth (1996)).

Dynamics of chromatographic behaviour

To ensure an effective chromatographic separation of two or more components of a mixture (i.e., a minimum overlapping of two consecutive zones) the retention times of the solutes should be sufficiently different from each other and the peaks should be as compact and sharp as possible. In other words, the selectivity of the column (which is a measure of the peak-to-peak separation time), the capacity and the efficiency of the column should be high in order to have a good resolution, R_s, of the solutes. The resolution of two zones (two components with subscripts 1 and 2) is given by

$$R_s = \frac{t_{R_2} - t_{R_1}}{0.5(W_1 + W_2)} = \frac{N^{0.5}}{4} \left(\frac{\alpha - 1}{\alpha} \right) \left(\frac{k_2}{1 + k_2} \right), \tag{1}$$

where α is the *selectivity*, k is the *capacity* and N is the *efficiency*; t_R is the *retention time* or *stoichiometric time* and W is the solute peak width.

The *selectivity* represents the ability of the chromatographic column to separate any two solutes and is given by

$$\alpha = \frac{k_1}{k_2} = \frac{(V_{R_1} - V_m)}{(V_{R_2} - V_m)}, \tag{2}$$

where V_R is the peak elution volume for each solute and V_m is the void volume of the column. The *capacity* is a measure of the column to retain a solute and is given by

$$k = K_d \frac{(1 - \varepsilon)}{\varepsilon} = \frac{(V_R - V_m)}{V_m},$$ (3)

where $K_d = q/C$ is the distribution or partition coefficient of the solute concentrations between the stationary (q) and the mobile (C) phases, and ε is the porosity of the bed. This retention capacity of the column can also be characterised by the *retardation factor*, or R-*factor*, as

$$R = \frac{V_m}{V_m + K_d V_s} = \frac{V_m}{V_R}.$$ (4)

The control of the capacity and selectivity is the same as the control of the retention times and is, therefore, related to the thermodynamic equilibrium of distribution of the solutes between the stationary and mobile phases. The separation of the peaks can, thus, be improved by an adequate selection of the stationary and mobile phases. In some cases an advantage can even be taken of specific interactions between some solutes and the stationary phases; however, if the solutes have similar structures it may be difficult to attain significant differences in the migration velocities following this approach.

The *efficiency* of the column is a measure of the zone broadening which results from diffusional and hydrodynamic effects and from limitations to the mass transfer of the solute between the mobile and the stationary phases (in fact, the chromatographic process proceeds in a non-equilibrium state). The performance can, thus, be further improved by controlling those operational parameters, mainly the eluent velocity and the particle diameter, that affect the zone broadening. An efficient separation can then be made in a shorter column with a better design and operated under better conditions.

The design and operation of chromatographic processes require, however, the knowledge of the theories of chromatography and the mathematical tools that describe them. Several theories have been proposed which can be grouped in two main categories: the plate theories or tanks-in-series models and the rate theory or the mass balance models. The so-called equilibrium theory is no more than a special case of the rate theories.

Discrete plate analysis

The plate theory assumes a discrete nature of the chromatographic column, which is considered as a series of N equally sized and well mixed contactors, each named as a theoretical plate. Considering that: (a) the sorption process is thermodynamically reversible; (b) the equilibrium of distribution of solutes is instantaneously attained, i.e., no resistances to mass transfer of solutes between the phases; (c) there is a continuous flow of eluent through plates; (d) there is no back-mixing between consecutive plates; (e) the equilibrium isotherms are linear (K_d = constant); and (f) the plates are all equivalent, i.e., V_s/V_m is constant (V_s and V_m are the volumes of the stationary and mobile phases in that stage), then a mass balance to plate j is

$$Q_e (C_{j-1} - C_j) = \left(\frac{V_m}{N} + \frac{V_s}{N} K_d \right) \frac{\partial C_j}{\partial t}$$ (5)

or

$$NR\left(C_{j-1} - C_j\right) = \frac{V_m}{Q_e}\frac{\partial C_j}{\partial t} \tag{6}$$

(1) In *elution chromatography* the sample is applied on the top of the column, in the first plate, before the elution is started (this is equivalent, in mathematical terms, to the introduction of an impulse of Dirac delta function, $\delta(t)$). Thus, the initial conditions are

$$C_{j \neq 0}(0) = 0,$$
$$C_{j=0}(t) = C_0\delta(t). \tag{7}$$

Equation (6) can, then, be easily integrated in the Laplace domain. The corresponding normalised solution for the last plate (i.e., the solute concentration leaving the column) is the Poisson distribution function

$$E(\theta) = \frac{C_N}{C_0} = (RN)^N \frac{1}{(N-1)!} \theta^{N-1} e^{(-RN\theta)} \tag{8a}$$

or

$$E(t) = \frac{C_N}{C_0} = \frac{1}{t_R}\left(\frac{t}{t_R}\right)^{(N-1)} \frac{N^N}{(N-1)!} e^{(-N(t/t_R))}, \tag{8b}$$

which is reduced to the Gauss distribution function without an appreciable error when N is large.

(2) In the case of *frontal analysis* the sample is applied continuously, as a step function ($C_{j=0} = C_0 H(0)$), where $H(t)$ is the Heaviside or unit step function, and the normalized response is

$$F(\theta) = \frac{C_N}{C_0} = 1 - e^{(RN\theta)}.\sum_{i=0}^{N-1}\frac{RN\theta^i}{i!} \tag{9a}$$

or

$$F(t) = \frac{C_N}{C_0} = 1 - e^{(-N(t/t_R))}.\sum_{i=0}^{N-1}\frac{N\left(\frac{t}{t_R}\right)^{(i-1)}}{R^{(i-1)}i!} \tag{9b}$$

(3) In *displacement chromatography*, which is particularly suitable for process scale applications, the sample is applied to the column under such conditions that all the solutes strongly bind to the stationary phases; these are, then, separated into adjacent bands by a displacer, a substance that has an higher affinity to the stationary phase. The corresponding inlet boundary conditions are for the solute i and the displacer n $C_{j=0}^i(0) = C_0^i\delta(t)$, $C_0^n(0) = C_0^n H(t - t_F)$, with $i = 1, 2, \ldots, (n-1)$ and t_F is the duration of the sample application.

Parameter estimation: determination of N and the concept of HETP

The parameter N (number of theoretical plates) in Equations (8–9b) can be estimated by different techniques but the method of moments is particularly well suited for this purpose. It is known from Statistics that the moment of order k of a normalised distribution E(x) is

$$\mu_k = \int_0^\infty x^k E(x)\, dx. \tag{10}$$

Since E(x) is a normalized function, $\mu_0 = 1$, μ_1 is the mean and $(\mu_2 - \mu_1^2) = \sigma^2$ is the variance of the distribution. If a tracer amount of solute is injected at the feed point and detected on the outlet of the column, the moments can then be estimated from the impulse response $E(\theta)$ or E(t) drawn from the detector signal in just one single experiment. For the response in the time domain we will have then

$$\mu_{t,1} = t_R,$$

$$\mu_{t,2} = t_R^2 \left(1 + \frac{1}{N}\right), \tag{11}$$

$$\sigma_t^2 = \mu_{t,2} - \mu_{t,1}^2 = \frac{t_R^2}{N}.$$

From this equation, the number of theoretical plates in a column of length L is estimated by

$$N = \frac{t_R^2}{\sigma_t^2} = 16\frac{t_R^2}{W^2}, \tag{12}$$

where $W = 4\sigma_t$ is the peak width, measured in time units on the baseline and can be determined directly from the experimental elution curves. Thus, the length of each plate, known as the Height Equivalent to a Theoretical Plate (HETP), is

$$HETP = L\frac{\sigma_t^2}{t_R^2}. \tag{13}$$

This is a well known parameter used in Chemical Engineering to characterize the effectiveness of interphase mass transfer in several unit operations. Notice that

$$E(\theta) = \frac{\partial F(\theta)}{\partial t} \tag{14}$$

and the number of theoretical plates can also be estimated in the frontal analysis mode by estimating the moments of the response to a step input of the solute. Equation (13) does not include either the operational conditions or the packing characteristics and some more explicit form should be derived.

Non-equilibrium and zone spreading

In real chromatographic processes, even if the isotherm of the solute partition is linear, zone spreading occurs due to: (i) limited rates of mass transfer and/or chemical reaction (e.g. in adsorption and immuno affinity processes) which is a factor of local non-equilibrium; (ii) molecular diffusion, which is particularly important for very low flow rates of the mobile phase; and (iii) turbulent or "eddy" diffusion. As shown by van Deemter *et al.* (1956), each of these factors contribute with a partial variance to the total variance of the impulse response, that is,

$$\sigma_t^2 = ((\sigma_{md}^2 + \sigma_{ed}^2) + \sigma_{ne}^2), \tag{15}$$

where the indexes refer to non-equilibrium (ne), and molecular diffusion (md) and eddy diffusion (ed), respectively. The plate theory models have, thus, to be further refined to accommodate also these effects.

Local non-equilibrium effects   Local non-equilibrium effects result from three main sources: external diffusion in a liquid film around the particles, internal diffusion within the particles and adsorption kinetics. For instance, in the simple case of limited rate of mass transfer of the solute through the liquid film around the particle and neglecting the mass transfer resistance inside the particles, the mass balance in each stage is

$$Q_e(C_{j-1} - C_j) = v_m \frac{\partial C_j}{\partial t} + k_L a_p v_s \left(C_j - \frac{q_j}{K_d} \right). \tag{16a}$$

A second equation is needed to relate q_j and C_j; this can be a mass balance of the solute in the stationary phase

$$k_L a_p v_s \left(C_j - \frac{q_j}{K_d} \right) = v_s \frac{\partial q_j}{\partial t}, \tag{16b}$$

where k_L is the liquid film mass transfer coefficient (ms^{-1}) and a_p is the specific interfacial area of the particles (m^2/m^3). Again, this system of two equations can be solved in the Laplace domain.

The moments of the impulse response are

$$\mu_1 = \tau(1 + k) = t_R, \tag{17}$$

$$\sigma_t^2 = \frac{t_R^2}{N} + \frac{2k}{(1 + k)} t_m t_R, \tag{18}$$

where $t_m = K_d/k_L a_p$ is the time constant for the mass transfer between the mobile and the stationary phases. If the intraparticle diffusion and adsorption kinetics are also non-negligeable then t_m is a global mass transfer time constant to comprise the sum of the external and the internal diffusion and the adsorption kinetics contributions: $t_m = t_{ef} + t_{id} + t_{ak}$, with $t_{ef} = K_d d_p/k_L$, $t_{id} = \mu d_p^2/D_i$, and $t_{ak} = \rho_p K_a/K_d k_a$; here, d_p is the particle diameter, μ is a shape factor characteristic of the particles, K_a the adsorption equilibrium constant, ρ_p is the density of the solid particles and k_a is an adsorption rate constant, $D_i (= D_{md}/T)$ is an effective diffusion coefficient of the solute inside the solid particles, and T is the tortuosity of the macropores ranging from 2 to 7. The second term of the right hand side in Equation (18) accounts for mass transfer limitations to equilibrium.

Axial diffusion   The axial dispersion and the consequent zone broadening resulting from the molecular and eddy diffusion were already considered in the simple plate theory model described in the section on Discrete plate analysis, when each plate was seen as a well mixed reactor. In a well packed column they will become less and less important when the HETP is smaller and smaller; a relationship between the number of plates and the axial dispersion, other effects being neglected, is

$$N = \frac{Pe}{2},$$ (19)

where $Pe = uL/D_{ax}$ is the axial Peclet number, u is the interstitial velocity of the eluent and D_{ax} is the axial dispersion coefficient.

Then, from Equations (15), (18) and (19), the contribution of the dispersion effects to the zone broadening is

$$\frac{\sigma_{md}^2 + \sigma_{ed}^2}{t_R^2} = \frac{2D_{ax}}{Lu}.$$ (20)

The dispersion in the axial direction, D_{ax}, includes both the molecular diffusion, D_m, accounting for $\sigma_{md}^2 = gD_{md}$, and the eddy (statistical) dispersion, D_{ed}, due to the changes in the flow direction near the particles, accounting for $\sigma_{ed}^2 = ud_p/Pe_p$, where $Pe_p = ud_p/D_{ax}$ is a particle Peclet number, ranging from 0.5 to 2 in liquid chromatography, and the factor g accounts for the irregular pattern (the tortuosity) inside the praticles.

Finally, from Equations (13), (18) and (20), the HETP is (also under non-equilibrium conditions)

$$HETP = L\frac{\sigma_t^2}{t_R^2} = \frac{2gD_{dm}}{u} + \frac{d_p}{Pe_p} + \frac{2k}{(1+k)^2}t_m u,$$ (21)

which has the form of the well known equation of van Deemter

$$HETP = \frac{A}{u} + B + Cu.$$ (22)

This equation shows a minimum value of HETP with the meaning of a theoretical "optimum" velocity $u_{opt} = (B/C)^{1/2}$ that maximizes the column efficiency.

Continuous description of chromatography

Continuous description is based on the continuity equations derived from differential mass balances, and involves the application of the conservation laws, equilibrium laws and kinetic laws of transport and reaction, together with boundary and initial conditions.

A mass balance to a solute in the flowing mobile phase in a differential length, dx, of column is

$$D_{ax}\frac{\partial^2 C}{\partial x^2} - u\frac{\partial C}{\partial x} = \frac{\partial C}{\partial t} + \frac{(1-\varepsilon)}{\varepsilon}\frac{\partial q}{\partial t}.$$ (23)

An additional relation between C and q is needed. In the more general case, the rates of mass transfer in each phase or the adsorption reaction kinetics have finite values and such a relation is the mass balance in the stationary phase

$$\frac{\partial q}{\partial t} = f(C, q, C^*, q^*) \tag{24}$$

which, if the resistances to mass transfer and adsorption are negligeable and an equilibrium is instantaneously established at the interface, is just replaced by the equilibrium law

$$q = q^* = f(C^*) = f(C) \tag{25}$$

where the asterisk (*) refers to the concentrations in the interface. Equation 24 lumps together the external and internal mass transfer resistances and adsorption kinetics as well as a sorption equilibrium isotherm. In the case of a non-homogeneous, porous particle the transport inside the pores has also to be considered. Therefore, for a porous particle, the interfacial mass transfer rate at the outer particle surface is

$$\frac{\partial q}{\partial t} = \frac{6k_L}{d_p}(C - C|_{r=R_p}) = \frac{6D_i\varepsilon_i}{d_p}\left(\frac{\partial C^P}{\partial r}\right)_{r=R_p}. \tag{26}$$

The continuity equation for the component inside the pores is

$$\varepsilon_i\frac{\partial C^P}{\partial t} + (1 - \varepsilon_i)\frac{\partial C^{Ps}}{\partial t} = \varepsilon_i D_i\left[\frac{1}{r^2}\frac{\partial}{\partial r}\left(r^2\frac{\partial C^P}{\partial r}\right)\right], \tag{27}$$

where C^P and $C^{Ps} = C^*$ are the solute concentrations in the stagnant liquid inside the pores and on the internal pore surface, respectively, and R_p is the particle radius.

Moreover, equations for the sorption isotherm and adsorption kinetics are required and can have different forms.

Then, given explicit forms for these equations, the solution $C(x,t)$ requires the definition of space and time boundary conditions (which depend on the type of operation: displacement, frontal analysis or elution chromatography) the type of sorption isotherm and the initial state of the eluent and the sorbent. However, these highly sophisticated mathematical equations conceived to describe real chromatographic processes are of unsurmountable complexity and only approximate solutions have been obtained for less complex situations on the basis of simple but reasonable assumptions.

Equilibrium models

Equilibrium without dispersive effects   One of the more frequent assumptions is that of an instantaneous adsorption equilibrium under isothermal and isocratic conditions and in the absence of longitudinal dispersion effects ($D_{ax} = 0$). Each zone would, then, migrate keeping the same shape during the entire percolation process on the additional condition of linear isotherm. In the more general case of non-linear isotherm zone spreading will occur. The solution $C(x,t)$ for the continuity equations depends not only on the appropriate boundary and initial conditions (namely the cases of frontal or elution analysis) but also on the type of isotherm. In the case of a favorable sorption isotherm (such as the Langmuir isotherm) higher concentrations C of solute move faster than lower solute concentrations and the front of the wave is compressive; if, on the contrary, the isotherm is unfavorable, e.g., the Freundlich isotherm, the front of the wave is dispersive as lower solute concentrations move faster than higher solute concentrations. These effects of front wave dispersion or compression are proportional to the migration length and the wave is said to have a *proportional pattern*.

Other types of isotherms such as the S-shaped B.E.T. or the bi-Langmuir isotherms have also been considered. Obviously, these assumptions of the equilibrium theory are a rather simplified picture of the actual chromatographic processes but give some important preliminary informations on the movement and broadening of the zone.

Equilibrium and dispersive effects   The compression of the wave front of Langmuiran solutes will be opposed by the axial dispersion effects (also proportional to the migration length) resulting from finite kinetic phenomena (such as sorption reaction or mass transfer) or from molecular or eddy diffusion. After a short transient time down the column a steady shape of the front develops and remains time-independent as it moves along the column; we say then that the wave has a *constant pattern*. It should be emphasized that the constant pattern develops only after a certain migration length (or time) down the column which depends on the equilibrium parameters (the degree of non-linearity of the isotherm) and operating variables that affect the mass transfer kinetics.

Rate theories

When the mass transfer between the phases and/or the sorption/desorption processes occur at a finite rate (the equilibrium models are just a special case where those processes occur with an infinitely large rate), then the zone spreading effects have to be considered in what are the so called rate models. Depending on the limiting step two classes of simplified models have been studied in more detail, one in which the (chemical) reaction kinetics is limiting and the other in which the mass transfer (physical) kinetics is the slowest and limiting process. Each of these two classes has a basic model around which many others have been built with either simplifications or extensions.

Chemical kinetics limiting – the Thomas model   The basic model for the concentration profile under chemical adsorption rate control was developed by Thomas (1944) and is based on the assumptions of the negligeable axial dispersion (mobile phase plug flow, $D_{ax} = 0$), a fast mass transfer rate in the liquid film around the particles and an isothermal operation. Then the mass balance equation is

$$u\frac{\partial C}{\partial x} + \frac{\partial C}{\partial t} + \frac{1-\varepsilon}{\varepsilon}\frac{\partial q}{\partial t} = 0. \tag{28}$$

Regarding the chemical resistances, the stoichiometry and the type of reaction (ionic exchange, covalent bonds, physical adsorption through van der Waal's or electrostatic forces) that occurs on the particle surface can be described by more complex equations and the total number of reaction sites (total surface area for reaction) depends also on the homogeneity and porosity of the particles. However, the Thomas approach was originally developed for ion exchange $(NA^+ + HR \Leftrightarrow H^+ + NaR)$ and the kinetic equation needed to relate q and C in such circumstances was

$$\frac{\partial q}{\partial t} = k_r \left[C(Q - q) - rq(C_0 - C) \right] . \tag{29}$$

The solution was given for the frontal analysis mode of operation, where Q is the maximum sorption capacity and r is the equilibrium parameter that equates the sorption isotherms in a dimensionless form. A similar approach was followed by Chase (1984) to simulate the performance of affinity chromatography assuming a monovalent adsorption of a protein P to a ligand L $(P + L \Leftrightarrow PL)$. Due to the simplicity of the result, Thomas' solution has been a very useful result despite the assumptions.

Physical (mass transfer) kinetics limiting – the Rosen model Another simplified approach to non-equilibrium was made by Rosen (1952) who assumed a limited rate of diffusion through the stagnant film around the particle and a resistance to mass transfer inside the particle, in addition to fluid plug flow $(D_{ax} = 0)$, fast sorption rate and isothermal operation. A solution was obtained for the case of frontal analysis when homogeneous structure of the particles and a linear isotherm were also assumed. A more simplified solution was obtained for the limiting case of no surface film resistance, that is, if the diffusion inside the particle is limiting. Analytical solutions were also obtained for other simple problems where external mass transfer resistance, coupled with linear isotherms, was the sole limiting factor (Anzelius, 1926). Rosen's work was extended and analytically solved by Rasmuson and Neretnieks (1980) who considered also external mass transfer resistance and axial dispersion.

General remarks

As said before, real chromatographic processes are often of much higher complexity than these ideal situations just described. Additional problems are then raised to solve the more sophisticated mathematical models developed to describe them. Linear isotherms have often been adopted in order to simplify the mathematical integration of the models, which may be acceptable in many cases where the concentration is low and no competition for the adsorption sites is exerted among the components to be resolved. Numerical methods have been developed and the Fast Fourier Transform appears to be the most suitable technique (Bellot and Condoret, 1991).

The cases of non-linear isotherms are more complex. When a set of differential equations is required to integrate axial dispersion and significant mass transfer resistances (particularly polymeric solutes, such as proteins) numerical solutions have to be developed; as reviewed by Bellot and Condoret (1991), the finite difference method and the orthogonal collocation method, eventually combined, are particularly suited for solving the non-linear problems in chromatography.

Equilibrium and adsorption kinetic data obtained for a single solute may be invalidated when competition for the active sites arise in multicomponent systems. Often, more than one kind of solute interaction with the particles also occurs. In non-isocratic elution, particularly in gradient non-linear chromatography, the equilibrium relationships change according to the gradient.

Particle sizes and pores sizes distributions add to the complexity of the problems. Recently, the importance of the convective transport inside the pores has been demonstrated (Rodrigues, 1991).

Radial velocity profiles may occur in the bed, particularly in preparative chromatography where the columns of larger diameter are used (Nicoud and Perrut, 1991).

It is impossible to deal with all these factors simultaneously and in practice the mathematical representation, necessary for scale-up and optimization of the operation conditions, has to be simplified, particularly in non-linear chromatography. The differential models will then be more and more used in the future, not only for column design but also for the operation automation.

However, the plate theory and the development of experimental protocols for the design of chromatographic separations, despite the drawback of considering the discrete nature of the column and being non-predictive, has remained useful and popular.

Scale-up

The development of a separation process has to proceed from the laboratory through the pilot plant to the safe commercial production scale, a problem that was well addressed by Sofer and Nyström (1989). First, the final product has to be characterised in terms of the activity, purity, formulation and stability, the possible contaminants that can be tolerated and the impurities (e.g., bacterial endotoxins, pyrogens or carcinogens) that have to be removed. In this respect, convenient assay methods have to be chosen.

Integration of chromatography with other up- and down-stream separation operations have to be carefully assessed. The samples to be chromatographed should be free of particles that can block up the bed. Protease activities must be reduced but certain additives may cause problems. Foaming resulting from the presence of tensioactive agents should also be avoided.

The chromatographic technique or a combination of techniques should be chosen depending on the most appropriate properties to be exploited: molecular weight for gel filtration, charge for ion exchange, hydrophobicity for hydrophobic interaction chromatography, affinity to other molecules in the case of affinity (or pseudo-affinity) chromatography. The choice should be made with a high selectivity in mind, but some attention should be given to the stability of the product under the chromatographic conditions (pH, ionic strength, etc). In accordance, the mobile (eluting buffer) and stationary phases should be selected and optimised.

The gel material, apart from the different affinities for the components to be resolved, should satisfy some important requirements: good physical stability, high chemical stability to withstand the agression of sterilizing and cleaning agents, non-biodegradability, inertness to the product, insoluble, high mechanical resistance and incompressibility to withstand the high pressure drops.

When enough data are collected the development proceeds with the optimization, still in a small scale, by manipulating the operational parameters that lead to improvements in the chromatographic efficiency, a high capacity and resolution in shorter columns and higher yields of recovery. To maximize the capacity factor the gel beads should have a macroporous structure while maximizing the resolution requires smaller bead sizes. The capacity of the separation media to adsorb the sample components has thus to be assessed.

Analytical scale optimization is not valid for process scale chromatography where the philosophy is the maximization of the product recovery with the specified purity (resolution) and of throughput (productivity) at reduced costs. Sample load (volume and concentration) should then be maximized. Recalling the van Deemter equation, the linear flow rate has also to be optimized to maximize the number of theoretical plates. The pressure drop in the column directly related to the linear flow rate, the mobile phase viscosity and the bed characteristics (length, bead size, porosity) through the Carman–Kozeny equation

$$\Delta P = K \frac{\mu uL}{d_p^2} \frac{(1 - \varepsilon)^2}{\varepsilon^3}, \tag{30}$$

K is a constant that accounts for the friction losses. These operational parameters should then be optimised to fix the maximum allowed pressure drop taking into account the pumping energy, the drag forces acting on the particles and the bed compressibility. Temperature can also be varied to reduce the buffer viscosity but only within the limits of thermal stability of the product, without neglecting the effects on the distribution equilibrium constant, and, in certain cases, the operation has even to be carried out in cold rooms. In the case of elution chromatography the gradient shape has also to be optimised.

Proceeding to the scale-up, the optimised column length, the linear velocity and the sample load per unit volume of the stationary phase are kept constant while the column diameter, the volumetric flow rate of the eluent buffer and the sample load increase proportionally. Fine adjustments can then be made in the fluid velocity, particle size and column length.

The scale-up of the column diameter, however, generates some other complexities. The bed compression increases and, as a consequence, the pressure drop is also increased if the flow rate is to be kept the same as in the smaller scale. A radial velocity profile in the mobile phase can eventually be observed, adding to increased zone broadening (Nicoud and Perrut, 1991). A similar effect results from the heterogeneities in the packing (Tallarek *et al.*, 1996).

Increased dispersion arise also in a scaled-up operation from the injection of a larger sample, that is more difficult to distribute over a larger section, and from the distributor itself.

Equipment

Apart from the chromatographic design, the mechanical design of the column and anxiliary equipment has to be made criteriously concerning the productivity, the throughput, the product purity, product hygiene and safety, containment, cleaning and sterilisation, automation, the contribution to the degree of zone broadening.

The columns   The heart of the system is the column. The materials of construction should be mechanically resistant and chemically inert, compatible with buffers, solvents and cleaning agents, and this applies to the seals, connectors, tubing, etc. Some plastics (occasionally, in low pressure systems), borosilicate glass and stainless steel are the materials of choice. The surface should be polished. The construction has to obey very tight tolerances and O-ring seals should be as thin as possible to avoid dead spaces. The flow distributors should be designed to spread the liquid uniformly and keep an even pressure distribution over the packing. Valves, tanks, pumps and tubing must follow the same criteria of hygienic design. Multiport valves should be used to minimise dead spaces. From an hygienic point of view, solenoid actuated diaphragm valves are the best choice. Pumps (such as the diaphragm) should also be easily dismantled for hygienisation, and introduce little pulsation in the flow; good maintenance of seals and rotating parts is essential. The number of tube connectors should be reduced to a minimum and have sanitary designs. The length of tubings should also be kept to a minimum in order to minimise extra-column dispersive effects (Nicoud and Perrut, 1991).

Column packing   Packing large scale chromatographic columns raises problems that are not found in analytical columns. It is much more difficult to pack sectionally homogeneous columns of larger diameter, the density of the packing varies and causes differential migrations and non-chromatographic dispersion. The conventional technique of slurry packing, consolidating the bed by a high velocity solvent stream gives poor reproducibility in the packing density, the bed is not always stable as is difficult to use in wide bore columns (Tallarek *et al.*, 1996). Bed consolidation using mechanical stresses such as axial compression is an alternative, but inhomogeneous distribution of mechanical stresses, the compressibility of the particles, low reproducibility of column-to-column packing density (Tallarek *et al.*, 1996) are just some of the problems that remain unsolved. The HETP and the velocity of the mobile phase are not constant, large discrepancies exist between the observed efficiency and the efficiency predicted by the most reliable existing methods, and new methods to assess the global efficiency of the column have to be developed.

Detectors and sensors   Different types of detectors are used for the detection of the peaks at the column outlet. For biomolecules the most frequently used are UV, conductivity, pH and refractive index (RI) detectors. They, generally, are of flow-through designs, and should be easily cleaned and sanitised, explosion proof and have available adjustable alarm systems. They should be sensitive, have a high signal-to-noise ratio and particular care should be exerted concerning the fouling of the sensor device (e.g., the pH electrode or the walls of the flow-through cell in UV detectors).

Air sensors in series with air traps should be placed upstream the column enabling the eluent pumps to be automatically switched-off to prevent air bubbles from entering the column. Pressure sensors should protect the column from overpressures. Flow meter/controllers of sanitary design should be sensitive to flow but insensitive to viscosity changes.

Fraction collectors   Fraction collectors are required to recover the product that was resolved in the column. Distinct from those used in the laboratory, fraction collectors for process scale have multiport or manifolds of two-way valves to recover a lower number (generally five or six) of different solutes (Sofer and Nyström, 1989).

Automation and control   Automation has several advantages and one is obviously the reduction of human error, therefore increased reproducibility of the process. By including sensors and alarms together with control systems and logic displays, the process can be remotely controlled. The labour costs are thus reduced. The specifications for the hardware and software depend on each case on the complexity of the system, the number of variables to be controlled and versatility and the functions to be performed (e.g., documentation, results evaluation, levels of security, ease of use by non-specialised people, etc.).

Process hygiene

The maintenance of a chromatographic system (columns and equipment) is fundamental in terms of process economics and safety. Among other things, this involves routine cleaning, sanitization and sterilization procedures. While cleaning operations are designed to remove and prevent the build-up of impurities, the goal of sanitization is the reduction of the number of microbial contaminants to acceptable levels, and that of sterilization is the complete removal of all forms of life. Cleaning and sanitization are usually performed after each run. The design of a cost effective chromatographic process should as a rule include the possibility of cleaning in place (CIP) procedures. The choice of the cleaning agent should take into account not only the nature of the impurities to be removed but also the compatibility with the equipment and chromatographic media. Impurities associated with the production of biologicals usually originate from the starting medium (e.g. viruses, additives, antifoams), the host cells (e.g. proteins, lipids, endotoxins, nucleic acids), the purification process (e.g. leachables from chromatographic media) and the product itself (multimeric and denatured forms).

Sodium hydroxide (up to 1 M) is one of the best cleaning agents for the removal of a variety of impurities such as nucleic acids, pyrogens (endotoxins), viruses and hydrophobic proteins. Non-ionic detergents like Tween 80 and organic solvents such as ethanol, isopropanol and acetonitrile are often used for the removal of lipids and in cases where hydrophobic interactions might be present. Additionally, some detergents display the ability to inactivate viruses. Cleaning procedures often alternate different chemical agents, improving the efficiency of the process. For instance, sodium hydroxide is often used in sequential washing procedures with acidic treatments (e.g. acetic acid), sodium chloride and water. Other agents such as formaldehyde, phenol, urea, peracetates and hypochlorites have been used in cleaning procedures. Some cleaning procedures may resort to higher temperatures in order to improve the effectiveness of the process. After cleaning, chemical agents are thoroughly removed from the columns and equipment by washing extensively with water or buffer.

Many of the above mentioned cleaning agents such as sodium hydroxide, ethanol, hypochlorite and peracetic acid have a sterilizing action. Sodium hydroxide, for instance, has proven to be an effective disinfectant for vegetative bacteria and yeast (Sofer and Nyström, 1989). Some chromatographic media can even withstand sterilization by steam, although it is hard to perform this operation in packed columns without destroying the packing. If the column is by-passed, steam can be used very effectively to sterilize the equipment in place. The effectiveness of the sterilizing agent depends on the organism, the agent concentration, the temperature and the contact time. The effectiveness of a certain procedure is usually tested with challenging studies where certain model microorganisms such as *Staphylococcus aureus, Escherichia coli, Aspergillus niger, Pseudomonas aeruginosa, Candida albicans* are deliberately introduced in the chromatographic system. Following sterilization, the number of surviving microorganisms is determined and the information obtained used for evaluating the effectiveness of the process. In extreme cases, when dealing with particularly hazardous agents, the chromatographic media may have to be sterilized and discarded after each run.

Validation

Validation, as defined by the US Food and Drug Administration (FDA), is the process of "Establishing documented evidence which provides a high degree of assurance that a specific process will consistently produce a product meeting its predetermined specification and quality attributes" (Sofer and Hagel, 1997). Validation should be considered and designed already at the design stage and before equipment purchase and system configuration (Beatrice, 1993). Benefits arising from validation include not only increased productivity but also reduced costs for utilities and systems/equipment maintenance. The validation process of a chromatographic operation must contemplate all aspects of the process, including raw materials, facilities, HVAC (heating, ventilation and air conditioning) systems, water, *equipment process performance* and maintenance (including cleaning and sterilization).

The validation activities relating to *equipment* involve, among other things, installation and operational qualification (IQ and OQ) which basically check if the equipment meets pre-determined specifications. In IQ, documentation should be generated that describes the equipment characteristics and parts, calibration, operation and maintenance procedures, process flow chart, standard operating procedures (e.g. for column packing and storage, buffer preparation), etc. In OQ, the function of components such as pumps, valves, alarms, detectors, controllers, recorders etc is checked. The quality of the chromatographic packing should also be verified, by determining parameters such as HETP and asymmetry factors using defined conditions (Sofer and Hagel, 1997).

Process qualification (PQ) is usually carried out at pilot scale and involves assessing if the chromatographic separation is performing the task it was designed for in a reproducible and reliable way. PQ will also provide the basis for setting acceptance limits for the process. These limits should be wide enough to accommodate scale-up. Several validation runs should be performed to assure that product can be obtained consistently, within specifications. Important aspects to be checked in each run include column performance, removal of process contaminants and impurities and column scale-up. Documentation on column performance (e.g. flow rate, pressure drop, chromatograms, product recovery and purity) is a valuable indicator of media deterioration and will ultimately determine when to repack. The consistency of the removal of contaminants and impurities (leachables, protein variants, endotoxins, viruses, DNA and microorganisms) during the chromatographic separation should be demonstrated analytically. Finally, the demonstration of the existence of product equivalency throughout the process of scaling-up from lab to pilot-scale to full-scale manufacturing is a fundamental aspect of validation which may originate adjustments in the process (Beatrice, 1993; Sofer and Hagel, 1997).

References

Anzelius, A. Z. (1926) "Uber Erwarming vermittels durchstromender Medien", *Z. Angew. Math. Mech.*, **6**, 291–94.

Beatrice, M. G. (1993) "Biotechnology Facility Design and Process Validation". In *Biotechnology, Vol 3: Bioprocessing*. H.-J. Rehm, G. Reed (eds) VCH, Weinheim, pp. 739–767.

Bellot, J. C. and Condoret, J. S. (1991) "Liquid Chromatography Modelling: A Review", *Process Biochemistry*, **26**, 363–376.

Chase, H. A. (1984) "Affinity Separations Utilising Immobilised Monoclonal Antibodies – A New Tool for the Biochemical Engineer", *Chem. Eng. Sci.*, 39, 1099–1125.

Freitag, R. and Horváth, C. (1996) "Chromatography in the Downstream Processing of Biotechnological Products" in *Adv. Biochem. Eng.*, A. Fiechter (ed.) Vol. 53, Springer-Verlag, Berlin.

Janson, J.-C. and Hedman, P. (1982) "Large Scale Chromatography of Proteins", in *Adv. Biochem. Eng.*, A. Fiechter (ed.) Vol.25, Springer–Verlag, Berlin.

Nicoud, R. M. and Perrut, M. (1991) "Operating Modes, Scale-up and Optimization of Chromatographic Processes", in *Chromatographic and Membrane Processes in Biotechnology*, C. A. Costa, J. S. Cabral (eds) NATO ASI Series, Kluwer Academic Publishers, Dordrecht.

Rasmuson, A. and Neretnieks, I. (1980) "Exact Solution of a Model for Diffusion in Particles and Longitudinal Dispersion in Packed Beds", *AIChE J.*, **26**, 686–690.

Rodrigues, A. E., Dias, M. M. and Lopes, J. B. C. (1991) "Theory of Linear and Nonlinear Chromatography", in *Chromatographic and Membrane Processes in Biotechnology*, C. A. Costa, J. S. Cabral (eds) NATO ASI Series, Kluwer Academic Publishers, Dordrecht.

Rosen, J. B. (1952) "Kinetics of a Fixed Bed System for Solute Diffusion into Spherical Particles", *J. Phys. Chem.*, **20**, 387.

Ruckenstein, E. and Lesins, V. (1988) "Classification of Liquid Chromatographic Methods Based on the Interaction Forces: The Niche of Potential Barrier Chromatography", in *Downstream Processes: Equipment and Techniques*, A. Mizrahi (ed.) Alan R. Liss, Inc., New York.

Sherwood, T. K., Pigford, R. L. and Wilke, C. R. (1975) *Mass Transfer*, McGraw-Hill, Inc., New York.

Sofer, G. K. and Hagel, L. (1997) *Handbook of Process Chromatography: A Guide to Optimization, Scale-up and Validation*, Academic Press, San Diego.

Sofer, G. K. and Nyström, L. E. (1989) *Process Chromatography – A Practical Guide*, Academic Press Ltd., London.

Tallarek, U., Albert, K., Bayer, E. and Guiochon, G. (1996) "Measurement of Transverse and Axial Apparent Dispersion Coefficients in Packed Beds", *AIChE J.*, **42**, 3041–3054.

Thomas, H. (1944) "Heterogeneous Ion Exchange in a Flowing System", *J. Amer. Chem. Soc.*, **66**, 1664.

Yang, C.-M. and Tsao, G. T. (1982) *Packed-Bed Adsorption Theories and Their Applications to Affinity Chromatography*, in *Adv. Biochem. Eng.*, A. Fiechter (ed.) Vol. 25, Springer-Verlag, Berlin.

van Deemter, J. J., Zuiderweg, F. J. and Klinkenberg, A. (1956) "Longitudinal diffusion and resistence to mass transfer as causes of nonideality in chromatography", *Chem. Eng. Sci.*, **5**, 271–289.

Villermaux, J. (1987) "Chemical Engineering Approach to Dynamic Modelling of Linear Chromatography. A Flexible Method for Representing Complex Phenomena from simple Concepts", *J. Chromatogr.*, **406**, 11–26.

Yamamoto, S., Nakanishi, K. and Matsuno, R. (1988) *Ion-Exchange Chromatography of Proteins*, Marcel Dekker, Inc., New York.

Chapter 18

Validation aspects in biochromatography

Charles Lutsch

Introduction

Chromatography is a highly selective separation technique commonly used for the isolation and purification of biologicals. In chromatography, a liquid mixture is passed through a column of packed particles. Because solutes in the mixture have different molecular size vis à vis the pore volume of the matrix beads or affinities for the sorbent, they partition differently in the stationary sorbent phase and in the mobile liquid phase. Those molecules of a smaller size or a greater affinity for the solid phase (i.e. due to the charge distribution, hydrophobicity, or hydrogen bonds) migrate slower than larger molecules or those attracted to the mobile phase, thus effecting resolution. The column based dynamic processes can, in some cases be replaced by a batch mode of retention based on the same principles.

A wide range of chromatographic techniques has been used for large scale bio-purification: Size Exclusion Chromatography and Adsorption chromatography as Ion Exchange, Hydroxyapatite, Affinity, and Hydrophobic Interaction Chromatography (HIC), and Reversed Phase Chromatography (RPC).

In the industrial context, the chromatographic procedures as applicable to a given product manufacture, should be validated and documented. In this chapter, we will describe a plan for the validation of chromatographic processes for biopharmaceuticals, in order for the product to move from the research to full scale process with the ultimate objective of being validated as a process at the time of product license submission.

Validation plan

The validation of the chromatographic process should be conducted in accordance with a defined protocol. It is a written plan stating how validation will be conducted including purification process description, production equipment, test parameters, product characteristics, and decision criteria on what consists acceptable test results.

Defining process and product [1–5]

Process objective [1]

The objectives of a chromatographic process must state exactly what the process is intended to do. In general, it removes unwanted substances from the desired products providing the end-product quality required for a given application. Because a chromatographic purification process contains in general several steps, it is necessary to qualify and quantify the substances that are being removed at each step. The major steps can be classified into two categories: primary and secondary.

Primary step: The primary step deals with products extraction, concentration and polishing. All these steps will target the removal of specific contaminants, which include host cell proteins, cell culture additives, antibiotics, nucleic acids and the modified or inactive forms of the product to be processed. Also, the contaminants resulting from the process such as reagents, chromatographic media products, leaking ligands, endotoxins and pyrogens either endogeneous from the cultures broth or resulting from the microbial contamination during the process, sometimes introduced by water or solvents.

The secondary steps target mainly the virus removal. Some quality concerns for cell derived biological products (i.e. mammalian, avian, insect) originate from the presence of adventitious viral contaminants. Recombinant DNA-derived products also raise quality concerns regarding the expression constructs contained in the cell substrate. Virus removal is more pertinent for products derived from *in vitro* cell culture (i.e. recombinant DNA-derived bioproducts including subunit vaccines, monoclonal antibodies from hybridomas), products derived from hybridoma cells grown *in vivo* as ascites and all bioproducts extracted from the mammalian body fluids.

Starting materials/feed stream

General composition and acceptance criteria for the product concentration of starting material, product activity and specific contaminant levels are established. Buffers and chromatographic media are described.

Purified product characteristics

The purified product should be defined in terms of its physical and biological characteristics. Acceptance criteria are defined: identity, purity, concentration and levels of product related and non related impurities have to be defined.

Equipment/hardware and software [3]

The chromatographic system should be described in the Installation Qualification (IQ) and the Operational Qualification (OQ) process in order to demonstrate that the process equipment or systems are capable of consistently operating within the established limits and tolerances. The IQ should include a detailed description of the column equipment, chromatography medium performance, specifications, and the vendor qualification data for both of those two elements. The OQ should verify the readiness of packed chromatographic columns for use. In addition, this IQ/OQ reveals that the compatibility of the equipment with the process was considered, and that the standard operating procedures (SOPs) for the equipment do exist.

Computerised (hardware and software) system validation should be introduced by documentation of installation, operation and performance parameters.

Process description [4,5]

When a potential bio-product has been identified, it may be cloned, characterized, isolated and purified. At this stage, process development starts with the selection of a production clone, suitable for production scale, and by choosing unit operations that are scalable and operable in manufacturing.

Laboratory scale downstream process development is then elaborated by choice of the suitable raw materials (i.e. chromatography media), chromatography media screening, rational process design, scale capabilities and reproducibility testing of the process. Critical control parameters (which affect product quality) and non-critical control parameters (product yield related) are identified at each step, and product characteristics are defined at intermediary stages using all available analytical techniques. A causal relationship between process, product structure and product function should be established.

During the process development, optimization of resolution/efficiency (=purity), speed, recovery and capacity are performed by: determination of the number of purification steps, bead size of media, sample load, buffer system, flow rate, gradient shape and volume, column length and volume, working temperature, regeneration, cleaning and sanitization, and close cooperation between laboratory and manufacturing personnel.

When a scale-up is considered, ranges of critical (e.g. product purity related parameters) and non-critical control parameters (e.g. product yield related parameters) should be examined during process robustness analysis in order to obtain consistent product quality and quantity.

DESCRIPTION OF THE CHROMATOGRAPHY STEP/PROCESS IN THE MANUFACTURING PROCESS

This describes the place of the chromatography process in the general manufacturing process.

DESCRIPTION AND JUSTIFICATION OF THE STANDARD CHROMATOGRAPHIC PROCEDURE (SCP) [4]

This describes and justifies the usage of a selected media and of the chromatographic conditions:

- Chromatographic media: When chromatographic media are chosen, give a preference to those having a Drug Master File – DMF or a Regulatory Support File – RSF.

  The DMF is confidential and filed with FDA. It includes full manufacturing procedures, QC test method and specifications for raw materials, processes and final products. When a chromatographic medium supported by a DMF is used for pharmaceutical bioproduct production, only the DMF number should be considered for the marketing approval file. In some circumstances, specific information from the DMF document could be provided from the matrix manufacturer.

In the European Union, the DMF is replaced by the RSF. This document, available for the user under confidentiality agreement, does not describe the detailed manufacturing procedure of the matrices but provides the information needed to answer the safety issues.

The separation chemistry, the base matrix and the bead size are described and acceptance criteria are documented.

The packing material should be treated like any other process raw material, i.e. quarantined upon receipt and released for use only after specified criteria are met (i.e. composition, functional group identity, particle size and distribution measurements, titration curves for anion exchanger media, separation of a standard protein mixture for size exclusion media, binding capacity for the adsorption media, bacterial endotoxin level etc.)

- Column geometry description

  - cross-sectional area, minimum and maximum bed heights,
  - column packing and determination of packing quality,
  - determination of pressure/flow rate to establish optimal packing for each lot of medium, and acceptability criteria as the height equivalent to a theorical plate value (HEPT) or the asymmetry factor (As).

- Chromatographic cycle: Description of column equilibration, loading and flow through, product recovery (eluate) and regeneration using physicochemical parameters:

  - sample volume, viscosity,
  - flow rates (total, linear), volumes, gradient shape,
  - contact times,
  - pressure,
  - working temperature,
  - buffers systems(nature, ionic strength, pH). Raw material used as buffer salts and water should have the consistent quality for the pharmaceutical production,
  - routine test parameters (including UV profile, osmolality and pH).

DESCRIPTION OF COLUMN MAINTENANCE PROCEDURES AND CRITERIA FOR ITS REUSE [5]

The chromatographic column maintenance conditions are described in order to show the efficacy of the cleaning procedure for the column:

- Regeneration/Cleaning (CIP) in order to reduce the risk of contamination of the product with potential harmful substances, to prolong the lifetime of the media and to reduce the frequency of repacking.

  - Routine regeneration after each run (cleaning reagents, contact time, temperature).
  - Occasional: cleaning of media every 5–10 cycles using a designed protocol (cleaning reagents, contact time, temperature, criteria for reuse).

- Sanitization (SIP)/aseptic maintenance: Column sanitization and storage conditions (time, temperature, pH, buffer, biosafety endotoxins) are defined and must be validated.
- Criteria for reuse of the column are determined: Column volume to remove storage solutions and to equilibrate, matrix characteristics (e.g. bead size), HEPT, peak symmetry, purity, and yield of product.

CRITERIA FOR COLUMN REPACKING OR REPLACEMENT

Describe when the chromatographic column has to be repacked or replaced and provide information on leakage from the media into the product:

- The column repacking frequency should be determined by: analysis of the modification of flow rate and/or pressure, elution and/or regeneration profiles and/or decreasing product yield.
- Medium life span should be evaluated by checking the leakage if any, from the media in the final product, and also after sanitization and storage using the assay methods described in the RSF document. The estimate of medium's useful life should complete this evaluation.

THE CAPACITY AND MEDIUM USEFUL LIFE ASSESSMENT (AGING MECHANISM DOCUMENTATION)

This assessment will provide information on the medium capacity for the product to be purified, and the shelf-life of the chromatographic media: the dynamic capacity and the efficiency studies (quality and recovery related to the product) should be performed in order to evaluate the useful life by performing numerous purification cycles using the same chromatographic columns.

SCALING UP [4]

Scale up should be followed in order to avoid deviations in product quality and recovery: maintain bed height, linear flow rate, sample concentration and sample/media volume ratio; increase sample load, volumetric flow rate and column diameter.

Process validation studies [2–15]

Validation studies of chromatographic processes are performed in order to demonstrate the consistency of the chromatographic process performance required for the quality, potency and safety of the product [11]. Process/Product performance can be defined by a combination of criteria, such as purity and recovery of the product, and is documented during Performance Qualification (PQ) of the chromatography process:

- Effectiveness of the purification process in removing impurities and cleaning specific contaminants (i.e. host cell proteins, endotoxins, nucleic acids, etc.) [12].
- Determination of process reproducibility (= consistency of the process).

- Consistency requires that processes demonstrate robustness i.e. an ability to tolerate reasonable variability. It follows that upper and lower control ranges for process parameters must be generated and such ranges subsequently validated, by determination of the range of chromatographic column operating parameters in the purification process, in order to obtain a defined purity, quality and recovery of the product.
- Determination of lifetimes and product capacity of chromatographic media.
- Determination of bioburden control.
- Chromatographic media are critical raw material having acceptance criteria.
- Critical process parameters, as cleaning, sanitization and storage routines must be validated using validated tests.

Validation of chromatographic processes requires that they have been adequately designed and controlled, and that the equipment is qualified. FDA states that each step of a GMP manufacturing process must be controlled to maximize the probability that the finished product meets all the quality and design specifications [11].

In order to demonstrate how and why the process was designed and to establish its reproducibility, the performance qualification of chromatographic processes requires testing of the product (initial product to be purified, in-process analysis of the intermediate products, and control at final purified stage). The validation study reports should document the variability in each process as it relates to final specifications and quality of the product.

The performance of chromatographic systems should be evaluated under the routine as well as "worst case" production conditions.

Standard performance qualification studies (concurrent/prospective/retrospective)

Validation studies establish documented evidence that a process does what it suppose to do: for concurrent studies, the information is being generated during ongoing implementation of the process. For retrospective studies, the historical information is reviewed and analyzed based upon accumulated manufacturing, testing and control data.

Prospective studies are performed in order to provide information before starting the manufacturing batches, based on a pre-learned protocol, as follows:

- Select routine or specific test parameters and analytical methods [13]. As the starting material, the flow-through or the eluate from the column, which contains the product, should be characterized and the yield of product measured (quality data are indicators of process step reproducibility):
  - activity (immunological or biological) and purity tests acceptance criteria,
  - concentration and yield acceptance criteria,
  - including UV elution profile (pH and conductivity profile should be provided),
  - sterility testing and bioburden.

- Perform successive purification runs (scale down runs or from 1 to all routine runs). A sampling plan (for starting material, flowthrough, eluates and regenerates, sanitization for each chromatographic steps) is established. Correct sampling for all chromatographic steps should be carefully considered and planned. The samples are evaluated according to the plan using validated or partially validated analytical (where identity recovery, linearity and reproducibility are demonstrated) and biological assays. It should be noted that the acceptance criteria are claimed only when the analytical tests are validated.

• Check compliance of results with product acceptance criteria for critical parameters or expected values for non-critical parameters. The collected data are analyzed in respect to the acceptance criteria and are summarized in the performance validation report.

A combination of process validation, validated in-process testing, and final product analysis can ensure the removal of undesired real or potential impurities to the levels suggested by the regulatory authorities.

Specific validation studies and worst-case conditions (prospective)

Perform, on scaled down laboratory columns, the spiking studies with process reagents, infectious biological agents, overload of product, radiolabelled products in set of conditions encompassing upper and lower chromatography processing limits including those within Standard Operation Procedures, when practical issues and safety make the production scale impractical and uneconomical.

These experiments will include an assessment of:

• Column dynamic capacity and usefull lifetime for the active ingredient. Quality assessment of the purified product when increasing the starting material load on the column.
• Column contaminant clearance by specific overload study, or cross-contamination (e.g.: host cell proteins, nucleic acids, etc.).
• Maximum contaminant clearance by specific overload study, or cross-contamination (e.g.: capacity for contaminant elimination, etc.).
• Consequence of SCP deviations within the normal operational range of critical process parameters such as buffer pH and ionic strength, amount of material applied per unit volume of the packing material, temperature, flow-rate [14].
• Abnormal conditions should be tested in order to evaluate the robustness of the process.
• Scaled-down procedure must itself be validated. Product yield and purity must be comparable to those obtained on a typical full scale. The protein load to column volume ratio, the column geometry, the flow rates, are all important factors to be considered.

Useful life of the chromatographic medium/efficacy of aged medium [15]

Standard validation (concurrent/retrospective) The most common way for validating the useful life of columns is to monitor their performance with pilot and production batches by collecting data using validated analytical and biological assays. The chromatographic profiles can also be monitored for consistency from run to run.

Prospective scale-down conditions (prospective)   Numerous scaled-down cycles should be done before registration in order to guarantee a reasonable production period.

Leakage components from the chromatographic media [15]

- Possible leaking components are known from DMF and RSF documentation.
- When possible, assess product contamination with fresh and aged medium.
- Measure leakage also in the discarded effluents using validated test protocols, often provided by the matrix manufacturers.
- Set up acceptable concentration limits of the leakage components (taking into account possible removal during subsequent steps of the process).
- Collect data from scaled-down (prospective) or full-scale experiments (concurrent/retrospective).

Validation of column maintenance procedures

The most common way for validating the cleaning and the sanitization of columns is to monitor the column performance on production batches by collecting data using validated analytical and biological assays.

Cleaning methods should preferably be validated by small scale studies where normal and "stressing" conditions could be tested in order to document:

- virucidal and bactericidal agents,
- removal of active and degradated products from the matrix,
- depyrogenation,
- storage,
- stability of chromatographic media exposed to cleaning, sanitization agents.

Viruses clearance validation of chromatographic processes (16–20)

When human/animal cells or tissues are used as substrates to produce a biopharmaceutical product, there is concern about the presence of viruses and other transmissible agents. As no single approach provides adequate levels of assurance, a combination of three complementary approaches should be adopted to control potential viral contamination of biologicals:

- Selecting and testing source material for the presence of detectable viruses (for cell lines see references [16] and [17]; for products derived from human, ovine, caprine and bovine tissues see reference [18]).
- Testing the capacity of the production processes to remove/inactivate viruses (viral clearance) [19,20].
- Testing the product at appropriate stages of production for total absence of detectable viruses.

Virus clearance of a chromatographic process should include both, removal and inactivation, and is measured by small scale spiking experiments. The virus clearance studies have to be done for all categories of medicinal biological products for human use, notably the products derived from characterized cell lines (for example, monoclonal antibodies, recombinant-DNA derived products including recombinant subunit vaccines) except the inactivated viral vaccines, all live viral vaccines containing self-replicating agents and engineered live vectors [19,20].

Validation of viral removal

- The studies should be conducted in the scale down spiking studies for viral removal by chromatography.
- The choice of viruses for validation should take into account their resemblance to the product and represent as wide a range of physico-chemical properties as possible (enveloped vs non-enveloped; DNA vs. RNA; small vs large; resistant vs non-resistant). The most resistant virus should be used when there is a choice between two viruses. An efficient, sensitive, reliable and validated infectivity assay is required for each virus.

When performing the viral clearance validation studies

- The studies should be done before testing the product in human subjects.
- First, the validation studies should use model viruses of the viruses that could contaminate the product.
- For registration of the bioproduct, a large spectrum of viruses should be used for the validation studies.
- Changes in the production process may necessitate a new validation study.

Changes in chromatography processes [1–2,21–26]

Improvement of chromatographic processes may be necessary for the following main reasons: process changes due to regulatory concerns, necessity of product quality, purity or yield enhancement, usage of more technologically advanced media and improved process economics.

During the process development of bioproducts, some changes relevant to chromatographic processes should be considered: chromatographic media and addition, deletion or change in order of the purification steps.

A change in chromatographic media requires a major revalidation effort in terms of evaluation of the product purity, yield, contaminant removal validation [1] but also physico-chemical characteristics as ion capacity, flow curves, pressure, bed height, elution position and peak shape.

When addition, deletion or change in order of purification steps is considered, product comparability should be performed using extensive analytical techniques in order to prove that the process modification has no major impact on the end product.

Before submission for regulatory approval, changing purification processes requires notification at the point at which the characteristics of batches involved in clinical studies have been defined.

The postmarketing approval changes should be reported as validation of a new system to demonstrate product comparability (in terms of efficacy, quality and safety) [25] supported by data for at least three consecutive batches [24]. It must be kept in mind, that validation of processes results in consistent production and prevents failed batches.

Study phasing

U.S. and European Union (EU) regulatory bodies actively encourage compiling quality information and validation data for chromatographic processes at an early stage in the development of a biopharmaceutical product. The existing regulatory guidelines provide the information necessary to build a validation plan for a defined process.

The time to start the validation studies is during product development on the laboratory scale. Process documentation is obtained at this stage where analytical parameters, acceptance criteria are established (see Table 18.1). At pilot scale, this documentation is continued under GMP conditions and is finally completed with "consistency full scale batches."

Some of the issues include:

- Initial purification scheme is developed at the laboratory scale using suitable raw materials and chromatographic media. Identification of critical parameters and analytical test development are followed by the first performance validation study.
- At pilot stage, the purification scheme is confirmed, critical and non-critical parameters are confirmed, test development is completed and performance qualification study is performed. Each time when scale-up occurs, the product is considered essentially as a "new" product and performance qualification study should be done. Description and justification of standard chromatographic procedures (SCP) and column maintenance procedures are required.
- For pharmaceutical grade material, in addition to the previous considerations, production equipment (IQ, OQ), bioburden control on chromatography media, criteria of column repacking, and media useful life should be considered. From this stage, the validation of analytical tests is performed. Limited validation studies are usually performed prior to the early clinical studies: scale-down validation of viral clearance, nucleic acids, cell contaminants clearance.
- For full scale consistency batches, once the full scale equipment is installed and validated, the process is then performed by manufacturing at the minimum three consecutive full scale batches that meet all the specifications for process parameters, process intermediates and products.

    - GMP documentation has to be established for products that are to be administered to humans. A validation master plan should be prepared, SOP's for production, quality assurance, quality control, batch records and facility management operations have to be established.
    - Full scale consistency material is produced in a dedicated production facility and the validation studies are usually completed. After installation and operational qualifications are completed, the performance qualifications are carried out using validated analytical methods. Full scale and scale-down validation studies are best performed at this stage with production feed-stream product. If the process changes occur in the production, the validation studies are performed.

Table 18.1 Chromatographic process validation study phasing; from process/product definition to process validation

Pre-development	Development	Consistency full scale
LABORATORY SCALE BATCHES	LABORATORY/PILOT SCALE BATCHES PHARMACEUTICAL GRADE BATCHES PRODUCED UNDER GMP'S	CONSISTENCY FULL SCALE BATCHES PRODUCED UNDER GMP'S AT FULL SCALE IN VALIDATED FACILITES
INITIAL PURIFICATION SCHEME DEVELOPED AT LABORATORY SCALE	CONFIRMATION AND OPTIMIZATION OF PURIFICATION SCHEME AT LABORATORY SCALE AND PILOT SCALE BATCHES REPRODUCIBILITY OF PURIFICATION PROCESS AT PILOT/LARGE SCALE	REPRODUCIBILITY OF PURIFICATION PROCESS AT FULL SCALE ON AT LEAST THREE CONSISTENCY BATCHES
Use of suitable raw materials and selection of chromatography media	Usage of well-documented chromatography media (RSF, DMF) and qualified raw materials	Usage of well-documented chromatography media (RSF, DMF) and qualified raw materials
IDENTIFICATION OF CRITICAL PARAMETERS (= product purity related parameters)	CONFIRMATION OF CRITICAL AND IDENTIFICATION/CONFIRMATION OF NON-CRITICAL PARAMETERS (= product yield related parameters)	CONFIRMATION OF CRITICAL AND NON-CRITICAL PARAMETERS
Text development for: • In process testing • Characterization of purified product	From test development completion to validation of analytical tests for critical parameters	All used analytical tests are validated using samples from consistency batches
CONSIDERATION OF PERFORMANCE QUALIFICATION STUDY:	PERFORMANCE QUALIFICATION STUDY OF DEFINED PROCESS ON ALL PILOT BATCHES	PERFORMANCE QUALIFICATION STUDY AT LEAST THREE FULL SCALE CONSECUTIVE BATCHES UNDER NORMAL PRODUCTION CONDITIONS
PROTOCOL • Place of the chromatographic step in the manufacturing process • Starting material characteristics (= specifications or expected values) • Specific contaminant removal: purity, activity, yield issued for each chromatograph step (= specifications or expected values)	Perform performance validation study (Protocol + Report) at each "scale up" change or process modification	Perform performance validation study (Protocol + Report)

Table 18.1 (Continued)

Pre-development	Development	Consistency full scale
• Characteristics of purified product (= specifications or expected values) • Set a sampling plan REPORT • Perform successive purification runs • Analysis of samples using partial validated or partial validated tests • Check compliance of results with specifications or expected values SCALING UP CONSIDERATIONS • Up scale abilities in process design		
	SCALING UP CONSIDERATIONS • Bed height • Linear flow • Sample concentration • Media volume ratio	FINAL SCALING UP • Bed height • Linear flow • Sample concentration • Media volume ratio
	DESCRIPTION, JUSTIFICATION OF STANDARD CHROMATOGRAPHIC PROCEDURES (SCP) (STARTED) • Chromatographic media • Column geometry • Chromatographic cycle • Chromatographic conditions (buffers, pH, temperature...)	STANDARD CHROMATOGRAPHIC PROCEDURES (COMPLETED AT FULL SCALE)
	DESCRIPTION OF COLUMN MAINTENANCE PROCEDURES (STARTED) • Regeneration (CIP) • Santization (SIP)	DESCRIPTION OF COLUMN MAINTENANCE PROCEDURES (COMPLETED)

Table 18.1 (Continued)

Pre-development	Development	Consistency full scale
	By monitoring the column performance on pilot batches By monitoring of bioburden control on chromatographic columns	
	CRITERIA FOR COLUMN REPACKING (STARTED) • flow rates • pressure • elution profiles	CRITERIA FOR COLUMN REPACKING AND MEDIUM LIFE SPAN (COMPLETED)
	CHROMATOGRAPHIC MEDIUM USEFUL LIFE ASSESSMENT/EFFICACY OF AGED MEDIUM (STARTED) • Documented from pilot scale batches or performed on specific scaled down studies	CHROMATOGRAPHIC MEDIUM USEFUL LIFE ASSESSMENT/EFFICACY OF AGED MEDIUM (COMPLETED)
	SPECIFIC VALIDATION STUDIES PERFORMED ON SCALED DOWN LABORATORY COLUMNS (STARTED) • Column capacity for the active ingredient • Column contaminant clearance • Robustness – consequence of SCP deviations (test of abnormal chromatographic conditions)	SPECIFIC VALIDATION STUDIES PERFORMED ON SCALED DOWN LABORATORY STUDIES (COMPLETED) • Using production feedstream material
	VIRUS CLEARANCE VALIDATION STUDIES (STARTED) • By small scale experiments • Started with representative model viruses	VIRUS CLEARANCE VALIDATION STUDIES (COMPLETED) • Using production feedstream material for spiking experiments • Using at least 4 model viruses (ARN vs ADN, enveloped vs non-enveloped)
	PRODUCTION EQUIPMENT (STARTED) • Installation Qualification (IQ) • Operational Qualification (QQ)	PRODUCTION EQUIPMENT (COMPLETED) • Installation Qualification (IQ) • Operational Qualification (QQ)

Documentation

The validation of the chromatographic process results and conclusions will be communicated in a report summarizing the execution of the protocol, results, and conclusions [27].

The installation qualification (IQ), operational qualification (OQ) and performance qualification (PQ) data are submitted as part of a new drug application (NDA), biologics license application (BLA) and in some cases as part of the investigational new drug (IND) application. Equivalent data are submitted as part of clinical trial exemption (CTX) and clinical trial certificate (CTC), and in marketing authorization applications (MAA) in Europe [22].

References

[1] US FDA. Guidance for Industry for the Submission of Chemistry, Manufacturing, and Controls Information for a therapeutic Recombinant DNA-Derived Product or a Monoclonal Antibody Product for *In Vivo* use. CBER/CDER, August 1996.

[2] Sofer G. and Zabriskie D. W. (2000) Biopharmaceutical process validation. Marcel Dekker Inc., New York, 382 p.

[3] Barry A. and Chojnacki R. (1994) Biotechnology Product Validation, Part 8. Chromatography media and column qualification. *BioPharm*, **7**(9), 43–47.

[4] Lugo N. (1998) Elements of Dowstream Bioprocess Validation. *BioPharm*, **11**(6), 18–26.

[5] Adner N. and Sofer G. (1994) Biotechnology Product Validation, Part 3. Chromatography cleaning validation. *BioPharm*, **7**(3), 44–48.

[6] US FDA. Process validation guidance. Draft global harmonization Task Force Study Group 3. FDA, June 1998.

[7] US FDA. Guidance for industry. Content and format of chemistry, manufacturing and controls; information and establishment; description information for a vaccine or related product. US Department of Health and Human Services. Center for Biologics Evaluation and Research (CBER), January 1999.

[8] Sofer G. and Hagel L. (1997) Handbook of Process Chromatography: A guide to Optimization, Scale-up, and Validation. Academic Press, London, 387 p.

[9] Parenteral Drug Association. (1992) Industry perspective on the validation of column-based separation processes for the purification of proteins. *Journal of Parenteral Science & Technology*, **46**, 87–97.

[10] Akers J., McEntire J. and Sofer G. (1994) Biotechnology Product Validation, Part 2. A logical plan. *BioPharm*, **7**(2), 54–56.

[11] US FDA: Guidelines on General Principles of Process Validation. Center for Drug and Biologics, Center for Devices and Radiological Health, Food and Drug Administration, 5600 Fishers Lane, Rockville MD 20857, May 1987.

[12] ICH-International Conference on Harmonisation; Specifications; test procedures and acceptance criteria for biotechnological/biological products. ICH Topic Q6B Document step 4 (March 10, 1999), CPMP/ICH/365/96.

[13] McEntire J. (1994) Biotechnology Product Validation, Part 5: Selection and validation of analytical techniques. *Pharmaceutical Technology Europe*, **6**, 48–55.

[14] Kelley B. D. *et al.* (1997) Demonstrating process robustness for chromatographic purification of a recombinant protein. *BioPharm*, **10**(10), 36–47.

[15] Seeley R. *et al.* (1994) Validation of chromatography resin useful life. *BioPharm*, **7**(7), 41–48.

[16] ICH-International Conference on Harmonisation; Note for Guidance on Quality of Biotechnological Products: Derivation and Characterization of Cell Substrates used for Production

of Biotechnological/Biological Products. ICH Topic Q5D Document step 2 (January 10, 1997).

[17] WHO. Requirements for the Use of Animal Cells as in vitro Substrates for the Production of Biologicals (Final Draft). Requirements for Biological Substances No. 50. WHO Expert Commitee on Biological Standardization, January 17, 1997.

[18] EMEA. Note for Guidance on Minimising the Risk of Transmitting Spongiform Encephalopathy Agents via Human and Veterinary Medicinal Products. EMEA/410/01-FINAL.

[19] EMEA. Note for Guidance on Virus Validation Studies: the Design, Contribution and Interpretation of Studies Validating the Inactivation and Removal of Viruses. CPMP Biotechnology working party. The European Agency for the Evaluation of Medicinal Products. CPMP/BWP/268/95, FINAL.

[20] ICH-International Conference on Harmonisation : Note for guidance on Quality of Biotechnological Products: Viral Safety Evaluation of Biotechnology Products Derived From Cell Lines of Human and Animal Origin. CPMP/ICH/295/95.

[21] US FDA. Guidance for Industry: Changes to an Approved Application for Specified Biotechnology and Specified Synthetic Biological Products. CBER/CDER, July 1997.

[22] Behizad M. and Baines D. (1998) Regulatory Aspects of Column Chromatography in Biopharmaceutical Manufacturing. U.S. and EU Regulatory Attitudes Toward Change. *BioPharm*, 11(5), 72–80.

[23] Talarico T. L. *et al.* (1999) Comparability analysis to support a manufacturing site change and process modifications for a biopharmaceutical. A regulatory submission case study. *BioPharm*, 12(1), 42–47.

[24] "Changes to Approved Applications (Final Rule), "Federal Register 62 (142) **39**, 889–39, 903, Docket No. 95N95N-0329, (24 July 1997).

[25] US FDA. "Use of compatibility protocols to evaluate and implement changes in analytical, method, facilities and manufacturing process for approved or licensed biotechnological/biological Drug products" PhRMA/BIO Compatibility Protocol Guidance (21 August 1997).

[26] EMEA. Note for Guidance on Comparability of Medicinal Products Containing Biotechnology-derived Proteins as Drug Substance. CPMP/BNP/3207/00.

[27] DeSain C. Documentation Basics: That Support Good Manufacturing Practices (ed.) Advanstar communications, Cleveland, 1993, 88 p.

Chapter 19

Biochromatography and biomedical applications

C. Legallais, Mookambeswaran A. Vijayalakshmi and Ph. Moriniére

Introduction

As it has been presented in other chapters, the applications of any type of biochromatography are numerous: different methods are available for the removal or recovery of many target molecules. These technologies have been also exploited for biomedical applications.

In a number of diseases, the administration of some drugs appears to be not efficient enough for the patient's safety. This is the case in familial hypercholesterolemia (Thompson *et al.*, 1976), preparation to graft (Agishi, 1996), autoimmune diseases (Nyddeger *et al.*, 1990). The extracorporeal removal of pathogenic substances appears then as an attractive alternative.

The first and now widely applied extracorporeal therapy is hemodialysis, for the treatment of acute or chronic renal failure. In the late 1970s, the development of microporous membranes allowed the use of plasmapheresis for the extracorporeal removal of pathogenic proteins. Removal of antibodies through plasma exchange after transplantation resulted in the graft's survival (Adams *et al.*, 1979). Unfortunately, plasmapheresis (i.e. replacement of plasma by a substitution fluid) results also in the loss of all patient's own plasma proteins. Replacing the patient's plasma by that of a donor may cause allergy, hypocalcemia, viral infections, etc. Therefore, it seems more appropriate to achieve a selective removal of the pathogenic molecules. In 1981, Agishi *et al.* proposed the use of cascade filtration (CF) for the selective removal of immunoglobulin G (IgG). However, this technique is only semi-selective, which constitutes one of its limits. To wit, not only IgGs and all the molecules larger than IgG, but also albumin to a certain extent, are removed from the patient's plasma.

It is of prime importance to develop techniques as specific as possible to avoid the side effects generated by the introduction of foreign substances into the blood. Some of the adsorption techniques described in this book appear to meet this challenge. Several devices based on these principles are already existing, at research levels or even in some commercial applications.

In this chapter, only the systems commercially available and clearly identified for removing pathogenic molecules are described in detail. Thus, the systems called by the clinicians "hemoperfusion" (Bonomini and Chang, 1982) are not considered. These systems rely on coated or uncoated activated charcoal or resins columns and are able to retain several plasma molecules, but the type of interactions and the real binding properties are ill defined. The same can be said about activated charcoal columns proposed for the treatment of hepatic failure (Ouchi *et al.*, 1978) or acute poisoning.

The purpose of this chapter is to demonstrate, through various examples, how a chromatographic column, originally designed for biotechnological applications, may be integrated into an extracorporeal circuit. It should be kept in mind that the constraints in term of efficiency, cost, etc. may be completely different for different applications. The biocompatibility issue of these systems, that is not a limiting factor in biochromatography, but essential in medical devices, will be specifically addressed.

Extracorporeal set ups

At the outset of this chapter, it is important to discuss the operational rules governing extracorporeal set ups, in order to appreciate the distinguishing features of biotechnological and medical applications of biochromatographic techniques.

The purpose of the extracorporeal circuit is to allow the contact between the target molecule and the adsorbent. Hence it is based on the classical circuit widely used in hemodialysis. Basic elements, such as pumps, pressure transducers, air bubble traps, alarm sensors etc., are found in all of these circuits. All of them are connected to the adequate monitor device which pilots the complete procedure. The blood is withdrawn from the patient via a peripheral venous access, at a flow rate of 80–100 ml/min. The coagulation is prevented with heparin or with acid citrate dextrose (ACD). The blood may then directly contact the adsorbent column (Fig. 19.1a) or be directed to the primary separation device (Fig. 19.1b). This device is a plasma filter in most cases, or a centrifuge bowl, where the plasma is separated from the blood cells (red blood cells, white blood cells, platelets) at a flow rate equivalent to 1/3 of the inlet blood flow rate. In the case illustrated in Fig. 19.1a, blood cells are in direct contact with the adsorbent and may be activated or altered. For biocompatibility reasons, the set up of Fig. 19.1b is more

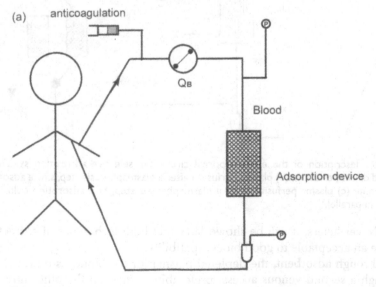

Figure 19.1 (Continued)

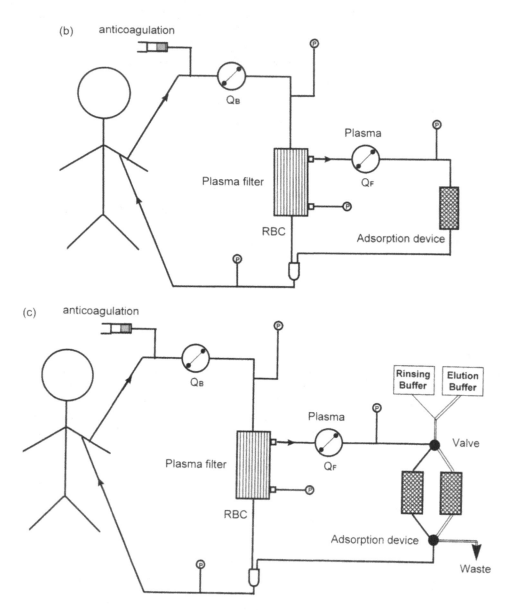

Figure 19.1 Schematic description of the extracorporeal circuit for selective adsorption systems: (a) blood direct perfusion; (b) plasma perfusion after a plasmapheresis step, single adsorption column; (c) plasma perfusion after a plasmapheresis step, two adsorption columns working in parallel.

often preferred. Nevertheless, it will be shown later that both techniques, if correctly executed, provide an acceptable to good biocompatibility.

After passing through adsorbent, the depleted plasma (or the blood) is returned to the patient through a second venous access, preferably located on the other arm so as to avoid recirculation. The effectiveness of both circuits is limited by the adsorbent column capacity. To circumvent this limitation, many manufacturers choose to make both columns work in parallel (Fig. 19.1c): when one column is loaded, the other one is being regenerated. This requires the handling of different solutions. The column is first rinsed with physiological buffer to pump back to the patient the plasma retained in the void volume. The elution is then performed under the optimal conditions (high ionic strength, low or high pH) according to the binding mechanism. Finally, the column is equilibrated with physiological buffer before the next loading procedure. Thanks to these rather involving operating conditions, the removal of target molecules is optimized. The number of cycles is determined by the physician. The treatment schedule depends on the type of disease to be treated. For example, LDL-apheresis is performed during 4 hours weekly or biweekly over years while acute syndromes are treated daily over a short period.

Adsorbents for biomedical applications

As can be seen in the foregoing chapters, the different chromatographic adsorbents could be incorporated into the extracorporeal devices. In fact, some of them are already being used in clinical practice while others are still tested in the laboratories. While the first category will be dealt in some detail in this chapter, the new possibilities will be only considered in general terms. Adsorbents under consideration could be described as involving: chemoadsorption, pseudobioadsorption and bioadsorption.

Chemoadsorption

"Chemoadsorption" is the name adopted by the clinicians to broadly describe the adsorption resulting from an interaction, mainly of ionic type, between the immobilized ligand and the target molecule. The negatively or positively charged ligand immobilized on the solid support is able to bind not only the target molecule of the opposite charge, but also all the molecules presenting the similar electrostatic properties. Chemoadsorption is thus a "group selective" albeit non specific procedure. In Table 19.1 are presented the different commercially available systems and their purposes, while Table 19.2 describes the operating conditions. Table 19.3 lists the clinical results. The main application for chemoadsorption is the treatment of familial hypercholesterolemia achieved by removal of low density lipoprotein (LDL) and lipoprotein(a) (Lp(a)). The negatively charged ligands bind the positive charges of the apolipoprotein B (ApoB) present on the surface of both molecules. Desorption is very simple to perform since the competition with salt (NaCl 4%) allows the release of adsorbed ApoB. Another application of chemoadsorption is the removal of endotoxins by immobilized polymyxin B. The three systems available nowadays are described in detail below.

Liposorber LA15 (Kaneka)

This system (Takada et al., 1987) has been widely used for LDL removal in Japan and in Europe. The extracorporeal circuit is based on the principle described in Fig. 19.1c. A screening procedure was carried out by Tani (1996) to identify the best polyanion to

Table 19.1 Blood purification systems based on chemoadsorption

Manufacturer	Trade name	Support	Ligand	Target molecule	Binding type (q_α, K_D)	Reference
Kaneka (Japan)	Liposorber LA15	Porous cellulose hard gel	Dextran sulfate MW: 10^3 Da	LDL-C LP(a)	Electrostatic $q_\alpha = 10\,mg/ml$ $K_D = 3.10^{-7}M$	Tani *et al.* (1996)
Fresenius (Germany)	DALI	Porous beads of polyacryl-amide	Polyacrylate	LDL-C Lp(a)	Electrostatic $q_\alpha = 12\,mg/ml$ $K_D = 10^{-5}\,M^*$	Bosch *et al.* (1993) Bosch *et al.* (1997) *Tani *et al.* (1996)
Toray (Japan)	PMX-20R	Polystyrene fibers	Polymyxin B	Endotoxin	Electrostatic $q_\alpha = 0.06\,\mu g/ml$	Toray brochure

Table 19.2 In vivo operating conditions for the blood purification systems based on chemoadsorption

Product	Column volume	Feed flow rate fluid type	Elution mode	Anticoagulation	Reference
Kaneka Liposorber LA15	$2 \times 150\,ml$	30 ml/min plasma	NaCl 4.1%	Heparin bolus: 2000 U+ 20 U/kg/h*	Olbricht (1996)
Fresenius DALI	480 ml	50 ml/min blood	No elution during the treatment	Heparin bolus: 40 U/kg* citrate: 2.5 ml/min continuously	Bosch *et al.* (1997)
Toray PMX-20R	50 m fibers packed into a 200 ml column	80–100 ml/ min blood	No elution during the treatment	Heparin or nafamostat mesilate	Aoki *et al.* (1994)

* U/kg = U/kg of body weight.

mimic the function of the LDL receptor. Dextran sulfate, with a molecular weight of 1000 Da, was selected because of its high affinity for ApoB and its low toxicity.

The clinical studies reported by Olbricht (1996) indicate that two small columns running in parallel achieve the set goals. The columns are switched between 6 and 10 times per treatment depending on the severity of the hypercholesterolemia and thus on the plasma volume to be processed. One session per week is necessary in order to maintain the patient LDL-cholesterol level below the acceptable threshold.

As expected, non specific binding at dextran sulfate to other positively charged molecules occurs (Ikonomov *et al.*, 1989). This may have either a deleterious or a beneficial effect on the patient. For instance, the reduction of plasma fibrinogen level (up to 25%) (Grützmacher *et al.*, 1990) could represent a positive aspect in the treatment of coronary lesions (Matsuda *et al.*, 1994).

Table 19.3 Clinical results obtained with the blood purification systems based on chemo-adsorption

Product	Removal rate of target molecules	Non-specific binding	Clinical outcome (long-term)	Reference
Kaneka Liposorber LA15	LDL: −70% Lp(a): −60% VLDL: −60%*	Fibrinogen coagulation factors some IgG	Regression and inhibition of progression of coronary lesions	Olbricht (1996) Tatami et al. (1992)
Fresenius DALI	LDL: −45% Lp(a): −43%	Fibrinogen Mg^{2+}, Ca^{2+} prevented by adequate prerinsing	Presumably the same as above	Bosch et al. (1997)
Toray PMX-20R	Endotoxin: −70%	Not described	Survival rate after a septic shock: more than 50%	Aoki et al. (1994), Kodama et al. (1995), Tani et al. (1998)

* This rate depends on the number of cycles achieved.

DALI (Fresenius)

LDL removal is achieved here with another anionic compound: polyacrylate. Its affinity for LDL is lower than that of dextran sulfate because of the absence of sulfonate or sulfate group, but its ionic characteristics are mainly the same. The main difference in the set up is the direct perfusion of the adsorption column by the blood, which makes it easier to operate (Bosch *et al.*, 1993). The adopted principle is the size exclusion chromatography: the ligands are located at the inner surface of the porous beads (diameter 100 nm) representing an available area of about 1200 m². The blood cells are hence excluded from the pores, where LDL are adsorbed, allowing only a minor ligand-cell interaction. Two drawbacks are nevertheless present: first, the use of a single column, although large, limits the LDL removal rate, and second, the huge anticoagulation results in an activated partial thromboplastin time (apTT) multiplied by a factor of four at the end of the treatment (Bosch *et al.*, 1997b).

Polymyxin B: PMX-F (Toray)

The immobilized polymyxin B targets endotoxins through an interaction between five positively charged amino groups and the mono- or diphosphate anionic group of Lipid A (Hanasawa *et al.*, 1988). Endotoxins are involved in the pathogenesis of septic shock ensuing poor prognosis. They need to be directly removed from the patient's. Polymyxin B is an antiendotoxic antibiotic peptide, however, it is also neurotoxic and nephrotoxic. Its immobilization on polystyrene fibers permits its use without the mentioned side effects. The initial clinical results are satisfactory (Aoki *et al.*, 1994), and the biocompatibility is high enough to apply the system in emergency cases, although not in the repeated ones. A recent study mentions an increase in the survival rate of patients with multiple organs failure caused by endotoxemia, after the application of this selective treatment (Tani *et al.*, 1998). It is commercially available only in Japan up to now (Toray).

Pseudobioadsorption

The term "pseudobioadsorption" covers the removal of target molecules by a pseudobiospecific ligand, as defined by Vijayalakshmi (1989) and described in detail in Chapter 8. The binding may be complex, involving hydrophobic, aromatic and ionic forces on a large recognition site between the immobilized ligand and the molecule to be removed. Table 19.4 lists the devices now commercially available. One is dedicated to immunoglobulin removal, and the other to beta$_2$-microglobulin (β_2-M) removal. The operating conditions and the clinical results are given in Tables 19.5 and 19.6, respectively.

Immusorba (Asahi)

In this case, the ligand is an amino acid: tryptophan or phenylalanine (Yamazaki *et al.*, 1989). Both amino acids are able to bind immunoglobulins and circulating immune complexes (CIC) via a combination of aromatic and hydrophobic interactions (Ikonomov *et al.*, 1992). In contrast to histidine (Bueno *et al.*, 1996), the binding is

Table 19.4 Blood purification systems based on pseudobioadsorption

Manufacturer	Trade name	Support	Ligand	Target molecule	Binding type (q_α, K_D)	Reference
Asahi (Japan)	Immusorba TR-350 PH-350	Spherical PVA gel particles	Tryptophan or phenyl-alanine	Ig	Pseudo-biospecific $q_\alpha = 20\,mg/ml$	Fadul et al. (1996) Haupt et al. (1996) Ikonomov et al. (1992)
Kaneka (Japan)	BM01	Porous cellulose beads	Hydrophobic hexadecyl-alkyl chain	β_2-M	Hydrophobic $q_\alpha = 3.5\,mg/ml$	Nakazawa et al. (1993)

Table 19.5 In vivo operating conditions for the blood purification systems based on pseudobioadsorption

Product	Column volume	Feed flow rate fluid type	Elution mode	Anticoagulation	Reference
Asahi Immusorba TR-350, PH-350	350 ml	20 ml/min plasma	No elution during the treatment	Heparin: bolus 2000 U + 1000 U/hr	Fadul et al. (1996) Shibuya et al. (1994)
Kaneka BM01	350 ml	120–200 ml/min blood	No elution during the treatment	Heparin: 1000 U/hr	Gejyo et al. (1995)

Table 19.6 Clinical results obtained with the blood purification systems based on pseudobioad-sorption

Product	Removal rate of target molecules	Non-specific binding	Clinical outcome (long-term)	Reference
Asahi Immusorba TR-350, PH-350	IgG: −50% IgM: −60%	Fibrinogen: −70% C₄: −70%	Depends on the disease: good for graft, rebound generally observed	Fadul et al. (1996) Haupt et al. (1996) Morosetti et al. (1994)
Kaneka BM01	β₂-M: −70% (including the effect of dialysis)	IL1β: −98% * IL1Ra: −98% * IL6: −83% * TNFα: −31% *	Improvement in daily life activity ↘ joint pain	Gejyo et al. (1995) Tsuchida et al. (1998)

* *In vitro* studies.

possible at the plasma ionic strength, because ionic interactions are not involved. Each amino acid finds specific applications: phenylalanine for the treatment of immunological diseases such as multiple sclerosis (MS), Guillain-Barré Syndrome and Systemic Lupus Erythematosus (SLE), and tryptophan for Myasthenia Gravis (MG). The single column is integrated in a circuit represented by Fig. 19.1b. The perfused plasma crosses a particle removal filter before returning to the patient, in order to prevent the possible release of complexes in the patient's circulation. These columns are not very specific, as shown in Table 19.6. Especially, fibrinogen and complement are adsorbed at the same rate as the immunoglobulins (Ikonomov *et al.*, 1992).

BM01 (Kaneka)

There is no detailed information about the immobilized ligand ("an hydrophobic hexadecylalkyl chain") used to bind β₂-M. This molecules accumulates in the plasma of long term hemodialysis patients and is responsible for amyloidosis. The single column made of cellulose beads is inserted in the dialysis extracorporeal circuit before the hemodialyser (Nakazawa *et al.*, 1993). It is then perfused with whole blood. The reduction of plasma β₂-M level is quite significant, but it should be noted that its removal also occurs by non-specific adsorption and filtration in the dialysis step. Moreover, although long term clinical study did not mention non-specific adsorption of other proteins displaying surface hydrophobicity (Gejyo *et al.*, 1995), recent data outlined concomitant removal of inflammatory cytokines (IL1-β, IL1-Ra, IL6 and TNFα in a lower extent) (Tsuchida *et al.*, 1998). The clinical outcome of the prolonged treatment has been the reduction of pain and the improvement in daily activities of the patient.

Bioadsorption

The term "bioadsorption" describes the use of biological ligands binding very specifically the target molecules. The term "immunoadsorption" is not employed in order to avoid any confusion between the adsorption of immunoglobulins (usually employed

Table 19.7 Blood purification systems based on bioadsorption

Manufacturer	Trade name	Support	Ligand	Target molecule	Binding type (q_α, K_D)	Reference
Excorim (Sweden)	Immunosorba	Sepharose beads	Protein A	Ig CIC	Biospecific $q_\alpha = 20\,mg/ml$ $K_D = 10^{-8}\,M$	Excorim brochure Gjörstrup *et al.* (1991)
IMRE (USA)	Prosorba	Silica beads	Protein A	Ig CIC	Biospecific $q_\alpha = $ 8 mg/bead $K_D = 10^{-8}\,M$	Balint (1996)
Therasorb (Germany)	Ig-Therasorb	Sepharose beads	Polyclonal anti human IgG from sheep	IgG	Ag–Ab $q_\alpha = 8\,mg/ml$	Therasorb brochure
Therasorb (Germany)	LDL-Therasorb	Sepharose beads	Polyclonal anti human ApoB from sheep	LDL-C	Ag–Ab $q_\alpha = 16\,mg/ml$ $K_D = 10^{-4} - 10^{-8}\,M$	Therasorb brochure Spaethe *et al.* (1996)

by physicians), and the binding of any type of molecules by their respective antibodies. The nature of the binding is complex, that is, based on the complementarity of charge, hydrophobicity, shape, etc., stronger than that observed in pseudobioaffinity. A complete description of the possible interactions is provided in Chapter 7 of this book. Table 19.7 lists the different systems commercially available. Immobilized Protein A is included here since it can be considered as a "super antigen" for all types of immunoglobulins. The other devices are based on antigen-antibody recognition. The respective operating conditions and clinical results are found in Tables 19.8 and 19.9.

Immobilized Protein A: Immunosorba (Excorim) and Prosorba (Imré)

Protein A is a cell-wall protein of Staphylococcus aureus with a molecular weight of 42 000 Da and a strong specific affinity for the Fc region of immunoglobulins. It is hence able to bind all types of Ig: IgG (IgG3 subclass excepted), IgA, IgM, IgE, and circulating immune complexes (CIC). The number of applications for the treatment of various diseases is large. A non-exhaustive list of possible treatments is provided in Table 19.10. The versatility of this system is apparent. The benefit of using Protein A columns is well established for immunomodulation in hyperimmunized patient expecting a graft (Balint *et al.*, 1996); even if the potentially responding patient needs to be clearly identified (Esnault *et al.*, 1990). Its use is less clear in the treatment of cancer. The use of Protein A was proposed to remove tumor-associated CIC but Fennelly *et al.*, (1995) did not find an increased level of CIC in the eluates compared to a control group. Moreover, the stage of cancer seems of importance in the success of the procedure. The Protein A use could also be a drawback since it results in hypogammaglobulinemia and consequently in an increased risk of infection (Esnault *et al.*, 1990).

Table 19.8 In vivo operating conditions for the blood purification systems based on bioadsorption

Product	Column volume	Feed flow rate fluid type	Elution mode	Anticoagulation	Reference
Excorim Immunosorba	2 × 62.5 ml	30 ml/min plasma	Glycine HCl pH = 2.2	Citrate	Excorim brochure Nilsson et al. (1993)
Imré Prosorba	2 × 125 silica beads	20 ml/min plasma	PBS pH = 11.5	Heparin	Balint et al. (1996)
Therasorb Ig-Therasorb	2 × 100 ml	25 ml/min plasma	Glycine HCl 1M pH = 2.8	Heparin: 1000 U/hr + ACD 1: 22	Knöbl et al. (1995)
Therasorb LDL-Therasorb	2 × 310 ml	25 ml/min plasma	Glycine HCl 1M pH = 2.8	Heparin: 2000 U/hr + ACD 1: 22	Gruber et al. (1993)

Table 19.9 Clinical results obtained with the blood purification systems based on bioadsorption

Product	Removal rate of target molecules*	Non-specific binding	Clinical outcome (long-term)	Reference
Excorim Immunosorba	IgG:−80%	Unknown	see Table 19.11	Esnault et al. (1990) Excorim brochure
Imré Prosorba	IgG: −70%	C$_4$, rheumatoid factor	see Table 19.11	Snyder et al. (1992) Snyder et al. (1991)
Therasorb Ig-Therasorb	IgG: −70%	No	Comparable to that of Protein A	Knöbl et al. (1995)
Therasorb LDL-Therasorb	LDL: −65% Lp(a): −65%	No	Regression and inhibition of progression of coronary lesions	Gruber et al. (1993) Richter et al. (1993)

* This rate depends on the number of cycles achieved.

Two different companies (Excorim, Sweden, and IMRE, USA) market immobilized Protein A columns. They may differ in the support, but the employed set ups are similar; they rely on the alternate adsorption using two columns in parallel (Fig. 19.1c). The elution is achieved either under very acidic or under very basic pH conditions. The efficiency of Protein A for total IgG and CIC removal is very high, but some non specific bindings are also detected (Ikonomov et al., 1992).

Table 19.10 Clinical applications for Protein A columns

Application / Disease	Molecule to be removed	Results	Comments	References
Immuno-modulation preparation to graft	AntiHLA antibodies	↗ survival rate of kidney or heart transplantation recipients	Need for a better definition of target patients	Agishi et al. (1996) Ross et al. (1993) Ruiz et al. (1994) Hiesse et al. (1992) Esnault et al. (1990)
Malignant diseases	Circulating immune complexes (CIC)	Not completely established transient effect	Depends on the tumor severity	Fennelly et al. (1995) Hakansson et al. (1984) Ray et al. (1982)
Autoimmune diseases: SLE, ITP etc.	Antiplatelet IgG RBC autoantibodies	About 50% success allows transfusion	Transient effect	Branda et al. (1986) Balint et al. (1996) Muroi et al. (1989) Snyder et al. (1992) Esnault et al. (1993)
Hemophilia	Antifactor VIII or IX	Allows efficient injection of factor VIII and IX		Nilsonn et al. (1995) Gjörstrup et al. (1991) Uehlinger et al. (1991)

Immobilized antibodies (Therasorb)

This device exploits the immobilized antibodies to specifically and reversibly bind their respective antigens. Thus, it represents the highest specificity in blood purification devices. The company Therasorb (Germany) proposes two devices based on polyclonal antibodies originating from sheep and developed against either ApoB or IgG (Stoffel *et al.*, 1981). They are not directed against a very specific molecule: LDL-Therasorb adsorbs VLDL, LDL and Lp(a) and Ig-Therasorb adsorbs all kinds of immunoglobulins. The applications are similar to those of Protein A or tryptophan columns for IgG removal. The columns perfused with plasma work in parallel (Fig. 19.1c). They are very expensive but a sterilization technique makes it possible to reuse them at least 20 times for Ig-Therasorb and 40 times for LDL-Therasorb. One set of columns is dedicated to a single patient.

Specific features pertinent in extracorporeal adsorbents

The different systems hitheto described represent not only a means for the removal of a target molecule, but also constitute therapeutic tools. In addition to their efficiency, other criteria need to be considered: cost/effectiveness, and most of all biocompatibility, which becomes an essential feature in biomedical applications.

Adequacy of the existing systems for a treatment

In addition to non-selective techniques (plasma exchange, cascade filtration), many modalities are proposed for blood purification. A certain number of criteria may be considered to compare the rationale for use of the different available systems. They are

Table 19.11 Comparison of the available methods for blood purification

Method	Specificity	Versatility	Cost	Multiple use device	Simplicity for use	Frequency of use	Comments
Plasma exchange	− − −	+ + +	+	No	+ + +	+ + +	Need for substitution fluid
Cascade filtration	−	+	+	No	+ +	+/−	
Chemo-adsorption	+	−	+/−	No	+/++(*)	+	Risk of ana-phylactic reactions
Pseudobio-adsorption	+ +	+ +	−	No	+	+/−	
Bioadsorption	+ + +	+/−	− − −	Yes/No	+	− −	Risk of leakage of bioactive substances

* DALI system.
+ + + → − − − From the best to the worst choice considering the criterion.

introduced in Table 19.11, with the evaluation of each device in respect to them. It is abundantly clear that the more specific the technique, the higher the cost. However, there is more than one way to amend it. To wit, an important way to reduce the cost of the process is its versatility. The production costs can be significantly decreased if the product has wide applications. Moreover, if the device is reusable, its cost per treatment may become much less than that of a single use product. Up to now, only the antibody-based sorbents are considered to be multiple use devices, because they can be sterilized. In non selective techniques based on filtration, the modules are rejected after each treatment because of the membrane fouling which affects their sieving properties. Dextran sulfate columns are also single use products because they can not be disinfected (Mabuchi *et al.*, 1987). Many other systems are also sold up to now as single use devices. Thus, the cost of treatment with antibody-based sorbent may be comparable or even less than that with Protein A, or with DSC columns.

Great attention should be also paid to how easy it is to handle the complete process. Even when sustained by a reliable monitor, a complicated technique may repel the user, i.e. the clinician and the nurse. For instance, the processes based on Fig. 19.1c are considered to be more difficult to use than those proposing direct hemoperfusion or non specific plasma treatment. The simplicity in use combined with the versatility may affect the frequency of use of a device.

All these considerations outline the difficulty in choosing the "best" method. It seems more suitable to adapt the treatment to the patient's disease and the available clinical facilities: in a small center, very versatile techniques such as cascade filtration could be preferred, while larger hospitals could employ many different devices. For the treatment of familial hypercholesterolemia, it is recognized that not only LDL-C and Lp(a) should be removed, but also fibrinogen (Malchesky *et al.*, 1995). Hence dextran sulfate columns, which are not too expensive, seem appropriate. On the other hand, a very specific treatment should preferably be chosen to remove an autoimmune IgG.

In fact, it appears that nowadays the choice depends more on the strategies of a particular country in terms of health insurance and governmental approval (Malchesky *et al.*, 1997): in the USA where it takes long time for a new product to obtain FDA approval, and where only plasma exchange is reimbursed, very few specific treatments are offered. To the contrary, the market is much more developed in Japan where selective or specific removal of pathogenic substances is given priority as compared to plasma exchange. This also probably explains why about half of the commercially available products come from Japan.

Biocompatibility aspects

Definitions

In extracorporeal circuits, blood flows in contact with different biomaterials (blood lines, membrane, etc.). The adsorption column is considered as a biomaterial and needs also to demonstrate its compatibility with the blood components. The absence of adverse reactions from the blood is often called biocompatibility. The most intense studies in the field of extracorporeal circuits have been conducted on hemodialysis modules. The Consensus Conference on Biocompatibility (Gurland *et al.*, 1993) proposes a standardization of the terminology and the methodologies to assess biocompatibility. The proposed definitions are also relevant to the blood purification systems described in this chapter. Biocompatibility is defined as "the ability of a material, device, or system to perform without a clinically significant host response in a specific application". Hence, it is important to prove that the proposed adsorption systems, which strongly interact with the blood components, are able to meet these requirements. In Table 19.12 are summarized the different reactions that may occur during the contact between the blood and the adsorption column, and the means to detect them. The most acute, but fortunately very uncommon, reaction from the patient during the treatment is the hypersensitivity towards the material, resulting in an anaphylactic shock. The common first response is the activation of the complement system, resulting in reactions possibly enhanced by the material itself. Holmes *et al.* (1995) describes in detail the biochemical mechanisms of reactions occurring in the blood contacting hemodialysers.

The adsorbents are different from dialysis membranes because their original surface (Sepharose, silica, etc.) is modified to couple the desired ligand. Vienken *et al.*, (1995) proposed to modify cellulosic or hydrophobic membranes by grafting additional compounds capable of improving their biocompatibility. The graft might also make the basic material less compatible, because hydrophobic or charged regions are introduced to their surface. In addition, the leakage of immobilized ligand into the extracorporeal circuit might also be responsible for acute reactions and ultimately for the synthesis of anti-ligand antibodies.

Most of the manufacturers propose to avoid the blood cells traversing the adsorbent column. This should minimize the host response, although the complement activation alone may induce reactions when the plasma is remixed with the cells before returning to the patient. Since the bioincompatibility is responsible for many short term and long term side effects, it is of prime importance to check all the parameters listed in

Table 19.12 Signs of bio(in)compatibility and methods of assessment

Potential activation factor	Immediate result	Detection	Consequences	
			Short term	Long term
Material (free OH groups, hydrophilic regions)	Complement activation	C3a, C5a	Activate circulating cells	—
Complement activation + material	Leukopenia	White Blood Cells count	—	Endothelial damage infections
Complement activation + material (hydrophobic and cationic regions)	Platelet activation	β-thrombo-globulin	Clotting	Atherosclerosis
Complement activation + material?	Monocyte activation	ILl β, IL6, TNFα	Pyrogenic reactions	Amyloidosis osteodystrophy
Material (anionic regions) unadapted anticoagulation	Coagulation (contact phase activation)	Thrombin-antithrombin III (TAT) partial thrombo-plastin time	Clotting / bleeding	—

Table 19.12, when developing a new device. It is nevertheless unrealistic to expect no changes in these parameters, since it is well known that the other components of the circuit (tubing, needles, bubble trap, etc.) also interact with the blood.

Usual assessment of biocompatibility

All the commercially available systems for specific blood purification are validated in the countries of use in terms of biocompatibility. It does not mean that these systems do not induce any of the response indicated in Table 19.12, but only that the patients' responses are considered to be tolerable. The observed reactions are described in Table 19.13. Significant complement activation was reported by Snyder et al. (1991) with Protein A columns, in a very large study including about 150 patients: C_{3a} and C_{5a} levels were multiplied by 27 at the end of the treatment. This increase was associated with multiple mild to moderate side effects such as chills, fever, etc., which stop in a few hours after the patient's disconnection. To prevent these reactions, most of the procedures tend to "overuse" anticoagulation: acid citrate dextrose (ACD) is often added to heparin in order to complex the Ca^{2+} and Mg^{2+} ions involved as the essential cofactors for the complement activation.

Generally, all the systems also exhibit a drop in the white blood cells count a few minutes after the beginning of a treatment. It usually normalizes within 30 to 60 minutes.

Table 19.13 Effective biocompatibility of the blood purification systems

Product	Biocompatibility	Side effects	References
Kaneka Liposorber LA15	↘ factors VIII, IX, XI minor complement activation	Anaphylactic reactions for patients with ACE inhibitors	Olbricht et al. (1996) Yamamoto et al. (1992)
Fresenius DALI	Mild complement activation all other parameters constant	See above	Bosch et al. (1997b)
Toray PMX-20R	Decrease in platelet count "acceptable" variations for the other parameters	Not described	Aoki et al. (1994) Hanasawa et al. (1989)
Asahi Immusorba TR-350, PH-350	Partial thromboplastin time multiplied by 3	No allergic reaction No bleeding	Fadul et al. (1996) Haupt et al. (1996)
Kaneka BM01	Slight ↘ of white blood cells	Not mentioned	Nakazawa et al. (1993)
Excorim Immunosorba	Not described	Not observed	Esnault et al. (1993)
Imré Prosorba	Increase of C3a, C5a transient leukopenia	Mild to moderate chills, fever	Snyder et al. (1991)
Therasorb Ig-Therasorb	Not described	No bleeding No side effects observed	Tribl et al. (1995) Leventhal et al. (1995)
Therasorb LDL-Therasorb	PTT multiplied by 3 slight ↗ C5a	Nothing serious fatigue	Richter et al. (1993)

A very acute reaction was described by Olbricht *et al.* (1992) in some patients submitted to DSC columns. These patients took angiotensin converting enzyme (ACE) inhibitors just before or during the extracorporeal treatment. In these specific cases, either the drug or the extracorporeal therapy had to be avoided. This same recommendation is valid for the DALI system, which certainly also increases, as a negatively charged particle, the generation of bradykinin.

Leakage problems

All the techniques presented derive their specificity from the ligands immobilized on the solid matrix. These molecules are, in principle, covalently attached to the support, activated usually via the cyanogen-bromide (CNBr) method.

However, the risk of the leakage should be always considered as a potential hazard of the systems. Indeed, troubles initially caused by Protein A came from these leakages (Messerschmidt *et al.*, 1984). Ligands are more or less toxic when released into the plasma or in the blood. Dextran sulfate and amino acids were for instance chosen because of their low toxicity. This is not the case with polymyxin B, which is neurotoxic and nephrotoxic when released. Protein A is also a very toxic molecule as a component of the membrane of Staphylococcus aureus. If immunoglobulins are released from the matrix, the risk for developing anti-animal antibodies is enhanced.

Ubricht *et al.* (1996) describe in detail the potential risk of leakage of immobilized antibodies in contact with blood and propose a screening of the behavior of different supports activated by various methods. During the extracorporeal treatment, the adsorbent is in contact with blood or plasma, but possibly also with different buffers when two columns operate in parallel. In the case of high affinity sorbents, the elution conditions need to be harsh. This enhances the risk of ligand shedding. Under physiological conditions, Ubricht *et al.* (1996) show that the immobilization is fairly stable, whatever the type of matrix and the activation method employed. To the contrary, under a very low pH necessary to protein desorption, the stability of the adsorbent is affected for all types of matrices, including Sepharose 4B activated with CNBr, employed in the Therasorb system. The progressive loss of bound ligand is probably the reason why the system can not be reused after 20 or 40 times.

Immune reactions

Even if the release of ligands into the blood is very low, there is a risk of production of anti-ligand antibodies by the patient. This was observed by Richter *et al.* (1993) and Spaethe *et al.* (1993) in hypercholesterolemic patients regularly treated with Therasorb columns. The level of sheep antibodies normally present in the plasma was multiplied by a factor of four after one year treatment. However, this increase did not apparently induce untoward side effects for the patients. Olbricht (1996) accepts the possibility of dextran sulfate shedding followed by the development of anti-DS antibodies, but states that no data are available so far.

Future perspectives

This chapter has described the systems based on the selective adsorption of pathogenic substances, developed and commercialized for the extracorporeal treatment of the patients. The aim was to show how techniques already well established in biotechnology could find other and new applications in the biomedical field. Through the examples presented here, it clearly appears that the constraints are much more rigid than those found in biotechnology. In the medical field, the economic aspects, generated by the health insurance policies, are the major determinant in the choice of a product. The most versatile, cheap and easy-to-use systems seem to be the most attractive for the implementation in human therapy.

Concerning the biocompatibility aspects, which constitute the last but the most severe constraint before the product's commercialization, the following conclusions may be addressed:

1   All commercially available systems show a certain level of bioincompatibility.
2   Depending on the severity of the disease, the occurrence of several side effects may be tolerated.
3   It is of prime importance to distinguish between acute treatments, when the blood contacts the biomaterial during few hours or few days, and long term treatments when the patient undergoes the treatment during a few hours per week but over years. In the first case, side effects and moderate reactions can be accepted for the

patient's safety. In the second one, the requirements need to be stronger in terms of biocompatibility.

The use of specific ligands in the extracorporeal treatment is at its very beginning. The idea of selectively removing the pathogenic molecule from the patient's blood could be applied to any type of a molecule, once it is identified. These techniques will certainly undergo a significant development in the future.

Highly specific ligands, directed only against one pathogen could be proposed for instance: anti-IgE to treat allergy (Adachi *et al.*, 1995, Gorchakov *et al.*, 1991), DNA to fix anti-DNA antibodies for systemic lupus erythematosus (SLE) patients (Gao *et al.*, 1995, Kong *et al.*, 1998). The use of these products will nevertheless be impeded by their high cost. To circumvent we could use the combination of wide specificity ligands (pseudobiospecific) with size exclusion, in a unique column. The sieving properties of the gel could prevent the contact between the immobilized ligand and the potential contaminants, such as albimum. This approach was developed by Vijayalakshmi *et al.* (1998) for the selective removal of β_2-microglobulin from ultrafiltrate for long-term dialysed patients.

Another important issue is the removal of heparin present in excess when cardiopulmonary bypass is performed. Different ligands are under study: immobilized protamine, a heparin antagonist that may, however, cause severe or even fatal cardiovascular response when intravenously injected (Byun *et al.*, 1995), or immobilized poly-L-Lysine (Vertrees *et al.*, 1994).

The solid support itself and the means to contact the target molecule with the ligand can play an important role: up to now, the ligands are mostly immobilized on beads packed into chromatographic columns. These devices present several drawbacks. First of all, they constitute an additional element in the extracorporeal circuit. Second, they decrease the blood or plasma flow rate that results in a prolonged treatment time. Third, the adsorption process itself is diffusion-limited. Some authors now project the use of functionalized membranes for a specific treatment. Klein *et al.* (1997) propose to employ ligand-immobilized microfiltration membrane. Bueno *et al.* (1996) had used histidine-linked plasma fractionation membrane for the *in vitro* removal of immunoglobulins from human plasma. Vallar *et al.* (1996) suggest to immobilize ligands directly on dialysis membrane for the concomitant dialysis and specific adsorption, of β_2-M for instance.

In the above cases, convection is employed in addition to diffusion to improve the probability that a target molecule meets the bullit (ligand) (Brandt *et al.*, 1988). Another means to improve the convective effects is to induce the motion of beads normally packed in a chromatographic column. The method proposed by Weber *et al.* (1994) consists in a plasmapheresis filter module in which the fluid on the permeate side is recirculated at very high speed in a closed loop circuit containing microspherical adsorbent particles. Due to backfiltration, the depleted plasma is directly remixed with the blood cells along the second half of the module. This system called "Microspheres based Detoxification System" (MDS) was tested *in vitro* for endotoxins and LDL-cholesterol removal, and for the adsorption of other proteins (Mullaney *et al.*, 1999).

Many more ideas are likely to arise from an enhanced collaboration among physicians, biochemists and biomedical engineers. Each of them may provide the others with his/her own experience of clinical aspects of the diseases, knowledge of ligands, chemistry and technological ingenuity in building up of a therapeutic device.

References

Adachi, T., Mogi, M., Harada, M. and Kojima, K. (1995) Selective removal of immunoglobulin E from rat blood by membrane-immobilized antibody. *J. Chromatogr. B*, **668**, 327–332.

Adams, M. B., Kauffman, J. Jr., Hebert, L. A., Hussey, C. V., Duquesnoy, A. and Tomasulo, A. (1979) Plasmapheresis in the treatment of renal allograft rejection. *Proc. Dial. Transplant. Forum*, **9**, 252–255.

Agishi, T. (1996) Extracorporeal immunomodulation relevant to organ substitution. *Artif. Organs*, **20**(8), 917–921.

Agishi, T., Kaneko, I., Hasuo, Y., Hayasaka, Y., Ota, K., Abe, M., Ono, T., Kawai, S. and Yamane, K. (1980) Double filtration plasmapheresis. *Trans. ASAIO*, **26**, 406–411.

Aoki, H., Kodama, M., Tani, T. and Hanasawa, K. (1994) Treament of sepsis by extracorporeal elimination of endotoxin using polymyxin B-immobilized fiber. *Am. J. Surg.*, **167**, 412–417.

Balint, J. P. Jr. (1996) Immune modulation associated with extracorporeal immunoadsorption treatments utilizing protein A/silica columns. *Artif. Organs*, **20**(8), 906–913.

Bonomini, V. and Chang, T. M. S. (1982) *Hemoperfusion*, Kärger, Basel.

Borberg, H., Kadar, J. and Oette, K. (1990) The current status of low-density-lipoproteins apheresis. In U. E. Nydegger (ed.) *Therapeutic apheresis in the 1990s*, Kärger, Basel (Switzerland), pp. 239–248.

Bosch, T., Schmidt, B., Blumenstein, M. and Gurland, H. J. (1993) Lipid apheresis by hemoperfusion: *in vitro* efficacy and *ex vivo* biocompatibility of a new low-density lipoprotein adsorber compatible with human whole blood. *Artif. Organs*, **17**(7), 640–652.

Bosch, T., Schmidt, B., Kleophas, W., Gillen, C., Otto, V., Passlick-Deetjen, J. and Gurland, H. J. (1997a) LDL hemoperfusion – a new procedure for LDL apheresis: first clinical application of a LDL adsorber compatible with human whole blood. *Artif. Organs*, **21**(9), 977–982.

Bosch, T., Schmidt, B., Kleophas, W., Otto, V. and Samtleben, W. (1997b) LDL hemoperfusion – a new procedure for LDL apheresis: biocompatibility results from a first pilot study in hypercholesterolemic atherosclerosis patients. *Artif. Organs*, **21**(10), 1060–1065.

Branda, R. F., Miller, W. J., Soltis, R. D. and MacCullough, J. J. (1986) Immunoadsorption of human plasma with protein A – sepharose columns. *Transfusion*, **26**(5), 471–477.

Brandt, S., Goffe, R. A., Kessler, S. B., O'Connor, J. L. and Zale, S. E. (1988) Membrane-based affinity technology for commercial scale purifications. *Bio/Technology*, **6**(July), 779–782.

Bueno, S. M. A., Legallais, C., Haupt, K. and Vijayalakshmi, M. A. (1996) Experimental kinetic aspects of hollow fiber membrane-based pseudobioaffinity filtration: process for IgG separation from human plasma. *J. Membrane Sci.*, **117**, 45–56.

Byun, Y., Yun, J. H., Han, I. S., Fu, Y., Shanberge, J. N. and Yang, V. C. (1995) A protamine filter for extracorporeal heparin removal: development, testing, blood compatibility evaluation, and future direction. *ASAIO J.*, **41**, M301–M305.

Du Moulin, A., Müller-Derlich, J., Bieber, F., Richter, W. O., Frei, U., Müller, R. and Spaethe, R. (1993) Antibody-based immunoadsorption as a therapeutic means. *Blood Purif.*, **11**, 145–149.

Esnault, V., Bignon, J. D., Testa, A., Preud'homme, J. L., Vergracht, A. and Soulillou, J. P. (1990) Effect of protein A immunoadsorption on panel lymphocyte reactivity in hyperimmunized patients awaiting a kidney graft. *Transplantation*, **50**(3), 449–453.

Esnault, V. L. M., Testa, A., Wayne, D. R. W., Soulillou, J. P. and Guenel, J. (1993) Influence of immunoadsorption on the removal of immunoglobulin G autoantibodies in crescentic glomerulonephritis. *Nephron*, **65**, 180–184.

Fadul, E. M., Danielson, B. G. and Wikström, B. (1996) Reduction of plasma fibrinogen, immunoglobulin G, immunoglobulin M concentration by immunoadsorption therapy with tryptophan and phenylalanine adsorbents. *Artif. Organs*, **20**(9), 986–990.

Fennelly, D. W., Norton, L., Sznol M. and Hakes, T. B. (1995) A phase II trial of extracorporeal immunoadsorption of patient plasma with PROSORBA columns for treating metastatic breast cancer. *Cancer*, 75(8), 2099–2102.

Gao, C. L., Li, B. A., Chen, C. Z., Yu, Y. T., Yuan, P. and Song, J. C. (1995) Clinical trials of immunoadsorbents in systemic lupus erythematosus therapy. *Artif. Organs*, 19(5), 468–469.

Gejyo, F., Homma, N. and Arakawa, M. (1988) Carpal tunnel syndrome and β_2-microglobulin related amyloidosis in chronic hemodialysis patients. *Blood Purif.*, 6, 125–131.

Gejyo, F.,Teramura,T., Ei, I.,Arakawa, M.,Nakazawa, R., Azuma, N., Suzuki, M., Furuyoshi, S., Nankou, T., Takata, S. and Yasuda, A. (1995) Long-term clinical evaluation of an adsorbent column (BM-01) of direct hemoperfusion type for β_2-microglobulin on the treatment of dialysis-related amyloidosis. *Artif. Organs*, 19(12), 1222–1226.

Gjörstrup, P., Berntorp, E., Larsson, L. and Nilsson, I. M. (1991) Kinetic aspects of the removal of IgG and inhibitors in hemophiliacs using protein A immunoadsorption. *Vox. Sang.*, 61(4), 244–250.

Gorchakov, V. D., Sakodynskii, K. I., Lebedin, Y. S. and Chuchalin, A. G. (1991) Immunoadsorbents for clinical use: *ex vivo* immunoglobulin E removal in allergy. *J. Chromatogr. B*, 563, 166–171.

Gruber, C., Swoboda, K., Pidlich, J., Gottsauner-Wolf, M., Sunder-Plassmann, G., Pamberger, P., Jansen, M., Derfler, K. and Widhalm, K. (1993) Reduction of lipoprotein(a) by immunospecific LDL apheresis. In A. M. Jr Gotto, M. Mancini, W. O. Richter and P. Schwandt, (eds). *Treatment of severe dyslipoproteinemia in the prevention of coronary heart disease*, Karger, Basel, pp. 219–222.

Grützmacher, P., Landgraf, H., Esser, R., Okon, J., Vlachojannis, J., Ehrly, A. M. and Schoeppe, W. (1990) *In vivo* rheologic effects of lipid apheresis techniques: comparison of dextran sulfate LDL adsorption and heparin induced LDL precipitation. *Trans. ASAIO*, 36, M327–330.

Gurland, H. J., Davison, A. M., Bonomini, V., Falkenhagen, D., Hansen, S., Kishimoto, T., Lysaght, M. J., Moran, J. and Valek, A. (1993) Definitions and terminology in biocompatibility. *Nephrol. Dial. Transpl.*, 9(2), 4–10.

Hakansson, L., Jonsson, S., Sôderberg, M., Eneström, S., Liedén, G. and Lindgren, S. (1984) Tumor regression after extracorporeal affinity chromatography of blood plasma across agarose beads containing staphylococcal protein A. *Eur. J. Cancer Clin. Oncol.*, 20(11), 1377–1388.

Hanasawa, K., Tani, T. and Kodama, M. (1989) New approach to endotoxic and septic shock by means of polymyxin B immobilized fiber. *Surg. Gynecol. Obstet.*, 168, 323–331.

Haupt, W. F., Rosenow, F., van der Ven, C., Borberg, H. and Pawlik, G. (1996) Sequential treatment of Guillain-Barré syndrome with extracorporeal elimination and intravenous immunoglobulin. *J. Neurol. Sci.*, 137(2), 145–149.

Hiesse, C., Kriaa, F., Rousseau, P., Farahmand, H., Bismuth, A., Fries, D. and Charpentier, B. (1992) Immunoadsorption of anti-HLA antibodies for highly sensitized patients awaiting renal transplantation. *Nephrol. Dial. Transplant.*, 7(9), 944–951.

Holmes, C. J. (1995) Hemodialyser performances: biological indices. *Artif. Organs*, 19(11), 1126–1135.

Ikonomov, V., Samtleben, W., Schmidt, B., Blumenstein, M. and Gurland, H. J. (1992) Adsorption profile of commercially available adsorbents: an *in vitro* evaluation. *Int. J. Artif. Organs*, 15, 312–319.

Klein, E., Yeager, D., Seshadri, R. and Baurmeister, U. (1997) Affinity adsorption devices prepared from microporous poly(amide) hollow fibers and sheet membranes. *J. Membrane Sci.*, 129, 31–46.

Knöbl, P., Derfler, K., Korninger, L., Kapiotis, S., Jäger, U., Maler-Dobersberger, T., Hörl, W., Lechner, K. and Pabinger, I. (1995) Elimination of acquired factor VIII antibodies by extracorporal antibody-based immunoadsorption. *Thrombosis and Haemostasis*, **74**(4), 1035–1038.

Kodama, M., Tani, T., Maekawa, K., Hirasawa, H., Otsuka, T., Takahashi, Y. and Kaneko, M. (1995) Endotoxin eliminating therapy in patients with severe sepsis – direct hemoperfusion using polymyxin B immobilized fiber column. *Nippon Geka Gakkai Zasshi*, **96**, 277–285.

Kong, D. L., Chen, C. Z., Lin, E. F. and Yu, Y. T. (1998) Clinical trials of type I and *in vitro* studies of type II immunoadsorbents for systemic lupus erythematosus therapy. *Artif. Organs*, **22**(8), 644–650.

Leventhal, J. R., John, R., Fryer, J. P., Wilson, J. C., Derlich, J. M., Remiszewski, J., Dalmasso, A. P., Matas, A. J. and Morton Bolman, R. (1995) Removal of baboon and human antiporcine IgG and IgM natural antibodies by immunoadsorption. *Transplant.*, **59**(2), 294–300.

Mabuchi, H., Michishita, I., Takeda, M., Fujita, H., Koizumi, J., Takeda, R., Takada, S. and Oonishi, M. (1987) A new density lipoprotein apheresis system using two dextran sulfate cellulose columns in an automated column regenerating unit (LDL continuous apheresis). *Atherosclerosis*, **68**, 19–25.

Malchesky, P. S., Bambauer, R., Horiuchi, T., Kaplan, A., Sakurada, Y. and Samuelsson, G. (1995) Apheresis technologies: an international perspective. *Artif. Organs*, **19**(4), 315–323.

Matsuda, Y., Malchesky, P. S. and Nosé, Y. (1994) Assessment of currently available low-density lipoprotein apheresis systems. *Artif. Organs*, **18**, 93–99.

Messerschmidt, G. L., Bowles, C. A., Henry, D. H. and Deisseroth, A. B. (1984) Clinical trials with Staphylococcus aureus and protein A in the treatment of malignant disease. *J. Biol. Response Mod.*, **3**, 325–329.

Morosetti, M., Meloni, C., Gallucci, M. T., Rossini, P. M., Felicioni, R., Palombo, G., Boccasena, P. and Casciani, C. U. (1994) Plasmapheresis versus plasma perfusion in acute Guillain-Barré syndrome. *ASAIO J.*, **40**, M638–M642.

Mullaney, M., Groth, T., Darkow, R., Hesse, R., Albrecht, W., Paul, D. and von Sengbush, G. (1999) Investigation of plasma protein adsorption on functionalized nanoparticles for application in apheresis. *Artif. Organs*, **23**(1), 87–97.

Muroi, K., Sasaki, R. and Miura, Y. (1989) The effect of immunoadsorption therapy by a protein A column on patients with thrombocytopenia. *Semin. Hematol.*, **26**(2) Suppl. 1, 10–14.

Nakazawa, R., Azuma, N., Suzuki, M., Nakatani, M., Nankou, T., Furuyoshi, S., Yasuda, A., Takata, S., Tani, N. and Kobayashi, F. (1993) A new treatment for dialysis-related amyloidosis with β_2-microglobulin adsorbent column. *Int. J. Artif. Organs*, **16**(12), 823–829.

Nilsson, I. M., Berntorp, E. and Freiburghaus, C. (1993) Treatment of patients with Factor VIII and IX inhibitors. *Thrombosis and Hemostasis*, **70**(1), 56–59.

Nydegger, U. E., Rieben, R. and Jungi, T. W. (1990) Synergy between plasma exchange and intravenous immunoglobulins. In U. E. Nydegger (ed.) *Therapeutic apheresis in the 1990s*, Kärger, Basel (Switzerland), pp. 31–50.

Olbricht, C. J., Schaumann, D. and Fischer, D. (1992) Anaphylactoid reactions, LDL apheresis with dextran sulfate, and ACE inhibitors. *Lancet*, **340**, 908–909.

Olbricht, C. J. (1996) Extracorporeal removal of lipids by dextran sulfate cellulose adsorption. *Artif. Organs*, **20**(4), 332–335.

Ouchi, K., Piatkiewicz, W., Malchesky, P. S., Carey, W. D., Hermann, R. E. and Nosé, Y. (1978) An efficient specific and blood compatible sorbent system for hepatic assist. *Trans. ASAIO*, **24**, 246–249.

Ray, P. K., Idiculla, A., Mark, R., Rhoads, J. E. Jr., Thomas, H., Bassett, J. G. and Cooper, D. R. (1982) Extracorporeal immunoadsorption of plasma from a metastatic colon carcinoma patient by protein A-containing nonviable Staphylococcus aureus: clinical, biochemical, serologic, and histologic evaluation of the patient's response. *Cancer*, **49**(9), 1800–1809.

Richter, W. O., Jacob, B. G., Ritter, M. M., Sühler, K., Vierneisel, K. and Schwandt, P. (1993) Three-year treatment of familial heterozygous hypercholesterolemia by extracorporeal low-density lipoprotein immunoadsorption with polyclonal apolipoprotein B antibodies. *Metabolism*, 42(7), 888–894.

Ross, C. N., Gaskin, G., Gregor-Macgregor, S., Patel, A. A., Davey, N. J., Lechler, R. I., Williams, G., Rees, R. J. and Pusey, C. D. (1993) Renal transplantation following immunoadsorption in highly sensitized recipients. *Transplantation*, 55(4), 785–789.

Ruiz, J. C., de Francisco, A. L., Vasquez de Prada, J. A., Pastor, J. M., Alcade, G. and Arias, M. (1994) Successful heart transplantation after anti-HLA antibody removal with Protein A immunoadsorption in a hyperimmunized patient. *J. Thorac. Cardiovasc. Surg.*, 107(5), 1366–1367.

Shibuya, N., Sato, T., Osame, M., Takegami, T., Doi, S. and Kawanami, S. (1994) Immunoadsorption therapy for myasthenia gravis. *J. Neurol. Neurosurg. Psychiatry*, 57(5), 578–581.

Snyder, H. W., Henry, D. H., Messerschmidt, G. L., et al. (1991) Minimal toxicity during protein A immunoadsorption treatment of malignant disease: an outpatient therapy. *J. Clin. Apheresis*, 6, 1–10.

Snyder, H. W. Jr., Cochran, S. K., Balint, J. P. Jr., Bertram, J. H., Mittelman, A., Guthrie, T. H. Jr, et al. (1992) Experience with protein A – immunoadsorption in treatment-resistant adult immune thrombocytopenic purpura. *Blood*, 79(9), 2237–2245.

Spaethe, R., du Moulin, A., Bieber, F. and Böhm, W. (1993) Principles of immunapheresis and specific elimination of plasma components. *Biomat., Artif. Cells, and Immob. Biotech.*, 21(2), 239–251.

Stoffel, W., Greve, V. and Borberg, H. (1981) Application of specific extracorporeal removal of low density lipoprotein in familial hypercholesterolemia. *Lancet*, 2, 1005–1007.

Takada, S., Tani, N., Oonishi, M., Kan, A. and Narisada, M. (1987) Automated continuous low density lipoprotein adsorption system. In T. Oda (ed.), *Therapeutic plasmapheresis*, Vol. VII, Schatteuer, New York, pp. 454.

Tani, N. (1996) Development of selective low-density lipoprotein (LDL) apheresis system: immobilized polyanion as LDL-specific adsorption for LDL apheresis system. *Artif. Organs*, 20(8), 922–929.

Tani, T., Hanasawa, K., Endo, Y., Yoshioka, T., Kodama, M., Kaneko, M., Uchiyama, Y., Akizawa, T., Takahasi, K. and Sugai, K. (1998) Therapeutic apheresis for septic patients with organ dysfunction: hemoperfusion using a polymixin B immobilized column. *Artif. Organs*, 22(12), 1038–1044.

Tatami, R., Inoue, N., Itoh, H., et al. (1992) Regression of coronary atherosclerosis by combined LDL apheresis and lipid lowering drug therapy in patients with familial hypercholesterolemia: a multicenter study. *Atherosclerosis*, 95, 1–13.

Terman, D. S. and Bertram, J. H. (1985) Antitumor effects of immobilized protein A and Staphylococcus products: linkage between toxicity and efficacy, and identification of potential tumoricidal reagents. *Eur. J. Cancer Clin. Oncol.*, 21, 1115–1122.

Thompson, G. R. and Myant, N. B. (1976) Low density lipoprotein turnover in familial hypercholesterolemia after plasma exchange. *Atherosclerosis*, 23, 371–377.

Tribl, B., Knöbl, P., Derfler, K., Kapiotis, S., Aspöck, G., Jäger, U., Hörl, W. and Lechner, K. (1995) Rapid elimination of a high-titer spontaneous factor V antibody by extracorporeal antibody-based immunoadsorption and immunosuppression. *Ann. Hematol.*, 71, 199–203.

Tsuchida, K., Takemoto, Y., Nakamura, T., Fu, O., Okada, C., Yamagami, S. and Kishimoto, T. (1998) Lixelle adsorbent to remove inflammatory cytokines. *Artif. Organs*, 22(12), 1064–1069.

Ubrich, N. and Rivat, C. (1996) Antibodies released from immunoadsorbents: effect of support, activation and elution conditions. *Art. Cells, Blood Subs. and Immob. Biotech.*, 24(1), 65–75.

Uehlinger, J., Button, G. R., McCarthy, J., Forster, A., Watt, R. and Aledort, L. M. (1991) Immunoadsorption for coagulation factor inhibitors. *Transfusion*, 31, 265–269.

Vallar, L. and Rivat, C. (1996) Regenerated cellulose-based hemodialyzers with immobilized proteins as potential devices for extracorporeal immunoadsorption procedures: an assessment of protein coupling capacity and *in vitro* dialysis performances. *Artif. Organs*, 20(1), 8–16.

Vertrees, R. A., Zwischenberger, J. B., McRea, J. C., Tao, W., Kurusz, M. and Conti, V. R. (1994) Reversal of anticoagulation without protamine using a heparin removal device after cardiopulmonary bypass. *ASAIO J.*, 40, M560–M564.

Vienken, J., Diamantoglou, M., Hahn, C., Kamusewitz, H. and Paul, D. (1995) Considerations on developmental aspects of biocompatible dialysis membranes. *Artif. Organs*, 19(5), 398–406.

Vijayalakshmi, M. A. (1989) Pseubiospecific ligand affinity chromatography. *Trends Biotechnol.*, 7(3), 71–76.

Vijayalakshmi, M. A., Pitiot, O., Legallais, C., and Moriniere, P. (1998), Gel with adsorptive size exclusion chromatography AdSEC: use for β_2 microglobulin gel dialysis, French patent, no 98.13655 with international extension PCT/FR 99/02635.

Wallukat, G., Reinke, P., Dörffel, W.V., Luther, H.P., Bestvater, K., Felix, S.B. and Baumann, G. (1996) Removal of autoantibodies in dilated cardiomyopathy by immunoadsorption. *Int. J. Cardiol.*, 54, 191–195.

Weber C., Rajnoch C., Loth F., Schima H. and Falkenhagen D. (1994) The Microspheres based Detoxification System (MDS). A new extracorporeal blood purification technology based on recirculated microspherical adsorbent particles. *Int. J. Artif. Organs*, 17(11), 595–602.

Yamamoto, A., Kojima, S., Shiba-Harada, M., Kawaguchi, A. and Hatanaka, K. (1992) Assessment of the biocompatibility and long term effect of LDL-apheresis by dextran sulfate–cellulose column. *Artif. Organs*, 16(2), 177–181.

Yamasaki, Z., Idezuki, Y., Inoue, N., Yoshigawa, H., Yamawaki, N., Inagaki, K. and Tsuda, N. (1989) Extracorporeal immunoadsorption with IM-PH or IM-TR column. *Biomater. Artif. Cells Artif. Organs*, 17, 117–124.

Index

Printed in the United States
By Bookmasters